Helicobacter pylori
Basic Mechanisms to Clinical Cure 2000

Helicobacter pylori
Basic Mechanisms to Clinical Cure 2000

Edited by

Richard H. Hunt
Professor of Medicine
Director, Division of Gastroenterology
McMaster University Medical Centre
1200 Main Street West
Hamilton, Ontario L8N 3Z5
Canada

Guido N. J. Tytgat
Professor, Department of
Gastroenterology and Hepatology
Academic Medical Centre
9 Meibergdreef
1105 AZ Amsterdam
The Netherlands

*The proceedings of a symposium organised by AXCAN PHARMA,
held in Bermuda, March 26–29, 2000*

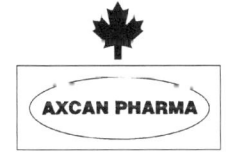

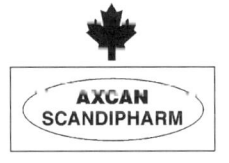

KLUWER ACADEMIC PUBLISHERS
DORDRECHT / BOSTON / LONDON

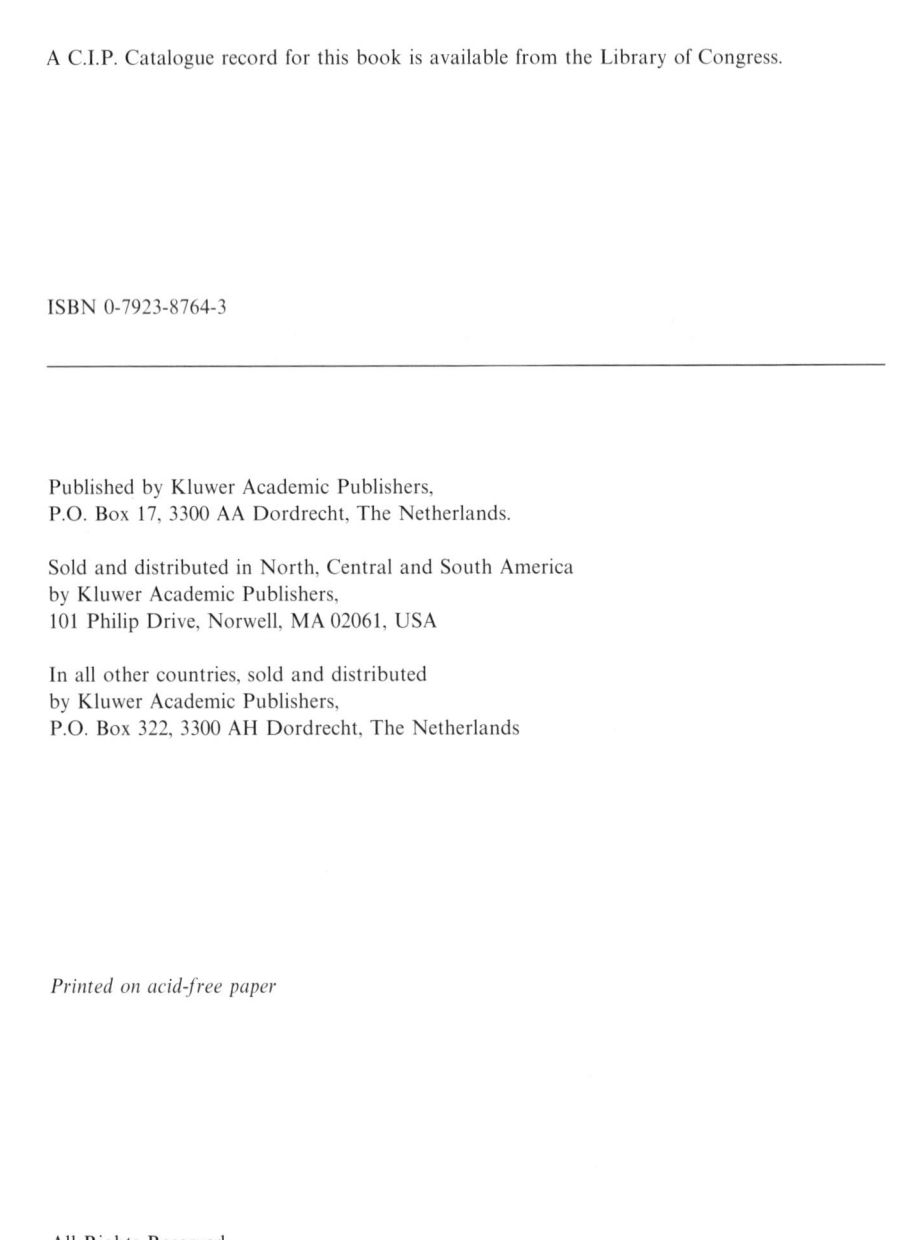

A C.I.P. Catalogue record for this book is available from the Library of Congress.

ISBN 0-7923-8764-3

Published by Kluwer Academic Publishers,
P.O. Box 17, 3300 AA Dordrecht, The Netherlands.

Sold and distributed in North, Central and South America
by Kluwer Academic Publishers,
101 Philip Drive, Norwell, MA 02061, USA

In all other countries, sold and distributed
by Kluwer Academic Publishers,
P.O. Box 322, 3300 AH Dordrecht, The Netherlands

Printed on acid-free paper

All Rights Reserved
© 2000 Kluwer Academic Publishers and Axcan Pharma
No part of the material protected by this copyright notice may be reproduced or
utilized in any form or by any means, electronic or mechanical, including photocopying,
recording or by any information storage and retrieval system, without written permission
from the copyright owners.

Printed and bound in Great Britain by Antony Rowe Limited.

Contents

List of Principal Contributors   ix

Preface   xix

Section I: *Helicobacter pylori* – The Organism

1   What are the biochemical and physiological implications of the new genetic information?
SL Hazell, MA Trend, GL Mendz   3

2   The urease system of *Helicobacter pylori*
DL Weeks, DR Scott, P Voland, EA Marcus, C Athmann, K Melchers, G Sachs   15

3   The amphibiotic relationship of *Helicobacter pylori* and humans
MJ Blaser   25

4   *Helicobacter pylori* is pathogenic flora
A Lee   31

5   Disease-specific *Helicobacter pylori* virulence factors: the role of *cagA*, *vacA*, *iceA*, *babA2* alone or in combination
Y Yamaoka, DY Graham   37

Section II: *Helicobacter pylori* – Epidemiology

6   Factors associated with disappearance of *Helicobacter pylori* in the West
J Parsonnet   45

7   Factors associated with disappearance of *Helicobacter pylori* in the Far East
JJY Sung   53

CONTENTS

8 Differences in prevalence of *Helicobacter pylori* and disease outcomes according to race/environmental factors in Southeast Asia
KL Goh
57

Section III: Novel *Helicobacters*

9 Infection with *Helicobacter heilmannii* (formerly *Gastrospirillum hominis*): characterization, epidemiology and therapy
P Malfertheiner, URM Bohr, T. Günther
73

10 Hepatobiliary *Helicobacters*: recognized animal pathogens with suspected pathogenic potential in humans
JG Fox
83

11 Novel *Helicobacter* species in the intestine
A Lee
105

Section IV: Diagnosis of *Helicobacter pylori* Infection

12 Diagnosis of *Helicobacter pylori* infection: faecal antigen determination
D Vaira, C Ricci, M Menegatti, C Acciardi, L Gatta, A Geminiani, M Miglioli
115

13 Pitfalls in *Helicobacter pylori* diagnosis
P Malfertheiner, A Leodolter, C Gerards
123

Section V: Inflammation and the Immune Response to *Helicobacter pylori* Infection

14 Overview of immune and inflammatory changes due to *Helicobacter* infection
A Hamlet, K Croitoru
141

15 Interaction of *Helicobacter pylori* with gastric epithelium
E Solcia, V Ricci, P Sommi, V Necchi, M Candusso, R Fiocca
151

16 *Helicobacter pylori* and the epithelial barrier: role of oxidative injury
S-Z Ding, SE Crowe
155

17 Immuno-inflammatory response to *Helicobacter pylori* in children
SJ Czinn, JC Eisenberg, JG Nedrud, TG Blanchard
169

18 Severity and reversibility of mucosal inflammation in children and adolescents infected with *Helicobacter pylori*
PM Sherman
175

CONTENTS

19 Elimination of *Helicobacter pylori* is dependent on a Th2 response
A Lee   187

20 Elimination of *Helicobacter pylori* is not dependent on a Th2 cytokine response
K Croitoru   193

21 The inflammatory activity in *Helicobacter pylori* infection is predominantly organism related
P Michetti   197

22 The inflammatory activity in *Helicobacter pylori* infection is predominantly host-related
PB Ernst   203

Section VI: *Helicobacter pylori* and Gastritis

23 *Helicobacter pylori* gastritis – a global view
Y Liu, CIJ Ponsioen, GJ Waverling, S-D Xiao, GNJ Tytgat, FJW Ten Kate   213

24 Unusual forms of gastric inflammation and their relationship to *Helicobacter pylori* infection
MF Dixon   221

25 Can atrophic gastritis be diagnosed in the presence of *Helicobacter pylori* infection?
RM Genta   229

26 Mechanisms involved in gastric atrophy
NA Wright   239

27 Intestinal metaplasia: types, mechanisms of origin, and role in gastric cancer histogenesis
E Solcia, O Luinetti, L Villani, P Quilici, C Klersy, R Fiocca   249

28 Long-term proton pump inhibitor therapy accelerates the onset of atrophic gastritis in *Helicobacter pylori*-positive patients
EJ Kuipers, SGM Meuwissen   255

29 Proton pump inhibitors do not accelerate the development of gastric atrophy in *Helicobacter pylori* gastritis
JW Freston   269

30 Autoimmune gastritis via mimicking does occur
M Stolte, S Rappel, H Müller   269

31 Autoimmune gastritis and antigenic mimicking
F Franceschi, RM Genta   289

32 Carditis and intestinal metaplasia of the cardia is reflux related
MB Fennerty   295

CONTENTS

33 Carditis and cardia intestinal metaplasia are *Helicobacter pylori*-related
WM Weinstein — 299

34 Is gastric metaplasia in *Helicobacter pylori* really gastric?
NA Wright — 307

Section VII: *Helicobacter pylori* and Clinical Consequences

35 Extragastric manifestations of *Helicobacter pylori* – are they relevant?
CW Howden, GI Leontiadis — 315

36 Peptic ulcer disease – the transitional zones are important
MF Dixon, A Lee, SJO Veldhuyzen van Zanten — 327

37 What causes *Helicobacter pylori*-negative non-NSAID-related ulcers?
CW Howden — 339

38 From the pump to the helix
IM Modlin, J Farhadi, M Kidd — 347

39 Mechanisms involved in the development of hypochlorhydria and pangastritis in *Helicobacter pylori* infection
KEL McColl, E El-Omar — 373

40 Effect of *Helicobacter pylori* infection on gastric acid control using proton pump inhibitors
PO Katz — 385

41 Rebound acid hypersecretion after acid-suppressive therapy
D Gillen, KEL McColl — 391

42 Gastric consequences of proton pump therapy and *Helicobacter pylori* eradication
G Sachs, G Athmann, D Weeks, D Scott — 397

Section VIII: *Helicobacter pylori*, Dyspepsia and NSAIDs

43 Current concepts of dyspepsia: the role of the nervous system
P Bercik, SM Collins — 411

44 How to explain outcome differences in dyspepsia studies
MB Fennerty, LA Laine — 421

45 *Helicobacter pylori* eradication for dyspepsia is clinically useful
D McNamara, C O'Morain — 427

46 Dyspepsia is no indication for *Helicobacter pylori* eradication
SJO Veldhuyzen van Zanten — 435

CONTENTS

47 Role of *Helicobacter pylori* infection in NSAID-associated gastropathy
J-Q Huang, R Lad, RH Hunt — 443

48 Role of *Helicobacter pylori* in NSAID gastropathy: can *Helicobacter pylori* infection be beneficial?
DY Graham — 453

49 *Helicobacter pylori* and non-steroidal anti-inflammatory drugs
CJ Hawkey — 461

Section IX: *Helicobacter pylori* and 'Test-and-Treat' Strategies

50 The impact of a 'test-and-treat' strategy for *Helicobacter pylori*: the United States perspective
DA Peura — 469

51 Test-and-treat strategy in dyspepsia – the European perspective
P Malfertheiner — 475

52 The impact of the 'test-and-treat' strategies for *Helicobacter pylori* infection – an Asian perspective?
JJY Sung — 483

Section X: *Helicobacter pylori* and Gastric Malignancy

53 Rodent models for *Helicobacter*-induced gastric cancer
JG Fox — 489

54 *Helicobacter pylori* and gastric cancer: the risk is real
D Forman — 507

55 *Helicobacter pylori* in gastric malignancy: role of oxidants, antioxidants and other co-factors
Z-W Zhang, MJG Farthing — 513

56 Gastric markers of pre-malignancy are not reversible
RM Genta, F Franceschi — 525

57 The case for the reversibility of gastric dysplasia/neoplasia
RH Riddell — 535

58 Evaluation of the long-term outcome of *Helicobacter pylori* related gastric mucosa-associated lymphoid tissue (MALT) lymphoma
M Stolte, A Morgner, B Alpen, Th Wündisch, C Thiede, A Neubauen, E Bayerdörffer — 535

Section XI: Treatment of *Helicobacter pylori* Infection

59 Current state-of-the-art management for *Helicobacter pylori* infection: global perspective
DA Peura — 551

CONTENTS

60 Guidelines for therapy of *Helicobacter pylori* infection – a world perspective
S-K Lam — 559

61 Bismuth triple and quadruple studies for *Helicobacter pylori* eradication in Canada
CA Fallone — 567

62 Approach to *Helicobacter pylori* infection in children
E Hassall — 575

63 What role for clarithromycin in the treatment of *Helicobacter pylori* infection?
R Clancy, T Borody, C Clancy — 587

64 What is the role of bismuth in *Helicobacter pylori* antimicrobial resistance?
SJO Veldhuyzen van Zanten, N Chiba — 593

65 Risk factors for failure of *Helicobacter pylori* eradication therapy
N Broutet, S Tchamgoué, E Pereira, F Mégraud — 601

66 Strategies for therapy failures: choice of 'back-up' regimen determined by primary treatment for *Helicobacter pylori* infection
WA de Boer — 609

67 Quadruple should be first-line therapy for *Helicobacter pylori* infection
TJ Borody — 623

68 Quadruple therapy should be secondline treatment for *Helicobacter pylori* infection
A Axon — 631

69 *Helicobacter pylori* infection: expectations for future therapy
CJ Hawkey — 637

70 A *Helicobacter pylori* vaccine is essential
S Banerjee, P Michetti — 643

Section XII: *Helicobacter* Infections and the Future

71 The agenda for the microbiologist
A Lee — 655

72 The agenda for the immunologist
PB Ernst — 663

73 The agenda for the histopathologist
RH Riddell — 669

74 *Helicobacter* infections in the new millennium: the challenge for the clinician
A Axon — 673

Index — 679

List of Principal Contributors

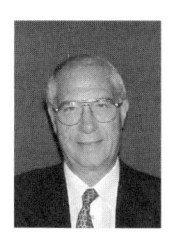

A. AXON
The Centre for Digestive Diseases
The General Infirmary at Leeds
Great George Street
Leeds LS1 3EX
UK

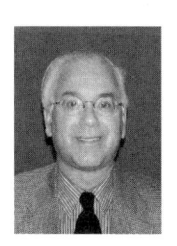

M. J. BLASER
Department of Medicine
New York University School of Medicine
550 First Avenue
New York, NY 10016
USA

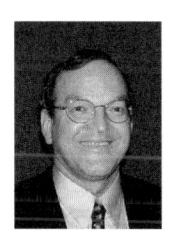

T. J. BORODY
Centre for Digestive Diseases
144 Great North Road
Five Dock, NSW 2046
Australia

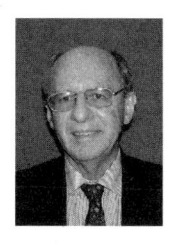

R. CLANCY
Discipline of Immunology and Microbiology
Faculty of Medicine and Health Sciences
David Maddison Clinical Sciences Building
Royal Newcastle Hospital
Newcastle, NSW 2300
Australia

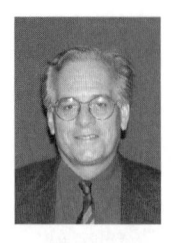

S. M. COLLINS
McMaster University Medical Centre
P.O. Box 2000, Station A
Hamilton, Ontario
L8N 8Z5
Canada

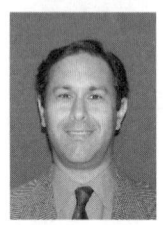

K. CROITORU
Intestinal Disease Research Program
McMaster University
1200 Main Street West, Room 4W8
Hamilton, Ontario
L8N 3Z5
Canada

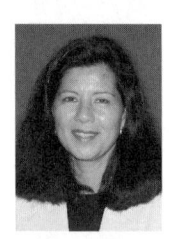

S. E. CROWE
Division of Gastroenterology
Department of Internal Medicine
4.106 McCullough Building
301 University Avenue
Galveston, TX 77555-0764
USA

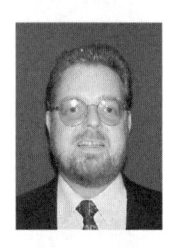

S. J. CZINN
Rainbow Babies and Children's Hospital
Division of Pediatric Gastroenterology and Nutrition
11100 Euclid Avenue
Cleveland, OH 44106
USA

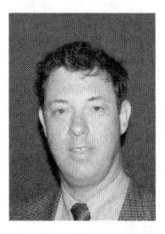

W. A. De BOER
Sint Anna Hospital
Ziekenhuis Bernhoven
Postbus 10
5340 BE Oss
The Nethelands

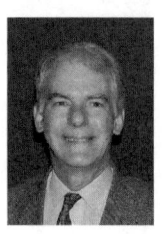

M. F. DIXON
Division of Pathological Sciences
University of Leeds and Centre for Digestive Diseases
General Infirmary at Leeds
Leeds, LS2 9JT
UK

LIST OF PRINCIPAL CONTRIBUTORS

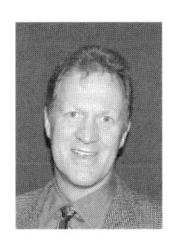

P. B. ERNST
Department of Pediatrics, Microbiology and Immunology and the
Sealy Centre for Molecular Sciences
University of Texas Medical Branch
Galveston, TX 77555-0366
USA

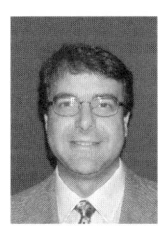

C. A. FALLONE
Division of Gastroenterology
Royal Victoria Hospital
687 Pine Avenue West
Montreal, Quebec
H3A 1A1
Canada

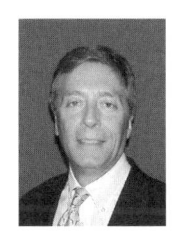

M. J. G. FARTHING
Digestive Diseases Research Centre
St Bartholomew's and The Royal London School of Medicine and Dentistry
London E1 2AT
UK

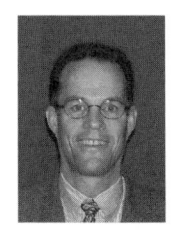

M. B. FENNERTY
Division of Gastroenterology, PV-310
Oregon Health Sciences University
3181 SW Sam Jackson Park Road
Portland, OR 97201-3098
USA

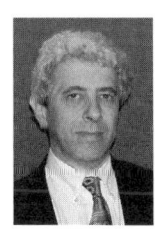

D. FORMAN
Centre for Cancer Research
University of Leeds
Arthington House
Cookridge Hospital
Leeds, LS16 6QB
UK

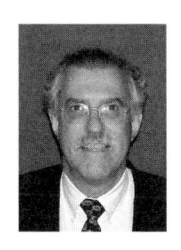

J. G. FOX
Division of Comparative Medicine
Massachusetts Institute of Technology
Building 16-825
77 Massachusetts Avenue
Cambridge, MA 02139-4307
USA

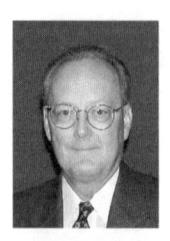

J. W. FRESTON
Office of Clinical Research, Building 20
University of Connecticut Health Center
263 Farmington Avenue
Farmington, CT 06030-2806
USA

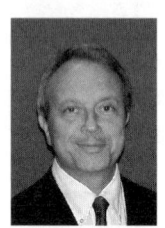

R. M. GENTA
Pathology – 113
Veterans Affairs Medical Center
2002 Holcombe Boulevard
Houston, TX 77030
USA

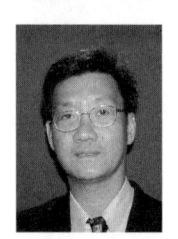

K. L. GOH
Department of Medicine
Faculty of Medicine
University of Malaya
50603 Kuala Lumpur
Malaysia

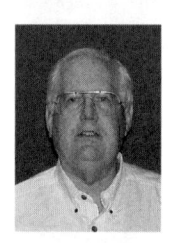

D. Y. GRAHAM
Baylor College of Medicine
Room 3A-320 (111D)
Veterans Affairs Medical Center
2002 Holcombe Boulevard
Houston, TX 77030
USA

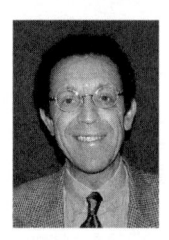

E. G. HASSALL
Division of Gastroenterology
B. C. Children's Hospital
4480 Oak Street
Vancouver, British Columbia
V6H 3V4
Canada

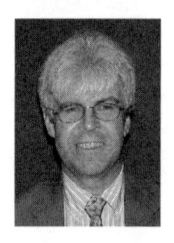

C. J. HAWKEY
Division of Gastroenterology
University Hospital Nottingham
Queen's Medical Centre
Nottingham NG7 2UH
UK

LIST OF PRINCIPAL CONTRIBUTORS

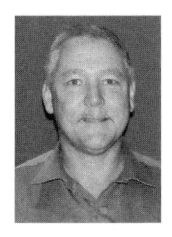

S. L. HAZELL
Centre for Microbiology and Molecular Biology in Medical and
Veterinary Science
Faculty of Informatics, Science and Technology
University of Western Sydney
Campbelltown Campus
P.O. Box 555
Campbelltown, NSW 2560
Australia

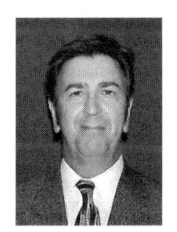

C. W. HOWDEN
Northwestern University
Northwestern Center for Clinical Research
680 N. Lakeshore Drive
Suite 1220
Chicago, IL 60611
USA

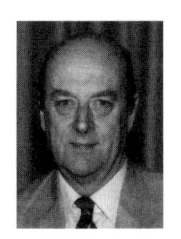

R. H. HUNT
Division of Gastroenterology
McMaster University Medical Center
1200 Main Street West, Room 4W8
Hamilton, Ontario
L8N 3Z5
Canada

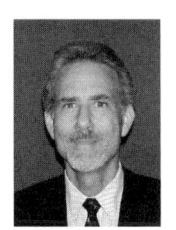

P. O. KATZ
1800 Lombard Street
Suite 501
Graduate Hospital
Philadelphia, PA 19146
USA

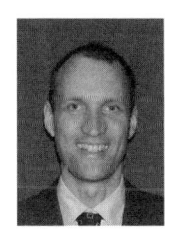

E. J. KUIPERS
Department of Gastroenterology
Free University Hospital
P.O. Box 7057
1007 MD Amsterdam
The Netherlands

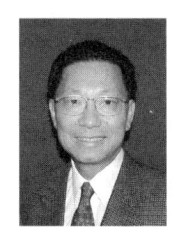

S.-K. LAM
Department of Medicine
University of Hong Kong
Queen Mary Hospital
Hong Kong
China

HELICOBACTER PYLORI 2000

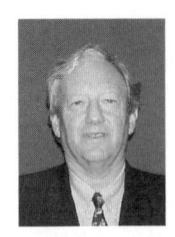

A. LEE
School of Microbiology and Immunology
The University of New South Wales
Sydney, NSW 2052
Australia

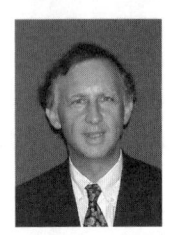

P. MALFERTHEINER
Otto-von-Guericke University Megdeburg
Department of Gastroenterology, Hepatology and Infectious Diseases
Leipziger Straße 44
39120 Magdeburg
Germany

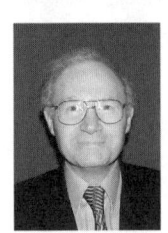

K. E. L. McCOLL
Department of Medicine and Therapeutics
University of Glasgow
Western Infirmary
Glasgow G11 6NT
UK

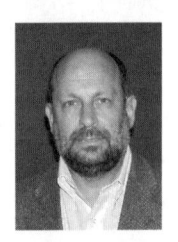

F. MÉGRAUD
C.H.U. de Bordeaux
Laboratoire de Bactériologie–Enfants
Hôpital Pellegrin
33076 Bordeaux Cedex
France

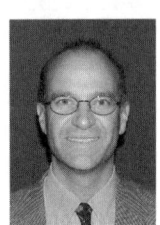

P. MICHETTI
Division of Gastroenterology, Dana 601
Beth Israel Deaconess Medical Center
330 Brookline Avenue
Boston, MA 02215
USA

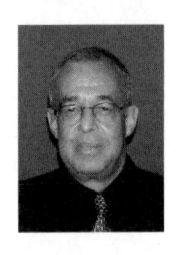

I. M. MODLIN
Yale University School of Medicine
333 Cedar Street
P.O. Box 208062
New Haven, CT 06520-8062
USA

LIST OF PRINCIPAL CONTRIBUTORS

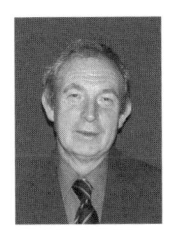

C. O'MORAIN
Adelaide and Meath Hospital
Trinity College
Dublin
Republic of Ireland

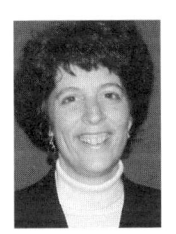

J. PARSONNET
Division of Infectious Diseases and Geographic Medicine
Room S156
Stanford University School of Medicine
Stanford, CA 94305-5107
USA

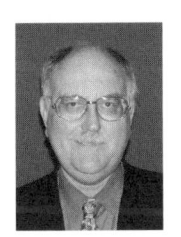

D. A. PEURA
Division of Gastroenterology and Hepatology
University of Virginia Health System
PO Box 800708
Charlottesville, VA 22908-0708
USA

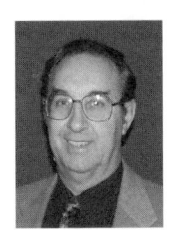

R. H. RIDDELL
Department of Pathology and Molecular Medicine
McMaster University Medical Center
1200 Main Street West
Hamilton, Ontario L8N 3Z5
Canada

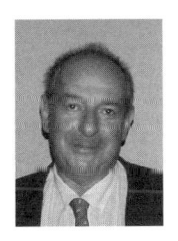

G. SACHS
CURE VA Medical Center-Wadsworth
Bldg. 113, Room 324
11301 Wilshire Boulevard
Los Angeles, CA 90073
USA

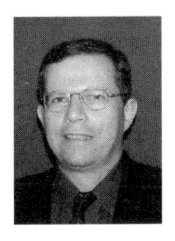

P. M. SHERMAN
Division of Gastroenterology and Nutrition
Room 8409
The Hospital for Sick Children
555 University Avenue
Toronto, Ontario
M5G 1X8 Canada

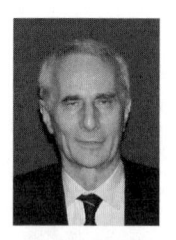

E. SOLCIA
Department of Human Pathology
University of Pavia and IRCCS Policlinico S. Matteo
Via Forlanini 16
I-27100 Pavia
Italy

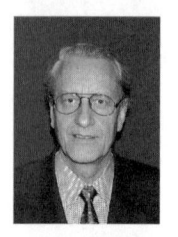

M. STOLTE
Institut für Pathologie
Klinikum Bayreuth
Preuschwitzer Straße 101
D-95445 Bayreuth
Germany

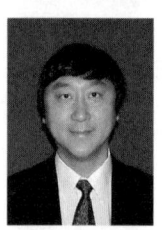

J. J. Y. SUNG
Department of Medicine
Prince of Wales Hospital
30–32 Ngan Shing Street
Sha Tin, N.T.
Hong Kong
China

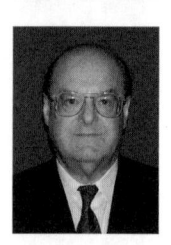

G. N. J. TYTGAT
Department of Gastroenterology and Hepatology
University of Amsterdam
Academic Medical Center
9 Meibergdreef
1105 AX Amsterdam
The Netherlands

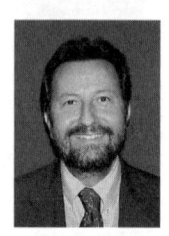

D. VAIRA
Clinical Medica I
Università di Bologna
Policlinico S. Orsola
Bologna
Italy

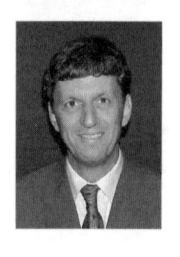

S. J. O VELDHUYZEN VAN ZANTEN
Queen Elizabeth II Health Sciences Center
Victoria General Hospital Site
Room 928, Centennial Building
1278 Tower Road
Halifax, Nova Scotia
B3H 2Y9 Canada

LIST OF PRINCIPAL CONTRIBUTORS

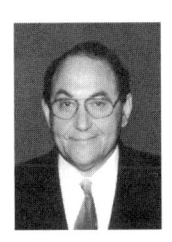

W. M. WEINSTEIN
Department of Medicine
Division of Digestive Diseases
UCLA Center for Health Sciences
10833 LeConte Ave
Los Angeles, CA
USA

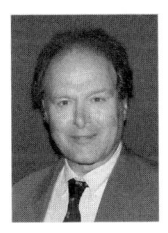

N. A. WRIGHT
Department of Histopathology
Hammersmith Hospital and Histopathology Unit
Imperial Cancer Research Fund
London
UK

Preface

The fourth meeting in the very successful series *Helicobacter pylori*: Basic Mechanisms to Clinical Cure was held on the island of Bermuda in late March 2000. This was only some two years after the third meeting in San Diego and it seemed hardly possible that there would be so much new information. However, as the contributions in this volume testify, there was plenty of exciting new information with important implications for both understanding this infection and for clinical management. Some of this information was of a fundamental nature, such as the role of the acid-sensitive ureI channel in regulating the influx of urea and the formation of ammonia transported back in the microbial periplasmic space to neutralize acid; the observation of genetic polymorphism of the IL-1β gene as an explanation of achlorhydria and gastric cancer risk in the first-degree relatives of gastric cancer patients; and the peculiar biochemical and physiological consequences of the genome of the microorganisms.

The format of the meeting, with short fifteen-minute state-of-the-art presentations by world experts closely involved in *Helicobacter* research followed by ample time for panel discussions, was again followed this year. Traditional aspects included detailed study of the microbial characteristics, the novel *Helicobacters*, the interaction with the human host, the peculiarities of the inflammatory immune response, the short and long-term mucosal consequences, the effects on acid secretion, the problem of gastric malignancy and the therapeutic possibilities.

However, a series of short debates was introduced to highlight controversial issues such as the pathogenic or commensal role of the organism, the role of virulence factors, the characteristics of the inflammatory immune response, the reversibility of mucosal atrophy and metaplasia, and the primary or secondary role of quadruple therapy, to name just a few. This provocative approach was very successful and provided fuel for further in-depth discussions. These debates have been included in this book in the form of conventional manuscripts in order to maintain the shortest possible production time for the publication of the proceedings.

Helicobacter pylori has come a long way since the first meeting in Amelia Island in 1993, and the science of this organism and the understanding of the consequences of the infection have advanced our knowledge fundamentally and revolutionized our thinking about gastrointestinal disease. We now recognize the existence of more than thirty *Helicobacter* species, some of which may play a significant role in human disease. The experience gained through our investigation of *H. pylori* promises to make a significant contribution to the future exploration of the possible role of *Helicobacter* species in hepatic, biliary and intestinal diseases.

The chapters published in these proceedings reflect the contributions of our speakers, whom we thank for their superb presentations and timely submission of their manuscripts. This allowed us to work closely with Phil Johnstone and his team at Kluwer Academic Publishers to achieve the fastest possible publication time. We believe that these manuscripts accurately incorporate the critical cutting-edge issues which formed the foundation of the presentations and debates in Bermuda.

Lastly, we would like to thank all our colleagues for their support in making this meeting work so well. Their enthusiastic participation and willingness to challenge and be challenged has created a forum at these meetings, which has continued to move us forward in this exciting field of gastroenterology. The vision of Léon Gosselin, President of Axcan Pharma, in supporting these meetings is much appreciated and we thank him and Diane Gosselin and the staff of Axcan for their continuing generous support and wonderful organization which made this meeting possible.

Richard H. Hunt
McMaster University Medical Centre
Hamilton, Ontario
Canada

Guido N. J. Tytgat
Academic Medical Centre
Amsterdam
The Netherlands

Scientific Organizers and Co-Chairmen, *Helicobacter pylori*: Basic Mechanisms to Clinical Cure, Bermuda, March 2000

Section I
Helicobacter pylori – The organism

1
What are the biochemical and physiological implications of the new genetic information?

S. L. HAZELL, M. A. TREND and G. L. MENDZ

INTRODUCTION

As an agent of disease *Helicobacter pylori* has a marked impact on the health and well-being of populations throughout the world[1-4]. In addition to being an important pathogen, *H. pylori* has the potential to be an important model pathogen, with genomic data and the tools necessary for functional analysis, including good animal models of human disease.

Microbial genomics have been at the forefront of a new era of whole cell molecular biology. *H. pylori* is one of over 20 microorganisms for which complete sequence data are publicly available[5,6]. The two *H. pylori* strains characterized (26695 and J99) contain about 1600 open-reading frames (ORFs). Of these ORFs, in the order of 58% have been assigned *putative* functions[5,6] Generally 18% of the ORFs encode products having homologues of *unknown* function in other species, while about 23% of the ORFs have no significant sequence similarity to publicly available genes[5,6]. Thus more than 40% of the genes in these strains encode products of *no known function*! In addition, in a comparison of the genomes of the two sequential strains of *H. pylori*, Alm *et al* noted that *each* contained strain-specific genes[6].

Genomic data provided a quantum leap in the genetic data available in relation to *H. pylori*. Prior to the release of the genomes, biochemical and physiological studies had revealed much about the primary metabolic systems of *H. pylori*[7,8]. The new genetic data confirmed much of what was known, and extended these findings to give a more complete overview of the primary metabolic systems of the bacterium[7,8]. While releasing vast amounts of genetic code, the genomes posed more questions, especially in terms of the huge amounts of genetic information that could not be categorized by functional type, or where biochemical data remain at odds with genetic inference[9-12]. Indeed, genetic data provide limited information on topics such as subcellular location, post-transitional modification, protein structure and domains[13]. Given what we *don't* know about *H. pylori*, a systematic exploration of the network of interactions of genes and gene products is an important challenge that must be met if we are to increase our awareness of the mechanisms contributing to microbial colonization, survival and disease processes. Indeed, many of the approximately 1600 putative genes within the *H. pylori* genome may be expressed only within the gastric environment, being regulated by environmental factors such as pH, availability of iron, surface interactions or the composition and flux of nutrients across the gastric mucosa.

METABOLIC PATHWAYS OPERATING IN *H. PYLORI*

The genomic and other genetic data have provided unique insights. For instance, the bacteria within the family Helicobacteriaceae have a fused *rpoB–rpoC* structure (RNA polymerase), which may be of evolutionary and functional significance[14]. Then there is the apparent absence of homologues to the transcription regulatory sigma factors σ^{32} (heat-shock) and σ^S (stationary-phase)[5,6], suggestive of an organism well adapted to life within a relatively constant gastric environment, where the bacterium is maintained in a semi-continuous culture system. We may add to this the apparent absence of an active stringent response in *H. pylori*. This is also suggestive of adaptation to a defined and limited niche[15]. This level of adaptation is also reflected in other aspects of the basic biochemistry and physiology of the organism.

H. pylori has limited capacity to metabolize carbohydrates, and appears to prefer amino acids and perhaps fatty acids as the carbon and energy source[16]. Amino acids may be deaminated and processed through the tricarboxylic acid (TCA) cycle to release energy. The limited range of carbohydrates utilized by the bacterium is reflected in the expression of a specific glucokinase (JHP1029, HP1103), rather than the broader spectrum hexokinase, in the phosphorylation of glucose[17,18]. Glucose-6-phosphate can be used in either the pentose phosphate pathway or the Entner–Doudoroff pathway, with the Entner–Doudoroff pathway being potentially the major pathway for glucose metabolism[19–22]. The presence or absence of glycolysis (Embden–Mayerhof–Parnas pathway) remains controversial, although it is probable that gluconeogenesis does occur[5,6,19,22]. Pyruvate generated by the Entner–Doudoroff pathway may be converted to acetyl-CoA or fermented, forming metabolic by-products that include lactate, acetate, formate, ethanol, succinate and alanine (via alanine transaminase)[21,23,24]. Such metabolic processes determined by classical techniques have been confirmed by the genome.

Adaptation to life in the stomach may also be reflected in the microaerobic growth requirements of the organism. *H. pylori* cannot grow anaerobically and requires oxygen. At oxygen concentrations approaching atmospheric concentration some strains are able to adapt to the higher than normal oxygen concentration but grow at a slower rate, while others are unable to adapt and fail to grow. The ideal growth conditions are an oxygen concentration of 5–15% and 10% carbon dioxde[25]. As carbon dioxide is essential for growth, *H. pylori* may be classed as capronophilic. Such growth conditions reflect the ecological niche in which the bacterium resides, where the oxygen tension may vary depending on the location of the bacterium in the stomach, the acidity and contents of the stomach. Despite this, *H. pylori* exhibits many biochemical attributes in common with anaerobic bacteria. This bacterium may use either oxygen or fumarate as a terminal electron acceptor in respiration[26].

The use of fumarate as a terminal electron acceptor can be related to the incomplete TCA cycle within the bacterium that operates in the oxidative direction from acetyl-CoA to α-ketoglutarate and in the reductive direction from oxaloacetate to succinate[22,27]. The organism does not have succinate dehydrogenase based on genomic data and confirmed by biochemical data[5,6,27]. Instead fumarate reductase (menaquinone:fumarate oxidoreductase) is used to reduce fumarate to succinate. The presence of both aerobic and anaerobic respiratory pathways is not an unusual occurrence, many bacterial species (facultative anaerobics) can adjust their metabolic status to changes in environmental conditions. A variety of anaerobic electron transport systems and fermentative processes can be introduced as the oxygen tension of the environment decreases, and according to the availability of substrates and electron acceptors[28]. What is unusual with *H. pylori* is that both aerobic and anaerobic metabolic pathways may be operative at the same time, with fumarate reduction and electron transportation to oxygen occurring in the same instance[5,6]. However, since the bacterium has menaquinone and appears to lack ubiquinone[29-31], it is possible that fumarate is the preferred electron acceptor. Indeed, the genomes revealed a putative NADH:ubiquinone oxidoreductase complex (NDH-I dehydrogenase) which may link the oxidation of NADH to the generation of a proton-motive force in aerobic respiration[5,6]. Yet NDH-I may be able to use menaquinone as an electron acceptor and thus link NADH oxidation with fumarate respiration[32]. Diane Taylor's goup has constructed an isogenic mutant in *frdA* which encodes one of the three subunits of the *H. pylori* fumarate reductase, being similar to the fumarate reductase of *Wolinella succinogenes*[33]. They demonstrated that fumarate respiration was not essential *in vitro*, although mutants grew more slowly. However, *in vivo* it is not known whether oxygen or fumarate is the preferred electron acceptor.

Another 'anaerobic' enzyme found in *H. pylori* is pyruvate:flavodoxin oxidoreductase[34]. Pyruvate:flavodoxin oxidoreductase performs a similar function to the pyruvate dehydrogenase of aerobic organisms, that is the generation of acetyl-CoA from pyruvate. The genomic data reveal four putative genes encoding components of a pyruvate:ferrodoxin oxidoreductase complex (*porGDAB*)[5,6]. The difference in terms of the specification of ferrodoxin or flavodoxin reflects the difference between predicted gene products based on similarity and specific biochemical data. Hughes and associates cloned and sequenced *porGDAB* and noted significant sequence similarity to the equivalent Archaeal genes. These data are suggestive of gene transfer between two distinct domains of life on earth, Bacteria and Archaea[35].

The presence of diverse aerobic and anaerobic systems within *H. pylori* raises issues of the internal redox potential of the bacterium, the processes leading to reduction of 5-nitroimidazole antibiotics and defence against oxidative damage to the cell.

THE GENERATION OF FREE RADICALS

Oxygen is the best electron acceptor available to living organisms. The reduction potential of oxygen allows for a large energy change to occur as hydrogen is introduced into the electron transport chain via NADH and succinate dehydrogenase. However, the electron transport chain in aerobic and microaerophilic organisms is not 'leak-proof' and free radical oxygen species are generated as electrons leak out of the transport chain[36]. The incidence of oxygen free radical generation is increased as the oxygen tension of the environment is increased and the likelihood of an electron encountering dioxygen dissolved in solution is increased. Reactive oxygen radical species can also be formed by chemical and radiation processes. In addition, organisms may be exposed to externally generated free radicals such as from the oxidative burst produced by polymorphonuclear leucocytes (PMNL). Infection with *H. pylori* induces an inflammatory response, which leads to an increase in the amount of reactive oxygen species in the gastric mucosa and the gastric juice[37–39].

Nitro compounds and quinones are present in a wide variety of agricultural, food and pharmaceutical products. The microbiota of the gastrointestinal tract can produce toxic products from non-toxic dietary components through hydrolytic and reductive enzyme activities[40]. Nitro and quinone compounds can undergo a one- or a two-electron reduction process. The one-electron reduction of nitro compounds leads to the formation of a nitro radical anion and a semi-quinone radical in the case of quinone compounds. Some of the reduction products are mutagenic, or their formation can lead to the generation of secondary free radicals, which include reactive oxygen species. The 5-nitroimidazole antibiotic metronidazole has a very low reduction potential and is activated by a one-electron reduction process. *H. pylori* is sensitive to metronidazole and other nitroheterocyclic compounds[41], which indicates that the bacterium has the capacity to reduce a wide range of nitro compounds.

OXYGEN, REDOX POTENTIAL AND THE REMOVAL OF TOXIC OXYGEN SPECIES

The oxidation–reduction state of cells can be defined in terms of the ratio of oxidized and reduced thiols present. The major free thiol in most organisms is glutathione (γ-glutamylcysteinylglycine). Oxidative stress leads to the generation of free radicals and an increase in the disulphide forms as proteins and non-protein compounds are oxidized. Reduced glutathione (GSH), which can act in a vast number of cellular processes, can scavenge a variety of free radical species, is important in maintaining the sulphydryl status of many proteins, can chemically react with DNA, and can act as a catalyst in several metabolic reactions. Oxidized glutathione (GSSG) is normally converted back to the reduced state by the enzyme glutathione reductase, with the cycling of glutathione having a critical detoxification role in many organisms. Yet the genome of *H. pylori* appears not to contain a homologue of a gene encoding a typical glutathione reductase[5,6]. In addition, our group has found that the major thiol compound in *H. pylori* is cysteine (unpublished data). The protozoa *Trichomonas vaginalis* and *Trichomonas foetus*, and the amitochondrial eukaryotes *Giardia duodenalis*, *G. intestinalis* and *Entamoeba histolytica* lack detectable levels of glutathione. These organisms are microaerophiles but are also able to grow in anaerobic conditions, and have cysteine as their major thiol[42-45]. In the presence of a metal catalyst, cysteine is oxidized at a much faster rate than glutathione in air. This is thought to account for the lack of cysteine in aerobic organisms. *H. pylori* appears to lack a 'cysteine reductase'; thus we must ask what keeps the cysteine in the bacterium in the reduced state. It has been proposed that in the case of *G. duodenalis* the free cysteine content is maintained in a reduced state via a broad-range thioredoxin-like reductase[46].

H. pylori possesses two genes encoding putative thioredoxin reductase and two genes encoding putative thioredoxin. Thioredoxin and thioredoxin reductase form a NADPH-linked thiol-dependent redox system that selectively reduces proteins. The protein encoded by HP0825 (JHP764) has the greatest similarity to typical thioredoxin reductase and that encoded by HP0824 (JHP763) to typical thioredoxins. HP0824 and HP0825 have been purified and cloned and shown to be the components of a thioredoxin system involved in the stress response[47]. Interestingly, *H. pylori* thioredoxin was able to reduce human IgG and IgA as well as soluble mucin[47].

The putative thioredoxin reductase encoded by HP1458 (JHP1351) and the putative thioredoxin encoded by HP1164 (JHP1091) may fulfil a similar role as the thioredoxin-like reductase in *G. duodenalis* in the maintenance of free cysteine. In addition, the genome reveals the presence of a putative thiol peroxidase (scavengase) (JHP991), a novel family of bacterial antioxidant enzymes possessing thioredoxin-linked thiol peroxidase activity[48]. Direct biochemical evidence for the existence of scavengase in *H. pylori* has been provided by an assay for antioxidant activity[49].

Another defence against oxidative stress is the management of the oxygen status of the cell. NADH oxidases are enzymes that are able to reduce molecular oxygen to hydrogen peroxide or water without the use of an intermediate electron acceptor. No gene encoding a typical NADH oxidase has been found in the *H. pylori* genome; however, NAD(P)H oxidase activity has been reported to be present in cytosolic fractions of *H. pylori*[41]. Sometimes, the NAD(P)H oxidase activity exhibited by an enzyme is not the primary reaction of the enzyme. This has been found to be the case for a number of flavoproteins. For example, alkyl hydroperoxide reductase[50], thioredoxin reductase[51-54], glutathione reductase[55], mercuric reductase[56] and dihydrolipoamide dehydrogenase[56]. The oxidase activity exhibited by these flavoproteins is thought to be due to electron leakage for the reduced flavin co-factor of the enzymes[50].

The redox status of a cell is very important, and this is especially true for the microaerophile *H. pylori*. Changing the environmental oxygen concentration can greatly affect metabolic processes and clinical outcomes. The use of the antimicrobial agent metronidazole in therapy leads to a high incidence of metronidazole-resistant *H. pylori*. These resistant bacteria have lost the capacity to reduce metronidazole under microaerophilic conditions. However, exposure of the bacterium to anaerobic conditions causes them to become sensitive to the drug[41,57]. Goodwin and associates identified a nitroreductase (RdxA) that appears to play an important role in the activation of metronidazole in *H. pylori*[58]. The beneficial or deleterious nature of nitroreductases and quinone reductases depends on the reduction process. A one-electron reduction process leads to the generation of radical species whereas a two-electron reduction process generates the nitroso and the quinol in the case of nitro compounds and quinone compounds, respectively. The best example of such an enzyme is NAD(P)H:(quinone-acceptor) oxidoreductase, known as DT-diaphorase, which is present in hepatocytes. This enzyme catalyses the two-electron reduction of quinones to quinols, without the formation of the toxic semi-quinone radicals. Therefore, the degree of free radical generation from non-toxic compounds depends on the balance of reductases that reduce these compounds by a one-electron reduction process compared with those which cause a two-electron reduction.

Organisms that use oxygen as an electron acceptor and thereby generate toxic oxygen species as a by-product have evolved defensive mechanisms. These include the enzymes superoxide dismutase, catalase, peroxidases and a variety of reductases. Some of these mechanisms are also found in organisms that do not use oxygen in their metabolic pathways but may occasionally encounter oxygen in the environment or exogenous toxic oxygen species.

Superoxide dismutase catalyses the dismutation of superoxide ions to hydrogen peroxide. The superoxide dismutase in *H. pylori* is a typical prokaryotic iron-containing enzyme[59], which consists of two identical subunits of 24 kDa. Catalase converts hydrogen peroxide to water and oxygen. The catalase in *H. pylori* is a typical catalase in that it contains iron-porphyrin and lacks peroxidase activity[60]. The enzyme is a tetramer with a subunit mass of 58 kDa based on the genome sequence and physical measurement[5,6,60]. Both superoxide dismutase and catalase may be expressed on the cell surface, with catalase also being expressed in the cytoplasm, and potentially within the periplasm[60-62]. Whereas surface expression may afford protection against extracellular oxidative damage, the genetic sequence for catalase does not encode a known amino acid signal sequence. Spontaneous and isogenic catalase negative mutants are viable, indicating that the enzyme is not essential for growth *in vitro*[63-65]; however, it is yet to be determined if such mutants are able to survive in the hostile environment of the gastric lumen. No genes encoding classical peroxidase have been found in the genomes of *H. pylori* strains 26695 and J99[5,6].

Another important enzyme system present in many bacteria is alkyl hydroperoxide reductase. This enzyme complex consists of two proteins, a large subunit (AhpF) and a small subunit (AhpC). An ORF encoding a homologue of *ahpC* is present in the genome of *H. pylori*; however there is no ORF encoding a homologue of *ahpF*. Baillon et al.[66] identified a homologue of *ahpC* in the microaerophile *Campylobacter jejuni*. Like *H. pylori*, *C. jejuni* appears not to contain *ahpF*, encoding the large subunit of alkyl hydroperoxide reductase. Importantly, however, insertional mutagenesis of *ahpC* in *C. jejuni* resulted in an increased sensitivity to oxidative stresses induced by cumene hydroperoxide and atmospheric air. These data suggest that it is possible that AhpC may be functional in *H. pylori*.

THE ROLE OF CARBON DIOXIDE

Another aspect of the microaerophile of *H. pylori* relates to CO_2. The requirement by *H. pylori* for CO_2 may relate to the abundance of CO_2/HCO_3^- derived from the degradation of urea. *H. pylori* expresses acetyl-CoA carboxylase which appears to form part of a multi-protein complex catalysing the first step in fatty acid biosynthesis, fixing HCO_3^- to form malonyl-CoA[34,67]. Consistent with the hypothesis that *H. pylori* has adapted to life with abundant CO_2/HCO_3^- the affinity of the enzyme for bicarbonate appears relatively low[34,67]. One of the subunits of acetyl-CoA carboxylase is a biotin containing protein of approximately 24 kDa[67]. Biotin is required by acetyl-CoA carboxylase for CO_2/HCO_3^- fixation and, within the genome, seven ORFs linked to biotin synthesis and associated functions have been identified[5,6]. These ORFs have homology with the biotin synthesis genes *bioABCDF*, *birA* (biotin operon repressor/biotin acetyl coenzyme A carboxylase synthetase) and *bisC* (biotin sulphoxide reductase) genes. In addition to the enzymes for fatty acid synthesis and related genes, the genome revealed two ORFs with 33.3% and 37.9% similarity to carbonic anhydrase (HP0004 and HP1186). Carbonic anhydrase catalyses the interconversion between CO_2 and carbonic acid (which dissociates into H^+ and HCO_3^-). The true functions and role of the product of these two ORFs remain to be determined.

ION TRANSPORT

As a defence against infection iron is sequestered by systems including transferrin and lactoferrin. Most pathogenic bacteria can abstract iron from the host by means of siderophores. The Institute for Genomic Research group identified a number of homologues of the siderophore-mediated iron-uptake *fec* system of *E. coli* (*fecADE*), a result confirmed by the Astra (AstraZeneca) group[5,6]. These *fec* homologues were not organized into a single operon. What were not identified were homologues of *E. coli fecR* and *fecI*, encoding regulatory proteins, and siderophore-related genes of *E. coli*, *fecB* and *fecC*. While some *E. coli fec* homologues were not present, there were three copies of *fecA*[5,6]. In addition, a homologue of *tonB*, which encodes a siderophore-mediated iron transport protein, was identified[5,6]. These data, while still requiring further study, are supported by the findings of Illingworth and associates in relation to the extracellular siderophores produced by *H. pylori*[68].

Five complete or truncated homologues of *frpB* (HP0876, HP0915, HP0916, HP1512, HP1511), encoding putative haem- or lactoferrin-binding proteins have been identified[5,6]. Husson et al. detected a surface receptor that would allow *H. pylori* to grow on human lactoferrin as the sole iron source[69], while Worst et al. identified haem-binding outer membrane proteins[70]. Further, Worst and associates[71] have demonstrated that for unrelated segments in the genome of *H. pylori* facilitate haem utilization. Such haem may be utilized either complete or as an iron source, together with human lactoferrin and iron abstracted by siderophores[72].

While the ability to abstract iron from haem and lactoferrin is biologically significant, the genome of *H. pylori* also contained a homologue of *feoB*, part of a system that with *feoA* in *E. coli* facilitates ferrous iron uptake system[73]; yet no *feoA* homologue was identified[5,6]. In addition, a homologue of the gene encoding the ferric uptake regulator, *fur* was present in the genome. Fur regulates individual genes in response to iron and other environmental signals[74]. Consensus sequences for Fur-binding boxes were found upstream of two *fecA* gene homologues, the three *frpB* gene homologues and the *fur* homologue[5,6]. A Fur-like binding box was also reported upstream of the *katA* gene by Odenbreit et al. and Manos et al.[63,64]

Ion transport is also intimately linked to urease activity. Urease was identified as a prominent enzyme early in the history of *H. pylori*[75]. Urease requires nickel as a prosthetic group, the metal ion being taken up into *H. pylori* by the high-affinity nickel transport protein (NixA)[76,77]. In addition, nickel may be imported by a non-specific metal ion transporter, a P-type ATPase[78]. While *H. pylori* is able to import necessary trace elements including nickel, accumulation of some metal ions is toxic. Thus, the bacterium needs to eliminate such toxic elements[79].

The genome uncovered a number of systems for the efflux of ion, including *copA*, *copP* and *czcA*. In *H. pylori* copper and mercuric ions may be selectively exported by means of the protein CopA, homologous with known copper-transporting P-type ATPases, and CopP[80–83]. Bayle and associates[84] determined the location of the ion-binding motif in CopA and proposed that the protein was a member of the CPX-type ATPase family binding predominantly to copper ion. Bayle et al. considered the CopP homologue of *H. pylori* to be a regulatory protein similar to the CopZ of *Enterococcus hirae*. The three homologues of the *Alcaligenes eutrophus* gene *czcA* (HP1328, HP1239, HP0969) are related to the three-protein complex (CzcABC) which acts as a cation–proton cobalt, zinc, and cadmium anti-port[85].

CONCLUSION

The literature is growing substantially with reports of studies into the function and nature of the gene products of *H. pylori*. Many of these studies have been made possible through access to the genomic data published by Tomb et al.[5] and Alm et al.[6]. Genomics and proteomics will provide further information in the coming years. We are entering an exciting period of discovery where we will gain an unprecedented understanding of the interaction of pathogens with their specific hosts. *H. pylori* will be in the vanguard of some of these developments.

References

1. IARC Monographs on the Evaluation of Carcinogenic Risks to Humans,. 1994, Vol. 61, pp. 177–240. Lyon: International Agency for Research on Cancer, World Health Organization.
2. Forman D. The etiology of gastric cancer. IARC Scientific Publications (Lyon) 1991;105:22–32.
3. Lee A, Fox J, Hazell S. Pathogenicity of *Helicobacter pylori* – a perspective. Infect Immun. 1993;61:1601–10.
4. Wotherspoon A *et al*. *H. pylori* associated gastritis and B-cell gastric lymphoma. Lancet. 1991;338:1175–6.
5. Tomb JF *et al*. The complete genome sequence of *H. pylori*. Nature. 1997;388:539–47.
6. Alm R *et al*. Genomic-sequence comparison of two unrelated isolates of the human gastric pathogen *H. pylori*. Nature. 1999;397:176–80.
7. Marais A, Mendz GL, Hazell SL, Megraud F. Metabolism and genetics of *Helicobacter pylori:* the genome era. MMBR. 1999;3:642–74.
8. Doig P *et al*. *Helicobacter pylori* physiology predicted from genomic comparison of two strains. MMBR. 1999;3:675–707.
9. Mendz GL, Jimenez BM, Hazell SL, Gero AM, O'Sullivan WJ. De novo synthesis of pyrimidine nucleotides by *Helicobacter pylori*. J Appl Bacteriol. 1994;77:1–8.
10. Mendz GL, Jimenez BM, Hazell SL, Gero AM, O'Sullivan WJ. Salvage synthesis of purine nucleotides by *Helicobacter pylori*. J Appl Bacteriol. 1994;77:674–81.
11. Mendz GL, Hazell SL. The urea cycle of *Helicobacter pylori*. Microbiology. 1996; 142:2959–67.
12. Cordwell, SJ. Microbial genomes and 'missing' enzymes: re-defining biochemical pathways? Arch Microbiol. 1999;172:269–79.
13. Urquhart BL, Cordwell SJ, Humphery-Smith I. Comparison of predicted and observed properties of proteins encoded in the genome of *Mycobacterium tuberculosis* H37Rv. Biochem Biophys Res Commun. 1998;253:70–9.
14. Zakharova N, Paster BJ, Wesley I, Dewhurst FE, Berg DE, Severinov KV. Fused and overlapping *rpoB* and *rpoC* genes in *Helicobacters*, *Campylobacters* and related bacteria. J Bacteriol. 2000;181:3857–9.
15. Scoarughi GL, Cimmino C, Donini P. *Helicobacter pylori:* a eubacterium lacking the stringent response. J Bacteriol. 1999;181:552–5.
16. Reynolds DJ, Penn CW. Characteristics of *Helicobacter pylori* growth in a defined medium and determination of its amino acid requirements. Microbiology. 1994;140:2649–56.
17. Burns B, Mendz GL, Hazell SL. Characterisation of the glucose transporters in *Helicobacter pylori*. Acta Gastro-Enterol Belg. 1993;56(S):44.
18. Mendz GL, Hazell SL. Glucose phosphorylation in *Helicobacter pylori*. Arch Biochem Biophys. 1993;300:522–5.
19. Mendz GL, Hazell SL, Burns BP. The Entner–Doudoroff pathway in *Helicobacter pylori*. Arch Biochem Biophys. 1994;312:349–56.
20. Mendz GL, Hazell SL. Evidence for a pentose phosphate pathway in *Helicobacter pylori*. FEMS Lett. 1991;84:331–6.
21. Chalk PA, Roberts AD, Blows WM. Metabolism of pyruvate and glucose by intact cells of *Helicobacter pylori* studied by C-13 NMR spectroscopy. Microbiology. 1994;140:2085–92.
22. Hoffman PS, Goodwin A, Johnsen J, Magee K, Veldhuyzen van Zanten SJO. Metabolic activities of metronidazole-sensitive and -resistant strains of *Helicobacter pylori* – repression of pyruvate oxidoreductase and expression of isocitrate lyase activity correlate with resistance. J Bacteriol. 1996;178:4822–9.
23. Mendz GL, Hazell SL, Burns BP. Glucose utilization and lactate production by *Helicobacter pylori*. J Gen Microbiol. 1993;139:3023–8.
24. Mendz GL, Hazell SL, Vangorkom L. Pyruvate metabolism in *Helicobacter pylori*. Arch Microbiol. 1994;162:187–92.

25. Hazell SL. Cultural techniques for the growth and isolation of *Helicobacter pylori*. In: Goodwin CS, Worsley BW, editors. *Helicobacter pylori*: Biology and Clinical Practice. Boca Raton, FL: CRC Press; 1993:273–83.
26. Mendz GL, Hazell SL. Fumarate catabolism in *Helicobacter pylori*. Biochem Mol Biol Int. 1993;31:325–32.
27. Pitson SM, Mendz GL, Srinivasan S, Hazell SL. The tricarboxylic acid cycle of *Helicobacter pylori*. Eur J Biochem. 1999;260:258–67.
28. Tseng CP, Hansen AK, Cotter P, Gunsalus RP. Effect of cell growth rate on expression of the anaerobic respiratory pathway operons *frdABCD*, *dmsABC*, and *narGHJI* of *Escherichia coli*. J Bacteriol. 1994;176:6599–605.
29. Goodwin CS, Collins MD, Blincow E. The absence of theroplasmaquinones in *Campylobacter pyloridis*, and its temperature and pH growth range. Microbiol Lett. 1986;32:137–40.
30. Moss CW, Lambert Fai MA, Nicholson MA, Guerrant GO. Isoprenoid quinones of *Campylobacter cryaerophila*, *C. cinaedi*, *C. fennelliae*, *C. hyointestinalis*, *C. pylori*, and '*C. upsaliensis*'. J Clin Microbiol. 1990;28:395–7.
31. Marcelli SW, Chang HT, Chapman T, Chalk PA, Miles RJ, Poole RK. The respiratory chain of *Helicobacter pylori* – identification of cytochromes and the effects of oxygen on cytochrome and menaquinone levels. FEMS Microbiol Lett. 1996;138:59–64.
32. Tran QH, Bongaerts J, Vlad D, Unden G. Requirement for the proton-pumping NADH dehydrogenase I of *Escherichia coli* in respiration of NADH to fumarate and its bioenergetic implications. Eur J Biochem. 1997;244:155–60.
33. Ge ZM, Jiang Q, Kalisiak MS, Taylor DE. Cloning and functional characterisation of *Helicobacter pylori* fumarate reductase operon comprising three structural genes coding for subunits C, A and B. Gene. 1997;204:227–34.
34. Hughes NJ, Chalk PA, Clayton CL, Kelly DJ. Identification of carboxylation enzymes and characterization of a novel four-subunit pyruvate:flavodoxin oxidoreductase from *Helicobacter pylori*. J Bacteriol. 1995;177:3953–9.
35. Hughes NJ, Clayton CL, Chalk PA, Kelly DJ. *Helicobacter pylori porCDAB* and *oorDABC* genes encode distinct pyruvate:flavodoxin oxidoreductase and 2-oxogluterate:acceptor oxidoreductase which mediate electron transport to NADP. J Bacteriol. 1998;180:1119–28.
36. Ksenzenko MY, Vygodina TV, Berka V, Rauge EK, Konstantinov AA. Cytochrome oxidase-catalyzed superoxide generation from hydrogen peroxide. FEBS Lett. 1992;297:63–6.
37. Davies GR, Simmonds NJ, Stevens TRJ, Grandison A, Blake DR, Rampton DS. Mucosal reactive oxygen metabolite production in duodenal ulcer disease. Gut. 1992;33:1467–72.
38. Davies GR, Banatvala N, Collins CE *et al*. Relationship between infective load of *Helicobacter pylori* and reactive oxygen metabolite production in antral mucosa. Scand J Gastroenterol. 1994;29:419–24.
39. Nalini S, Ramakrishna BS, Mohanty A, Balasubramanian KA. Hydroxyl radical formation in human gastric juice. J Gastroenterol Hepatol. 1992;7:497–501.
40. Goldin BR, Gualtieri LJ, Moore RP. The effect of *Lactobacillus* GG on the initiation and promotion of DMH-induced intestinal tumors in the rat. Nutr Cancer. 1996;25:197–204.
41. Smith MA, Edward DI. Redox potential and oxygen concentration as factors in the susceptibility of *Helicobacter pylori* to nitroheterocyclic drugs. J Antimicrob Chemother. 1995;35:751–64.
42. Fahey RC, Newton GL, Arrick B, Overdankbogart T, Aley SB. *Entamoeba histolytica*: a eukaryote without glutathione metabolism. Science. 1984;224:70–2.
43. Smith NC, Bryant C, Boreham PFL. Possible roles for pyruvate:ferredoxin oxidoreductase and thiol-dependent peroxidase and reductase activities in resistance to nitroheterocyclic drugs in *Giardia intestinalis*. Int J Parasitol. 1988;18:991–7.
44. Brown DM, Upcroft JA, Upcroft P. Cysteine is the major low molecular weight thiol in *Giardia duodenalis*. Mol Biochem Parasitol. 1993;61:155–8.
45. Ellis JE, Yarlett N, Cole D, Humphreys MJ, Lloyd D. Antioxidant defences in the microaerophilic protozoan *Trichomonas vaginalis*: comparison of metronidazole-resistant and sensitive strains. Microbiology. 1994;140:2489–94.
46. Brown DM, Upcroft JA, Upcroft P. A thioredoxin reductase-class of disulphide reductase in the protozoan parasite *Giardia duodenalis*. Mol Biochem Parasitol. 1996;83:211–20.
47. Windle HJ, Fox A, Eidhin DN, Kelleher D. The thioredoxin system of *Helicobacter pylori*. J Biol Chem. 2000;275:5081–9.

48. Zhou Y, Wan XY, Wang HL, Yan ZY, Hou YD, Jin DY. Bacterial scavengase p20 is structurally and functionally related to peroxiredoxins. Biochem Biophys Res Commun. 1997;233:848–52.
49. Wan XY, Zhou Y, Yan ZY, Wang HL, Hou YD, Jin DY. Scavengase p20: a novel family of bacterial antioxidant enzymes. FEBS Lett. 1997;407:32–6.
50. Calzi ML, Poole LB. Requirement for the two AhpF cystine disulfide centers in catalysis of peroxide reduction by alkyl hydroperoxide reductase. Biochemistry. 1997;36:13357–64.
51. Arnér ESJ, Bjornstedt M, Holmgren A. 1-Chloro-2,4-dinitrobenzene is an irreversible inhibitor of human thioredoxin reductase – loss of thioredoxin disusulfide reductase activity is accompanied by a large increase in NADPH oxidase activity. J Biol Chem. 1995:270:3479–82.
52. Nordberg J, Zhong L, Holmgren A, Arner ESJ. Mammalian thioredoxin reductase is irreversibly inhibited by dinitrohalobenzenes by alkylation of both the redox active selenocysteine and its neighboring cysteine residue. J Biol Chem. 1998;273:10835–42.
53. Lin S, Cullen WR, Thomas DJ. Methylarsenicals and arsinothiols are potent inhibitors of mouse liver thioredoxin reductase. Chem Res Toxicol. 1999;12:924–30.
54. Zhang Z, Hillas PJ, de Montellano PRO. Reduction of peroxides and dinitrobenzenes by *Mycobacterium tuberculosis* thioredoxin and thioredoxin reductase. Arch Biochem Biophys. 1999;363:19–26.
55. Carlberg I, Mannervik B. Oxidase activity of glutathione reductase effected by 2,4,6-trinitrobenzenesulfonate. FEBS Lett. 1980;115:265–8.
56. Carlberg I, Sahlman L, Mannervik B. The effect of 2,4,6-trinitrobenzenesulfonate on mercuric reductase, glutathione reductase and lipoamide dehydrogenase. FEBS Lett. 1985; 180:102–6.
57. Cederbrant G, Kahlmeter G, Ljungh A. Proposed mechanism for metronidazole resistance in *Helicobacter pylori*. J Antimicrob Chemother. 1992;29:115–20.
58. Goodwin A, Kersulyte D, Sisson G, Veldhuyzen van Zanten SJO, Berg DE, Hoffman PS. Metronidazole resistance in *Helicobacter pylori* is due to null mutations in a gene (rdxA) that encodes an oxygen-insensitive NADPH nitroreductase. Mol Microbiol. 1998;28: 383–93.
59. Spiegelhalder C, Gerstenecker B, Kersten A, Schiltz E, Kist M. Purification of *Helicobacter pylori* superoxide dismutase and cloning and sequence of the gene. Infect Immun. 1993;61:5315–25.
60. Hazell SL, Evans DJJ, Graham DY. *Helicobacter pylori* catalase. J Gen Microbiol. 1991;137:57–61.
61. Hazell SL. Urease and catalase as virulence factors of *Helicobacter pylori*. In: Menge H, Gregor M, Tytgat GNJ, Marshall BJ, McNulty CAM, editors. *Helicobacter pylori* 1990. Berlin: Springer-Verlag; 1991:3–12.
62. Phadnis SH, Parlow MH, Levy M *et al*. Surface localization of *Helicobacter pylori* urease and a heat shock protein homolog requires bacterial autolysis. Infect Immun. 1996; 64:905–12.
63. Odenbreit S, Wieland B, Haas R. Cloning and genetic characterization of *Helicobacter pylori* catalase and construction of a catalase-deficient mutant strain. J Bacteriol. 1996;178: 6960–67.
64. Manos J, Kolesnikow T, Hazell SL. An investigation of the molecular basis of the spontaneous occurrence of a catalase-negative phenotype in *Helicobacter pylori*. Helicobacter. 1998;4:1–7.
65. Westblom TU, Phadnis S, Langenberg W, Yoneda K, Madan E, Midkiff BR. Catalase negative mutants of *Helicobacter pylori*. Eur J Clin Microbiol Infect Dis. 1992;11:522–6.
66. Baillon ML, van Vliet AH, Ketley JM, Constantinidou C, Penn CW. An iron-regulated alkyl hydroperoxide reductase (AhpC) confers aerotolerance and oxidative stress resistance to the microaerophilic pathogen *Campylobacter jejuni*. J Bacteriol. 1999;181:4798–804.
67. Burns BP, Hazell SL, Mendz GL. Acetyl-CoA carboxylase activity in *Helicobacter pylori* and the requirement of increased CO_2 for growth. Microbiology. 1995;141:3113–18.
68. Illingworth DS, Walter KS, Griffiths PL, Barclay R. Siderophore production and iron-regulated envelope proteins of *Helicobacter pylori*. Zbl Bakt-Int J Med Microbiol. 1993;280:113–19.
69. Husson MO, Legrand D, Spik G, Leclerc H. Iron acquisition by *Helicobacter pylori* – importance of human lactoferrin. Infect Immun. 1993;61:2694–7.

70. Worst DJ, Otto BR, Degraaff J. Iron-repressible outer membrane proteins of *Helicobacter pylori* involved in heme uptake. Infect Immun. 1995;63:4161–5.
71. Worst DJ, Maaskant J, Vandenbroucke-Grauls CM, Kusters JG. Multiple haem-utilization loci in *Helicobacter pylori*. Microbiology. 1999;145:681–8.
72. Dhaenens L, Szczebara F, Van Nieuwenhuyse S, Husson MO. Comparison of iron uptake in different *Helicobacter* species. Res Microbiol. 1999;150:475–81.
73. Kammler M, Schon C, Hantke K. Characterisation of the ferrous iron uptake system of *Escherichia coli*. J Bacteriol. 1993;175:6212–19.
74. Litwin CM, Calderwood SB. Role of iron in regulation of virulence genes. Clin Microbiol Rev. 1993;6:137–49.
75. Hazell SL, Lee A, Brady L, Hennessy W. *Campylobacter pyloridis* and gastritis: association with intercellular spaces and adaption to an environment of mucus as important factors in colonization of the gastric epithelium. J Infect Dis. 1986;153:658–63.
76. Mobley HLT, Garner RM, Bauerfeind P. *Helicobacter pylori* nickel-transport gene nixA: synthesis of catalytically active urease in *Escherichia coli* independent of growth conditions. Mol Microbiol. 1995;16:97–109.
77. Bauerfeind P, Garner RM, Mobley HLT. Allelic exchange mutagenesis of nixa in *Helicobacter pylori* results in reduced nickel transport and urease activity. Infect Immun. 1996;64:2877–80.
78. Melchers K, Weitzenegger T, Buhmann A, Steinhilber W, Sachs G, Schafer KP. Cloning and membrane topology of a P type ATPase from *Helicobacter pylori*. J Biol Chem. 1996; 271:446–57.
79. Silver S. Bacterial resistances to toxic metal ions: a review. Gene. 1996;179:9–19.
80. Ge ZM, Hiratsuka K, Taylor DE. Nucleotide sequence and mutational analysis indicate that two *Helicobacter pylori* genes encode a P-type ATPase and a cation-binding protein associated with copper transport. Mol Microbiol. 1995;15:97–106.
81. Beier D, Spohn G, Rappuoli R, Scarlato V. Identification and characterization of an operon of *Helicobacter pylori* that is involved in motility and stress adaptation. J Bacteriol. 1997;179:4676–83.
82. Ge ZM, Taylor DE. *Helicobacter pylori* genes hpcopA and hpcopP constitute a cop operon involved in copper export. FEMS Microbiol Lett. 1996;145:181–8.
83. Ge ZM, Taylor DE. Sequencing, expression, and genetic characterization of the *Helicobacter pylori* FtsH gene encoding a protein homologous to members of a novel putative ATPase family. J Bacteriol. 1996;178:6151–7.
84. Bayle D, Wangler S, Weitzenegger T et al. Properties of the P-type ATPase encoded by the copAP operons of *Helicobacter pylori* and *Helicobacter felis*. J Bacteriol. 1988;180:317–29.
85. Nies DH. The cobalt, zinc, and cadmium efflux system CzcABC from *Alcaligenes eutrophus* functions as a cation–proton antiporter in *Escherichia coli*. J Bacteriol. 1995;177:2707–12.

2
The urease system of *Helicobacter pylori*

D. L. WEEKS, D. R. SCOTT, P. VOLAND, E. A. MARCUS,
C. ATHMANN, K. MELCHERS and G. SACHS

THE HABITAT OF GASTRIC *HELICOBACTER* SPP

The habitation of the human and other mammalian stomachs by gastric *Helicobacter* spp. requires specific explanation since they are all Gram-negative neutralophiles. All infected human stomachs acquire gastritis due to the infection, although only 20% of these achieve the distinction of peptic ulcer disease. Specific regions of the stomach can be inhabited by the organism, such as the antrum, the transition zone, or the fundus. In the latter situation atrophic gastritis can ensue, in the former sites either duodenal or gastric ulcer, respectively. The theme of this brief review is that the explanation for denizenic ability, gastritis and locale of habitation depends on a balance between acidity, urea concentration and activity of intrabacterial urease.

H. pylori synthesizes urease constitutively, dedicating up to 15% of its protein synthetic effort to making this enzyme. Clearly, the organisms think that it is very important to make this protein at a higher level than any other known organism[1]. Since urease hydrolyses urea to form ammonia and carbon dioxide, and ammonia can absorb acid to form ammonium, it is natural to suspect that this dedication to make urease has a relationship to survival and growth in the stomach. This suspicion has been confirmed many times in animal models where infection of mice, ferrets and pigs requires the presence of urease[2-4]. It is not certain that the requirement for urease is for colonization as well as for infection.

There is a dispute as to the acidity of the environment that the organism inhabits. Many think that there is a large pH gradient from gastric contents to the surface of the mucosa. When the pH of contents is >2.0, epithelial cell surface pH may be as high as 6.0. This is based on data using open-tip pH microelectrodes to measure surface pH[5]. There is some evidence that this may not be the case, however, since confocal microscopy using pH-sensitive fluorescent dyes does not show such a gradient[6]. However, even microelectrodes show that the pH gradient disappears when gastric contents have a pH < 2.0^5; and median 24 hour intragastric pH in the human stomach is 1.4! This suggests that *H. pylori* must be able to live in a highly acidic environment, not just at a close to neutral pH on the gastric surface.

ACID ACTIVATION OF INTRABACTERIAL UREASE

The pH at which *H. pylori* colonizes the stomach bears a relationship to the pH at which urease works best or at all. The pH optimum of the urease made by gastric *Helicobacter* is neutral, meaning it has high activity at pH 7.5–8.5 and no activity at pH < 4.5. One would therefore conjecture that intrabacterial urease is what is being used for acid resistance by these organisms. Unfortunately, this idea is muddied by the finding that the organism also has urease on its surface, albeit much less than in its interior. Surface urease is also inactive at pH < 4.5. There is continuing dispute as to whether this urease is secreted or released by lysis of the organism[7,8]. Since there is no signal sequence in either urease subunit (A or B), and there are no proteins capable of type III secretion in the genome of *H. pylori*, one is left with type IV secretion as the only means of exteriorizing urease without lysis[9,10]. Type IV secretion, however, is restricted to placement of bacterial proteins into host cells. Putting urease into gastric cells would not be helpful to the bacteria. Further, to exteriorize active folded heterodimeric urease is beyond the capacity of type IV secretion and to exteriorize six members of the urease gene cluster and nickel to assemble active urease is even more unlikely. The perspective of this review is that the external urease of *H. pylori* that is on its surface is there because of lysis. Given its absence of activity at pH 4.5, it performs no useful function in resistance to gastric acidity or indeed colonization of the stomach, except that, at pH 4.5 or greater, it has neutralizing activity. Perhaps this prevents or reduces extra gastric infection and prevents a more robust antigenic response.

This leaves intrabacterial urease as the only candidate for significant acid resistance. If this is the case, one should see intrabacterial urease activity under acidic pH conditions for production of neutralizing ammonia, NH_3, that will form NH_4^+ in acid. In contrast to surface or free urease, measurement of intrabacterial urease activity at different pH values, either by release of $^{14}CO_2$ from labelled urea, or by measurement of the rate of alkalinization as a function of pH in a microphysiometer[1,11], shows low urease activity at neutral pH, rapid increase between pH 6.0 and 5.0 and steady activity down to a pH of 2.5 but still present at pH 2.0 as illustrated in Figure 1 and ref. 11.

The 10-fold activation of urease between pH 6.5 and 5.5 is striking. Using pH-metry in a microphysiometer, where there is little buffering, activation of intrabacterial urease is closer to 20-fold.

BUFFERING OF THE PERIPLASM BY INTRABACTERIAL UREASE

The consequence of the activity profile of intrabacterial urease is that the intact organism is able to generate NH_3 in acid; just what is necessary to

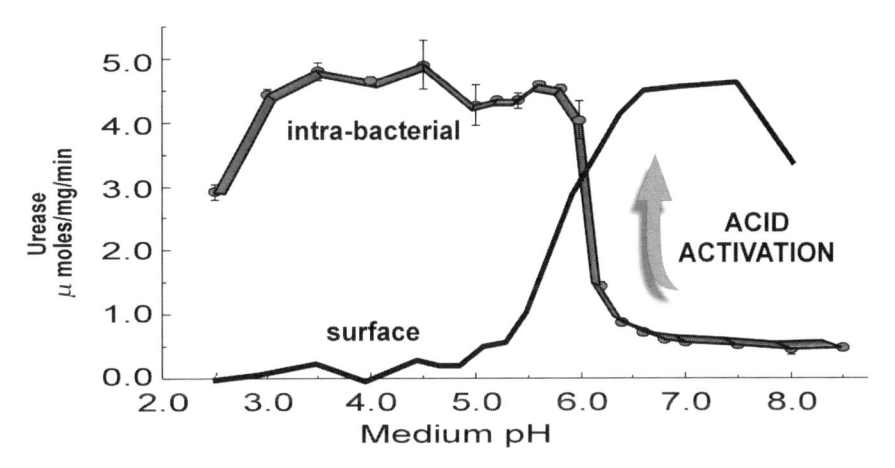

Figure 1. pH activity profile of surface and intrabacterial urease under strong buffering conditions, showing loss of activity in acidic medium of surface urease and a steep increase in intrabacterial urease between pH 6.5 and 5.5, with steady activity until pH 2.5. The activity of intrabacterial urease at acidic pH is the same as urease activity of a homogenate or a detergent-treated preparation at neutral pH.

combat gastric acidity. The concentration of urea in the normal gastric juice is about 1–2 mM. It is there due to diffusion across the epithelium without the presence of a specific transporter for urea as found in the kidney or red blood cells[12] (N. Zeng, unpublished). Gastric juice can contain as much as 100 mM HCl; 1 mM urea, no matter how efficiently utilized, is not sufficient to combat this acidity if it is trying to do this in the external environment of the organism. However, the periplasm that lies between the inner and outer membrane of this Gram-negative bacterium has a very small volume, in the order of a fraction of a femtolitre, and has some degree of protection from acid due to the outer membrane and cell wall. The periplasm would also be the first space, external to the cytoplasm, to see the NH_3 produced in the cytoplasm. The periplasm would therefore seem the only region where NH_3 generated intrabacterially could possibly enable gastric acid resistance. There are two lines of evidence for this: indirect and direct.

The membrane potential across the inner membrane is a function of the pH gradient between the periplasm and the cytoplasm. As the periplasm becomes more acidic, thereby increasing the pH gradient inward, the membrane potential will decrease, to maintain a constant driving force for proton flux across the ATP synthase, F_1F_0. This is the proton motive force, the bioenergetic basis of life, and must be kept high for bacteria to survive[13]. In the case of *H. pylori*, at pH 7.0 it is composed of about 1.4 pH units inward and -140 mV negative inside to give a total of about -220 mV, that is maintained between pH 4.0 and 8.0. It is irreversibly lost at pH < 4.0 in the absence of urea[14].

However when ~ 1 mM urea is added between pH 3.0 and 5.0 the potential rapidly increases to a constant value of ~ -100 mV. This happens even in the presence of strong buffer, emphasizing the buffering ability of intrabacter-

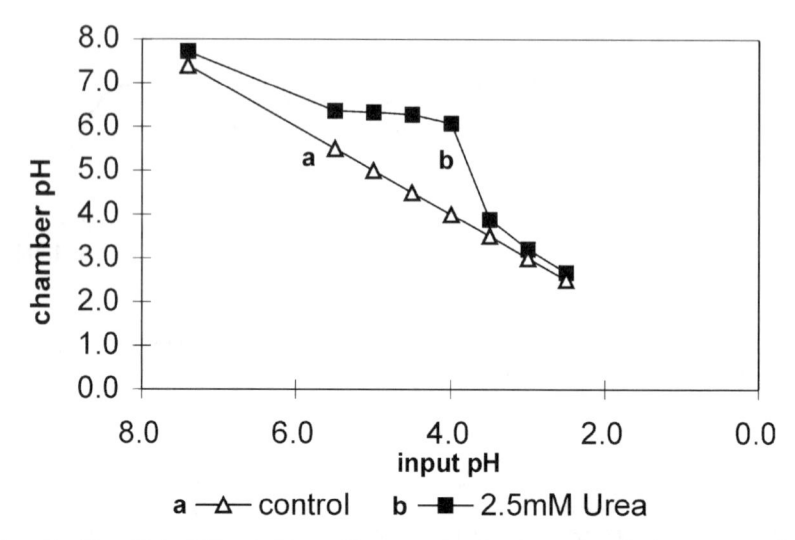

Figure 2. The effect of *H. pylori* in a pH sensor chamber in a microphysiometer superfused without and with urea. Between pH 6.0 and 4.0 urease activity sets chamber pH to ~6.2, the same pH as predicted for the periplasm using measurement of membrane potential[1].

ial urease in acid[1]. The simplest explanation for this finding is that intrabacterial urease has produced NH_3 and that efflux of NH_3 has buffered the periplasm to a pH of ~6.2. Certainly, urease activity is responsible for this, and it is intrabacterial urease, not surface urease, since high concentrations of the selective urease inhibitor, flurofamide, are necessary to blunt the response and this does not happen in urease-negative organisms.

When *H. pylori* is placed in a pH sensor chamber, and the pH of the chamber at steady state is measured in the presence of urea at different initial pH values, the bacteria in the presence of urea increase chamber pH to 6.2 at a pH between 3.0 and 5.5 even during perfusion, the same value as calculated from changes in membrane potential[14]. This is shown in Figure 2.

A direct demonstration of the elevation of periplasmic pH is possible using confocal microscopy. In *H. pylori*, co-cultured with the gastric AGS cell line, the bacteria adhere well and are immobilized to allow relatively convenient high-magnification microscopy. The fluorescent pH dye, BCECF, is impermeant across the inner membrane of the organism but not the outer membrane, which contains porins that are helical membrane proteins permeable to negatively charged molecules such as ATP. The dye signals elevation of pH by an increase in fluorescence and so should be able to define a change in the pH of the periplasm upon the addition of urea. With *in-vivo* microscopy, as illustrated below, the periplasm is defined by an elevation of pH in a restricted space immediately adjacent to the bacteria. If this were external to the outer membrane no such restriction would be evident, due to the rapid diffusion of NH_3 in solution.

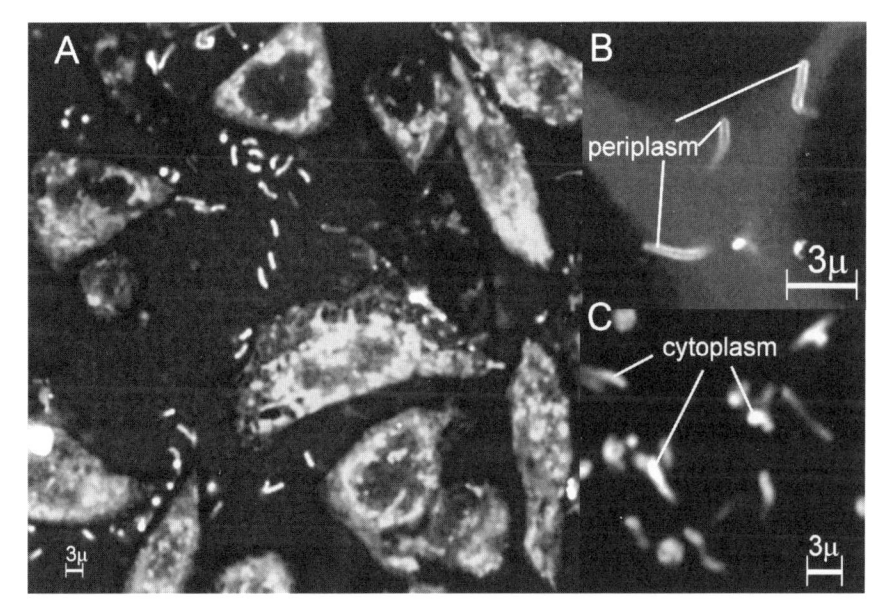

Figure 3. Visualization of *H. pylori* and site of pH elevation in a AGS co-culture system. On the left (**A**) is a confocal image of AGS cells that have taken up the mitochondrial potential probe, $DiSC_3(5)$ and peribacterial fluorescence using the impermeant pH probe, BCECF free acid, immediately following the addition of 5 mM urea. At the top right (**B**) is a higher magnification of this experiment showing that it is the periplasm of the organism that is showing the pH increase due to urea addition and intrabacterial urease activity. At the bottom right (**C**) is an experiment following treatment with 0.01% $C_{12}E_8$, a non-ionic detergent, and then addition of urea, showing that membrane permeabilization has allowed entry of BCECF and also urea with consequent alkalinization of the cytoplasm.

The initial change in pH upon urea addition is in the periplasm and then in the medium in intact organisms. These changes are shown in Figure 3A and B. The large panel shows AGS cells stained with a mitochondrial potential dye and the organisms increasing peribacterial BCECF fluorescence upon addition of urea at pH 5.5. This shows that peribacterial pH is increasing following urea addition at this pH. At neutral pH there is no such change, consistent with the lack of activation of intrabacterial urease at neutral pH. The higher magnification on the upper right (B) shows the increase of the pH in the periplasm first and then the medium as shown by the different intensities of green fluorescence. These data show that the organisms do buffer their periplasm first in acidic pH using their intrabacterial urease activity[15]. This does not happen in *ureI*-negative organisms. Addition of detergent permeabilizes the membrane and allows BCECF penetration into the cytoplasm. In this case, addition of urea results in alkalinization of the cytoplasm as shown in the bottom right panel of Figure 3. This also occurs in *ureI* mutants.

KINETIC MECHANISM OF ACTIVATION

From the pH activity curve of intact bacteria (Figure 1), it would appear that there is a mechanism for activation of the urease inside *H. pylori* that

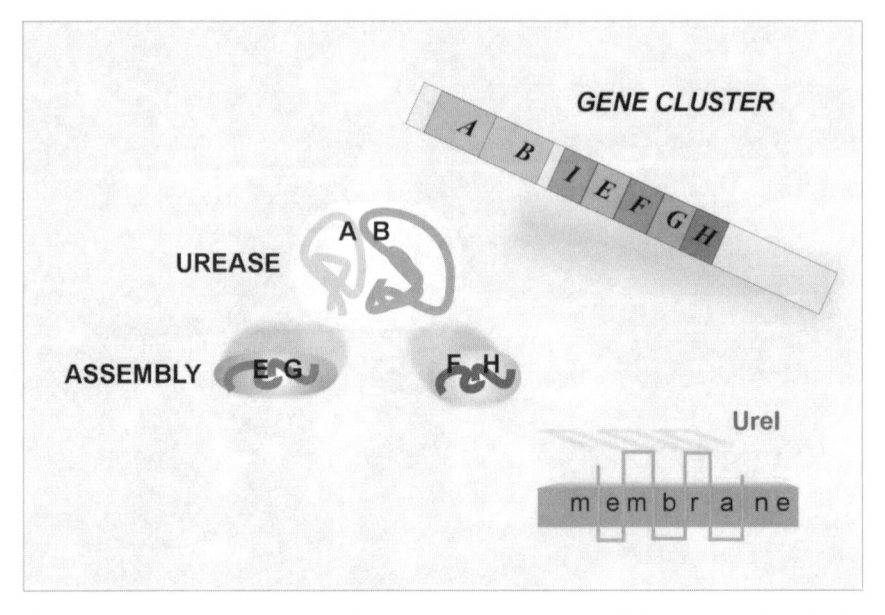

Figure 4. The urease gene cluster of *H. pylori* showing that six of the genes are invovled in urease activity and assembly with the interaction of *UreE* and *G* and *F* and *H* illustrated, as well as their interaction with *UreB*. Distinct from these is *ureI*, which encodes a six-transmembrane segment inner integral membrane protein..

has a set point of $\sim$pH 6.0. The $K_{m,app}$ of free urease is 0.7 mM. In intact bacteria at neutral pH the $K_{m,app}$ is >200 mM. This shows that there is a restriction on intrabacterial urease activity that is most easily interpreted as being due to a non-saturable process such as urea diffusion across the inner membrane. At acidic pH, where there is full activity of urease, the $K_{m,app}$ becomes that of free urease, i.e. 0.7 mM. The limitation on intrabacterial urease activity has disappeared. The simplest explanation for this kinetic behaviour of intrabacterial urease is that the permeability of the inner membrane of the organism for urea is increased at acidic pH. At neutral pH, urease activity is limited by slow penetration of urea, and urea concentrations inside the organism never reach close to $K_{m,app}$ levels, except at very high and non-physiological concentrations. In acid, the permeability of the inner membrane to urea is increased so that the rate of entry of urea from the bulk medium is fast enough, allowing saturation of urease activity[1]. Evidently there is an efficient mechanism for enablement of urea access to the intrabacterial urease.

UreI, AN AMIDOPORIN

There are seven genes in the urease gene cluster of *H. pylori*, as shown in Figure 4[16]. Two of these genes, *ureA* and *ureB*, encode the structural subunits. These form a dimer that then requires Ni^{2+} insertion to form active urease. This is carried out by the concerted action of four accessory genes, three of which are essential for the synthesis of active urease. These genes ureE, F, G and H are assembled as pairs, shown by yeast two hybrid analysis, E pairing with G and F pairing with H. Further UreE and UreH associate with UreB[17]. After ureB there is a promoter sequence immediately followed by *ureI* and then E, F, G, H. The sequence encoding UreI is unique in this cluster in that it predicts a polytopic, integral membrane protein of ~21 kDa. There is no signal peptide predicted and therefore it is a putative inner membrane protein, a candidate for participating in the mechanism regulating urea flux across the inner membrane.

Several types of experiments have defined the properties of UreI. Firstly, the protein is expressed in every gastric *Helicobacter* but in none of the non-gastric *Helicobacters* that we have examined[18]. Thus, it seems important for living in the mammalian stomach. Deletion of *ureI* results in loss of acid activation of intrabacterial urease. Addition of low concentrations of detergent to the mutant results in full urease activity at neutral pH, suggesting that acidity activates urea transport through UreI. The deletion mutants show normal urease activity in lysates and are complemented by *ureI*-containing vectors, showing that the deletion mutants are non-polar. The mutants are also unable to survive a pH < 4.0 even in the presence of 2.5 mM urea, whereas wild-type organisms readily do. This indicates that UreI is essential for acid survival of the organism and that urea interacts with UreI to allow this survival. Again, all these data point to activation of urea transport as the function of UreI. *In-vitro* transcription/translation showed that the protein has six membrane-inserted segments[19], as predicted from a variety of hydropathy algorithms[20,21].

Given the high intrabacterial urease activity, an adequate rate of access of urea to the bacterial cytoplasm would be achieved by placing a urea channel in the bacterial inner membrane. Then intrabacteial urease activity would maintain a large inward urea gradient sufficient to meet the requirements for NH_3 generation by *H. pylori* in acid. Measurement of urea transport in intact bacteria without highly specialized equipment is very difficult. Urea permeability at room temperature across an unmodified bilayer is 4×10^{-6} cm/s. Given the large surface area to volume ratio of a bacterial cell that measures 2.5×0.5 μm and a volume of 5.8×10^{-15} ml, urea would equilibrate in a fraction of a second if it were passively distributed. The high intrabacterial urease would make it unnecessary to expend energy on urea accumulation provided there was an adequate rate of transport of urea.

Hence *Xenopus* oocytes were used as a means of defining UreI function. These have a volume about one billion times greater than that of bacteria, with a several thousand-fold smaller surface to volume ratio. These are the cells of choice for analysis of a passive transport system expressed by bacteria. cRNA encoding UreI is injected and transport function with respect to [^{14}C]urea measured. In the series of experiments illustrated, uptake of urea was determined as a function of pH. It can be seen in Figure 5 that there is a remarkable resemblance to the pH of activation curve seen for urease in intact bacteria. The pH at which there is 50% enhancement of maximal uptake is 6.0, the same pH as calculated for the steady state achieved in the periplasm with the addition of urea at acidic pH[11].

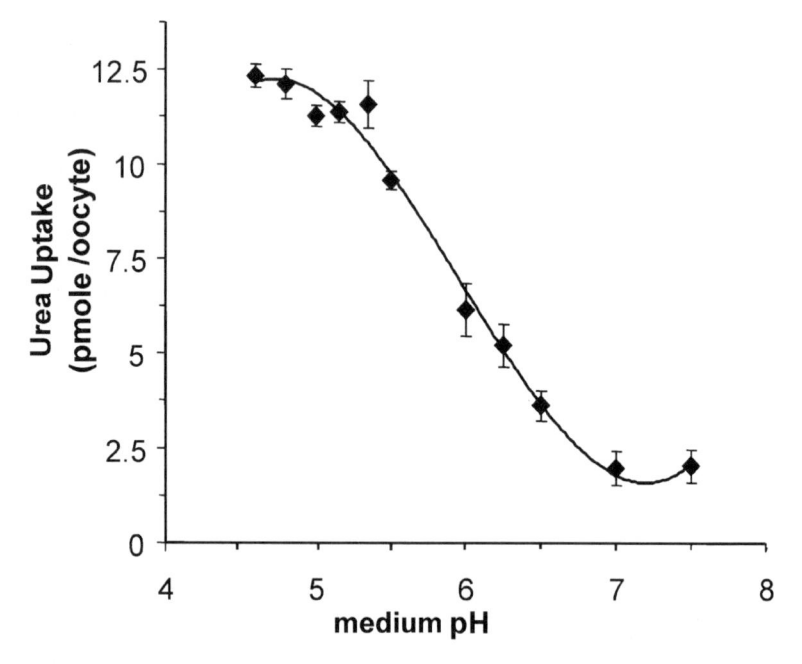

Figure 5. The pH profile of activation of urea entry into *Xenopus* oocytes following injection of *ureI* cRNA.

The transition pH suggests that there are one or more histidines that must be protonated to activate urea transport. Mutation of histidines in the first periplasmic loop had no effect on urea transport into oocytes at acidic pH, whereas mutation of the C-terminal histidine and the two histidines in the second periplasmic loop abolished acid activation of transport. This second loop is therefore part of the gate that opens on histidine protonation, as illustrated in Figure 6.

The transport of urea at acidic pH is essentially temperature-independent and non-saturable. This means that, after activation, there is virtually no conformational change or specific interaction of urea with the walls of the pore. UreI therefore demonstrates properties consistent with a proton-gated urea channel. Its properties determined thus far are illustrated in Table 1.

There is preliminary evidence that UreI is an oligomer, perhaps a dimer or a higher form. Crucial to our understanding of the structure–function of this transporter will be the availability of three-dimensional crystals at high resolution. It may also be able to transport NH_3 outward, helping to prevent cytoplasmic alkalinization due to intrabacterial urease activity and to ensure a rapid periplasmic pH response[22].

The protein has homology to putative amide transporters, a function suggested because they are a component of an amidase gene cluster[20]. However, it appears to be a unique protein only able to transport urea, not thiourea, oxamide or mannitol, for exmaple. It should be considered as a member of a family of amidoporins with analogy to the aquaporin known

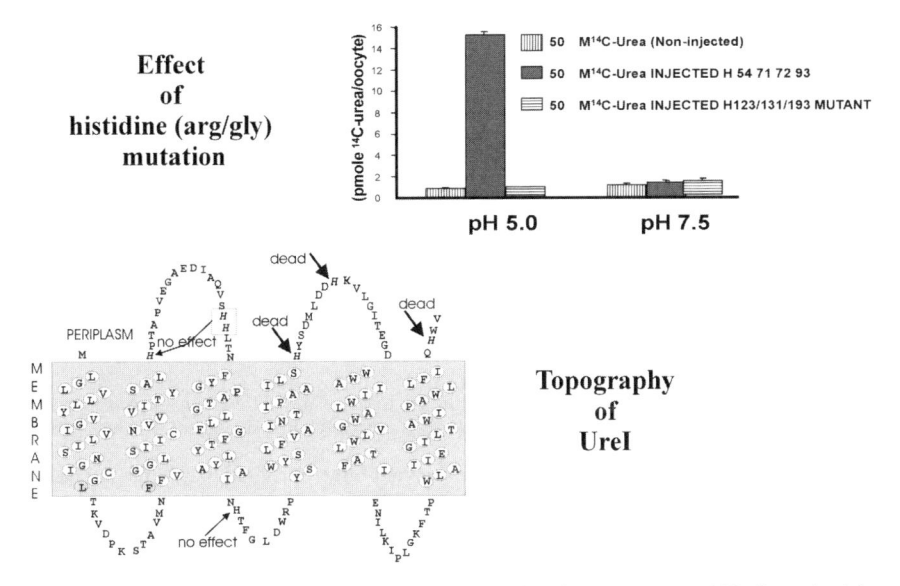

Figure 6. The experimentally determined two-dimensional arrangement of UreI on the left and, on the right, uptake of urea into oocytes injected with the cRNA of various histidine mutants in the first periplasmic loop and the second intracytoplasmic loop that do not affect acid activation of urea entry (bar graph on left) and then the two histidines in the second periplasmic loop and in the C terminus that abolish acid activation when mutated to gly or arg.

Table 1. A summary of the properties of UreI

- Six membrane segment inner membrane protein
- Urea-selective, non-saturable, temperature-independent
- Acid-activated with $pH_{50} = 6.2$
- Proton-gated urea channel
- Gating due to histidine protonation in 2nd loop
- Accelerates urea uptake 300-fold in acid
- Enables intrabacterial urease in acid
- Prevents alkalinization at neutral pH
- Allows gastric colonization at 1 mmol/L urea
- Unique oligomeric amidoporin

to be present in *E. coli*. As such, the protein should be a unique target for monotherapeutic eradication of *H. pylori*. Inhibition of urea transport at pH < 4.0 should be rapidly lethal to the organism. If a drug is developed, it has the benefit of not requiring entry across the bacterial inner membrane. The properties of UreI account for the finding that *ureI* deletion prevents colonization of the mouse stomach[21].

Acknowledgement

This work was supported in part by USVA SMI and NIH grants DK40615, 41301 and 17294.

References

1. Scott DR, Weeks D, Hong C, Postius S, Melchers K, Sachs G. The role of internal urease in acid resistance of *Helicobacter pylori*. Gastroenterology. 1998;114:58–70.
2. Tsuda M, Karita M, Morshed MG, Okita K, Nakazawa T. A urease-negative mutant of *Helicobacter pylori* constructed by allelic exchange mutagenesis lacks the ability to colonize the nude mouse stomach. Infect Immun. 1994;62:3586–9.
3. Andrutis KA, Fox JG, Schauer DB et al. Inability of an isogenic urease-negative mutant stain of *Helicobacter mustelae* to colonize the ferret stomach. Infect Immun. 1995;63:3722–5.
4. Eaton KA, Brooks CL, Morgan DR, Krakowka S. Essential role of urease in pathogenesis of gastritis induced by *Helicobacter pylori* in gnotobiotic piglets. Infect Immun. 1991; 59:2470–5.
5. Schade C, Flemstrom G, Holm L. Hydrogen ion concentration in the mucus layer on top of acid-stimulated and -inhibited rat gastric mucosa. Gastroenterology. 1994;107:180–8.
6. Chu S, Tanaka S, Kaunitz JD, Montrols MH. Dynamic regulation of gastric surface pH by luminal pH. J Clin Invest. 1999;103:605–12.
7. Phadnis SH, Parlow MH, Levy M et al. Surface localization of *Helicobacter pylori* urease and a heat shock protein homolog requires bacterial autolysis. Infect Immun. 1996; 64:905–12.
8. Vanet A, Labigne A. Evidence for specific secretion rather than autolysis in the release of some *Helicobacter pylori* proteins. Infect Immun. 1998;66:1023–7.
9. Alm RA, Trust TJ. Analysis of the genetic diversity of *Helicobacter pylori*: the tale of two genomes. J Mol Med. 1999;77:834–46.
10. Odenbreit S, Puls J, Sedlmaier B, Gerland E, Fischer W, Haas R. Translocation of *Helicobacter pylori* CagA into gastric epithelial cells by type IV secretion. Science. 2000; 287:1497–1500.
11. Rektorschek M, Weeks D, Sachs G, Melchers K. Influence of pH on metabolism and urease activity of *Helicobacter pylori*. Gastroenterology. 1998;115:628–41.
12. Hediger MA, Smith CP, You G, Lee WS, Kanai Y, Shayakul C. Structure, regulation and physiological roles of urea transporters. Kidney Int. 1996;49:1615–23.
13. Kashket ER. The proton motive force in bacteria: a critical assessment of methods. Annu Rev Microbiol. 1985;39:219–42.
14. Meyer-Rosberg K, Scott DR, Rex D, Melchers K, Sachs G. The effect of environmental pH on the proton motive force of *Helicobacter pylori*. Gastroenterology. 1996;111:886–900.
15. Athmann C, Zeng N, Kang T et al. Sites of pH elevation due to NH_3 generation by the intra-bacterial urease of *Helicobacter pylori* co-cultured with gastric cells. J Clin Invest. 2000 (Submitted).
16. Mobley HL, Island MD, Hausinger RP. Molecular biology of microbial ureases. Microbiol Rev. 1995;59:451–80.
17. Voland P, Sachs G. Identification of interactions of proteins of the *H. pylori* urease gene cluster using the yeast-two hybrid system. Gastroenterology. 2000 (abstract) (In press).
18. Scott DR, Marcus EA, Weeks DL et al. Expression of the *Helicobacter pylori ureI* gene is required for acidic pH activation of cytoplasmic urease. Infect Immun. 2000;68:470–7.
19. Weeks DL, Eskandari S, Scott DR, Sachs G. A H^+-gated urea channel: the link between *Helicobacter pylori* urease and gastric colonization. Science. 2000;287:482–5.
20. Chebrou H, Bigey F, Arnaud A, Galzy P. Amide metabolism: a putative ABC transporter in *Rhodococcus* sp. R312. Gene. 1996;182:215–18.
21. Skouloubris S, Thiberge J, Labigne A, De Reuse H. The *Helicobacter pylori* UreI protein is not involved in urease activity but is essential for bacterial survival *in vivo*. Infect Immun. 1998;66:4517–21.
22. Scott DR, Marcus EA, Sachs G. Urease and UreI of *H. pylori* form a membrane complex enabling selective periplasmic pH regulation. Gastroenterology. 2000 (abstract) (In press).

3
The amphibiotic relationship of *Helicobacter pylori* and humans

M. J. BLASER

INTRODUCTION

Medical science, as with most organized human activities, is subject to fashion and fad. The major scientific advances in the first half of the twentieth century, encompassed by the development of microbiology and improvements in public health, led to a marked reduction in the morbidity and mortality due to infectious diseases. Following the discovery and widespread use of antibiotics, society had become complacent about the role of infectious diseases as threats to humankind. However, the plagues of the acquired immunodeficiency syndrome (AIDS), and the development of multiply-resistant *Mycobacterium tuberculosis*, among others, have led to a sea-change in our attitudes about infectious diseases. Now we are at 'war' against microbes, and concerned about killer strains ('flesh-eating bacteria', for example), and distant epidemics. The threat of infectious diseases, once thought to be under control, clearly is not gone.

Much of this concern is appropriate, and yet we are in danger of losing an important perspective. Eminent biologists, including Carl Woese and Stephen Jay Gould, remind us of how dependent we humans are, as are all plants and animals, on the bacteria that in essence dominate the biosphere. For humans this is of particular significance, since the number of bacterial cells that we carry, in our indigenous biota (about 10^{14}) is about 10-fold more numerous than our own human cells[1], and mitochondria, originally bacteria, are endosymbionts, present within most human cells. The particular organisms carried are not determined by accident, but these relationships have roots deep in our evolution, extending back millions of years. In fact, carriage of indigenous microbiota dates back at least 800 million years to the point at which our ancestors diverged from those of earthworms, and for mitochondria, over a billion years. These microbes provide many services for the hosts that feed and shelter them. The relationships between *Vibrio fischeri* and squid[2], or rhizobia and leguminous plants[3] provide outstanding examples of cooperation between entirely unrelated genomes. Thus, in addition to our microbial enemies, higher organisms have microbial friends as well. In humans a succession of organisms colonize particular niches, indicating the non-random temporal development of the indigenous biota in its usual habitat[4-6].

The goal of this chapter is to examine the relationship of humans with the gastric colonizer, Helicobacter pylori. Since its initial isolation in 1982 it has become clear that carriage of H. pylori is associated with increased risk of peptic ulcer disease, non-cardia gastric adenocarcinoma, and an uncommon malignancy, non-Hodgkin's B-cell lymphoma of the stomach[7]. Are only the pathogenic features of H. pylori relevant to medical scientists, or may the organisms have benefits as well?

WHAT IS A PATHOGEN?

Despite the many advances in molecular biology and genetics, there are no simple definitions of what is a pathogen. About a century ago, building on the precepts of Henle, Robert Koch formulated criteria that can be used to determine whether or not an organism is a pathogen[8]. Even with adaptation of these precepts to the modern knowledge and tools of molecular biology[9], they remain insufficient to establish pathogenicity with certainty across broad classes of organisms. An important limitation is our attempt to divide microbes into those that are pathogens and those that are not, without recognizing that there might be overlap between these entities[10].

Microbes have classically been considered to have either parasitic (pathogenic) or symbiotic relationships with their hosts. However, circumstances arise in which either of these relationships can occur between a given host and microbe, depending on context. This concept, which was termed 'amphibiosis' by Theodore Rosebury in 1962[11], has great utility. The indigenous microbial biota of humans provide numerous examples of the phenomenon of amphibiosis[12]. The indigenous biota, innocuous *in situ*, may be lethal when introduced to other tissues after a human bite wound[13]. In another example, ordinarily, the α-haemolytic streptococci present in the oral cavity provide important functions, such as protection against high-grade and potentially lethal pathogens, including group A β-haemolytic streptococci. However, α-streptococci often migrate across the mucosal surface and are transiently present in the blood stream. In particular hosts this bacteraemia leads to subacute bacterial endocarditis, which was a uniformly lethal condition before the advent of antibiotic treatments. Since these organisms and (all?) other indigenous (commensal) microbiota have both symbiotic and pathogenic properties, *depending on context*, usage of the term 'amphibiotic relationship' is appropriate. The paradigm involving α-haemolytic streptococci also illustrates how a microbe can be a symbiont early in life, for example, when group A streptococcal infections are most common, but have its major expression as a pathogen, for example, causing endocarditis or increasing risk for dental caries, later in life. This time dimension is especially important to consider, since the most substantial natural selection for particular phenomena occurs early in life, before the end of reproductive age.

H. PYLORI AS INDIGENOUS BIOTA IN THE HUMAN STOMACH

There is increasing evidence that *H. pylori* has colonized the gastric mucosa of humans since time immemorial, just as other *Helicobacter* and related species colonize the stomachs of all mammalian hosts studied to date[14]. Such colonization is not accidental, but reflective of well-established modes of transmission and coexistence. There is also substantial evidence that, during the twentieth century, the prevalence of *H. pylori* colonization in human populations has progressively declined[15], concomitant with improving living standards, and probably accelerated by the widespread use of antibiotics (reviewed in ref. 16). This shift represents a major change in human ecology, and parenthetically probably reflects other similarly massive but still-hidden shifts in our micro-ecology.

BENEFITS TO HUMANS OF *H. PYLORI* COLONIZATION

From numerous studies it is clear that carriage of *H. pylori* has cost to humans, chiefly in the form of ulcer disease, and gastric malignancies, all of which predominantly occur after reproductive age (reviewed in refs 7 and 14). The potential benefits of *H. pylori* colonization are also emerging, in the course of contemporary research. Especially interesting is the concept that *H. pylori* may provide benefits against (lethal) diarrhoeal diseases in childhood due to enteric pathogens. In any niche the indigenous bacteria play important roles in preventing other bacteria from proliferating by outcompeting foreign bacteria for nutrients, occupying the available space, and/or producing antibacterial substances. Mechanisms by which *H. pylori* may protect include heightening of the gastric acid barrier[17], priming of the immune response in the stomach and systemically[18], and by production of direct antibacterial substances[19]. *H. pylori* colonization also appears to decrease the risk of gastro-oesophageal reflux disease, and especially its pre-malignant and malignant sequelae[16].

Thus, as with other indigenous organisms of humans[20,21], carriage of *H. pylori* appears to have both costs and benefits, consistent with an amphibiotic role. The major protective effect is by cag^+ strains[16], which concurrently have the greatest association with both peptic ulcer disease and gastric cancer[22–25]. How can this apparent paradox be explained? It now is clear that cag^+ strains are more interactive with their human hosts than are cag^- strains[26]. Based on our present understanding of gastric pathophysiology, cag^- strains are more inert in the gastric lumen, behaving more like silent commensals. One of the major factors affecting risk of oesophagogastroduodenal diseases is the extent of atrophic gastritis; colonization by cag^+ strains is associated with, and increases risk for, the development of atrophic gastritis[27]. This phenomenon helps explain both the increased risk of adenocarcinoma of the antrum and body of the stomach, and the decreased risk for adenocarcinoma of the oesophagus and gastric cardia associated with cag^+ strains (Figure 1).

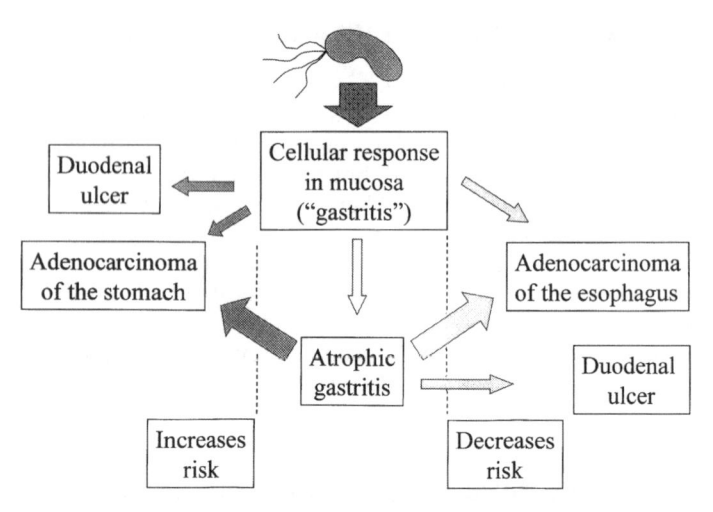

Figure 1. Schematic of the effects of *H. pylori* colonization on upper gastrointestinal disease in humans. *H. pylori* colonization induces a normal host response with cellular infiltration of the mucosa, which increases the risk for the later development of atrophic gastritis. Both the cellular response and atrophic gastritis can affect the risk of disease, on the one hand, increasing risk for adenocarcinoma of the stomach, and on the other hand decreasing the risk for adenocarcinoma of the oesophagus. For duodenal ulceration the normal host response to *H. pylori* increases risk, whereas the development of atrophic gastritis decreases the risk.

CONCLUSIONS

The central feature of physiological systems is homeostasis, as described more than a century ago by Claude Bernard and others; perturbations are transient, and equilibrium is restored. The similarities from individual to individual are the basis for the study of physiology. But no two individuals are alike, including their genetic composition and their environmental exposures. This polymorphism determines their daily conduct and ultimate fate. It is therefore critical to recognize that, with few profound exceptions, the variations between humans in their genetic polymorphisms are far less than the variation in the organisms that they carry and to which they are exposed. Habitation of the human stomach by *H. pylori* is a model of the complex interactions between host and persisting colonizer.

In examining the consequences of *H. pylori* colonization it is not sufficient to determine whether or not *H. pylori* is present, but the characteristics of the colonizing population. These include allelic differences such as *vac*A genotype, and the presence or absence of the *cag* island[28]. However, the emerging concept that *H. pylori* populations in a given host represent a quasispecies[29], most fit for the varied microniches in particular hosts, represents another dimension that must be considered in our view of the biological roles of the organism. The enormous variation in *H. pylori* reflects the diversity observed in other colonized niches of the human body[30–32].

Health or disease reflects gastric physiology, and the interactions of diverse hosts with varied *H. pylori* populations, in niches and microniches. The equilibria reached in the stomach in the presence of varied *H. pylori* populations[33], or in their absence, is the key to both health and disease[28]. Understanding that *H. pylori* has an amphibiotic relationship with humans provides the framework for dissecting out the specific and critical pathophysiological determinants in each host[34].

References

1. Savage DC. Microbial ecology of the gastrointestinal tract. Annu Rev Microbiol. 1977;31:107–33.
2. Ruby EG. Lessons from a cooperative, bacterial–animal association: the *Vibrio fischeri–Euprymna scolopes* light organ symbiosis. Annu Rev Microbiol. 1996;50:591–624.
3. McFall-Ngai MJ. The development of cooperative associations between animals and bacteria: establishing détente among domains. Am Zool. 1998;38:593–608.
4. Long SS, Swenson RM. Determinants of the developing oral flora in normal newborns. Appl Environ Microbiol. 1976;32:494–7.
5. McClellan DL, Griffen AL, Leys EJ. Age and prevalence of *Porphyromonas gingivalis* in children. J Clin Microbiol. 1996;34:2017–19.
6. Hill GB, St Claire KK, Gutman LT. Anaerobes predominate among the vaginal microflora of prepubertal girls. Clin Infect Dis. 1995;20(Suppl. 2):S269–70.
7. Blaser MJ. Science, medicine, and the future: *Helicobacter pylori* and gastric diseases. Br Med J. 1998;316:1507–10.
8. Evans AS. Causation and disease: the Henle–Koch postulates revisited. Yale J Biol Med. 1976;49:175–95.
9. Fredricks DN, Relman DA. Sequence-based identification of microbial pathogens: a reconsideration of Koch's postulates. Clin Microbiol Rev. 1996;9:18–33.
10. Hill AB. The environment and disease: association or causation. President's address; Proceedings of the Royal Society of Medicine Meeting, 14 Jan 1965, Section of Occupational Medicine, pp. 295–300.
11. Rosebury T. Microorganisms Indigenous to Man. New York: McGraw Hill; 1962:1–8.
12. Mackowiak P. The normal microbial flora. N Engl J Med. 1982;307:83–93.
13. Goldstein EJC, Citron DM, Wield B et al. Bacteriology of human and animal bite wounds. J Clin Microbiol. 1978;8:667–72.
14. Blaser MJ. *Helicobacters* are indigenous to the human stomach: duodenal ulceration is due to changes in gastric microecology in the modern era. Gut. 1998;43:721–27.
15. Kosunen TU, Aromaa A, Knekt P et al. *Helicobacter* antibodies in 1973 and 1994 in the adult population of Vammala, Finland. Epidemiol Infect. 1997;119:29–34.
16. Blaser MJ. The changing relationships of *Helicobacter pylori* and humans: implications for health and disease. J Infect Dis. 1999;179:1523–30.
17. El-Omar E, Penman I, Dorrian CA, Ardill JE, McColl KE. Eradicating *Helicobacter pylori* infection lowers gastrin mediated acid secretion by two thirds in patients with duodenal ulcer. Gut. 1993;34:1060–5.
18. Mattsson A, Lonroth H, Quiding-Jarbrink M, Svennerholm AM. Induction of B cell responses in the stomach of *Helicobacter pylori*-infected subjects after oral cholera vaccination. J Clin Invest. 1998;102:51–6.
19. Putsep K, Branden CI, Boman HG, Normark S. Antibacterial peptide from *H. pylori*. Nature. 1999;398:671–2.
20. Sutter VL. Anaerobes as normal oral flora. Rev Infect Dis. 1984;6(Suppl. 1):S62–6.
21. Rolfe RD. Interactions among microorganisms of the indigenous intestinal flora and their influence on the host. Rev Infect Dis. 1984;6(Suppl. 1):S73–9.
22. Covler TL, Dooley CP, Blaser MJ. Characterization and human serologic response to proteins in *Helicobacter pylori* broth culture supernatants with vacuolizing cytotoxin activity. Infect Immun. 1990;58:603–10.
23. Crabtree JE, Taylor JD, Wyatt JL et al. Mucosal IgA recognition of *Helicobacter pylori* 120 kDa protein, peptic ulceration, and gastric pathology. Lancet. 1991;338:332–5.
24. Blaser MJ, Pérez-Pérez GL, Kleanthous H et al. Infection with *Helicobacter pylori* strains possessing *cag*A associated with an increased risk of developing adenocarcinoma of the stomach. Cancer Res. 1995;55:2111–15.

25. Parsonnet J, Friedman GD, Orenterich N, Vogelman H. Risk for gastric cancer in people with CagA positive or CagA negative *Helicobacter pylori* infection. Gut. 1997;40:297–301.
26. Blaser MJ. The interaction of *cag*$^+$ *Helicobacter pylori* with their hosts. In: Hunt RH, Tytgat GNJ, editors. *Helicobacter pylori*, Basic Mechanisms to Clinical Cure. Dordrecht: Kluwer; 1998;27–32.
27. Kuipers EJ, Pérez-Pérez GI, Meuwissen SGM, Blaser MJ. *Helicobacter pylori* and atrophic gastritis: importance of the *cag*A status. J Natl Cancer Inst. 1995;87:1777–80.
28. Blaser MJ. Ecology of *Helicobacter pylori* in the human stomach. J Clin Invest. 1997;100:759–62.
29. Kuipers EJ, Israel DA, Kusters JG *et al.* Quasispecies development of *Helicobacter pylori* observed in paired isolates obtained years apart in the same host. J Infect Dis. 2000; 181:273–82.
30. Kroes I, Lepp PW, Relman DA. Bacterial diversity within the human subgingival crevice. Proc Natl Acad Sci USA. 1999;96:14547–52.
31. Croucher SC, Houston AP, Bayliss CE, Turner RJ. Bacterial populations associated with different regions of the human colon wall. Appl Environ Microbiol. 1983;45:1025–33.
32. Bartlett JG, Polk BF. Bacterial flora of the vagina: quantitative study. Rev Infect Dis. 1984;6(Suppl. 1):S67–72.
33. Odenbreit S, Puls J, Sedlmaier B, Gerland E, Fischer W, Haas R. Translocation of *Helicobacter pylori* CagA into gastric epithelial cells by type IV secretion. Science. 2000; 287:1497–500.
34. Feldman M, Cryer B, Sammer D, Lee E, Spechler SJ. Influence of *H. pylori* infection on meal-stimulated gastric acid secretion and gastroesophageal acid reflux. Am J Physiol. 1999;277:1159–64.

4
Helicobacter pylori is pathogenic flora

A. LEE

INTRODUCTION

To counter the arguments that *Helicobacter pylori* is commensal flora, what better quotes can be those by Blaser: '*Helicobacter* species may have been part of the indigenous gastric biota of humans and our prehuman ancestors from our earliest times'[1], and 'to date no benefits of *H. pylori* infection have been identified'[2]. This was followed only 3 years ago with the assertion that 'the author is unaware of any direct evidence that infection with *H. pylori* or with any specific subset of *H. pylori* carries any benefits to humans'[3].

However, subsequently Blaser has asserted that '*H. pylori* can thus be regarded as indigenous or "normal flora"'[4]; but it is our belief that '*H. pylori* USED to be indigenous or "normal flora"'. This is then the major argument in this debate in which it is our contention that *H. pylori* is pathogenic flora.

IN THE BEGINNING – THE PRIMORDIAL HELICOBACTERS

In the beginning, as the first primordial beasts roamed the earth, there were primitive intestinal tracts. The early microorganisms would have been exposed post-ingestion to the primitive gut and so began the millennia of evolution of the genus *Helicobacter*. First, the bacteria acquired their spiral morphology that enabled them to adapt to lower bowel mucus. Then, 300 million years ago, the first acid-secreting stomachs appeared. Acid was an effective antibacterial defence and, unlike the lower bowel, the primitive stomach remained bacteria-free. Such is the nature of evolution, *Helicobacter* species adapted to survive in the hostile acid milieu via subtle modifications of the enzyme urease which it was no longer required for nitrogen assimilation but rather allowed survival over a relatively narrow pH range. As the Sachs group has so elegantly shown, the acid-dependent urea channel controlled by the gene *UreI* permits survival in the human stomach[5].

To facilitate nutrient availability from the gastric mucosa the bacterium in the human stomach, now *H. pylori*, acquired genes that induced inflammation. However, no symptomatic disease was apparent, ulcers were not caused and the gastritis induced no long-term consequences as the lifespan of the human of the time was so short. *H. pylori* was normal flora, although this was not a symbiotic relationship in contrast to lower bowel flora. The immense complexity of the lower bowel meant that the similarly highly adapted bacterial flora could play a beneficial role by protecting the gut from invading potential pathogens by occupying all available niches. These pathogens could not survive in the stomach, whether *H. pylori* was present or not, as they had no acid defence mechanisms.

THE TRANSITION TO PATHOGENICITY

Then things changed. Diseases, now known without debate to be caused by *H. pylori*, began to appear; first gastric ulcer and then duodenal ulcer. Life expectancy increased and so gastric cancer, one of the great killing cancers, appeared in larger numbers. While *H. pylori* survived for thousands, if not millions, of years as a mere commensal, from about 150–200 years ago it became a pathogen. What changed? Some have suggested the bacterium changed and became more virulent. Yet there is no evidence for this hypothesis. Certainly the acquisition of the *cag* pathogenicity island was a major evolutionary step, enabling the bacterium to be much more pro-inflammatory[6].

However, this gene acquisition happened in pre-history long before the great *H. pylori* transition to pathogen status. The change is in the host.

As ulcer disease developed in relatively recent times, the correlation was with increases in socioeconomic status. The *H. pylori*-associated diseases were 'diseases of civilization'. How could the host change as a country or people developed? One obvious factor is diet. Processed foods, excess meat, etc. could certainly impact on the host's physiology.

Likewise, increased levels of nutrition would change the status of the host. Loss of a parasitic burden could change the immunology of the host response, as has been recently suggested[7]. It is our opinion that the most likely change, discussed in detail elsewhere, is in gastric acid secretion. The behaviour of *H. pylori* is critically dependent on the local acid environment as this is the ecological determinant to which it is uniquely adapted[8–10]. There is a logic to increased acid load. Chronic bacterial and parasite infection could be acid suppressive through IL-1. Reduction in parasite burdens could result in increased acid secretion. There is also direct evidence in Japan that acid output in the population is increasing over time[11,12]. This correlates with the change in *H. pylori*-associated disease that is now occurring in Japan, as it did in the West 50 years ago. Whatever the reason for the change in the human host, the direct consequence is that this benign gastric inhabitant has turned feral and is now a major pathogen.

Does anyone dispute that this bacterium causes up to 95% of duodenal ulcers, about 70% of gastric ulcers and nearly 100% of low-grade MALT lymphomas? The evidence is equally overwhelming that without this bacterial infection, gastric adenocarcinoma is highly unlikely. This organism is a pathogen. It is not an argument against the bacterium as pathogen that most infections are asymptomatic. Polio virus causes the debilitating central nervous system lesions that result in the disease polio in only 1% of those persons infected. *Mycobacterium tuberculosis* causes symptomatic disease in only 10% of those infected. Does anyone doubt that the polio virus and the tubercle bacillus are true pathogens? How could *H. pylori* be classified any differently? This is not a pathogen of minor consequence. In the US alone in 1998 nearly 13 000 died of gastric cancer and nearly 5000 succumbed to peptic ulcer disease. This compares with 1000 for TB, 5000 for viral hepatitis and 13 000 for HIV[13].

Even in its years as a supposed commensal, it is possible that *H. pylori* infection could have had negative impacts; certainly no positive ones as Blaser attests. A recent paper confirms an earlier suggestion that *H. pylori* infection may predispose children to cholera, and thus, presumably other gastrointestinal diseases due to the hypochlorhydria that accompanies each infection[14,15]. Also, *H. pylori* infection was found in 15% of children without iron deficiency anaemia, whereas 31% of those with the deficiency were infected[16]. This was consistent with studies where cure of infection reduced anaemia and resulted in increased blood counts and ferritin levels[17]. As iron deficiency anaemia is the most prevalent micronutrient deficiency in the world, affecting an estimated 2 billion people worldwide, should even a small percentage be attributable to *H. pylori* infection this would be yet another burden of *H. pylori* as pathogen.

H. PYLORI AS THE GOOD BACTERIUM

Recently, based on the false assumption that an evolved inhabitant of a vacant ecological niche must of necessity be of benefit, Blaser has suggested that 'It is certainly possible that in addition to "bad" and "very bad" *H. pylori*, "neutral" or "good" ones exist as well'[3]. Indeed it was also suggested that, in the future, physicians will be giving selected patients selected strains of *H. pylori* to reduce risks for particular diseases[18]. These ideas have arisen from observations that the decline in *H. pylori* infection worldwide has correlated with an increase in reflux oesophagitis and cancer of the cardia[19]. The latter disease remains at the very low prevalence of 4 per 100 000, and is mainly restricted to the white American male. Many markers of socioeconomic development could probably be correlated with the increase in oesphagitis, such as the toothbrush or the refrigerator.

EVEN IF *H. PYLORI* WERE PROTECTIVE OF REFLUX – IS THIS RELEVANT?

Reflux oesophagitis and the increased risk of cardia cancer that it brings could be considered an end-stage progression of the increase in acid output discussed above. There is a possibility that infection with *H. pylori* could result in a reduction of acid secretion and reduction in oesophagitis. The white American males who are at increased risk of cardia cancer will inevitably lose their *H. pylori* infection as they are usually in the privileged socioeconomic class. Should they have not lost *H. pylori* this is the group that would have at least a 10% chance of developing an ulcer in their lifetime compared to a 4 in 100 000 chance of cancer of the cardia, should this association be real. Even if it were, does this matter? What should be done? Should steps be taken to leave this population with their *H. pylori* and their ulcers. Should they be fed a culture of *H. pylori* so they would now be at risk of duodenal ulcer? I think not.

THE NEGATIVE CONSEQUENCES OF THE 'SAVE THE HELICOBACTER' CAMPAIGN

There is great satisfaction and stimulation in the debate as to whether *H. pylori* is normal flora or a pathogen. However, there is a downside to this intellectual exercise. Blaser has published his speculative articles in a range of influential journals, including the *British Medical Journal*, *Gut*, *Lancet* and the *Annals of Medicine*. Those who do not understand the complexity and fragility of the hypotheses proposed by Blaser are doubting whether they should intervene against *H. pylori* infection, even in patients in whom it would clearly be of benefit, e.g. a young Japanese with atrophy who is *H. pylori*-positive at endoscopy.

There are hundreds of millions of individuals in the developing world who will benefit from intervention against *H. pylori* infection, once acceptable strategies such as a vaccine become available. These intervention strategies will happen only if there is a demonstrated need and demand. Doubt caused by suggestions that *H. pylori* could be 'good for you' stifle that argument. Any serious cost benefit would suggest that not treating *H. pylori* infection diagnosed at endoscopy for the reason of protecting against a very rare cancer is neither cost-effective or life-effective. In most areas of the world the relative risk of *H. pylori* infection causing disease is much more than the likelihood of *H. pylori* protecting against disease. Those populations at risk of cardia cancer will inevitably have lost their *H. pylori* infection due to their higher socioeconomic status. As stated above, if they had retained the organism they are at considerable risk of peptic ulcer

CONCLUSION

H. pylori, each year, kills more than a million people and causes considerable discomfort to tens of millions. The cost of this bacterium to health-care budgets is enormous. Despite its origins as a benign fellow-traveller this fascinating spiral organism is now an unwanted inhabitant of our gastric mucosa. By any criteria applied, *H. pylori* is pathogenic flora.

References

1. Blaser MJ. *Helicobacters* are indigenous to the human stomach – duodenal ulceration is due to changes in gastric microecology in the modern era. Gut. 1998;43:721–7.
2. Blaser MJ, Parsonnet J. Parasitism by the 'slow' bacterium *Helicobacter pylori* leads to altered gastric homeostasis and neoplasia. J Clin Invest. 1994;94:4–8.
3. Blaser MJ. *Helicobacter pylori* eradication and its implications for the future. Aliment Pharmacol Ther. 1997;11(Suppl. 1):103–7.

4. Blaser MJ. Science, medicine, and the future – *Helicobacter pylori* and gastric diseases. Br Med J. 1998;316:1507–10.
5. Weeks DL, Eskandari S, Scott DR, Sachs G. A H^+-gated urea channel: the link between *Helicobacter pylori* urease and gastric colonization. Science. 2000;287:482–5.
6. Covacci A, Telford JL, Del Giudice G, Parsonnet J, Rappuoli R. *Helicobacter pylori* virulence and genetic geography. Science. 1999;284:1328–33.
7. Fox JG, Beck P, Dangler CA et al. Concurrent enteric helminth infection modulates inflammation and gastric immune responses and reduces helicobacter-induced gastric atrophy. Nature Med. 2000;6:536–42.
8. Danon SJ, O'Rourke JL, Moss ND, Lee A. The importance of local acid production in the distribution of *Helicobacter felis* in the mouse stomach. Gastroenterology. 1995;108:1386–95.
9. Lee A, Dixon MF, Danon SJ et al. Local acid production and *Helicobacter pylori*: a unifying hypothesis of gastroduodenal disease. Eur J Gastroenterol Hepatol. 1995;7:461–5.
10. Lee A, Mellgard B, Larsson H. Effect of gastric acid on *Helicobacter pylori* ecology. In: Hunt RH, Tytgat GNJ, editors. *Helicobacter pylori*: Basic Mechanisms to Clinical Cure 1996. Dordrecht: Kluwer; 1996:50–63.
11. Kinoshita Y, Kawanami C, Kishi K, Nakata H, Seino Y, Chiba T. *Helicobacter pylori* independent chronological change in gastric acid secretion in the Japanese. Gut. 1997;41:452–8.
12. Lee A, Van Zanten SV. The aging stomach or the stomachs of the ages – commentary. Gut. 1997;41:575–6.
13. Anon. National Vital Statisitics Reports. 1999;47:27–9.
14. Clemens J, Albert MJ, Rao M et al. Impact of infection by *Helicobacter pylori* on the risk and severity of endemic cholera. J Infect Dis. 1995;171:1653–6.
15. Shahinian ML, Passaro DJ, Swerdlow DL, Mintz ED, Rodriguez M, Parsonnet J. *Helicobacter pylori* and epidemic *Vibrio cholerae* 01 infection in Peru. Lancet. 2000;355:377–8.
16. Choe YH, Kim SK, Hong YC. *Helicobacter pylori* infection with iron deficiency anaemia and subnormal growth at puberty. Arch Dis Child. 2000;82:136–40.
17. Annibale B, Marignani M, Monarca B et al. Reversal of iron deficiency anemia after *Helicobacter pylori* eradication in patients with asymptomatic gastritis. Ann Intern Med. 1999;131:668–72.
18. Blaser MJ. In a world of black and white, *Helicobacter pylori* is gray. Ann Intern Med. 1999;130:695–7.
19. El-Serag HB, Sonnenberg A. Opposing time trends of peptic ulcer and reflux disease. Gut. 1998;43:327–33.

5
Disease-specific *Helicobacter pylori* virulence factors: the role of *cagA*, *vacA*, *iceA*, *babA2* alone or in combination

Y. YAMAOKA and D. Y. GRAHAM

INTRODUCTION

A number of putative virulence factors for *Helicobacter pylori* have been identified including CagA, VacA, IceA, and BabA. One of the problems separating putative virulence factors from true virulence factors has been the lack of criteria for establishing a true virulence factor, especially with regard to disease specificity. The criteria for a true virulence factor include meeting the tests of biological plausibility and epidemiological consistency (Table 1).

cagA

The cytotoxin VacA was the first putative disease-associated virulence factor described; shortly thereafter it was followed by the cytotoxin-associated gene product, CagA, which is now known to be the product of one of the genes in the *cag* pathogenicity island[1]. The pathogenicity island is a type IV secretory apparatus that injects CagA into the host cell, where it undergoes tyrosine phosphorylation[2–5]. CagA is involved in the cytoskeletal changes that occur (e.g. pedestal formation) when a *cagA*-positive isolate adheres to a host cell[2]. Two putative tyrosine phosphorylation motifs in CagA are located just before and after the 3' repeat regions[4]. This site may be important as differences in the 3' repeat regions have been associated with differences in pH susceptibility among *H. pylori* strains as well as in gastric histology[6].

Table 1. Criteria for a disease-specific virulence factor

The mechanism of action must be biologically plausible
The disease associations must be consistent both experimentally and epidemiologically

The *cag* pathogenicity island is involved in the induction of cytokine expression in gastric epithelial cells, which is seen as a marked increase in interleukin 8 (IL-8) secretion[1]. Cytokine induction associated with the *cag* pathogenicity island is independent of CagA[1]. The signal transduction pathway is thought to be through nuclear factor κB (NF-κB) and activator protein 1 (AP-1)[7-11]. Before activation, NK-κB resides in the cytoplasm and upon activation translocates to the nucleus, where it binds to DNA at κB sites and up-regulates IL-8 gene transcription.

Individuals infected with *H. pylori* that have a functional *cag* pathogenicity island have elevated mucosal levels of IL-8, marked neutrophilic infiltration into the gastric mucosa, and an increased risk of developing a symptomatic outcome such as peptic ulcer or gastric cancer. However, the relationship between the presence of the *cag* pathogenicity island and outcome is not consistent among the different geographic regions, especially in East Asia where more than 90% of isolates possess the *cag* pathogenicity island, irrespective of the outcome[12,13]. In Western countries, where *H. pylori* strains lacking the *cag* pathogenicity island are found in a higher percentage than in Asian countries, the increased likelihood of a symptomatic outcome can be seen. Thus, although the *cag* pathogenicity island lacks disease specificity, it does connote increased virulence.

The primary factor associated with the intensity of neutrophilic inflammation is the density of *H. pylori* organisms containing a functional *cag* pathogenicity island. The hypothesis that *cagA*-positive *H. pylori* strains grew to greater density than *cagA*-negative ones[14] has not been confirmed[15,16]. The original observation is now known to have been the result of comparing the density of *H. pylori* in the antrum of patients with duodenal ulcer with patients with simple *H. pylori* gastritis and *cagA*-negative infections[14]. Controlling for the disease presentation showed that there were no differences in the density of *cagA*-positive and *cagA*-negative *H. pylori* strains in *H. pylori*-infected individuals without duodenal ulcer disease[15,16]. Nevertheless, the mean density of *H. pylori* organisms in the antrum in duodenal ulcer is greater than in the antrum of patients with *H. pylori* gastritis. The fact that acid secretion might play a critical role in this difference is shown by the observation that the density of *H. pylori* organisms is higher in the corpus of patients with *H. pylori* gastritis than in those with duodenal ulcer[15,16].

The presence of a functional *cag* pathogenicity island is associated with increased inflammation. It is likely that any factor that results in an increase in inflammation will also increase the risk of a symptomatic outcome. Nevertheless, the presence of a functional *cag* pathogenicity island has no predictive value regarding current or future clinical presentation. *H. pylori* strains lacking a functional *cag* pathogenicity island are not commensal as they are also found in patients with peptic ulcer or gastric cancer, only at lower frequency.

iceA

*ice*A is a gene that is *I*nduced by *C*ontact with *E*pithelium[17]. The gene product is unknown but it appears to be a bacterial restriction enzyme. The initial studies showed that there were two variants of the *iceA* gene, *iceA*1 and *iceA*2, and suggested that *iceA*1 was highly correlated with disease presentation (i.e. the frequency of *iceA*1 was about 50% in duodenal ulcer patients and very rare in non-ulcer patients)[17,18]. However, both the initial study and a second one were small and, although the conclusions were similar, the results were not consistent (e.g. in the first report non-ulcer cases were associated with *iceA*1 in only 4%[17] and in the second in 50%[18]).

The hypothesis that *iceA* was associated with a particular clinical presentation was subsequently tested in a large study investigating the presence of *iceA*1 in duodenal ulcer, gastric ulcer, gastric cancer and simple gastritis in four different countries (US, Colombia, Japan and Korea)[13]. The inclusion of different countries was done to avoid the known problem of regional variation in *H. pylori* genes. The results failed to confirm an association between *iceA*1 and clinical outcome.

The conclusion about *iceA* as a potential virulence factor is that the original data were weak. The hypothesis that *iceA* has disease specificity has not been confirmed, and there is currently no known biological or epidemiological evidence for a role for *iceA* as a virulence factor in *H. pylori*-related disease.

vacA

vacA, the gene for the vacuolating cytotoxin, has been subtyped, and it was hypothesized that genotyping might show disease-specific associations[19,20]. The original hypothesis was that the s1 genotype was associated with duodenal ulcer disease and the s2 genotype had low ulcerogenic potential. It was also suggested that there were differences in cytotoxin production between the genotypes[20]. These hypotheses were derived from an evaluation of 42 *H. pylori vacA*-positive strains, 31 of which were in the original description of *vacA* genotypes[12]. A number of prospective studies have been undertaken to investigate the value of *vacA* genotyping[12]. A compilation of studies involving approximately 1500 isolates from Europe, the USA and Asia has not substantiated the original hypothesis[12] and the data are now overwhelming that *vacA* genotyping is not useful to predict symptoms, presentation, response to therapy or degree of inflammation. *vacA* genotyping is useful to predict *cagA* status.

World-wide, the majority of *vacA* s1 genotype strains are also *cagA*-positive. In East Asia the link with *cagA*-positivity is at least 95%. The *vacA* s1 genotype can be considered as a surrogate for the presence of the *cag* pathogenicity island. VacA was linked to changes in intracellular ERK activation[21], but that observation has also not been confirmed[10,22].

Current data do not support the notion that *vacA* is a virulence factor in its own right, or that it is additive with *cagA*. Overall, the hypothesis that *vacA* genotyping might prove clinically useful, for example to predict presentation such as duodenal ulcer, has been proven wrong.

TRIPLE-POSITIVE: cagA+, vacA s1, babA2

The blood group antigen-binding adhesin, BabA, is an outer membrane protein, which appears to be involved in adherence of *H. pylori* to Lewis-b

```
        100 ┐    95.5%
              ┌──────┐
         80 ┤  │      │   82.3%
              │      │ ┌──────┐
              │      │ │      │   70.1%
         60 ┤  │      │ │      │ ┌──────┐
              │      │ │      │ │      │
         40 ┤  │      │ │      │ │      │
              │      │ │      │ │      │
         20 ┤  │      │ │      │ │      │
              │      │ │      │ │      │
          0 ┴──┴──────┴─┴──────┴─┴──────┴
               Japan     USA    Colombia
```

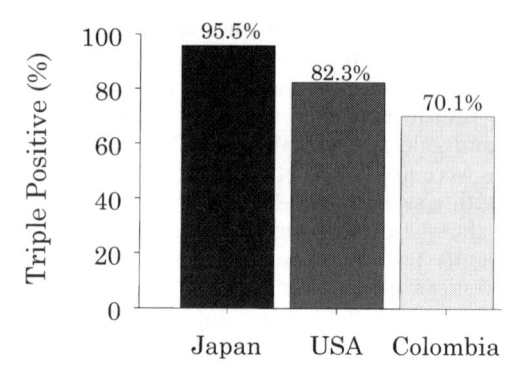

Figure 1. The prevalence of triple-positive (for $cagA+$, $vacA$ s1, $babA2$) *H. pylori* in duodenal ulcer patients in Japan ($n = 73$), USA ($n = 92$) and Colombia ($n = 67$).

(Le^b) blood group antigens on gastric epithelial cells[23]. Functional BabA adhesin is encoded by the *babA2* gene. The *babA2* gene is identical to the *babA1* gene, with the exception of an insert of 10 base pairs with a repeat motif in the signal peptide sequence, which results in the creation of a translational initiation codon and Le^b binding ability. Based on a small sample (e.g. 23 with duodenal ulcer, 35 with gastritis, and 27 with adenocarcinoma), it was suggested that triple positive for $cagA+$, $vacA$ s1, $babA2$ might be correlated with duodenal ulcer (100%). The association with gastric cancer was 74.1% and only 43% of those with gastritis[24]. We tested this hypothesis, and the proportion of duodenal ulcer patients in Japan ($n = 73$), USA ($n = 96$) and Colombia ($n = 67$) that were triple-positive was considerably lower (Figure 1) and was not significantly different in Japan or Colombia (e.g. $p = 0.467$ in Colombia) (Yamaoka *et al.*, unpublished observations). The fact that the proportion of duodenal ulcer patients with triple-positivity was as low as 70% in Colombia, and that triple-positivity was found in 87% (113/129) of those with gastritis in Japan suggests that triple-positivity is another example of a data-derived hypothesis using a small sample that was subsequently unsubstantiated in larger studies.

HOST FACTORS

There is now evidence to suggest that virulence of *H. pylori* is largely host-dependent. The pattern of gastritis has withstood the test of time for its relation to different *H. pylori*-related diseases (e.g. antral predominant gastritis with duodenal ulcer disease). The primary factors responsible for the different patterns of gastritis in response to an *H. pylori* infection are environmental (e.g. diet) with the *H. pylori* strain playing a lesser role[16,25].

SUMMARY

Although disease-specific associations have been hypothesized there are now sufficient data to state conclusively that none of these putative virulence factors has disease specificity. Future studies should exclude regional, geographic, or ethnic associations related to common strains circulating in regions rather than to the presentation. Studies must also control for both the presence of the factor and for the disease association. It is also important to address whether the new factor is really a surrogate for another marker (e.g *vacA* s1 for *cagA*). Only the *cag* pathogenicity island has passed the tests of biological plausibility (increased inflammation) and experimental and epidemiological consistency as an important virulence factor increasing the risk of a symptomatic outcome but without disease specificity.

References

1. Censini S, Lange C, Xiang Z et al. cag, a pathogenicity island of *Helicobacter pylori*, encodes type I-specific and disease-associated virulence factors. Proc Natl Acad Sci USA. 1996; 93:14648–53.
2. Segal ED, Cha J, Lo J, Falkow S, Tompkins LS. Altered states: involvement of phosphorylated CagA in the induction of host cellular growth changes by *Helicobacter pylori*. Proc Natl Acad Sci USA. 1999;96:14559–64.
3. Stein M, Rappuoli R, Covacci A. Tyrosine phosphorylation of the *Helicobacter pylori* CagA antigen after cag-driven host cell translocation. Proc Natl Acad Sci USA. 2000;97:1263–8.
4. Odenbreit S, Puls J, Sedlmaier B, Gerland E, Fischer W, Haas R. Translocation of *Helicobacter pylori* CagA into gastric epithelial cells by type IV secretion. Science. 2000;287:1497–500.
5. Asahi M, Azuma T, Ito S et al. *Helicobacter pylori* CagA protein can be tyrosine phosphorylated in gastric epithelial cells. J Exp Med. 2000;191:593–602.
6. Yamaoka Y, El-Zimaity HMT, Gutierrez O et al. Relationship between subtypes of the *cagA* 3′ repeat region, gastric histology, and susceptibility to low pH. Gastroenterology. 1999; 117:342–9.
7. Aihara M, Tsuchimoto D, Takizawa H et al. Mechanisms involved in *Helicobacter pylori*-induced interleukin-8 production by a gastric cancer cell line, MKN45. Infect Immun. 1997;65:3218–24.
8. Keates S, Hitti YS, Upton M, Kelly CP. *Helicobacter pylori* infection activates NK-kappa B in gastric epithelial cells. Gastroenterology. 1997;113:1099–109.
9. Glocker E, Lange C, Covacci A, Bereswill S, Kist M, Pahl HL. Proteins encoded by the *cag* pathogenicity island of *Helicobacter pylori* are required for NF-kappaB activation. Infect Immun. 1998;66:2346–8.
10. Keates S, Keates AC, Warny M, Peak RM Jr, Murray PG, Kelly CP. Differential activation of mitogen-activated protein kinases in AGS gastric epithelial cells by *cag+* and *cag−* *Helicobacter pylori*. J Immunol. 1999;163:5552–9.
11. Naumann M, Wessler S, Bartsch C et al. Activation of activator protein 1 and stress response kinases in epithelial cells colonized by *Helicobacter pylori* encoding the *cag* pathogenicity island. J Biol Chem. 1999;274:31655–62.
12. Yamaoka Y, Kodama T, Kita M, Imanishi J, Kashima K, Graham DY. Relationship of *vacA* genotypes of *Helicobacter pylori* to *cagA* status, cytotoxin production, and clinical outcome. Helicobacter. 1998;4:241–53.
13. Yamaoka Y, Kodama T, Gutierrez O, Kim JG, Kashima K, Graham DY. Relationship between *Helicobacter pylori iceA*, *cagA* and *vacA* status and clinical outcome: studies in four different countries. J Clin Microbiol. 1999;37:2274–9.
14. Atherton JC, Tham KT, Peek RM, Cover TL, Blaser MJ. Density of *Helicobacter pylori* infection *in vivo* as assessed by quantitative culture and histology. J Infect Dis. 1996;174:552–6.
15. Yamaoka Y, Kodama T, Kita M, Imanishi J, Kashima K, Graham DY. Relation between clinical presentation, *Helicobacter pylori* density, interleukin-1β and -8 production and *cagA* status. Gut. 1999;45:804–11.
16. Graham DY, Yamaoka Y. Disease-specific *Helicobacter pylori* virulence factors: the unfulfilled promise. Helicobacter. 2000;5:S3–9.

17. Peek RM, Thompson SA, Donahue JP *et al.* Adherence to gastric epithelial cells induces expression of a *Helicobacter pylori* gene, *iceA*, that is associated with clinical outcome. Proc Assoc Am Phys. 1998;110:531–44.
18. van Doorn LJ, Figueriedo C, Sanna R *et al.* Clinical relevance of the *cagA*, *vacA*, and *iceA* status of *Helicobacter pylori*. Gastroenterology. 1998;115:58–66.
19. Atherton JC, Cao P, Peek RM, Tummuru MKR, Blaser MJ, Cover TL. Mosaicism in vacuolating cytotoxin alleles of *Helicobacter pylori*. J Biol Chem. 1995;270:17771–7.
20. Atherton JC, Peek RM, Tham KT, Cover TL, Blaser MJ. Clinical and pathological importance of heterogeneity in *vacA*, the vacuolating cytotoxin gene of *Helicobacter pylori*. Gastroenterology. 1997;112:92–9.
21. Pai R, Wyle FA, Cover TL, Itani RM, Domek MJ, Tarnawski AS. *Helicobacter pylori* culture supernatant interferes with epidermal growth factor-activated signal transduction in human gastric KATO III cells. Am J Pathol. 1998;152:1617–24.
22. Wessler S, Hocker M, Fischer W *et al. Helicobacter pylori* activates the histidine decarboxylase promoter through a mitogen-activated protein kinase pathway independent of pathogencity island-encoded virulence factors. J Biol Chem. 2000;275:3629–36.
23. Ilver D, Arnquist A, Ögren J. *et al. Helicobacter pylori* adhesin binding fucosylated histoblood group antigens revealed by retagging. Science. 1998;279:373–7.
24. Gerhard M, Lehn N, Neumayer N *et al.* Clinical relevance of the *Helicobacter pylori* gene for blood-group antigen-biding adhesin. Proc Natl Acad Sci USA. 1999;96:12778–83.
25. Graham DY. *Helicobacter pylori* infection in the pathogenesis of duodenal ulcer and gastric cancer: a model. Gastroenterology. 1997;113:1983–91.

Section II
Helicobacter pylori – Epidemiology

6
Factors associated with disappearance of *Helicobacter pylori* in the West

J. PARSONNET

INTRODUCTION

Helicobacter pylori is an extraordinarily common pathogen that has coexisted with humans since prehistoric times[1]. Yet the organism's ascendancy in the human stomach may soon be at an end. Increasing evidence from industrialized Western nations indicates that human *H. pylori* infection is disappearing at a dramatic rate. In longitudinal studies from the US, Europe and Japan, *H. pylori* prevalence has demonstrated precipitous drops, at rates exceeding 25% per decade[2-7]. These decreases appear to have been more precipitous in children than in adults. Anecdotally, many paediatric gastroenterologists claim *H. pylori* to be a rarity among their patients. At our own hospitals at Stanford, *H. pylori* infection is harder and harder to find. In parallel with this drop in *H. pylori* infection are corresponding decreases in gastric cancer and in duodenal ulcer disease.

Why should an organism that survived so successfully in humans for millennia, begin on a road to extinction? Without a better understanding of its mode of transmission it is impossible to say. Yet reasons can be deduced from understanding of infectious diseases epidemiology in general. Disease incidence depends on three factors: the number of susceptible individuals in the population, the number of infected individuals, and the ease with which an organism is transmitted from one person to another (the transmission parameter, β)[8]. A decrease of sufficient size in any one of these factors can produce an accelerating decline in an infection's incidence and prevalence until it spirals to extinction. For the case of *H. pylori* I shall address each of these three factors individually.

SUSCEPTIBILITY TO *H. PYLORI*

Even in countries where *H. pylori* infection is extremely common, not all individuals have chronic *H. pylori* infection. It is not known what protects these fortunate few from infection. It could be that they were never exposed. Yet if 80% of a given region's population harbours the organism, it is hard to envision that any could escape exposure. It seems plausible, then, that some people are intrinsically resistant to *H. pylori* infection.

Little is known about the determinants of protective immunity against *H. pylori* infection or, indeed, whether protective immunity occurs at all. Infection does not prevent superinfection with a second organism; nor does eradication of infection prevent reinfection[9,10]. Thus, our immune system may not have the tools to combat this organism from finding its niche. Despite our inadequate immune defenses, some individuals lose *H. pylori* during the acute stages of infection. This has been most evident with endoscopy-related infections; in several of these cases, *H. pylori* has disappeared spontaneously following a period of acute inflammation[11]. Loss of acute infection has also been observed with experimental ingestion of the organism[12]. Finally, there is circumstantial evidence that infants and toddlers may gain and lose infection recurrently in the first few years of life[13]. One possible explanation for some of the decrease in *H. pylori* infection, then, rests in an improved ability to combat its initial assault.

To date, however, there are no data to support or refute changes in host susceptibility over time. In the absence of data, two hypotheses have been proffered. First, it has been suggested that improvements in nutrition in Western countries may decrease susceptibility to infection, both by improving immune response and by increasing gastric acidity. In support of this hypothesis, it has been known for decades that malnourished children are hypochlorhydric[14]. Unfortunately, the role of *H. pylori* in this hypochlorhydria has never been investigated; thus, we cannot distinguish whether *H. pylori* is the cause or the effect of this phenomenon. Moreover, there is little supportive data that the risk for other infections increases in the setting of malnutrition, although outcome of these infections may be worse. A second hypothesis for decreasing susceptibility over time posits that coincident infections that increase risk for *H. pylori* infection are also disappearing[15]. Again, no data support or refute this theory.

The best way to ensure decreased host susceptibility on a population level is through vaccination. So far, no vaccine exists for *H. pylori*, although several are in various stages of human trials. Thus, while decreasing susceptibility over time is probably not the reason for *H. pylori*'s current decline, this mechanism may be the ultimate key to the organism's elimination.

DECREASED NUMBERS OF INFECTED HOSTS

Since the advent of penicillin in the 1940s, the use of antimicrobial agents worldwide has skyrocketed. Although relatively unusual combinations of antimicrobial agents are typically required to eliminate *H. pylori* infection, single antibiotics can achieve success in a small number of patients. Thus, the escalating use of antimicrobial agents for various purposes, as an unintended consequence, could have hastened *H. pylori*'s disappearance.

Some data challenge the notion that antibiotic use has caused significant decreases in *H. pylori* prevalence, however. For example, investigations of

H. pylori indicate that its disappearance dates back to early in the 20th century, before antimicrobial agents were commonly used[7,16]. Of course, this does not mitigate against antimicrobial agents contributing to the process but it does not appear *necessary* to impute antimicrobial agents in the decline of *H. pylori* prevalence. Furthermore, longitudinal studies in adults demonstrate consistent maintenance of *H. pylori* in the stomach despite sporadic courses of antimicrobial agents for other purposes[2]. Conversely, it is possible that the widespread use of single antimicrobial agents is diminishing our ability to eradicate *H. pylori* infection. For example, data worldwide suggest that *H. pylori* infection is becoming increasingly resistant to clarithromycin and to metronidazole – two of the mainstays of triple and quadruple therapies – presumably due to the widespread use of these antibiotics for other purposes[17,18].

Thus, there are reasons to doubt that antibiotic use in adults has altered the epidemiology of *H. pylori* infection. Most antibiotics in the United States, however, are given to children, a group in whom *H. pylori* infection appears to be most plastic. It remains to be seen whether sporadic antibiotic use in childhood reverses early infection. This topic warrants further attention.

EXTRINSIC BARRIERS TO INFECTION

Neither decreased susceptibility to infection nor increased eradication of *H. pylori* seems a likely explanation for the loss of *H. pylori* in populations, although neither can be definitively excluded. More plausible is the possibility that barriers to *H. pylori* transmission have increased. The leading hypothesis for *H. pylori* transmission is person-to-person spread via contact with either gastric or faecal contents. A recent study demonstrates large quantities of culturable organisms in both vomitus and cathartic stools of normal, healthy, infected adults[19]. In this study, after vomiting, *H. pylori* was also readily culturable from the majority of saliva samples, and during vomiting it was culturable from the air. In other studies, *H. pylori* has also been cultured from the vomitus of infected children and from diarrhoeal stools of children and adults[20,21]. *H. pylori* has few regulatory genes, causing suspicion that it cannot survive well outside its human host[22]. Taken together, these data lend strong support to the large volume of epidemiological data indicating a high probability of person-to-person transmission among close contacts (e.g. within families or community homes). Although other forms of *H. pylori* transmission have been posited (e.g. from flies, from animals and from water), none of these hypotheses has yet attained the force of evidence as the person-to-person transmission theory[23]. Yet, as with other infections transmitted predominantly from person to person by the faecal–oral route, other modes of transmission (e.g. water, food and flies) are inevitably occasional culprits.

Some clues as to mechanisms of *H. pylori* transmission may be gleaned by comparing the features of its epidemiology with those of other infectious agents. The decline of *H. pylori* infection in developed countries mimics the decline of another enteric pathogen – *Shigella*. *Shigella*, like *H. pylori*, is strictly a primate pathogen that is transmitted through the faecal–oral route, usually by direct contact[24]. Transmission is particularly common within families, with very high secondary attack rates when the infected host is a young child (bacterial infections of humans). As hygienic conditions improve within communities, *Shigella* disappears in parallel. No specific interventions have targeted *Shigella*, host susceptibility has not diminished, and, indeed, enteric infections that have non-primate hosts and a higher proportion of food-borne transmission (e.g. *Salmonella* and *Campylobacter*) are on the increase. However, numerous barriers of faecal–oral spread have been imposed over the 20th century including: access within homes to piped water for toilets and for washing, universal availability of soap, decreased family size and household crowding with improved childhood survival, and disappearance of night soil use for fertilization. Additionally, the education of women – an important factor in preventing childhood diseases[25] – would serve to interrupt infection transmission. Numerous studies dating back half a century correlate with the demise of *Shigella* with these changes in hygiene[24]. These very same factors appear to have favoured *H. pylori's* demise.

Infectious agents that live a relatively short time in their host – such as *Shigella* – must transmit themselves efficiently to maintain their endemicity[8]. To do this the organism should optimally have a low infectious dose and be excreted in large quantities. *Shigella* certainly holds claim to both of these requirements: as few as 10 organisms have been known to cause disease and up to 10^8 organisms are shed per gram of stool[24]. In contrast, *H. pylori* is thought to have a relatively high infectious dose (at least 10^5 organisms are required in monkeys; personal communication from Jay Solnick) and to be rarely excreted in normal stools or oral secretions.[19] However, *H. pylori* is carried throughout the host's life. This lifelong carriage of infection provides *H. pylori* with decades of opportunity to exit the host and infect others – it just requires the right window of opportunity.

Understanding the window *H. pylori* requires for transmission may provide the key to its diminishing prevalence. A window of opportunity that I favour is gastroenteritis. As mentioned above, *H. pylori* is rarely excreted in normal stools but is commonly found in diarrhoeal stools and in vomitus. Throughout life, each person can be expected to have hundreds of episodes of gastroenteritis, each episode potentially shedding *H. pylori* in large quantities into the environment. In developing countries the rates of diarrhoea are considerably higher, providing even greater opportunity for transmission. Moreover, from developing countries there is a small amount of data suggesting that *H. pylori* may foster gastroenteritis. Specifically, *H. pylori* has been linked to severe cholera and to incident diarrhoea in children in developing countries[26–28]. Although this relationship has not been proved to be one of cause and effect, it makes teleological sense. It would be advantageous for *H. pylori* to be permissive of gastroenteritis since, by doing so, it would promote its own propagation throughout populations (Figure 1).

Thus, *H. pylori's* disappearance appears to be an unintended consequence of socioeconomic development. This conclusion provides reason for both optimism and pessimism. If *H. pylori* infection has disappeared from many countries worldwide without specific intervention, then it is almost certain

```
        H. pylori infection ←
               │         ╲
              ( 1 )      ( 4 )
               │          ╲
               │          H. pylori shedding
               ▼            ╲
        Hypochlorhydria      ╲
               ╲             ( 3 )
                ╲             ╲
               ( 2 )            ╲
                  ╲              ╲
Pathogen ──────────→ Gastroenteritis
exposure
```

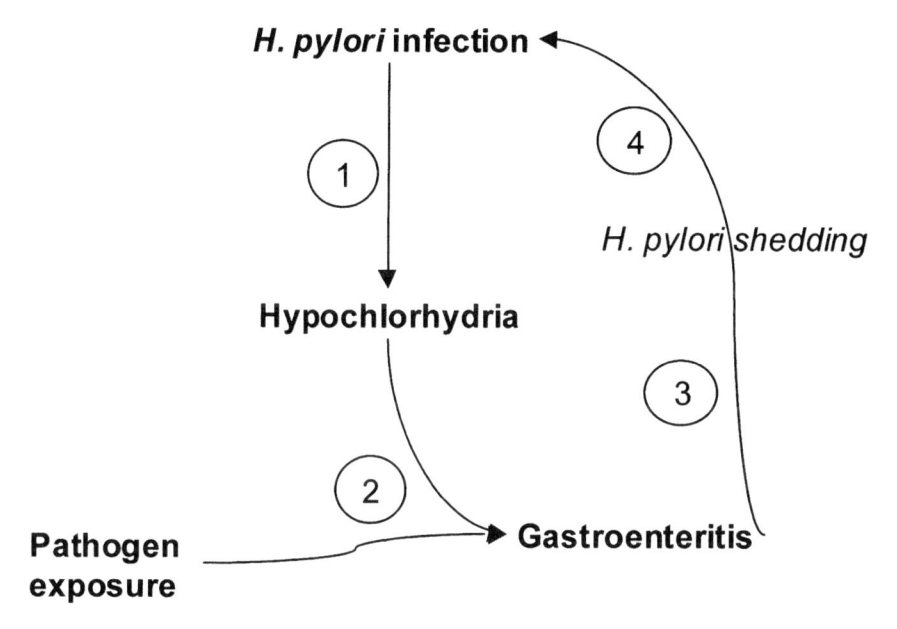

Figure 1. Hypothetical cycle of *H. pylori* transmission: In step one, *H. pylori* causes hypochlorhydria, either in the setting of acute infection or in the setting of atrophic gastritis. The resulting decrease in gastric acid is then permissive of infection with acid-sensitive gastroenteritis pathogens such as *Salmonella* and *Campylobacter* (step 2). When gastroenteritis occurs, *H. pylori* is shed into the environment, either in vomitus or stools (step 3). This shedding provides the opportunity for new infection of a susceptible host (step 4). A cycle such as this provides an overarching explanation of the parallel decline in *H. pylori* infection and diarrhoeal diseases.

that this can be recapitulated in current high prevalence areas as socioeconomic conditions improve. Yet the converse is also true: one can expect increases in *H. pylori* infection when governments destabilize, when wars destroy the infrastructure for sanitation and hygiene, and when economies collapse. Without a vaccine, the balance of what will happen to *H. pylori* throughout the world, then, depends on the stability of human society.

SUMMARY

H. pylori infection is disappearing rapidly from industrialized populations, most likely because of instituted barriers to transmission. In particular, changes in sanitation and hygiene appear to have decreased transmission both directly, by eliminating the organism from the environment, and indirectly by preventing gastroenteritis, thereby limiting shedding of the organism by infected hosts. Together, these changes have caused a spiralling decline in the incidence of infections. Institution of a vaccine into industrialized populations would be expected to accelerate the demise of *H. pylori*, but is not necessary to largely eliminate the organism from the population (M. T. Rupnow, personal communication). Unless our imposed battlements collapse, it seems unlikely that *H. pylori* infection will again threaten industrialized populations.

References

1. Covacci A, Telford JL, Del Giudice G, Parsonnet J, Rappuoli R. *Holicobacter pylori* virulence and genetic geography. Science. 1999;284:1328–33.
2. Parsonnet J, Blaser MJ, Perez-Perez GI, Hargrett-Bean N, Tauxe RV. Symptoms and risk factors of *Helicobacter pylori* infection in a cohort of epidemiologists. Gastroenterology. 1992;102:41–6.
3. Sipponen P. *Helicobacter pylori* gastritis – epidemiology. J Gastroenterol. 1997;32:273–7.
4. Roosendall R, Kuipers EJ, Buitenwerf J et al. *Helicobacter pylori* and the birth cohort effect: evidence of a continuous decrease of infection rates in childhood. Am J Gastroenterol. 1997;92:1480–2.
5. Replogle ML, Kasumi W, Ishikawa KB et al. Increased risk of *Helicobacter pylori* associated with birth in wartime and postwar Japan. Int J Epidemiol. 1996;25:210–14.
6. Haruma K, Okamoto S, Kawaguchi H et al. Reduced incidence of *Helicobacter pylori* infection in young Japanese persons between the 1970s and the 1990s. J Clin Gastroenterol. 1997;25:583–6.
7. Gause-Nilsson I, Gnarpe H, Gnarpe J, Lundborg P, Steen B. *Helicobacter pylori* serology in elderly people: a 21-year cohort comparison in 70-year-olds and a 20-year longitudinal population study in 70–90-year-olds. Age Ageing. 1998;27:433–6.
8. Anderson RM, May RM. Infectious Diseases of Humans: dynamics and control. New York: Oxford University Press; 1991.
9. Mitchell HM, Hu P, Chi Y, Li YY, Hazell SL. A low rate of reinfection following effective therapy against *Helicobacter pylori* in a developing nation (China). Gastroenterology. 1998;114:256–61.
10. Berg DE, Gilman RH, Lelwala-Guruge J et al. *Helicobacter pylori* populations in Peruvian patients. Clin Infect Dis. 1997;25:996–1002.
11. Morai T, Hirahara N. Clinical course of acute gastric mucosal lesions caused by acute infection with *Helicobacter pylori* [letter]. N Engl J Med. 1999;341:456–7.
12. Marshall BJ, Armstrong JA, McGeche DB, Glancy RJ. Attempt to fulfill Koch's postulates for pyloric *Campylobacter*. Med J Aust. 1985;142:436–9.
13. Klein PD, Gilman RH, Leon-Barua R, Diaz F, Smith EO, Graham DY. The epidemiology of *Helicobacter pylori* in Peruvian children between 6 and 30 months of age. Am J Gastroenterol. 1994;89:2196–200.
14. Viteri FE, Schneider RE. Gastrointestinal alterations in protein–calorie malnutrition. Med Clin N Am. 1974;58:1487–505.
15. Graham DY. *Helicobacter pylori* infection in the pathogenesis of duodenal ulcer and gastric cancer: a model. Gastroenterology. 1997;113:1983–91.
16. Parsonnet J. The incidence of *Helicobacter pylori* infection. Aliment Pharmacol Ther. 1995;9 (Suppl. 2):45–52.
17. Wreiber K, Olsson-Liljequist B, Engstrand L. Development of resistant *Helicobacter pylori* in Sweden. Tendency toward increasing resistance to clarithromycin. Lakartidningen. 1999;96:582–4.
18. van der Wouden EJ, Van Zwet AA, Vosmaer GD, Oom JA, de Jong A, Kleibeuker JH. Rapid increase in the prevalence of metronidazole-resistant *Helicobacter pylori* in the Netherlands. Emerg Infect Dis. 1997;3:395–9.
19. Parsonnet J, Shmuely H, Haggerty T. Fecal and oral shedding of *Helicobacter pylori* from healthy, infected adults. J Am Med Assoc. 1999;282:2240–5.
20. Leung WK, Sung, JY, Siu KLK, Kwok KL, Cheng AFB, Sung R. Isolation of *H. pylori* from vomitus in children. Gastroenterology. 1998:114 (abstract).
21. Thomas JE, Gibson GR, Darboe MK, Dale A, Weaver LT. Isolation of *Helicobacter pylori* from human faeces. Lancet. 1992;340:1194–5.
22. Tomb JF, White O, Kerlavage AR et al. The complete genome sequence of the gastric pathogen *Helicobacter pylori* [see comments]. Nature. 1997;388:539–47.
23. Mégraud F. Transmission of *Helicobacter pylori*: fecal–oral vs. oral–oral route. Aliment Pharmacol Ther. 1995;9(Suppl. 2):85–91.

24. Keutsch GT, Bennish ML. Shigellosis. In: Evans AS, Brachman PS, editor. Bacterial Infections of Humans: Epidemiology and Control. New York: Plenum; 1998:631–56.
25. Desai S, Alva S. Maternal education and child health: is there a strong causal relationship? Demography. 1998;35:71–81.
26. Clemens J, Albert MJ, Rao M *et al*. Impact of infection by *Helicobacter pylori* on the risk and severity of endemic cholera. J Infect Dis. 1995;171:1653–6.
27. Passaro D, Taylor D, Meza R, Cabrera L, Gilman R, Parsonnet J. Acute *Helicobacter pylori* infection in Peruvian children is followed by an increase in diarrheal disease. Program and Abstracts, IDSA '98, Denver, 79. 1998 (abstract).
28. Shahinian ML, Passaro DJ, Swerdlow DL, Mintz ED, Rodriguez M, Parsonnel J. *Helicobacter pylori* and epidemic *Vibrio cholerae* O1 infection in Peru. Lancet. 2000;355:377–8.

7
Factors associated with disappearance of *Helicobacter pylori* in the Far East

J. J. Y. SUNG

The question of whether *Helicobacter pylori* is disappearing in the Far East has very little data to support with the exception of one study in Japan. Fujisawa *et al.* reported the seroepidemiology of 766 samples from the National Institute of Infectious Disease in Tokyo collected over two decades[1]. The overall prevalence of *H. pylori* infection has dropped by almost half (from 72.7% to 39.3%) during the period of study. While the prevalence of infection increases with age in the three cohorts of 1974, 1984 and 1994, a clear cohort shift towards the right has been demonstrated. This study also shows that acquisition of *H. pylori* infection in Japanese infants and children has dramatically reduced in the past 20 years.

If *H. pylori* infection is disappearing, one would expect *H. pylori*-related gastroduodenal diseases also to decline. Data from the gastrointestinal bleeding registry from Hong Kong, which included 8628 patients with peptic ulcer bleeding, revealed a rapidly declining incidence of duodenal ulcer (DU) bleeding from 1990 to 1997[2]. The drop in DU bleeding incidence was more dramatic in patients under the age of 40 years. On the other hand, the incidence of gastric ulcer (GU) bleeding and DU bleeding in older patients (above 60 years) remains unchanged. As *H. pylori* infection is more closely related to DU than GU, especially for young patients who consume less NSAIDs and aspirin, the changing pattern of ulcer disease provides circumstantial evidence for a decline in *H. pylori* infection. Among other genetic and environmental factors, *H. pylori* infection has also been related to the development of gastric cancers. Data from various countries indicate that age-adjusted stomach cancer death rates have been steadily decreasing since World War II[3]. In Japan gastric cancer mortality increased after World War II, reaching 70 per 100 000, and then declined in the 1960s. Changes in dietary habit and the availability of fresh fruits may have a major impact on gastric cancer incidence. The decline in *H. pylori* infection may also have contributed to the changing epidemiology. Finally, gastro-oesophageal reflux disease (GERD) has been reported to show a rising trend[4]. Medical reports of 23 870 patients who underwent gastroscopy during the periods from 1975 to 1977, 1985 to 1987 and 1995 to 1997 were reviewed. Reflux oesophagitis has increased by 3-fold from 0.76% to 2.31% in this series. Although the incidence is still low compared to data from Western countries, and most patients have mild (Los Angeles Grade A/B) oesophagitis, the rapidly rising trend is alarming. In Hong Kong patients with GERD were shown to have a substantially lower prevalence of *H. pylori* infection when compared to controls[5]. Thus, the changing pattern of gastro-duodenal diseases, especially over the past two decades, lends strong support to the notion of disappearing *H. pylori* infection in the Far East.

What factors might be associated with the disappearance of *H. pylori* infection? There is ample evidence to suggest that person-to-person transmission is common, although few investigations clearly discriminate between direct interpersonal transmission or a common source of infection associated with overcrowding. Acquisition of *H. pylori* infection occurs in early childhood in China, especially in urban areas[6]. Density of living in the family environment will also increase the risk of acquiring the infection. In a family study using the [^{13}C] urea breath test conducted in the Shangdong province of China, Ma *et al.* reported that infected parents are strongly associated with childhood infections[7]. In families with at least one infected parent, 85% of children were *H. pylori*-positive, compared to 22% of children infected in families with both parents uninfected. The risk of transmitting the infection among siblings has recently been highlighted in a study involving 684 children in Colombia[8]. The risk of acquiring *H. pylori* infection was found to increase with the number of siblings in the household aged 2–9 years. Younger siblings are more likely to be infected if the older brother or sister is infected. A similar effect of the number of siblings on the risk of *H. pylori* infection has previously been shown in Taiwan[9].

The route of *H. pylori* transmission is still unclear. Hulten *et al.* analysed water samples from Peru using immunomagnetic separation and polymerase chain reaction (PCR), with successful detection of *H. pylori* in drinking water[10]. The quality of water supplies in some Asian countries may potentially be a source for transmission of the infection. However, studies from Southern China show no correlation between faecal contamination of the water supply and the prevalence of *H. pylori* infection[6]. However, the Chinese practice of boiling all drinking water and storing it in vacuum flasks prior to ingestion may account for this negative finding. Faecal–oral transmission of *H. pylori* infection has not gained support from Hazell's study comparing the seroprevalence of *H. pylori* to the prevalence of antibody to hepatitis A in certain rural and urban areas of China[11]. Leung *et al.* studied the vomitus of 18 children aged between 1 and 14 years, including four with a positive *H. pylori* serology[12]. Among them, *H. pylori* was isolated from vomitus by culture in one and by PCR in two. An 18-month-old girl with negative serology had *H. pylori* detected in vomitus by PCR and seroconverted 6 months later. Gastro-oral transmission could be an important route of infection, especially among children.

The most important factor associated with the falling incidence of *H. pylori* infection in the Far East is likely to be improved socioeconomic and sanitary conditions in the region. Although Asia still constitutes over 50% of the world's population, population growth in this region slowed down in the twentieth century[13]. The size of Asian families has become smaller with government policies promoting birth control. With the rapidly booming economy in the Far East over the past 30 years, many Asian countries have reported the highest growth in GNP per capita. Improvements in socioeconomic circumstances and standards of living have been reflected in the low infant mortality rate and prolonged life expectancy in this region. Since the decline in *H. pylori* infection actually preceded the discovery of the organism in 1982, improvement in living conditions is far more important than any other factor in contributing to the control of this infection.

Recurrence of *H. pylori* infection has been reported in the range of 0–14% in Asia. In most Asian countries, however, the re-infection rate is very low (probably below 5%). In a study designed to investigate the re-infection rate following effective therapy in China, Mitchell *et al.* followed 184 patients for up to 24 months using the urea breath test[14]. Only four patients were re-infected, giving an annual recurrence rate of 1.08%. Ulcer relapse occurred only in six patients (3.2%). Leung *et al.* investigated whether eating with chopsticks increased the risk of re-infection[15]. Among 32 patients, *H. pylori* was detected in the saliva in 10 cases, but on the chopsticks in only one.

In conclusion, there is circumstantial evidence to suggest that *H. pylori* infection is disappearing in the Far East. The most important contributing factor to the control of this infection is the improvement in socioeconomic conditions in Asia and the reduction of population growth. After successful eradication of *H. pylori* infection, recurrence is uncommon, even in Asia.

References

1. Fujisawa T, Kumagai T, Akamatsu T, Kiyosawa K, Matsunaga Y. Changes in seroepidemiological pattern of *Helicobacter pylori* and hepatitis A virus over the last 20 years in Japan. Am J Gastroenterol. 1999;94:2049–9.
2. Ng EKW, Chan A, Lee D *et al*. Time trend analysis of peptic ulcer bleeding over an 8-year period in Hong Kong. Gastroenterology. 1999;116:A1010.
3. Aoki K. Epidemiology of stomach cancer. In: Nishi M, Ichikawa H, Nakajima T, Maruyama K, Tahara E, editors. Gastric Cancer. Springer-Verlag; 1993:2–15.
4. Manabe N, Haruma K, Mihara M *et al*. The increasing incidence of reflux esophagitis during the past 20 years in Japan. Gastroenterology. 1999;116:A1061.
5. Wu JCY, Sung JJY, Ng EKW *et al*. Prevalence and distribution of *H. pylori* in gastroesophageal reflux disease: a study from the East. Am J Gastroenterol. 1999;94:1790–4.
6. Mitchell HM, Li YY, Hu PJ *et al*. Epidemiology of *Helicobacter pylori* in Southern China: identification of early childhood as the critical period for acquisition. J Infect Dis. 1992;166:149–53.
7. Ma JL, You WC, Gail MH *et al*. *Helicobacter pylori* infection and mode of transmission in a population at high risk of stomach cancer. Int J Epidemiol. 1998;27:570–3.
8. Goodman KJ, Gorrea P. Transmission of *Helicobacter pylori* among siblings. Lancet. 2000;355:258–62.
9. The BH, Lin JT, Pan WH *et al*. Seroprevalence and associated risk factors of *Helicobacter pylori* infection in Taiwan. Anticancer Res. 1994;14:1389–92.
10. Hulten K, Han SW, El-Zaatari FAK *et al*. Detection of *Helicobacter pylori* in Peruvian water sources by two PCR assays based on independent genes. Lancet. 1991;227:15–23.

11. Hazell SL, Mitchell HM, Hedges M et al. Hepatitis A and evidence against the community dissemination of *Helicobacter pylori* via feces. J Infect Dis. 1994;170:686–9.
12. Leung WK, Siu KLK, Kwok, CKL, Chan SY, Sung R, Sung JJY. Isolation of *Helicobacter pylori* in vomitus of children: implications in gastro-oral transmission. Am J Gastroenterol. 1999;94:2881–4.
13. World Bank. www.worldbank.org.
14. Mitchell HM, Hu PJ, Chi Y, Chen MH, Li YY, Hazell SL. A low rate of reinfection following effective therapy against *Helicobacter pylori* in a developing nation (China). Gastroenterology. 1998;114:256–61.
15. Leung WK, Sung JJY, Ling TKW, Siu SLK, Cheng AFB. Does the use of chopsticks for eating transmit *Helicobacter pylori*? Lancet. 1997;350:31.

8
Differences in prevalence of *Helicobacter pylori* and disease outcomes according to race/environmental factors in Southeast Asia

K. L. GOH

INTRODUCTION

Although *Helicobacter pylori* is believed to infect more than half the world's population, marked differences in prevalence exist between different countries and between different communities or regions within the same country. 'Developed countries' have lower prevalence rates compared to 'developing countries'. This difference appears to be related to the socioeconomic status of the country[1].

Ethnicity has been thought to be an important risk factor for *H. pylori* infection. In a study by Graham et al.[2], carried out in the metropolitan area of Houston, black Americans were found to have a significantly higher *H. pylori* prevalence compared to whites. This racial difference remained after adjustment for age and socioeconomic factors. However, while both whites and blacks with low income had high *H. pylori* prevalence, and the prevalence declined with increasing income among whites, the prevalence among blacks did not show a similar trend. Malaty et al.[3] performed a case–control seroepidemiological study in which Hispanics were matched with whites and blacks with respect to age and socioeconomic status. In this study the authors showed significantly higher prevalence rates among Hispanics and blacks compared to whites. The authors speculated, however, that this increased prevalence could be reflective of low socioeconomic status during childhood, rather than at that current point in time – a 'generational cohort' phenomenon, in blacks and Hispanics.

The Southeast Asian countries have an interesting ethnic mix of three major Asian races: Malays, Chinese and Indians. Racial differences in

H. pylori prevalence have been observed in the Southeast Asian countries for several years now[4,5]. The Malays have been shown to have a consistently low prevalence compared to the Indians and Chinese. While the Malays are considered to be the indigenous population, the Chinese and Indians are migrant races who moved to these countries in large numbers at the turn of the nineteenth century. While social integration, particularly among the Chinese and the local population, has taken place in Thailand and the Philippines, Chinese and Indians have remained socially, and racially, distinct in Malaysia, Singapore and Indonesia.

Differences in upper gastrointestinal disease patterns have also been observed between the major ethnic groups in Malaysia for a long time. This has particularly been noted with regard to peptic ulcer disease and cancer of the stomach[6-9]. These differences are intriguing because they allow for inferences to be made as to the mechanisms of disease operative in the local population with respect to the role of H. pylori and other environmental factors. This chapter reviews studies that have been performed in Malaysia over the past 10 years, and highlights several important observations made in these studies.

PREVALENCE OF H. PYLORI

Seroepidemiological studies (Table 1)

Several seroepidemiological studies were incorporated in an extensive seroprevalence survey performed in several parts of the country[10,11]. Geographical and racial differences in H. pylori prevalence have been noted. Serological assay using a standard commercial ELISA kit (HEL-p II test, AMRAD, Australia), which had been previously validated[12] and found to have a sensitivity of 96.7% and a specificity of 94.2%, was used for all the serological studies.

Consistently in every study, where the prevalence of the three major races can be compared, the Malays have the lowest prevalence rates compared to the Chinese and Indians. The highest overall prevalence rate of 55.0% was recorded among blood donors in Kota Kinabalu, Sabah, East Malaysia. In this study the Chinese had a prevalence rate of 49.3% and the Malays a prevalence of 29.2%. The indigenous population had a high prevalence rate of 65.3%. The differences in H. pylori prevalence between the indigenous population vs Malays ($p < 0.001$) and Chinese vs Malays ($p < 0.028$) were statistically significant. In another study, carried out among healthy volunteers and blood donors from Sibu in East Malaysia[11], a prevalence rate of 24.6% was reported among the Malays while a prevalence rate of 42.9% was found among the Chinese and 55.0% among the native races. The differences in prevalence of H. pylori infection between Chinese vs Malays and Native races vs Malays were statistically significant ($p < 0.001$).

In a study[11] on 548 blood donors from Kuala Lumpur on the West coast of West Malaysia, Malays were found to have a prevalence of 11.9%, Chinese 26.7% and Indians 49.4%. The differences in prevalence rates between Chinese vs Malays and Indians vs Malays were statistically significant

PREVALENCE OF H. PYLORI AND RACE/ENVIRONMENTAL FACTORS

Table 1. Summary of seroepidemiological studies: *H. pylori* prevalence according to gender, race and age-group and level of education

	H. pylori-positive				
	Kuala Pilah, West Malaysia (n = 626)	Kuala Lumpur, West Malaysia (n = 548)	Kota Baru, West Malaysia (n = 323)	Kota Kinabalu, East Malaysia (n = 373)	Sibu, East Malaysia (n = 512)
All subjects	199 (31.6)	145 (26.4)	85 (26.4)	205 (55.0)	221 (43.2)
Age (years)					
0–44	132/486 (27.1)	129/513 (25.1)	77/296 (26.0)	194/347 (40.3)	185/449 (41.2)
≥45	67/140 (47.9)	16/35 (45.7)	8/26 (30.8)	11/26 (42.3)	36/63 (57.1)
Gender					
Female	103/355 (29.0)	18/81 (22.2)	3/10 (30.0)	20/46 (43.5)	87/191 (45.5)
Male	96/271 (35.4)	127/467 (27.2)	82/312 (26.3)	185/327 (56.6)	134/321 (41.7)
Race					
Malay	61/380 (16.1)	16/135 (11.9)	69/282 (24.5)	14/48 (29.2)	29/118 (24.6)
Chinese	104/181 (57.5)	88/330 (26.7)	16/40 (40.0)	36/73 (49.3)	88/205 (42.9)
Indian	34/65 (52.3)	41/83 (49.4)	0/1	—	—
Indigenous native races	—	—	—	126/193 (65.3)	100/185 (54.0)
Immigrants	—	—	—	29/59 (49.2)	—
Education level					
High	—	45/180 (25.0)	4/27 (14.8)	42/72 (58.3)	9/30 (30.0)
Middle	—	74/293 (25.2)	64/251 (25.4)	25/45 (55.5)	139/356 (39.0)
Low	—	26/75 (34.6)	17/44 (38.6)	138/256 (53.9)	73/126 (57.9)

($p < 0.001$). In Kota Baru, on the East Coast of West Malaysia[10], prevalence rates among the Malays were 25.2%, and among the Chinese 40.0% ($p = 0.037$). In a community serological survey carried out in Kuala Pilah, a rural area on the West Coast of West Malaysia[10], Malays recorded a prevalence rate of 16.1%, Chinese 57.5% and Indians 52.3%. The differences in *H. pylori* prevalence between Chinese vs Malays ($p < 0.001$) and Indians vs Malays ($p < 0.001$) were statistically significant.

Multivariate analysis using multiple logistic regression analysis was performed on all these studies. Where comparisons could be made, Chinese and Indian races were determined as significant risk factors, vs Malays, for *H. pylori* infection, with odds ratios ranging from 2.1 to 7.4 (Table 2).

Survey of children

Racial differences in prevalence rates were already obvious in childhood. In a study performed at the University Hospital, Kuala Lumpur, 514 healthy children were screened for *H. pylori* infection over a 2-year period from January 1995 to 1997[13]. An overall prevalence rate of 10.3% (53/514) was noted. The prevalence rates by race were: Malay 6.5%, Chinese 10.4% and Indians 17.8%,. There was a significant difference in prevalence rates between Indian and Malay children ($p = 0.001$). The *H. pylori* prevalence was higher among Chinese compared to Malays, but this was not statistically significant ($p = 0.071$).

Endoscopic survey of asymptomatic volunteers

In a survey of 159 asymptomatic volunteers[14] who were endoscoped at the University Hospital, Kuala Lumpur, 28 (17.6%) were found to be *H. pylori*-positive. When the prevalence of *H. pylori* infection was analysed according to racial group, Indians were found to have an overwhelmingly higher prevalence rate of 46.1% (15/32). Chinese had a prevalence rate of 19.6% (9/46) and Malays a prevalence rate of 4.9% (4/81). The mean ages of all three racial groups were similar. The differences between Malays vs Chinese ($p = 0.013$) and Indian vs Malays ($p < 0.001$) were statistically significant.

Endoscopic surveys of dyspeptic patients

In an early study performed in 1988[4], 399 patients with dyspepsia who underwent endoscopy were investigated for the presence of *H. pylori* infection. Two hundred and two patients (50.6%) were found to be *H. pylori*-positive; 87.8% of duodenal ulcers (DU) and 87.5% of gastric ulcers (GU) and 39.3% of non-ulcer dyspepsia (NUD) patients were found to be infected with *H. pylori*. Of the four patients with cancer of the stomach, three were found to be *H. pylori*-positive (75%). Among the different races, Chinese had the highest prevalence of 56.4%. Indians had a similarly high prevalence of 51.9% while Malays were found to have a prevalence of 31.4%. The differences between Chinese and Indians versus Malays were highly significant ($p < 0.001$). The prevalence of *H. pylori* was noted to increase significantly with age: <39 years 41.1%, 40–59 years 57.6% and >60 years 75.0% ($p < 0.001$).

Table 2. Adjusted odds ratio of risk factors for *H. pylori* infection according to place of study

Variable	Odds ratio with (95% confidence intervals)				
	Kuala Pilah, West Malaysia	Kuala Lumpur, West Malaysia	Kota Baru, West Malaysia	Kota Kinabalu, East Malaysia	Sibu, East Malaysia
Age (years)					
0–44	1.0	1.0	1.0	1.0	1.0
≥45	2.6 (1.7, 4.1)	1.9 (0.6, 2.0)	1.0 (0.4, 2.6)	0.6 (0.3, 1.4)	1.8 (1.0, 3.3)
Gender					
Female	1.0	1.0	1.0	1.0	1.0
Male	1.0 (0.8, 1.2)	1.1 (0.6, 2.0)	1.0 (0.2, 4.3)	1.6 (0.8, 3.1)	0.8 (0.6, 1.3)
Race					
Malay	1.0	1.0	1.0	1.0	1.0
Chinese	7.4 (4.9, 11.2)	2.6 (1.4, 4.6)	2.1 (1.0, 2.3)	2.6 (1.2, 5.7)	2.2 (1.3, 3.7)
Indian	5.5 (3.1, 9.8)	6.7 (3.4, 13.2)	—	—	—
Indigenous/native races	—	—	—	4.8 (2.4, 9.8)	3.8 (2.3, 6.4)
Immigrants	—	—	—	2.6 (1.1, 5.9)	—
Education level					
High	—	1.0	1.0	1.0	1.0
Middle	—	1.0 (0.6, 1.5)	1.9 (0.6, 5.7)	1.0 (0.6, 1.7)	1.5 (0.6, 3.4)
Low	—	1.9 (0.9, 3.9)	3.6 (1.0, 12.7)	0.8 (0.4, 1.3)	2.9 (1.2, 7.1)

H.pylori prevalence %

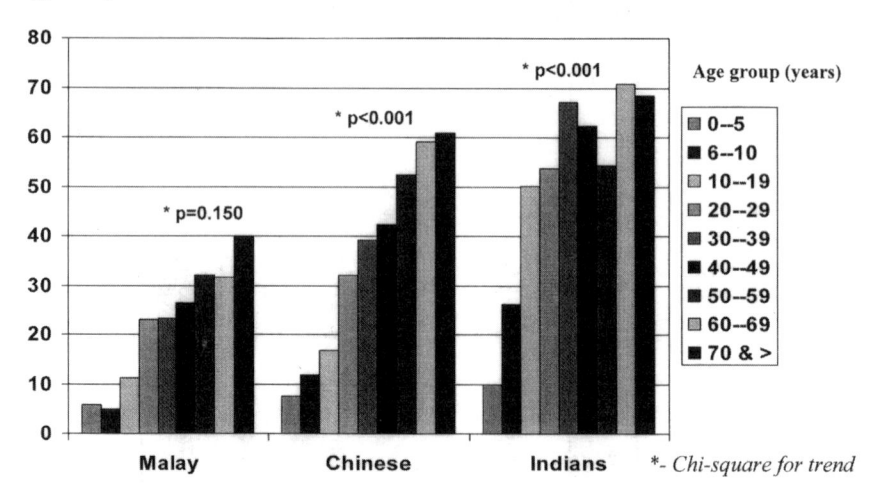

Figure 1. Prevalence of *H. pylori* by age group and according to races.

From January 1994 to July 1995 a large cross-sectional survey was performed on consecutive patients presenting with dyspepsia undergoing upper gastrointestinal endoscopy[15]. All patients had gastric biopsies taken for a rapid urease test. This test has been previously validated locally and found to have a high diagnostic accuracy[16].

One thousand and sixty patients were studied; 690 (65.1%) were diagnosed to have functional dyspepsia or NUD, 220 (20.8%) DU, 108 (10.2%) GU, 17 (1.6%) combined DU and GU, and 12 (1.1%) cancer of the stomach.

Analysis of *H. pylori* prevalence was carried out on the three major races: Malays, Chinese and Indians. Patients belonging to other races constituted a small group ($n = 17$) and were excluded from further analysis. Indians had the highest prevalence – 61.8% (193/314), Chinese 48.5% (269/555) and Malays 16.4% (45/174). The differences between Indians vs Malays ($p < 0.001$), Chinese vs Malays ($p < 0.001$) and Indians vs Chinese ($p < 0.001$) were highly significant. The data were also analysed separately for diagnoses of functional dyspepsia, duodenal ulcer and gastric ulcer (Figure 1). Multivariate analyses using multiple logistic regression analyses revealed that Indian race (OR: 4.9 (3.2, 7.5), 7.8 (4.3, 14.4)) and Chinese race (OR: 2.5 (1.7, 3.7), 2.5, (1.3, 4.6)), vs Malay race, were independent risk factors for *H. pylori* infection (OR for the overall and the functional dyspepsia group respectively).

H. pylori prevalence by age and racial group (Figure 1)

Overall, *H. pylori* prevalence increases with age (χ^2 for trend, $p < 0.001$). When *H. pylori* prevalence was analysed according to race, the *H. pylori* prevalence for Malays did not increase with age (χ^2 for trend, $p = 0.150$).

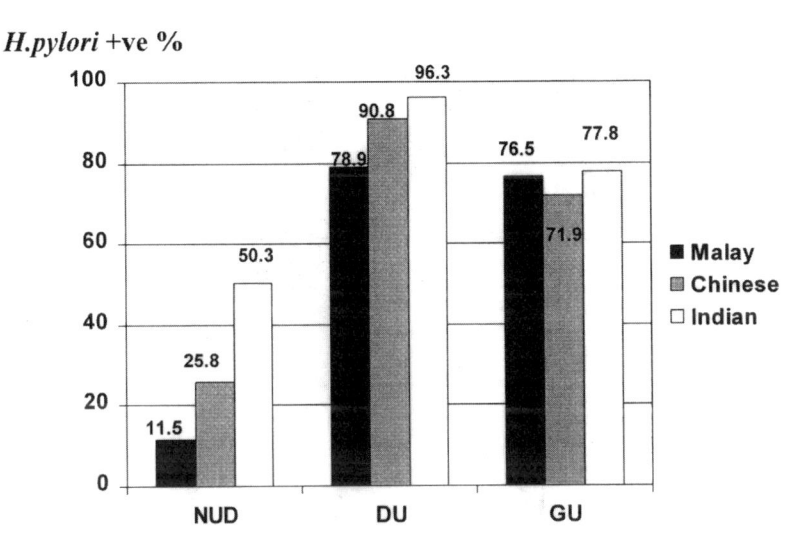

Figure 2. *H. pylori* prevalence according to race and ulcer status.

PEPTIC ULCER DISEASE

In the endoscopy survey on dyspeptic patients[15], we obtained an overall DU:GU ratio of 2.0:1 (220/108). The DU:GU ratio according to races are: Malay 1.1:1 (19:17), Chinese 2.2:1 (142:64), Indian 2:1 (54:27).

Distribution of peptic ulcer disease among races

Chinese had the highest proportion of dyspeptics with DU and GU, with percentages of 25.6% and 11.7%, respectively; Indians 17.2% and 8.6%, respectively and Malays 10.9% and 9.8%, respectively. These differences were statistically significant (Chinese vs Malays, $p < 0.001$, Chinese vs Indians, $p < 0.001$). The majority of ulcers in all racial groups were *H. pylori*-positive. The prevalence in both Malay DU and GU patients was lower compared to Chinese and Indians (Figure 2), although this was not statistically significant.

An intriguing observation was made when *H. pylori*-positive patients were analysed separately (Figure 3). Of the Chinese *H. pylori* positive patients 67.3% had peptic ulcers; of the Malay *H. pylori*-positive patients 65.1% had peptic ulcers while of the Indians only 39.9% had peptic ulcers. These differences in the proportion of ulcer and non-ulcer patients in *H. pylori*-positive patients between Chinese and Malays versus Indian patients were highly significant ($p < 0.001$). Multivariate analysis showed that Indian race remained a significant negative predictive factor with an odds ratio of 0.3 (0.2, 0.7) for ulcer disease in *H. pylori*-positive patients.

GASTRIC CANCER

In a retrospective survey of gastric cancer, seen over a 10-year period from 1987 to 1997 at the University Hospital, Kuala Lumpur, 675 cases were

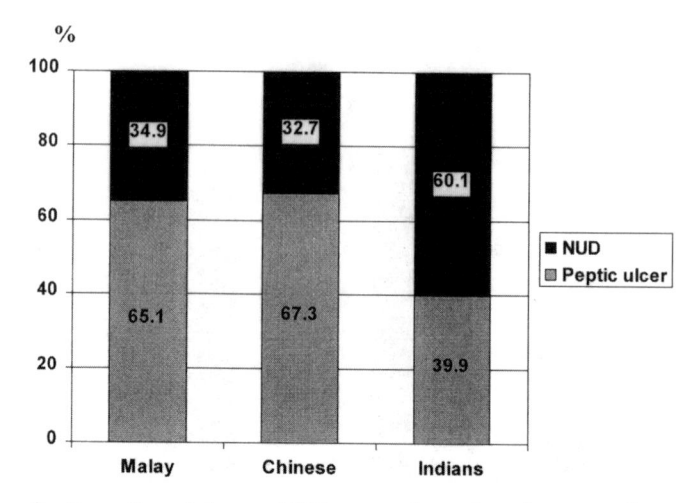

Figure 3. Proportion of ulcers vs NUD among dyspeptic patients according to race.

Table 3. Prevalence of gastric cancer according to race

	Chinese (n = 519)	Malay (n = 48)	Indian (n = 107)
Male:female	294:225	29:19	64:43
Age (years)			
Mean	62.6	58.0	60.5
Median	63	62	61
Range	21–96	28–90	29–90
Prevalence per 100 000 hospital admissions per race (95% CI)	397.1 (363–431)	24.0 (17.2–30.8)	116.4 (94.4–138)
Male	478.4 (424–533)	57.4 (36.5–78.4)	155.7 (118–194)
Female	325.0 (283–367)	12.7 (7.0–18.4)	84.7 (59.4–110)

diagnosed[17]. The prevalence in each racial group calculated per 100 000 hospital admissions for the particular racial group is shown in Table 3. Chinese had the highest prevalence of 397.1 per 100 000 Chinese hospital admissions compared to Malays and Indians with rates of 24.0 and 116.4 per 100 000 hospital admissions, respectively. In all racial groups the frequency of cancer was higher among men compared to women.

In an age- and sex-matched hospital-based, case–control study performed at the University Hospital, Kuala Lumpur[18], cases were matched to controls in a ratio of 1:2. The control patients were frequency-matched with respect to a 10-year age period. As there was no individual matching the numbers of cases and controls were not strictly defined in a 1:2 ratio. There were 86 cases of histologically confirmed adenocarcinoma and 160 controls. The mean age of controls was 58.5 years and cases 61.4 years. Fifty-four (62.8%) were found to involve the distal part of the stomach, 14 (16.3%) total involvement of the stomach and 18 (20.9%) the corpus and cardia of the stomach. Of 76 cases in which the adenocarcinoma was subtyped according

Table 4. Significant risk factors for gastric cancer following multivariate analysis

	OR	95% CI
Chinese race (vs Malay)	9.7	2.7, 34.4
Low education (vs high)	8.3	1.7, 41.9
Smoking	2.5	1.2, 5.1
High intake of fresh fruits/vegetables (vs low)	7.7	1.6, 37.9
High salt intake (vs low)	5.2	1.3, 20.5
H. pylori infection	2.2	1.0, 5.1

to Lauren's classification, 39 (51.3%) were of the intestinal type and 37 (48.7%) were of the diffuse type.

Chinese race, versus Malays, was found to be a significant risk factor for adenocarcinoma of the stomach with an adjusted odds ratio, following multiple logistic regression analysis, of 9.7 (2.7, 34.4) as was *H. pylori* infection, OR: 2.2 (1.0, 5.1). Other risk factors identified included smoking, odds ratio of 2.5 (1.2, 5.1), intake of salted vegetables and fish 5.1 (1.3, 20.5), low intake of fresh fruits and vegetables 7.7 (1.6, 37.8) and low level of education 8.4 (1.7, 41.9) (Table 4).

PATTERNS OF GASTRITIS

The pattern of gastritis in 75 *H. pylori*-positive patients with non-ulcer dyspepsia was studied[35]. In all patients at least four biopsies each were taken from the antrum and corpus. Among Chinese patients 14 of 28 (50.0%) were found to have antral-predominant gastritis. A similar proportion of Malay patients was also found to have antral gastritis – six of 11 (54.5%) while, on the contrary, only five of 31 (13.8%) of Indian patients had antral gastritis. The difference in the proportion of Chinese and Malay patients with antral gastritis versus Indian patients was statistically significant ($p = 0.001$ and $p = 0.017$, respectively). The difference in mean ages of all three groups were Chinese 36.1 years, Indians 33.2 years and Malays 39.0 years was not statistically significant ($p = 0.357$).

DISCUSSION

The prevalence of *H. pylori* infection shows an interesting distribution in a diverse country such as Malaysia. We have shown clearly the ethnic as well as geographical distribution of the infection. Other workers have documented the low prevalence in the Malays compared to the Chinese and Indians. Ethnic differences in neighbouring Singapore have been observed in an endoscopic and serological survey by Kang et al.[4,19]. In a report from Kelantan, in the northeast part of West Malaysia, an inordinately low prevalence of *H. pylori* was observed among the Malays[20]. In our seroepidemiological studies, and in our large endoscopic survey, Chinese and Indian race remained as independent predictive factors for *H. pylori* infection, after adjusting for possible confounding factors such as social class and age.

The reasons for the racial predilection are not entirely clear. Genetic factors may of course account for these differences. However, among the native and indigenous races of Sarawak and Sabah, East Malaysia, who belong to the same racial stock as the Malays, the *H. pylori* prevalence is, on the contrary, very high.

Racial differences may be a surrogate marker for different environmental exposures within the community. Environmental factors within the ethnic group and/or sociocultural practices peculiar to a racial group may perpetuate and encourage the spread of infection within the group. For instance, bedsharing among certain racial groups such as Pacific Island and Maori families, where *H. pylori* infection is high, is more common compared to the whites in New Zealand who have a low *H. pylori* prevalence[21]. Chow and colleagues[22] reported that the use of chopsticks may be a risk factor for *H. pylori* infection. Furthermore, most Asian Oriental races use common bowls for food during meals, which may presumably encourage the spread of an infection through an oral–oral route. Premastication is another cultural practice that is still carried out among the Chinese, where it is not uncommon for a mother or a grandmother to premasticate food before feeding a child. In contrast, use of common bowls and premastication do not appear to be common practices among the Malays and Indians in Malaysia. The role of environmental factors in *H. pylori* infection is also well shown in an important study from southern China[23]. Rural Guangdong was shown to have a lower *H. pylori* prevalence compared to urban Guangzhou, even though the latter is more affluent and with better public amenities. The authors suggested that the difference in prevalence rates points to overcrowding as an important factor in transmission of the infection.

We have proposed a *racial cohort theory* to explain the racial differences in Malaysia, in that the Malays started off with a low reservoir of infection while the Chinese and Indians had a high reservoir of infection. We know that the prevalence rates of *H. pylori* in southern India[24] and China[25] are high. *H. pylori* is an infection which is not highly contagious and requires close proximity, as within families and within a community, for spread. The races in Malaysia, although coexisting for close to two generations, have remained fairly separate and distinct as racial integration, and specifically intermarriages between ethnic groups, have not been commonplace. It is important to note that racial differences in *H. pylori* prevalence are already present during childhood in our Malaysian population, and are also obvious in asymptomatic healthy volunteers. Another interesting observation is that not only is the prevalence of *H. pylori* low among the Malays, but there is also an absence of a significant rise in prevalence with age among this racial group. Following the age-cohort theory this would mean that the reservoir of infection among the Malays was low even 60–70 years ago.

Confinement of *H. pylori* infection to racial cohorts has been well noted in other groups. Reports of high infection rates have been noted in Tibetan monks[26], Maoris and Pacific Islanders[21] and Eskimos[28]. Chow *et al.*[22] have noted differences in prevalence rates between Chinese immigrants from Malaysia/Singapore, Indochina and China compared to the local white population in Melbourne.

This racial cohort phenomenon has an analogy in another common infection in southeast Asia: hepatitis B infection. Transmission of hepatitis B infection occurs predominantly in the Far East during the perinatal and neonatal period, through mother to child transmission and leads to lifelong carriage of the virus. In Malaysia the Chinese have significantly higher hepatitis B carrier rates compared to the Indians and Malays[28]. Hepatitis B is another infection, apart from parenteral spread, which requires close contact between family members, particularly during the neonatal period and childhood, for spread of infection.

H. pylori infection is closely related to peptic ulcer disease and one would expect that the frequency of peptic ulcer disease is proportional to *H. pylori* prevalence. This is, however, not the case with the different races in Malaysia and Singapore. The low prevalence of peptic ulcers in Malays could be explained by the low *H. pylori* prevalence. The Indians, however, have a high *H. pylori* prevalence comparable or higher than the Chinese, and yet have a lower prevalence of peptic ulcers. This point is underlined in *H. pylori*-positive patients in whom the proportion of Indian patients with ulcer disease is significantly lower compared to the Chinese and Malays[15].

Differences in the incidence of peptic ulcer disease have been observed for a long time in Malaya and Singapore. Yeoh[6], in an analysis of consecutive cases seen and treated in a surgical unit in Singapore reported a preponderance of Chinese patients and a paucity of Malay patients. Alhady[7] reported similar ethnic differences in Malaya. Even allowing for the fact that, at that point in time, Malays tended not to seek treatment in hospitals compared to the other races, the differences noted were marked. Differences in acid secretion and pattern of gastritis may account for differences in the clinical outcome of *H. pylori* infection. We have shown significant differences in the proportion of patients with antral and pangastritis among *H. pylori*-positive non-ulcer dyspepsia patients between the three major races. The preponderance of pangastritis in Indians is in keeping with our previous findings that *H. pylori*-positive Indian patients were less likely to have ulcers compared to the other two races. Further studies need to be performed to determine if differences in acid secretion are responsible for the different proportion of patients with antral versus pangastritis. The role of diet, particularly with regard to the protective effect of chili, has been postulated. Kang et al.[29] and Yeoh et al[30] have shown that chilis protect against experimental gastric mucosal damage in both animal models and humans. Differences in *H. pylori* strains with different virulence, clustered within different races, has been reported by Campbell et al.[31] in New Zealand. Although differences in peptic ulcer incidence were not shown in this study, it is plausible that this may account for differences in peptic ulcer prevalence in other parts of the world.

The differences in the prevalence of cancer of the stomach between races have also been observed previously. In an early report[9], Chinese were found to have the highest prevalence of cancer of the stomach, with Malays and Indians having relatively lower prevalence. The lower prevalence of cancer among the Indians, who have a high prevalence of *H. pylori* infection is again an enigma. The findings of low gastric cancer incidence among Indians compared to Chinese are well shown in respective cancer registries in India and China[32]. Rates of above 30 per 100 000 are commonly reported in China compared to rates of below 10 per 100 000 recorded in India[32]. No cancer registry is, as yet, available in Malaysia. In neighbouring Singapore the racial distribution of cancer of the stomach follows a similar pattern. In the most recent National Cancer Registry Report[33], the age-specific standardized ratios for Chinese males and females were 29.3 and 13.6 per 100 000 population, respectively; for Indian males and females were 9.9 and 7.9 per 100 000, respectively; and for Malay males and females, 8.7 and 5.5 per 100 000, respectively.

In our case–control study[18] we found that Chinese race in particular was a highly significant independent predictive factor for gastric cancer. *H. pylori* infection was found to be only just significant. The reason for this relatively low odds ratio could be explained by the high mean age of both cases and controls, and because the *H. pylori* prevalence of controls was also high at this age. Another reason was that *H. pylori* serology was taken at the time of diagnosis of cancer, by which time many patients may have 'lost' the infection with the occurrence of pre-neoplastic changes, accompanied by a drop in *H. pylori* titres to undetectable levels. Gastric cancer is a multifactorial disease. In our study we identified high intake of salted vegetable and foods as a risk factor, as well as smoking and low social class.

The differing outcome between Indians and Chinese with regard to gastric cancer is puzzling. If we postulate that Indians acquire infection early in life with the development of pangastritis and a reduction in acid-secretory capacity, we would then expect a high prevalence of gastric cancer among the Indians. Studies are on-going to determine the prevalence of intestinal metaplasia and gastric atrophy in our patients. The cause of gastric cancer is multifactorial, and genetics and other exogenous factors such as a high salt intake may explain these racial differences. More intriguingly is the possible role of protective dietary factors: chilis, onions and turmeric are commonly used in the cooking of Malay and Indian foods, in contrast to Chinese food. In a review of the epidemiology of gastric cancer in India, Mohandas and Nagral[34] have suggested that this could indeed be an important factor for the lower gastric cancer rates among the local population in India.

Acknowledgements

The studies in this chapter were principally funded by the Government of Malaysia IRPA Research vote 06-02-03-0311. I acknowledge the contribution of my colleagues, in particular Professors N. Parasakthi and P. L. Cheah, in the studies carried out above.

References

1. Graham DY. *Helicobacter pylori*: its epidemiology and its role in duodenal ulcer disease. J Gastroenterol Hepatol. 1991;6:105–13.
2. Graham DY, Malaty HM, Dolores GE, Evans DJ Jr, Klein PD, Adam E. Epidemiology of *Helicobacter pylori* in an asymptomatic population in the United States. Gastroenterology. 1991;100:1495–501.

3. Malaty HM, Evans DG, Evans DJ Jr, Graham DY. *Helicobacter pylori* in Hispanics: comparison with blacks and whites of similar age and socioeconomic class. Gastroenterology. 1992;103:813–16.
4. Goh KL, Peh SC, Wong NW, Parasakthi N, Puthucheary S. *Campylobacter pylori* infection – experience in a multiracial population. J Gastroenterol Hepatol. 1990;5:277–80.
5. Kang JY, Wee A, Math MV et al. *Helicobacter pylori* and gastritis in patients with peptic ulcer and non-ulcer dyspepsia: ethnic differences in Singapore. Gut. 1990;31:850–3.
6. Yeoh GS. Peptic ulcers – an analysis of 700 cases seen and treated in the surgical Professorial unit, General Hospital, Singapore from the year 1948 to 1960. Sing Med J. 1961;2:127–37.
7. Alhady SA. The incidence of peptic ulceration in the 3 main races of Malaya. Proceedings of the 2nd Malaysian Congress of Medicine. 1965;2:146–8.
8. Kang JY, Labrooy SJ, Yap I et al. Racial differences in peptic ulcer frequency in Singapore. J Gastroenterol Hepatol. 1987;2:239–44.
9. Kang JY. Surgery for gastric cancer in Singapore, 1951–1980, with particular reference to racial differences in incidence. Aust NZ J Med. 1988;18:661–4.
10. Goh KL. Prevalence of *H. pylori* in various population groups in Malaysia. In: *Helicobacter pylori* infection in Malaysia. Doctor of Medicine thesis, 1996, University of Malaya: 46–77.
11. Goh KL, Ng OC, Zulkarnain A, Parasakhti N, Wong SY. Prevalence of dyspepsia and *Helicobacter pylori* amongst blood donors and healthy subjects in Sibu, Sarawak. J Gastroenterol Hepatol. 1998;13:A91 (abstract).
12. Goh KL Parasakthi N. Validation and determination of a cut-off level of a commercial ELISA serological kit for *Helicobacter pylori* diagnosis in a local Asian population. J Gastroenterol Hepatol. 1997;12(Suppl.):A241 (abstract).
13. Boey CCM, Goh KL, Lee WS, Parasakthi N. Seroprevalence of *Helicobacter pylori* in Malaysian Children – evidence for ethnic differences. J Paediatr Child Health. 1999; 35:151–2.
14. Goh KL, Parasakthi N, Cheah PL. Distinct racial differences in *Helicobacter pylori* prevalence in healthy asymptomatic Malaysian volunteers undergoing endoscopy. J Gastroenterol Hepatol. 1998;13:A92 (abstract).
15. Goh KL. Prevalence of and risk factors for *Helicobacter pylori* in a multiracial population undergoing endoscopy. J Gastroenterol Hepatol. 1997;12:S29–35.
16. Goh KL, Parasakthi N, Peh SC, Puthucheary SD, Wong NW. The rapid urease test in the diagnosis of *Helicobacter pylori* infection. Sing Med J. 1994;35:161–2.
17. Goh KL, Ranjeev P, Ong KT. Evidence for marked racial differences in the incidence of cancer of the stomach between racial groups in Malaysia. Med J Mal. 1999;54:16(Suppl. B) (abstract).
18. Goh KL, Noorafidah MD, Cheah PL, Parasakthi N. Risk factors for gastric cancer in Malaysian patients – a case–control study. J Gastroenterol Hepatol. 2000;18:B55 (abstract).
19. Kang JY, Yeoh KG, Ho KY et al. Racial differences in *Helicobacter pylori* seroprevalence in Singapore: correlation with differences in peptic ulcer frequency. J Gastroenterol Hepatol. 1997;12:655–9.
20. Uyub AM, Raj SM, Visvanathan R et al. *Helicobacter pylori* infection in North-Eastern Peninsular Malaysia – evidence for an unusually low prevalence. Scand J Gastroenterol. 1994;29:209–13.
21. Fraser AG, Scragg R, Metcalf P, McCullough S, Yeates NJ. Prevalence of *Helicobacter pylori* infection in different ethnic groups in New Zealand children and adults. Aust NZ J Med. 1996;26:636–51.
22. Chow TKF, Lambert JR, Wahlqvist ML, Hsu-Hage BHH. *Helicobacter pylori* in Melbourne Chinese immigrants: evidence for oral–oral transmission via chopsticks. J Gastroenterol Hepatol. 1995;10:562–9.
23. Mitchell HM, Li YY, Hu PJ et al. Epidemiology of *Helicobacter pylori* in Southern China: identification of early childhood as the critical period for acquisition. J Infect Dis. 1992; 166:149–53.
24. Graham DY, Adam E, Reddy GT et al. Seroepidemiology of *Helicobacter pylori* infection in India. Dig Dis Sci. 1991;3 6:1084–8.
25. Li YY, Hu PJ, Du GG, Hazell SL. The prevalence of *Helicobacter pylori* infection in the People's Republic of China. Am J Gastroenterol. 1991;86:446–9.
26. Katelaris PH, Tippett HK, Norbu P, Lower DG, Brennan R, Farthing MJG. Dyspepsia, *Helicobacter pylori* and peptic ulcer in a randomly selected population in India. Gut. 1992;33:1462–6.

27. Yip R, Limburg PJ, Ahlquist DA *et al.* Pervasive occult gastrointestinal bleeding in an Alaska Native population with prevalent iron deficiency – role of *Helicobacter pylori*. J Am Med Assoc. 1997;277:1135–9.
28. Lopez CG, Duraisamy G, Govindasamy S. Prevalence of hepatitis B infection as determined by 3rd generation tests in the Malaysian population. Mal J Pathol. 1978;1:91–5.
29. Kang JY, Teng CH, Wee A, Cheng FC. Effect of capsaicin and chilli on ethanol-induced gastric mucosal injury in the rat. Gut. 1995;36:664–9.
30. Yeoh KG, Kang JY, Yap I, Guan R, Tan CC. Chili protects against aspirin-induced gastroduodenal mucosal injury in humans. Dig Dis Sci. 1995;40:580–3.
31. Campbell S, Fraser A, Holliss B, Schmid J, O'Toole PW. Evidence for ethnic tropism of *Helicobacter pylori*. Infect Immun. 1997;65:3708–12.
32. Parkin DM, Muir CS, Whelan CS, Ferlay J, Raymond L, Young J. Cancer Incidence in Five Continents, 1997. Lyon: IARC Scientific Publication 143.
33. Chia KS, Lee HP, Sow A, Shanmugaratnam K. Trends in Cancer Incidence in Singapore 1968–1992. Singapore Cancer Registry Report No. 4, 1996.
34. Mohandas KM, Nagral A. Epidemiology of digestive tract cancers in India. II. Stomach and gastrointestinal lymphomas. Ind J Gastroenterol. 1998;17:24–7.
35. Goh KL, Tan YM, Cheah PL. Topography of gastritis amongst young non-ulcer dyspeptics in the different races in Malaysia. Med J Mal. 2000;55:17(abs)(Suppl. A).

Section III
Novel *Helicobacters*

9
Infection with *Helicobacter heilmannii* (formerly *Gastrospirillum hominis*): characterization, epidemiology and therapy

P. MALFERTHEINER, U. R. M. BOHR and T. GÜNTHER

HISTORY

Following the discovery of *Helicobacter pylori* a second *Helicobacter* species was detected in human gastric mucosa which is now named *H. heilmannii*. In 1987 Dent *et al.* were the first to describe this spiral organism in the gastric antrum[1]. McNulty in 1989 extended the report to six further cases and described the bacterium as Gram-negative, up to 7.5 µm long and approximately 0.9 µm wide, twice as large as *H. pylori* and with up to 12 flagella at each pole[2]. It closely resembled the spiral bacteria originally described and illustrated by Bizozzero (1893) in the stomach of dogs[2]. Based on morphology, site of colonization and host species the original name proposed was *Gastrospirillum hominis*[3]. Heilmann and Borchard (1991) described in a comprehensive way the histological pattern of the infected gastric mucosa and reported on 31 patients infected with *Gastrospirillum hominis*[4]. Subsequently Solnick *et al.* (1993), by analysis of the 16S ribosomal RNA, proved that *Gastrospirillum hominis* belongs to the genus *Helicobacter*[5] Based on this finding the name *H. heilmannii* was proposed instead of *Gastrospirillum hominis*. Comparison of the 16S rRNA sequence of different *H. heilmannii* strains, however, shows that the sequences are highly homologous but not identical[5,6]. It was concluded that the individual strains, which all matched the criteria proposed by McNulty and colleagues, are likely to be several different *Helicobacter* species. Minor morphological differences in individual *H. heilmannii* strains were also observed by electron microscopy[7]. Currently the epithet '*H. heilmannii*' is used as a working designation for unculturable gastric bacteria lacking an exact microbiological determination.

Table 1. Key features of *Helicobacter heilmannii*

Strains	*Helicobacter heilmannii* type 1
	Helicobacter heilmannii type 2
	Helicobacter heilmannii strain AF53
	Helicobacter suis = *Gastrospirillum suis* (probably identical to *H. heilmannii* type 1)
Morphology	Gram-negative spiral bacterium with four or more turns
Ultrastructure	Up to 7.5 μm long and approximately 0.9 μm wide, up to 12 bipolar flagella
Hosts	Human, cat, dog, pig
Transmission	Zoonosis, oral–oral transmission most likely
Pathology	Chronic (active) gastritis, predisposition for gastric and duodenal ulcer, MALT lymphoma, gastric cancer
Diagnostics	Histology, electron microscopy, touch cytology, 16S rRNA analysis
Therapy	*Mono therapy:* bismuth salts*
	Dual therapy: bismuth salts and antibiotic*
	Triple therapy: two antibiotics (tetracycline, amoxycillin, metronidazole) and acid suppression (PPI or H_2 inhibitor)*

*All forms of therapy shown to be effective in case reports; no controlled studies available up to now.

MICROBIOLOGY

Based on sequence comparison of 16S rRNA currently there are three types of *H. heilmannii*: *H. heilmannii* type 1 (L10079), *H. heilmannii* type 2 (L10080) and *H. heilmannii* strain AF53 (Y18028)[5,6,8]. *H. heilmannii* types 1 and 2 were shown to be transmissible from mouse to mouse in experimental settings. They have not been cultured *in vitro*. *H. heilmannii* strain AF53 up to now has been the only type that was cultured *in vitro*[9,10]. It grows under microaerobic conditions between 36°C and 41°C on 7% lysed, defibrinated horse blood agar plates within 3–7 days in small translucent colonies. *H. heilmannii* strain AF53 is, like *H. pylori* and *H. felis*, motile, oxidase, catalase, nitrite, nitrate, and urease positive, and produces alkaline phosphatase and arginine arylamidase. Like *H. pylori* and *H. felis* it is sensitive to cephalothin (30 μg disc), resistant to nalidixic acid (30 μg disc), and sensitive to most other antibiotics[6]. The other *H. heilmannii* types have not yet been cultured *in vitro*. However, *H. heilmannii* types 1 and 2 can be cultured *in vivo* by experimental infection of laboratory mice[11,12].

Other uncultured, tightly spiral microorganisms, similar to *H. heilmannii*, were detected in the stomach of pigs[13]. For this bacterium associated with gastric ulcers in pigs the provisional name *H. suis* was proposed. *H. suis* was later found to have a homology of greater than 99% to *H. heilmannii* type 1, which was found in humans, suggesting that the two bacteria are one species[14].

Together with *H. felis*, *H. bizzozeronii*, *H. salmonis*, *H. nemestrinae*, *H. acinonyx*, and *H. pylori* the *H. heilmannii* strains belong to a subgroup of genetically highly homologous gastric *Helicobacter* species. All of these *Helicobacter* species are involved in the development of gastric pathology in their mammalian hosts.

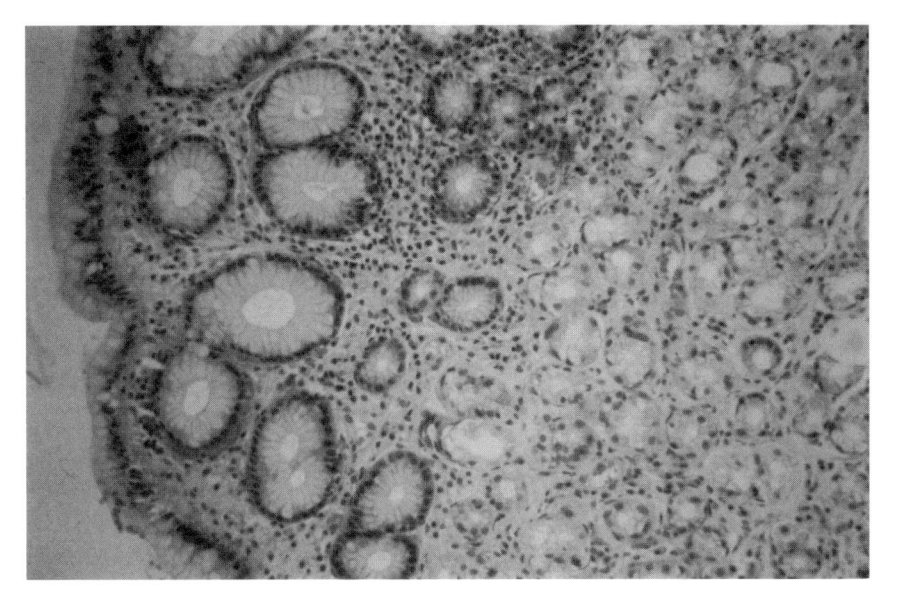

Figure 1. H&E stain showing the mild inflammatory reaction induced by *H. heilmannii*.

PATHOLOGY

H. heilmannii infection causes chronic gastritis[2,4,16,17], and was reported in association with gastroduodenal diseases[18–20], gastric cancer[17,21] and MALT lymphoma[17]. Chronic gastritis is reversible after eradication of *H. heilmannii*[4,7,19].

Currently best characterized is the chronic *H. heilmannii*-associated gastritis. A large matched control study involving 404 patients, that compared *H. heilmannii* gastritis with *H. pylori* gastritis, was published by Stolte and co-workers in 1997[17]. Their data, obtained from 202 patients with *H. heilmannii* gastritis, allow a reliable morphological characterization of *H. heilmannii* infection in the stomach. Although both bacteria cause gastritis, *H. heilmannii* gastritis generally shows a less acute inflammation, independent of topographical distribution in the stomach (Figure 1). The degree of chronic inflammation is also less than *H. pylori*-induced gastritis[17]. Since inflammation in *H. heilmannii* gastritis is often very mild or even absent histologically, there is a substantial risk of not recognizing *H. heilmannii* infection histologically. Failure of detection is increased by the fact that colonization by *H. heilmannii* is less dense compared with the diffuse distribution of *H. pylori* on the surface and foveolar epithelium. *H. heilmannii* is mostly recognized focally and in small groups in the foveola (Figure 2), primarily in the antrum of the stomach[17]. A specific feature is that *H. heilmannii* maintains a greater distance to the surface epithelium[9], as compared to *H. pylori*, which is adhesive to the epithelial cells[4]. Despite the lack of adhesion it was shown that *H. heilmannii* is able to invade parietal cells. This observation was made both in the gastric mucosa of dogs and

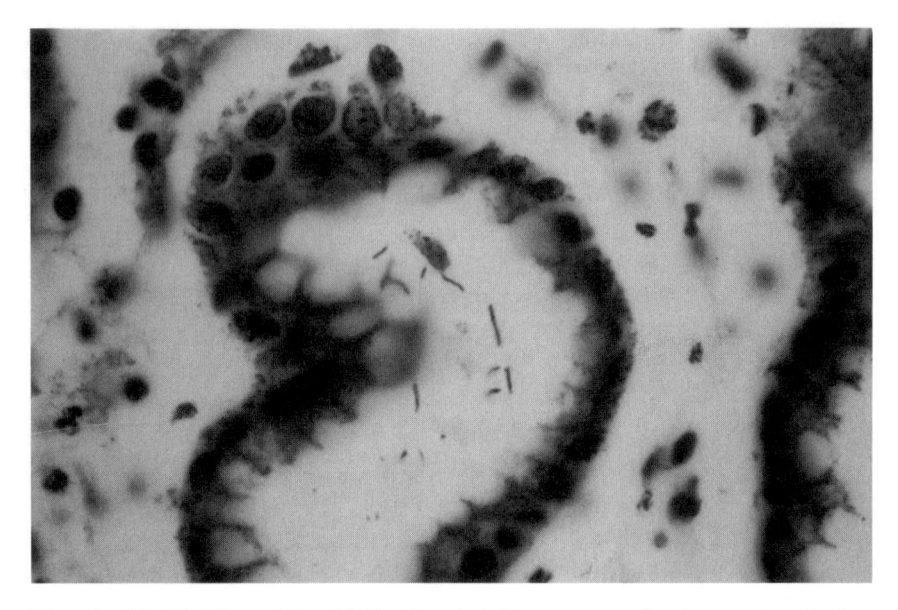

Figure 2. Warthin–Starry stain with the characteristic appearance of corkscrew non-adhering *H. heilmannii*.

cats[7], as well as in human mucosa[4]. With regard to further grading parameters according to the Updated Sydney System[22], there are considerable differences between *H. pylori* and *H. heilmannii* gastritis. Intestinal metaplasia in *H. heilmannii*-induced gastritis is seen in a few cases[17]. Lymphoid follicles and aggregates are also seen less frequently in *H. heilmannii* gastritis compared to *H. pylori* gastritis. In the patient groups examined by Stolte *et al.* (1997), mucosal atrophy played a role neither in *H. pylori*-infected nor in *H. pylori*-uninfected patients. Lee *et al.* (1993), however, found an association between *H. heilmannii* infection and atrophy of the gastric mucosa in an animal model[12]. Flejou *et al.* (1990) also described mild atrophy in some human patients[16].

The association between *H. heilmannii* infection and other diseases of the gastrointestinal tract is mostly in the form of case reports. Goddard *et al.* (1997)[19] described successful therapy of a patient with duodenal ulcer by eradication of *H. heilmannii*. Jhala *et al.* (1999)[28] also found *H. heilmannii* infection in patients with duodenal ulcer. In another report a link between *H. heilmannii* infection and gastric ulcers was described by Debongnie and co-workers (1998). In addition *H. heilmannii* in relation to gastric neoplasms has been the subject of interest in many case reports. Stolte *et al.* (1997) found an association between *H. heilmannii* infection with MALT lymphoma of the stomach in 3.4% of their cases[17]. This association was strengthened by the remission of low-grade gastric MALT lymphoma after eradication of *H. heilmannii* infection in six patients[23,24]. Yang *et al.* (1995) and Morgner *et al.* (1995) demonstrated *H. heilmannii* infections in patients with gastric carcinoma[21,25]. The question of whether a *H. heilmannii* infection is, in fact, associated with a higher risk of gastric carcinoma cannot be answered at present, because the number of cases reported to date is too low.

EPIDEMIOLOGY

Morphological criteria are most frequently used to differentiate between *H. heilmannii* and *H. pylori* in human mucosa samples. Typically, *H. pylori* assumes a curved, rod-like or short spiral morphology with up to three turns, while *H. heilmannii* is larger and grows as a long spiral bacterium with four or more turns. Additional differences can be detected by electron microscopy. Ultrastructurally, *H. heilmannii* has sheathed flagella at each pole while *H. pylori* has flagella at one pole only.

The prevalence of *H. heilmannii* in the Asian population was found to be 1.9–6.2% by microscopic studies[26,27]. In Europe the prevalence of *H. heilmannii* is lower with 0.25–0.49% in gastric biopsies[16,28]. In duodenal ulcer patients 0.7% were found to have *H. heilmannii* infection[18]. The prevalence in healthy volunteers was found to be 1.1%[29]. The frequency of *H. heilmannii* in symptomatic children is reported to be 0.3%[30].

The prevalence of the *H. heilmannii* infection is influenced to a considerable extent by the quality of the diagnostic tests used. Touch cytology can increase the sensitivity compared to histological examinations[31,32]. A comparison in 50 pigs of the urease test, microscopy and the inoculation of gastric mucus into the stomach of mice, showed the inoculation of gastric mucus into the stomach of mice to be the most sensitive, with 62.0% positive as compared to 8% in the histological examination of the gastric mucosa and 6% in the rapid urease test[33]. In pigs *H. heilmannii* was detected with histological examination in 58% and with polymerase chain reaction (PCR) in 80%[8]. *Helicobacter*-like organisms detected by Gram staining, Warthin–Starry staining were similarly sensitive to the rapid urease test and ^{13}C-urea breath testing in 79%, 77%, 78%, and 85% of cases, respectively. PCR analysis revealed that 78% of the cats were infected by *H. heilmannii* species, while one cat was infected with *H. pametensis*. Using all tests 91% of the pet cats were found to be *Helicobacter*-positive while in only 79% were the diagnostic tests concordant[34]. These data show the limits of histological methods to detect *H. heilmannii* infection in animals. Studies in humans, all based on microscopic techniques, probably underestimate the incidence of *H. heilmannii* infection. Morphology of *H. pylori* can change under certain culture conditions to a *H. heilmannii*-like phenotype and this may additionally be a possible pitfall in the diagnosis of *H. heilmannii* infection[35] as a change in phenotype of *H. pylori* infection could be misinterpreted as a *H. heilmannii* infection. No data exist on the phenotypic changes of *H. heilmannii*, or whether they exist. Immunochemical staining does not help to differentiate between *H. pylori* and *H. heilmannii* because of the high antigen similarity, which results in antibody cross-reaction between both bacteria[28]. The most reliable tool to differentiate *H. heilmannii* and its individual strains is based on DNA sequencing.

TRANSMISSION AND RESERVOIRS OF *H. HEILMANNII*

H. heilmannii may infect different host species and, therefore, is not host-specific. Simultaneous infections of an individual host with more than one *Helicobacter* species or with *H. pylori* and *H. heilmannii*[36,37], or with more than one *H. heilmannii* strain[38], have been described. *H. heilmannii* transmission is a characteristic example of a zoonosis. *H. heilmannii* is transmitted to humans from animals most probably by an inter-oral route rather than faecal oral route[39,40]. Dieterich *et al.* reported on a patient with acute gastric erosions infected with several *H. heilmannii* strains. One of the two cats in contact with the patient was infected by the same *H. heilmannii* strain, while the other cat and two unrelated cats were infected by different *H. heilmannii* strains[38]. In a large comparative study in 202 patients with histologically diagnosed *H. heilmannii* gastritis and 600 randomly selected patients with *H. pylori* gastritis the questionnaire revealed that contact with pigs, cats, and dogs leads to a significant risk of *H. heilmannii* infection (OR of 4.990, 1.710, 1.462)[41]. Pigs, cats, and dogs have a high incidence of *H. heilmannii* infection and appear to be reservoirs in the transmission of *H. heilmannii*[7,8,33,34,42].

DIAGNOSIS

Currently, diagnosis of *H. heilmannii* infection remains based on the characteristic morphological appearance in histology in conjunction with a positive urease test. There are no studies on the accuracy of the urease breath test. Only recently, ELISA has been used for serological detection of *H. heilmannii* infection in patients with associated MALT lymphoma, but this would need to be validated in a large study before applicable in routine clinical practice.

THERAPY

H. heilmannii infection was shown to be transient in some cases[32,43]. The disappearance of *H. heilmannii* is associated with a regression of gastritis[43], and in some patients this was paralleled by a resolution of symptoms[4]. Also, healing of gastric and duodenal ulcer[19,43] and very recently low-grade MALT lymphoma after eradication of *H. heilmannii*, has been reported[23,24]. For eradication, various therapies were successful[19,44–46]. Heilmann and Borchard (1991) found *H. heilmannii* responsive to monotherapy with bismuth salts[4]. Successful bismuth monotherapy also was described by Lavelle *et al.* (1994)[47]. Antisecretory drugs (ranitidine or omeprazole) alone were also shown to eliminate *H. heilmannii* in eight of 10 patients within 3 months but this, as known for *H. pylori*, was only apparent due to the different distribution of *H. heilmannii* in the stomach due to acid suppression and loss of detectable *H. heilmannii*. Most therapy data were obtained from case reports. Dual therapy with a combination of bismuth salts and antibiotics has been reported[39]. Triple therapy with an H_2-receptor antagonist, metronidazole and amoxycillin for 4 weeks eradicated *H. heilmannii* in both of two cases[48]. In a patient not successfully treated with PPI triple therapy, a second attempt to eradicate *H. heilmannii* with quadruple therapy for 2 weeks was effective[19]. Controlled eradication studies for *H. heilmannii* are lacking, but from the available reports therapies designed to eradicate *H. pylori* are also successful for the treatment of *H. heilmannii*. In contrast to human *Helicobacter* infections, it is more difficult to achieve a definitive long-term cure in cats naturally infected with *H. heilmannii*[49]. Nevertheless, *H. heilmannii* therapy should include domestic animals in the household of the infected person to prevent reinfection[39].

CONCLUSION

H. heilmannii infection is rare in humans, and may be associated with various complications such as peptic ulcer and MALT lymphoma. The histological pattern of gastritis is distinct from *H. pylori* gastritis, presenting with a mild acute and chronic inflammatory reaction. Diagnosis of *H. heilmannii* is still based on histological detection of the bacterium with characteristic morphological appearance. Therapy appears to be effective with bismuth salt monotherapy, but a proton pump inhibitor triple therapy, such as is used for *H. pylori* is preferred.

References:

1. Dent JC, McNulty CA, Uff JC, Wilkinson SP, Gear MW. Spiral organisms in the gastric antrum. Lancet. 1987;2:96.
2. Bizzozero G. Über die schlauchförmigen Drüsen des Magendarmkanals und die Beziehungen ihres Epithels zu dem Oberflächenepithel der Schleimhaut. Arch mikr Anat. 1893;42:82–152.
3. McNulty CA, Dent JC, Curry A, et al. New spiral bacterium in gastric mucosa. J Clin Pathol. 1989;42:585–91.
4. Heilmann KL, Borchard F. Gastritis due to spiral shaped bacteria other than *Helicobacter pylori*: clinical, histological, and ultrastructural findings. Gut. 1991;32:137–40.
5. Solnick JV, O'Rourke J, Lee A, Paster BJ, Dewhirst FE, Tompkins LS. An uncultured gastric spiral organism is a newly identified *Helicobacter* in humans. J Infect Dis. 1993;168:379–85.
6. Andersen LP, Boye K, Blom J, Holck S, Norgaard A, Elsborg L. Characterization of a culturable '*Gastrospirillum hominis*' (*Helicobacter heilmannii*) strain isolated from human gastric mucosa. J Clin Microbiol. 1999;37:1069–76.
7. Wegmann W, Aschwanden M, Schaub N, Aenishanslin W, Gyr K. Gastritis associated with *Gastrospirillum hominis* – a zoonosis? Schweiz Med Wochenschr. 1991;121:245–54.
8. Cantet F, Magras C, Marais A, Federighi M, Megraud F. *Helicobacter* species colonizing pig stomach: molecular characterization and determination of prevalence. Appl Environ Microbiol. 1999;65:4672–6.
9. Holck S, Ingeholm P, Blom J et al. The histopathology of human gastric mucosa inhabited by *Helicobacter heilmannii*-like (*Gastrospirillum hominis*) organisms, including the first culturable case. Apmis. 1997;105:746–56.
10. Andersen LP, Norgaard A, Holck S, Blom J, Elsborg L. Isolation of a '*Helicobacter heilmanii*'-like organism from the human stomach. Eur J Clin Microbiol Infect Dis. 1996;15:95–6.
11. Fox JG, Lee A. Gastric *Campylobacter*-like organisms: their role in gastric disease of laboratory animals. Lab Anim Sci. 1989;39:543–53.
12. Lee A, Chen M, Coltro N et al. Long-term infection of the gastric mucosa with Helicobacter species does induce atrophic gastritis in an animal model of *Helicobacter pylori* infection. Zentralbl Bakteriol. 1993;280:38–50.

13. Mendes EN, Queiroz DM, Rocha GA, Moura SB, Leite VH, Fonseca ME. Ultrastructure of a spiral micro-organism from pig gastric mucosa ('*Gastrospirillum suis*'). J Med Microbiol. 1990;33:61–6.
14. De Groote D, van Doorn LJ, Ducatelle R *et al.* 'Candidatus *Helicobacter suis*', a gastric *Helicobacter* from pigs, and its phylogenetic relatedness to other gastrospirilla. Int J Syst Bacteriol. 1999;49:1769–77.
15. Mendes EN, Queiroz DM, Coimbra RS, Moura SB, Barbosa AJ, Rocha GA. Experimental infection of Wistar rats with '*Gastrospirillum suis*'. J Med Microbiol. 1996;44:105–9.
16. Flejou JF, Diomande I, Molas G *et al.* Human chronic gastritis associated with non-*Helicobacter pylori* spiral organisms (*Gastrospirillum hominis*). Four cases and review of the literature. Gastroenterol Clin Biol. 1990;14:806–10.
17. Stolte M, Kroher G, Meining A, Morgner A, Bayerdorffer E, Bethke B. A comparison of *Helicobacter pylori* and *H. heilmannii* gastritis. A matched control study involving 404 patients. Scand J Gastroenterol. 1997;32:28–33.
18. Borody TJ, George LL, Brandl S *et al. Helicobacter pylori*-negative duodenal ulcer. Am J Gastroenterol. 1991;86:1154–7.
19. Goddard AF, Logan RP, Atherton JC, Jenkins D, Spiller RC. Healing of duodenal ulcer after eradication of *Helicobacter heilmannii*. Lancet. 1997;349:1815–6.
20. Nakshabendi IM, Peebles SE, Lee FD, Russell RI. Spiral shaped microorganisms in the human duodenal mucosa. Postgrad Med J. 1991;67:846–7.
21. Yang H, Li X, Xu Z, Zhou D. '*Helicobacter heilmannii*' infection in a patient with gastric cancer. Dig Dis Sci. 1995;40:1013–4.
22. Dixon MF, Genta RM, Yardley JH, Correa P. Classification and grading of gastritis. The updated Sydney System. International Workshop on the Histopathology of Gastritis, Houston, 1994. Am J Surg Pathol. 1996;20:1161–81.
23. Regimbeau C, Karsenti D, Durand V *et al.* Low-grade gastric MALT lymphoma and *Helicobacter heilmannii* (*Gastrospirillum hominis*). Gastroenterol Clin Biol. 1998;22:720–3.
24. Morgner A, Lehn N, Anderson LP *et al. Helicobacter heilmannii*-associated primary gastric low-grade MALT lymphoma – complete remission after curing the infection. Gastroenterology. 2000 (In press).
25. Morgner A, Bayerdorffer E, Meining A, Stolte M, Kroher G. *Helicobacter heilmannii* and gastric cancer. Lancet. 1995;346:511–2.
26. Yang H, Goliger JA, Song M, Zhou D. High prevalence of *Helicobacter heilmannii* infection in China. Dig Dis Sci. 1998;43:1493.
27. Yali Z, Yamada N, Wen M, Matsuhisa T, Miki M. *Gastrospirillum hominis* and *Helicobacter pylori* infection in Thai individuals: comparison of histopathological changes of gastric mucosa. Pathol Int. 1998;48:507–11.
28. Jhala D, Jhala N, Lechago J, Haber M. *Helicobacter heilmannii* gastritis: association with acid peptic diseases and comparison with *Helicobacter pylori* gastritis. Mod Pathol. 1999;12:534–8.
29. Mazzucchelli L, Wilder-Smith CH, Ruchti C, Meyer-Wyss B, Merki HS. *Gastrospirillum hominis* in asymptomatic, healthy individuals. Dig Dis Sci. 1993;38:2087–9.
30. Oliva MM, Lazenby AJ, Perman JA. Gastritis associated with *Gastrospirillum hominis* in children. Comparison with *Helicobacter pylori* and review of the literature. Mod Pathol. 1993;6:513–5.
31. Debongnie JC, Mairesse J, Donnay M, Dekoninck X. Touch cytology. A quick, simple, sensitive screening test in the diagnosis of infections of the gastrointestinal mucosa. Arch Pathol Lab Med. 1994;118:1115–8.
32. Debongnie JC, Donnay M, Mairesse J. *Gastrospirillum hominis* ('*Helicobacter heilmanii*'): a cause of gastritis, sometimes transient, better diagnosed by touch cytology? Am J Gastroenterol. 1995;90:411–16.
33. Mendes EN, Queiroz DM, Moura SB, Rocha GA. Mouse inoculation for the detection of non-cultivable gastric tightly spiralled bacteria. Braz J Med Biol Res. 1998;31:373–6.
34. Neiger R, Dieterich C, Burnens A *et al.* Detection and prevalence of *Helicobacter* infection in pet cats. J Clin Microbiol. 1998;36:634–7.
35. Fawcett PT, Gibney KM, Vinette KM. *Helicobacter pylori* can be induced to assume the morphology of *Helicobacter heilmannii*. J Clin Microbiol. 1999;37:1045–8.
36. Queiroz DM, Cabral MM, Nogueira AM, Barbosa AJ, Rocha GA, Mendes EN. Mixed gastric infection by *Gastrospirillum hominis* and *Helicobacter pylori*. Lancet. 1990;336:507–8.

37. Ierardi E, Monno R, Mongelli A et al. *Gastrospirillum hominis* associated chronic active gastritis: the first report from Italy. Ital J Gastroenterol. 1991;23:86–7.
38. Dieterich C, Wiesel P, Neiger R, Blum A, Corthesy-Theulaz I. Presence of multiple '*Helicobacter heilmannii*' strains in an individual suffering from ulcers and in his two cats. J Clin Microbiol. 1998;36:1366–70.
39. Thomson MA, Storey P, Greer R, Cleghorn GJ. Canine–human transmission of *Gastrospirillum hominis*. Lancet. 1994;343:1605–7.
40. Lee A, Fox JG, Otto G, Dick EH, Krakowka S. Transmission of *Helicobacter* spp. A challenge to the dogma of faecal–oral spread. Epidemiol Infect. 1991;107:99–109.
41. Meining A, Kroher G, Stolte M. Animal reservoirs in the transmission of *Helicobacter heilmannii*. Results of a questionnaire-based study. Scand J Gastroenterol. 1998;33:795–8.
42. Norris CR, Marks SL, Eaton KA, Torabian SZ, Munn RJ, Solnick JV. Healthy cats are commonly colonized with '*Helicobacter heilmannii*' that is associated with minimal gastritis. J Clin Microbiol. 1999;37:189–94.
43. Debongnie JC, Donnay M, Mairesse J, Lamy V, Dekoninck X, Ramdani B. Gastric ulcers and *Helicobacter heilmannii*. Eur J Gastroenterol Hepatol. 1998;10:251–4.
44. Wack RF, Eaton KA, Kramer LW. Treatment of gastritis in cheetahs (*Acinonyx jubatus*). J Zoo Wildl Med. 1997;28:260–6.
45. Yamamoto T, Matsumoto J, Shiota K et al. *Helicobacter heilmannii* associated erosive gastritis. Intern Med. 1999;38:240–3.
46. Tanaka M, Saitoh A, Narita T et al. *Gastrospirillum hominis*-associated gastritis: the first reported case in Japan. J Gastroenterol. 1994;29:199–202.
47. Lavelle JP, Landas S, Mitros FA, Conklin JL. Acute gastritis associated with spiral organisms from cats. Dig Dis Sci. 1994;39:744–50.
48. Fenjvesi A, Naumov B, Kovac I. *Helicobacter heilmanni* (*Gastrospirillum hominis*) as a new cause of gastritis-case report. Med Pregl. 1999;52:275–7.
49. Neiger R, Seiler G, Schmassmann A. Use of a urea breath test to evaluate short-term treatments for cats naturally infected with *Helicobacter heilmannii*. Am J Vet Res. 1999;60:880–3.

10
Hepatobiliary *Helicobacters*: recognized animal pathogens with suspected pathogenic potential in humans

J. G. FOX

INTRODUCTION

Since the discovery of *Helicobacter pylori* it is becoming increasingly clear that the genus *Helicobacter* is composed of numerous species, many of which can produce serious disease in their respective hosts. The genus now includes 20 named species and at least 30 unnamed species. This number will undoubtedly increase as culture methods improve for these fastidious microaerobes. Importantly, more novel *Helicobacters* will be recognized as well as their pathogenic potential realized, as the index of suspicion increases that these organisms can indeed cause a plethora of gastrointestinal diseases. The enterohepatic helicobacters (EHS) are distinct phylogenetically from the gastric helicobacters and also, as the name implies, are capable of colonizing the lower bowel and hepatobiliary tissue, but rarely the stomach (Table 1). The purpose of this chapter is to discuss the various EHS, particularly those infecting hepatobiliary tissue and, where known, detail their host range, epidemiology and pathogenic potential. The best known of the EHS, *H. hepaticus*, will be reviewed in greater detail, with the prediction that many of the salient features of this newly recognized pathogen will also be relevant to our evolving understanding of the EHS in general.

H. hepaticus hepatitis and associated liver cancer

An active chronic hepatitis was detected in the early 1990s in several inbred strains of mice originating from a barrier-maintained facility. The liver lesions advanced with age from a mild focal necrosis consisting of a mononuclear cell inflammation to more extensive liver involvement including hepatocytomegaly, bile duct hyperplasia, and a peribiliary inflammatory response. This disease entity, defined by a distinctive morphological pattern

Table 1. Non-gastric *Helicobacter* species and their hosts (as of 2000)

Species	Hosts	Primary site	Other sites	References
*H. bilis**	Mice, rats, dog, gerbils, cats	Intestine	Liver (mice), gall bladder (humans)	57, 70
H. canadensis	Human	Intestine		84
*H. canis**	Dog, cat, human	Intestine	Blood (humans)	79, 80
			Liver (dog)	
H. cholecystus	Hamster	Bile		35
*H. cinaedi**	Hamster, human	Intestine	Blood, soft tissue, joints (humans)	63, 99
H. fennelliae	Human	Intestine	Blood	1000
H. hepaticus	Mice	Intestine	Liver	1, 2
H. muridarum	Mice, rat	Intestine	Stomach (mice)	101, 102
H. pametensis	Bird, swine	Intestine		103, 104
*H. pullorum**	Chicken, human	Intestine	Liver (chicken)	81
'*H. rappini*'*	Sheep, dog, mice, human	Intestine	Blood (humans), liver (sheep), stomach (dogs)	66, 69, 75, 105
H. rodentium	Mice	Intestine		106
H. trogontum	Rat	Intestine		107
H. typhlocionus	Mice	Intestine		108, 109
		Liver		
H. westmeadii	Humans	Blood		110

*Some data suggest zoonotic potential.

of liver damage, had not been previously identified in mice from any other location worldwide, or produced experimentally by any previously known infectious agent[1]. This novel form of chronic active hepatitis was also recognized histologically in mouse hepatitis virus-negative A/JCr mice that were being used as controls for a carcinogenesis study. A striking increase in liver tumour incidence above the low prevalence previously characteristic of this mouse strain was noted in association with the hepatitis[1]. Because of the necrotic, focal nature of the liver lesions, pathologists interpreted the lesion as a 'toxic hepatitis'. Liver tissues from affected mice were then analysed for toxic substances, but none was found. Special tissue stains were subsequently utilized on the liver tissues in an attempt to identify possible infectious aetiological agents responsible for the hepatitis. Using a modified Steiner's silver stain, spiral-like organisms were clearly observed in the liver[1].

Infected mice were then sent to our laboratory for characterization and diagnostic evaluation. A microaerobic bacterium was isolated, and it had strong urease activity and spiral morphology. We hypothesized that the bacteria might be a *Helicobacter* species. By biochemical, ultrastructural, and molecular methodologies these bacteria were confirmed to represent a new *Helicobacter* species, which we named *H. hepaticus*[2]. We have now demonstrated that *H. hepaticus* has a worldwide distribution in academic and commercial mice[3].

To analyse whether *H. hepaticus* persisted in specified ecological niches, to determine whether biomarkers of infection exist, and to analyse the influence of *H. hepaticus* on hepatocyte proliferation, a longitudinal study of *H. hepaticus*-infected A/JCr mice was undertaken[4]. A/JCr mice were serially euthanized from 3 through 18 months and surveyed by ELISA and bacterial culture of liver, colon, and caecum. Histology and electron microscopy were conducted, and hepatocyte proliferation indices were determined by using BrdU. Measurement of the liver enzyme alanine aminotransferase (ALT) was also done. In infected animals throughout the 18-month study, *H. hepaticus* was consistently isolated from the lower bowel, but only sporadically from the liver. Thus, like other *Helicobacter* species, its normal ecological niche is the csaecum and colon where, in some instances, particularly in immune dysregulated mice, *H. hepaticus* causes inflammatory bowel disease (IBD)[5,6]. By electron microscopy, *H. hepaticus* was noted infrequently in the liver, and then only in bile canaliculi. Infected mice, particularly males, showed chronic inflammation, oval cell, Kupffer cell, and Ito cell hyperplasia, hepatocytomegaly, and bile duct proliferation. The inflammatory and necrotizing lesions were progressive and involved the hepatic parenchyma, portal triads, and intralobular venules. A distinct vasculitis was also present. Hepatic tumours were noted only in male mice, whereas BrdU proliferation indices were markedly increased in both sexes, but especially in males, compared with control A/J mice[4]. Infected mice also develop sustained anti-*H. hepaticus* serum IgG antibody responses and elevated ALT levels[4].

H. hepaticus induces a Th1 immune response

The relationship between development of hepatitis and the immune response of A/JCr mice to *H. hepaticus* infection has also been investigated. This was accomplished by associating the degree of hepatitis with the post-infection serum IgG and secretory IgA responses in faeces and bile, and production of cytokines and proliferative responses of splenic mononuclear cells to *H. hepaticus* antigens[7]. Secretory IgA and systemic IgG developed by 4 weeks post-infection and persisted through 12 months, but the antibody responses were ineffective in preventing chronic infection or hepatitis. *H. hepaticus*-infected mice produced predominantly IgG2, a serum antibody, which is consistent with a Th1 immune response as reported for *H. pylori*-infected humans and for the *H. felis* mouse model. Also characteristic of a Th1 response, splenocytes from infected mice proliferated and produced more IFN-γ than IL-4 or IL-5 in an antigen-specific manner to *H. hepaticus* outer membrane proteins[7]. Infected mice developed progressively severe lesions consisting of lympho-histiocytic and plasmacytic infiltrates in the hepatic parenchyma and surrounding the vessels and bile ducts. The characterization of non-protective humoral and cell-mediated Th1 immune response to *H. hepaticus* infection in the A/JCr mouse should prove valuable for developing regimens which manipulate the host response to *Helicobacter*, alter the balance between Th1 and Th2 cell-mediated immune responses, and influence severity and course of hepatocellular carcinogenesis[7]. *H. hepaticus* associated IBD in IL-10$^{\pm}$ and Rag-2 knockout mice are associated with a Th1 immune response, which is characterized by high levels of IFN-γ and the presence of activated macrophages[8,9].

FULFILLING KOCH'S POSTULATES

H. hepaticus was orally inoculated into axenic, outbred female mice, and the mice were studied longitudinally to fulfil Koch's postulates and to ascertain the pathogenic potential of the organism under defined germfree conditions[10]. Cage contact mice were also housed in the same germfree isolator to study transmission patterns, and germfree mice were maintained in separate isolators as controls. Female mice serially euthanized from 3 weeks though 24 months post-inoculation (PI) were surveyed by culture and PCR for *H. hepaticus* in liver and intestinal tissues. Inoculated mice and cage contact mice were persistently infected with *H. hepaticus* as identified by culture and PCR, in both the intestine and, less frequently, the liver, for the duration of the 2-year study. All infected animals developed persistent, chronic hepatitis. Hepatocellular carcinoma was diagnosed in one *H. hepaticus*-infected mouse. *H. hepaticus* serum antibody was highest in experimentally infected mice at 12–18 months PI; this corresponded in general to the time interval when the highest levels of ALT were recorded[10].

H. HEPATICUS CONFOUNDS MOUSE CARCINOGENESIS STUDIES

In a long-term rodent bioassay evaluating the carcinogenicity of triethanolamine, there was equivocal evidence of carcinogenic activity in male B6C3F$_1$ mice, based on a marginal increase in hepatocellular adenomas and hepatoblastomas. Interpretation was complicated by the presence of *H. hepaticus* in selected silver-stained liver sections which also had histological evidence of karyomegaly and oval cell hyperplasia[11]. An increase in liver tumours, as evidence of carcinogenic activity, was also noted in female mice. A retrospective analysis of 51 liver tissue samples from the original carcinogenicity study was conducted to determine the incidence of *H. hepaticus* infection, and to evaluate different diagnostic approaches for assessing the presence of *H. hepaticus* in livers lacking characteristic lesions[11]. The results of *H. hepaticus* culture and *H. hepaticus*-specific PCR concurred in 84% of the cases. Microscopic detection of immunofluorescence-labelled or silver-stained bacteria in liver sections was relatively insensitive, compared to either culture or PCR detection.

These findings prompted National Toxicology Program pathologists to undertake an extensive survey of 62 bioassay studies conducted to test compounds for carcinogenicity. Nine studies were confounded because of the presence of *H. hepaticus*. There was a statistically increased liver tumour burden in control males when compared to contemporary control groups with no *H. hepaticus* infection[12]. These studies clearly demonstrate the negative impact which this chronic liver infection has on long-term mouse studies.

HOST SUSCEPTIBILITY TO *H. HEPATICUS*-INDUCED HEPATITIS

Why some mouse strains appear more susceptible to the development of liver lesions is unknown, but our initial studies indicated that susceptibility was related to host genotype. We and others determined that A/JCr, C3H/HeNCr, and SJL/NCr mice were susceptible to infection whereas C57BL mice were not[10,13]. Given that B6C3F1 mice are produced by interbreeding susceptible C3H and resistant C57BL strains of mice, the finding of severe liver disease and tumour induction in B6C3F1 infected with *H. hepaticus* infers that genetic susceptibility to *H. hepaticus* induced neoplasia has a dominant pattern of inheritance. This is similar to a recent study reported by Sutton *et al.* which showed, by interbreeding two inbred strains of mice, one resistant and the other susceptible to *Helicobacter*-induced gastric inflammation, that the gastric inflammation phenotype also has a dominant pattern of inheritance[14]. Furthermore, it is well known that genetic background is often one of the determinants in conferring resistance or susceptibility to a number of infectious agents as well as carcinogens[15–17].

Recombinant inbred (RI) strains of mice are an important and useful tool for analysing genetic traits in mice. RI sets are derived by crossbreeding two parental inbred strains of mice, and then developing a set of inbred lines from the F2 generation of that cross. As a consequence the genetic composition of each strain in the RI set is a unique combination of genetic material from the parental strains, representing approximately 50% of each parental genome. Therefore, a genetic marker recognized in either of the parental strains will have a characteristic strain distribution pattern (SDP) among the RI strains. If a single gene is responsible for a trait with differing phenotypes in the parental strains the gene can be mapped to a chromosomal region using linkage analysis to compare the SDP of a particular phenotype

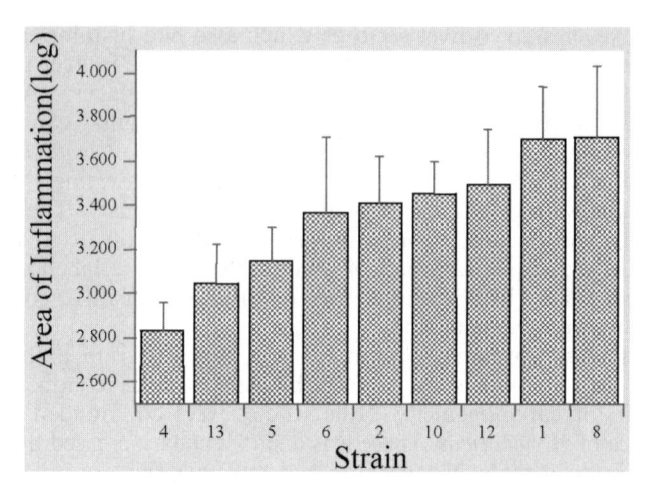

Figure 1. Hepatic inflammation scores in AXB recombinant inbred strains infected with *H. hepaticus*[18].

with the SDPs of all the known genetic markers. The AXB RI set utilized to study *H. hepaticus* genetic susceptibility was derived from parental A/J and C57BL/6J inbred strains[18]. It is one of the best-characterized of the RI panels, typed for over 400 genetic markers spanning the entire genome, and has been used extensively to study host-related mechanisms of immunity to infectious agents[19–21].

We recently characterized the phenotypes exhibited in response to chronic *H. hepaticus* infection among nine of the AXB recombinant inbred strains and determined that the most discriminating of the phenotypes was extent and severity of hepatic inflammation scored morphometrically (Figure 1). Five males and five females from each of the nine AXB RI strains were inoculated by gavage with *H. hepaticus* at 10 weeks of age and sacrificed 14 months PI[18]. Microscopic evaluation of haematoxylin and eosin-stained liver sections revealed lesions consisting of inflammation and necrosis of the hepatic parenchyma, intralobular veins, and portal areas that varied in severity for different strains. AXB strains 1 and 12 had the most severe changes, while strains 4 and 13 were the least affected. Morphometric scoring was done on all liver sections for every mouse in the study. Total area counted was standardized for each mouse by dividing the area affected with inflammation by the number of portal areas in the sections scored. A log transformation was performed on the data so that it had a normal distribution for statistical analyses. The morphometric scores for inflammation reflected these strain differences (Figure 1). The variation in hepatic inflammation between strains was statistically significant, and the continuous, rather than bimodal, distribution of inflammation scores among the strains was indicative of a multigenic trait[18]. Linkage analysis suggested that foci on chromosome 19 (D19Mit34 and D19Mit36) may contribute, in part, to *Helicobacter*-induced disease in AXB RI mice. Interestingly, a number of immunologically important genes are located on chromosome 19, including

CD5, which has been shown to be a phenotypic marker of autoreactive B lymphocytes in mice[22].

Bile ductule and oval cell hyperplasia were present in some severely affected portal areas, and occasionally dysplasia of biliary epithelium was present. Proliferative lesions ranging from nodular hyperplasia to hepatocellular adenomas and carcinomas were present in several cases with severe, chronic inflammation[18]. An additional significant finding was the presence of oval cell hyperplasia in susceptible AXB RI strains. Typically, oval cell proliferation has been linked to chronic, ongoing hepatic damage, usually from carcinogens[23]. More recently, however, pro-inflammatory cytokines produced by leucocytes have been recognized as important mitogens for oval cells[24]. In *H. hepaticus*-induced hepatitis, both direct cell damage and inflammatory cell-derived cytokines probably contributed to oval cell proliferation. This constellation of lesions is consistent with lesions seen in A/JCr mice that were similarly inoculated with *H. hepaticus*. In contrast, A/JCr mice that were not inoculated had minimal or no lesion and, as expected, all C57BL/6J mice, whether or not infected with *H. hepaticus*, had minimal or no lesions.

Notably, two mice from the AXB RI strain 12 developed lymphosarcoma that involved the liver, mesenteric lymph nodes, and large intestine, and both neoplasms were of B-cell origin, as are *H. pylori*-associated MALT lymphomas in humans[25,26].

H. hepaticus: possible mechanisms of tumour induction

The inbred strain A/J normally has a low incidence and multiplicity of liver tumours. Thus, their susceptibility to *Helicobacter hepaticus*-induced hepatitis and development of hepatocellular tumours has provided a unique opportunity to dissect *Helicobacter*-associated tumorigenesis. Our laboratory, and subsequently others, demonstrated that marked hepatocyte proliferation, strongly linked to tumour promotion, and presumably the result of *H. hepaticus*-induced chronic inflammation, is in part responsible for the increased rates of hepatocellular tumours in male A/J mice[4,18,27]. However, these histological features are expressed only in certain inbred strains of mice and not in other inbred strains (e.g. C57BL/6). These strain differences in *H. hepaticus* susceptibility also suggest a mechanism such as tumour promotion, because it is known that tumour promotion in the mouse liver is influenced strongly by the genetics of the host[28,29]. In addition, a tumour promotion mechanism is supported by a lack of mutagenic response in the Ames' assay, as well as lack of demonstrated mutations in H-, K-, and N-ras and p53 tumour suppressor genes in liver tumours of A/J mice infected with *H. hepaticus*[30-32]. Furthermore, the presence of a long-term chronic inflammatory response that precedes tumour development in *H. hepaticus*-infected mice supports this hypothesis[4,11].

We had previously shown that *H. mustelae*, a natural gastric pathogen in ferrets, strongly promotes carcinogenesis initiated by the gastric carcinogen MNNG[33]. Others demonstrated that liver fluke infection in hamsters also strongly promoted nitrosodimethylamine (NDMA)-initiated bile duct cancer[34]. It is interesting to speculate as to whether these hamsters were

Table 2. Characteristics which classify *H. hepaticus* as a tumor promotor

Strain susceptibility
Long-term inflammatory state with increased reactive oxygen species prior to tumour formation
Increased hepatocyte proliferation
Lack of mutations in *ras* and *p53* genes
Negative Ame's assay
H. hepaticus promotion of tumours initiated by hepatocarcinogens

also infected with *H. cholecystus*, a novel *Helicobacter* known to colonize the bile of hamsters[35]. In a recent study, male A/J infant mice infected with *H. hepaticus* were given a single intraperitoneal dose of NDMA and developed a statistically higher incidence of hepatocellular adenomas at two timepoints (31–36 weeks and 51–64 weeks PI) than in uninfected mice similarly treated with the carcinogen[31]. There was also a 4-fold increase in the multiplicity of adenomas at 31–36 weeks PI and a 5-fold increase in both incidence and multiplicity of carcinomas after 50 weeks. These data indicate that *H. hepaticus* not only stimulates the growth of tumours from initiated cells, but also enhances progression to malignancy[31]. Liver tumour promotion by *H. hepaticus* is also consistent with the observation of increased hepatic levels of reactive oxygen species (ROS); elevated 8-hydroxy deoxyguanosine (8-oxo-dG) was noted in *H. hepaticus*-infected livers, as well as formazan precipitates after liver perfusion with nitroblue tetrazolium[36]. These factors in combination suggest that *H. hepaticus* exerts a tumour-promotion liver effect in A/J mice (Table 2).

H. hepaticus may predispose the liver to develop cancer through the induction of apoptosis and proliferation

Several studies have shown that *H. pylori* infection leads to an increased proliferative index, and that the effect on proliferation may be one of the earliest identifiable abnormalities in the progression to gastric cancer[37]. The factors which lead to an increased proliferation rate have not been clearly delineated, although possibilities which have been studied include direct bacterial factors (e.g. adherence) and chronic inflammation with release of cytokines and growth factors. Apoptosis, or programmed cell death, is the primary mechanism for cell loss in the gastric mucosa[38], and the rate of apoptosis is normally closely aligned with the proliferative rate in the gastric mucosa. In the setting of *H. pylori* gastritis, apoptotic rates are markedly increased. Moss et al. showed that the mean apoptotic rate rose from 2.9% in uninfected patients to 16.8% in *H. pylori*-infected patients[39]. Changes in the apoptotic rate are normally matched by changes in the rate of proliferation; thus the induction of apoptosis by *H. pylori*, and possibly *H. hepaticus*, could be the stimulus for the increases in proliferation.

Preliminary studies performed on naturally *H. hepaticus*-infected A/JCr and B6C3F$_1$ mice also indicate that proliferation and apoptosis may be linked to progression of hepatitis to tumours in mice[4,12]. This observation suggested that growth-promoting factors, which increase the proliferative rate, might also lead to increases in the rate of apoptosis. The induction of apoptosis appears to be mediated by direct effects of *H. hepaticus*, with significant contributions by cytokines. Several groups have now shown that infection of gastric cancer cell lines with *H. pylori* leads to dose-related increases in the apoptotic rate, which is increased in a synergistic manner through co-incubation with interferon-gamma (IFN-γ) or tumour necrosis factor-alpha (TNF-α)[40,41]. Interestingly, increased levels of IFN-γ are also noted in A/J mice infected with *H. hepaticus*[7]. Thus, previous work has suggested that both direct bacterial effects and immune responses may induce apoptosis, which may be a possible stimulus for increased epithelial proliferation. The combination appears to lead – through unknown mechanisms – to altered differentiation and progression to cancer.

Biomarkers of oxidative stress and cytotoxicity in *H. hepaticus*-associated hepatitis

In addition to alterations in cell kinetics in the liver of mice infected with *H. hepaticus*, there is now good evidence for the presence of elevated levels of oxidative stress in *H. hepaticus*-associated hepatitis. Certainly in *H. pylori*-associated gastritis it is well recognized that the chronic–active inflammation is characterized by elevated levels of pro-inflammatory cytokines, including IL-1, IL-6, IL-8, TNF-α, and IFN-γ[42–44]. The inflammatory responses engendered by this cytokine milieu do not confer protective immunity, but instead promote inflammation and an elevated level of reactive oxygen species (ROS) in the gastric mucosa[45]. The elevated level of ROS is coincident with increased nitric oxide (NO) production by inducible nitric oxide synthase (iNOS)[46]. NO reacts with ROS to form additional reactive species. A major fate of NO is reaction with superoxide anion to yield peroxynitrite, which is even more reactive than NO itself. Importantly, the formation of NO and superoxide does occur simultaneously in activated inflammatory cells[47], and nitrotyrosine, a specific marker for peroxynitrite formation, is present in *H. pylori*-associated gastritis[46]. In addition to nitrotyrosine, the oxidation and nitration products of DNA, 8-oxo-dG and 8-nitrodeoxyguanosine (8-nitro-dG), are considered useful biomarkers for monitoring promutagenic DNA damage. The role of 8-oxo-dG in mutagenesis and carcinogenesis has been widely investigated, and several studies have shown a correlation between the formation of 8-oxo-dG and increased cancer risk[48].

Recently it has been demonstrated that there is a time-dependent increase in 8-oxo-dG in the liver of *H. hepaticus*-infected A/JCr mice compared to uninfected, age-matched controls[36]. In this study the source of the ROS was determined to be the hepatocytes, as evidenced by formazan deposition following perfusion of NBT. Immunohistochemistry revealed an increased number of cells expressing cytochrome P450 (CYP), and co-localization of formazan and the 2A5 isoform of the enzyme (CYP2A5) suggested a possible mechanism for the production of ROS. In addition, immunohistochemistry for glutathione *S*-transferase indicated that the hepatocytes were attempting to produce increased amounts of reduced glutathione (GSH). GSH is involved in protecting cells from killing by NO and by ROS, and both *de-novo* synthesis of GSH and reduction of oxidized glutathione (GSSG) are important responses to increased oxidative stress[49]. Therefore, TNF-α,

IFN-γ, iNOS, nitrotyrosine, 8-oxo-dG, and GSH should serve as useful biomarkers for oxidative stress and cytotoxicity in H. hepaticus-associated hepatitis.

H. hepaticus is a non-genotoxic carcinogen

Cancer development in the liver is incompletely understood. The major pathway to the development of hepatocellular carcinoma involves altered hepatic foci and hepatic nodules. Foci of altered hepatocytes can be recognized histologically; the foci show increased eosinophilia or basophilia, and they may appear vacuolated due to the accumulation of glycogen. Growth of these foci leads to hepatic nodules. Nodules are distinguished from foci by size, although they show tinctorial properties that are similar to foci. As in other organ systems, the mechanism of tumour induction in the liver is considered to be a two-step process involving initiation followed by promotion. The initiation phase is thought to result from an irreversible effect of genotoxic agents on DNA, while promotion occurs as a result of proliferation of the initiated cells. Agents that work through the stage of promotion are often called epigenetic or non-genotoxic carcinogens. There is no requirement for mice to be exposed to genotoxins for neoplasia to result; animals appear to have, within the liver, a population of spontaneously initiated cells. As animals age, an increasing number of altered foci are seen. It has been suggested that this indicates that initiation occurs spontaneously, either as a consequence of low-level exposure to genotoxins, or due to inherent metabolic processes leading to free radical formation[50]. Following exposure to genotoxic agents the initial biochemical lesions may be considered premutagenic. The functions of the ensuing mutations are poorly understood. Tumours that develop in C3H and B6C3F$_1$ mice show a high incidence of mutation at codon 61 of the H-ras oncogene, although there is some question as to whether such mutations are a cause of transformation or a result of it. Genetic analysis of recombinant inbred strains of mice derived from C57BL and C3H mice has indicated that susceptibility to neoplastic development may be controlled by two genetic loci, one of which plays a predominant (85%) role. This difference relates to the promotional stage, and susceptible strains have a more rapid growth of altered foci[51,52]. PCR and single-stranded conformation polymorphism (SSCP) have been used to examine DNA from H. hepaticus-associated hepatocellular tumours for the presence of H-, N-, and K-ras mutations, as well as mutations in the tumour suppressor gene p53[32]. In this study, mutations were not observed. These findings support the hypothesis that H. hepaticus infection causes liver tumours through a promotion-like mechanism.

Chronic hepatitis and lower bowel inflammation in H. hepaticus-infected SCID mice

Hepatitis, proliferative typhlitis and colitis were recently characterized in male and female SCID/NCr mice naturally infected with H. hepaticus[53]. Significant hepatitis and proliferative typhlitis were observed in all mice of varying age and sex. Hepatic lesions were most severe in older males and included multifocal to coalescing coagulative hepatocyte necrosis with minimal to mild monocytic and neutrophilic infiltration. Prominent pleomorphism of hepatocytes was noted along with numerous Warthin–Starry-positive helical organisms within the liver parenchyma and bile canaliculi. In comparison to susceptible immunocompetent mice, most of the *H. hepaticus*-infected SCID/NCr mice had higher numbers of *H. hepaticus* in the liver and only a moderate index of inflammation with, as expected, no serum IgG titre against *H. hepaticus*. Proliferative typhlitis was characterized by moderate to marked mucosal epithelial cell hyperplasia with mild monocytic and neutrophilic infiltration of the caecal wall. Minimal to mild colitis was present in all mice, with a trend for increased severity in older males. Proliferative changes in the colon were most severe in older males. The results suggested that an intact immune response may limit colonization of the liver and that, in contrast to the suggestion that *Helicobacter* infection may promote autoimmunity given that *H. hepaticus* and HSP 70 share cross-reactive epitopes[54], chronic lesions associated with *H. hepaticus* can develop in the absence of T and B cell-dependent immune responses[53].

Eradication of *H. hepaticus* from mice

H. hepaticus is known to persistently colonize the caecum and colon of mice, and causes serious disease in susceptible strains. Eradication of the organism from infected mouse colonies is therefore desirable. Treatment modalities that have been utilized for eradication of *H. hepaticus* from the gastrointestinal system have consisted of the oral administration of various antibiotic combinations previously evaluated for eradication of experimental *H. felis* gastric infection in mice. In one study, A/JCr mice naturally infected with *H. hepaticus* were divided into six treatment groups of 10 animals each. Animals received monotherapy of amoxicillin, metronidazole, or tetracycline or triple therapy of amoxicillin–metronidazole–bismuth (AMB) or tetracycline–metronidazole–bismuth (TMB). All medications were administered by oral gavage three times daily for 2 weeks. One month after the final treatment, mice were euthanized and liver, caecum, and colon were cultured for *H. hepaticus*. All untreated control animals had *H. hepaticus* isolated from the caecum and/or colon. *H. hepaticus* was not recovered from the liver, caecum, or colon of the AMB or TMB treatment groups. All animals receiving the various antibiotic monotherapies had *H. hepaticus* isolated from the caecum and colon[55]. Similar treatment strategies were used in a subsequent study in which the antibiotics were placed in drinking water or impregnated into a nutritionally complete food wafer, which served as the sole food source during the course of antibiotic treatment[56]. At the specified doses and the route of administration evaluated, AMB and TMB triple therapies can be effective for eradication of *H. hepaticus* in mice[55,56]. Also rederivation of mice by embryo transfer can ensure *Helicobacter*-free status of mice being used for experimental studies.

Thus, with effective eradication strategies, and use of assured *Helicobacter*-free mice as controls, studies can now be conducted which can determine at what stage *H. hepaticus* must be eradicated to interrupt the carcinogenic process.

ISOLATION AND IDENTIFICATION OF OTHER NOVEL MURINE HELICOBACTERS

H. bilis is associated with hepatitis in mice

A fusiform bacterium with three to 14 multiple bipolar sheathed flagella and periplasmic fibres wrapped around the cell was isolated from the liver, bile, and lower intestine of aged, inbred mice. The bacteria grew at 37°C and 42°C under microaerobic conditions, rapidly hydrolysed urea, were catalase- and oxidase-positive, reduced nitrate to nitrite, did not hydrolyse indoxyl acetate or hippurate, and were resistant to both cephalothin and nalidixic acid but sensitive to metronidazole. On the basis of 16S rRNA gene sequence analysis the organism was classified as a novel *Helicobacter*, *H. bilis*. This new *Helicobacter* which colonized the bile and liver was also associated with multifocal chronic hepatitis[57]. This bacterium has also been isolated from the stomach of dogs and intestine of gerbils, and is capable of inducing IBD in nude rats and ICR SCID mice[58,59]. Male CB17 SCID mice in addition to IBD also develop hepatitis when experimentally infected with *H. bilis*[60]. Importantly, *H. bilis* has been identified in the gallbladder tissue of humans with chronic cholecystitis[61] and from livers of humans with primary sclerosing cholangitis PSC[62] (see below).

H. CHOLECYSTUS COLONIZES BILIARY TRACT OF HAMSTERS

H. cholecystus was recently isolated from the bile of hamsters with cholangiofibrosis and centrilobular pancreatitis[35]. It is likely that this bacterium also colonizes the intestinal tract of hamsters, but it is unknown whether the bacterium plays a role in the pathogenesis of hepatobiliary and pancreatic disease in hamsters or colonizes and causes disease in other hosts. For example, *H. cinaedi* has also been isolated from the intestinal tract of hamsters and has been suggested to cause zoonotic disease including sepsis[63,64].

A NOVEL *HELICOBACTER* SP. COLONIZES WOODCHUCK LIVERS INFECTED WITH WOODCHUCK HEPATITIS VIRUS

Given the background incidence of hepatitis in woodchucks, unrelated to woodchuck hepatitis virus (WHV) infection, a study was undertaken to determine whether woodchucks' livers were infected with *Helicobacter* sp. Twenty woodchuck livers, 10 with WHV-associated hepatic tumours and 10 without tumours, were cultured using microaerobic techniques and analysed by using genus-specific *Helicobacter* PCR primers[65]. In 12 livers a 1200 bp *Helicobacter* spp. specific amplicon was observed. Southern hybridization confirmed the specific identity of the PCR products. Nine of the 10 livers with tumours had positive *Helicobacter* spp. identified by PCR, whereas only three of the livers without tumours were positive. In one case, a urease, catalase and oxidase positive bacterium was isolated from liver tissue. By 16S rRNA analysis the organism was classified as a novel *Helicobacter* sp. Using 16S rRNA-based primers specific to this novel

Helicobacter, the original 12 liver samples remained positive and an additional four liver samples had positive PCR amplicons, for an overall prevalence of 80%. Further studies are required to ascertain if this novel *Helicobacter* sp. plays a tumour promotion role in hepadnavirus-associated tumours in woodchucks, and to determine whether *Helicobacter* spp. could play a similar role in virally induced hepatitis in humans.

HEPATOBILIARY *HELICOBACTERS* IN BIRDS AND LARGER MAMMALS, INCLUDING HUMANS

'*H. rappini*' infects multiple hosts

A fusiform organism with periplasmic fibres and multiple bipolar sheathed flagella was first cultured from aborted ovine fetuses, and Bryner gave it the provisional name '*Flexispira rappini*'[66,67]. '*F. rappini*' can cross the placenta in pregnant sheep, induce abortions, and cause acute hepatic necrosis in sheep fetuses[66,68]. Experimentally, *F. rappini* causes abortions and necrotic hepatitis in guinea pigs[66,68,69]. This bacterium has also been isolated from the faeces of asymptomatic mice and identified on a morphological basis, as well as being cultured from the stomach of dogs[70–72]. By 16S rRNA analysis these closely related organisms belong in the genus *Helicobacter* and are composed of at least 10 closely related taxa[73].

The bacterium was first isolated in humans from a diarrhoeic patient; in the household the same bacterium was isolated from the faeces of a young clinically normal dog[74]. Although '*H. rappini*' is associated with gastroenteritis in humans, its causal role in diarrhoeal disease in humans requires further study[69,74]. More recently several immunocompromised patients and children have had '*H. rappini*' isolated from their blood[75–77]. Many of the patients also suffered from diarrhoeal episodes. Whether '*H. rappini*' can cause liver disease in humans is unknown. However, given the organism's ability to penetrate intestinal mucosa and cause bacteraemia this argues that the organism can colonize the liver and cause hepatitis.

H. CANIS INFECTS PETS AND HUMANS

H. canis was isolated from the faeces of a child suffering from gastroenteritis[78]. *H. canis* is differentiated from *H. fennelliae* by its ability to grow at 42°C, its failure to produce catalase and its marked tolerance to bile. This bacterium has also been isolated from the faeces of normal and diarrhoeic dogs and cats[13,79]. Morphologically the bipolar, sheathed flagella of *H. canis* are similar to those in *H. cinaedi* and *H. fennelliae*, and are useful in characterizing the organism as a helicobacter. We also cultured *H. canis* from the liver of a puppy diagnosed as having an active, multifocal hepatitis[80]. Whether this organism is capable of experimentally inducing hepatitis in dogs, or occurs as a natural liver infection in humans, requires further study. This possibility, however, is strengthened by isolation of *H. canis* from bacteraemic humans[67,80].

Additional investigations will be required to ascertain whether *H. canis* in dogs and cats constitutes a potential reservoir for zoonotic transmission to humans, and whether it can cause hepatitis. The fact that other microaerophilic bacteria, i.e. *Campylobacter jejuni* and *C. coli*, are associated with zoonotic transmission, especially children handling young puppies and kittens, strengthens the zoonotic argument[79].

H. PULLORUM, AN EMERGING ENTERIC PATHOGEN IN HUMANS

H. pullorum has been isolated from the caeca of asymptomatic chickens, the livers and intestinal contents of chickens with hepatitis, and faeces of humans with gastroenteritis[81]. It belongs to the urease-negative EHS, but can be distinguished from most other helicobacters by lack of sheathed flagella. *H. pullorum* is also tolerant to bile. The potential of *H. pullorum* to cause serious gastrointestinal disease is evidenced by isolation of the organism from two young adults, a man and a woman, both of whom suffered from chronic diarrhoea of 1 month's duration[82]. The young man also had elevated liver enzymes and hepatomegaly. Human cases of *H. pullorum*-associated gastroenteritis are increasingly reported and may in the future also play a role in bacterial-associated hepatobiliary disease[83]. The recent finding that some strains previously classified as *H. pullorum* are indeed another novel helicobacter, *H. canadensis*, highlights the importance of careful phenotypic, biochemical and molecular analysis when defining EHS, and ascribing their epidemiological and pathogenic potential[84]. Zoonotic transmission of *H. pullorum* from infected chickens seems a distinct possibility, but further studies are needed to firmly establish *H. pullorum's* zoonotic potential.

Virulence determinants of enterohepatic *Helicobacter* species

H. pylori has documented putative virulence determinants which have been implicated in the ability of the organism to colonize the host and to cause disease. Virulence determinants are less well characterized for the non-gastric species of *Helicobacter*, including *H. hepaticus*. However, several candidate virulence determinants have been proposed on the basis of their homology to virulence determinants of *H. pylori*, some of which may also be important for pathogenicity in EHS. The urease of *H. pylori* is one of the most abundant proteins produced by the bacterium. Urease helps protect bacteria from acid by the production of ammonia. *In-vivo* studies have shown that isogenic mutant strains which do not produce urease fail to colonize the stomach, even when acid secretion is suppressed[85]. These studies indicate a role for urease in pathogenesis, and suggest that ammonia liberated from urea may serve as an important nitrogen source. In the ferret model, isogenic mutants of *H. mustelae* that lack urease activity fail to colonize, whereas the wild-type strain can colonize and persist[86].

Like gastric helicobacters, *H. hepaticus* possesses a high level of urease activity. The role of this enzyme in colonization and pathogenic potential of EHS is not known. In parallel with the development of a *H. hepaticus* genomic library, PCR was used to amplify a portion of the urease structural genes from *H. hepaticus* genomic DNA[87]. Amplified DNA fragments were cloned and the nucleotide sequence was determined. The deduced amino acid sequence of the partial *H. hepaticus* ureA gene product was found to exhibit 60% identity and 75% similarity to the predicted *H. pylori* UreA. The deduced amino acid sequence of a partial *H. hepaticus* ureB gene product exhibited 75% identity and 87% similarity to the predicted *H. pylori* UreB. Diversity among *H. hepaticus* isolates was evaluated by means of a restriction fragment length polymorphism (RFLP) assay. The 1.6-kb fragments within the ureAB open reading frames, amplified from 11 independent isolates, were digested with the restriction endonuclease HhaI. Three distinct RFLP patterns were observed. Identical RFLP profiles were noted in sequential isolates of one strain of *H. hepaticus* during an 18-month *in-vivo* colonization study, suggesting that the urease genes of *H. hepaticus* are stable. The urease genes among *H. hepaticus* strains were also well conserved, sharing 98.8–99% nucleotide sequence identity among three isolates analysed[87]. Whether urease is important for *H. hepaticus* colonization will require *in-vivo* experiments with isogenic mutants. However, both urease-positive and urease-negative EHS can colonize livers and induce hepatitis.

Motility of these spiral microorganisms is also essential for colonization. Isogenic mutants of *H. pylori* lacking flagella fail to colonize the gnotobiotic piglet[88]. The essential role of flagella in long-term, persistent colonization by *H. mustelae* has also been demonstrated[89]. Undoubtedly flagella are important for colonization by lower bowel *Helicobacters*, but experiments to prove this point are thus far lacking.

A novel *H. hepaticus* toxin that causes vacuoles and granule formation in a murine liver cell line has been described[90]. The granulating cytotoxin is a heat-labile secreted protein with a molecular weight of >100 kDa that is distinct from the *H. pylori* cytotoxin. Young *et al.* have described another toxin in *H. hepaticus*[91]. This cytolethal distending toxin (CDT) causes cell cycle arrest in HeLa cells and is closely related to CDT of *Campylobacter* spp. and *Shigella* spp., as well as several other enterohepatic helicobacters[92]. The pathogenic potential of both of these toxins is unknown and further studies are warranted.

Enterohepatic *Helicobacters* – do they cause hepatobiliary disease in humans?

Cancer of the gallbladder is the number one cause of cancer mortality in Chilean women. Incidence rates for this tumour vary widely on a worldwide basis, being approximately 30 times higher in high-risk than in low-risk populations, suggesting that environmental factors such as infectious microorganisms, carcinogens, and nutrition play a role in its pathogenesis. Because several *Helicobacter* spp. colonize the livers of animals and induce hepatitis, the aim of this study was to determine whether *Helicobacter* infection was associated with cholecystitis in humans[61]. Bile or resected gallbladder tissue from 46 Chileans with chronic cholecystitis undergoing cholecystectomy were cultured for *Helicobacter* spp. and subjected to PCR analysis using helicobacter-specific 16S ribosomal RNA primers. Recovery of *Helicobacter* spp. from frozen specimens was unsuccessful. However, by PCR analysis, 13 of 23 bile samples and nine of 23 gallbladder tissues were positive for *Helicobacter* spp. Eight of the helicobacter-specific PCR amplicons were sequenced and subjected to phylogenetic analysis. Five sequences represented strains of *H. bilis*, two strains of '*H. rappini*' (ATCC 49317), and one strain of *H. pullorum*. These data support an association of bile-resistant *Helicobacter* spp. with gallbladder disease. Further studies are needed to ascertain whether similar *Helicobacter* spp. play a causative role in the development of gallbladder cancer[61].

Primary sclerosing cholangitis (PSC) is another chronic cholestatic liver disease of unknown aetiology. Pathological lesions consist of persistent inflammation with destruction and fibrosis of intrahepatic and extrahepatic bile ducts. The high correlation of PSC and ulcerative colitis has raised the hypothesis that chronic portal bacteraemia may initiate inflammation and promote subsequent hepatobiliary damage. A study was therefore undertaken to ascertain whether *Helicobacter* spp. known to cause hepatobiliary disease in animals were present in PSC patients[93]. Liver biopsies and bile were obtained from eight patients with PSC. Trypticase soy agar with 5% sheep blood, TVP and CVA medium were used for *Helicobacter* spp. isolation. The primers chosen for PCR amplification recognized conserved regions of the 16S rRNA specific for all known *Helicobacter* spp. and produced an amplified product of 1220 bp. For confirmation of the PCR-amplified fragment, Southern blot hybridization was performed with a *Helicobacter*-specific PCR-generated probe. A PCRTM II vector was used for cloning of PCR products. Although *Helicobacter* spp. were not cultured, *Helicobacter* spp. were identified by PCR amplification and Southern hybridization using a *Helicobacter*-specific probe in five of eight patients[92]. In three of these patients a 1200 bp PCR-amplified product was successfully cloned and sequenced. Analysis of the sequences indicated high homology to the 16S rRNA sequences of a cluster of *Helicobacter* spp. previously isolated from animals, i.e. *H. rodentium*, *H. rappini*, and *H. pullorum*[93]. Nilsson *et al.* have recently found *Helicobacter* spp. (including *H. pylori*) by using *Helicobacter* spp.-specific PCR in livers of PSC patients as well as patients with primary biliary cirrhosis, another idiopathic biliary disease. Interestingly, *Helicobacter* spp. were not identified in control patients' livers or in patients with non-cholestatic liver disease[93].

Case reports have also suggested that *H. pylori*, detected by PCR assays, can infect biliary and hepatic tissues[94,95]. Three of seven bile samples collected by percutaneous transhepatic cholangiodrainage were positive for *H. pylori* by PCR of the urease A gene[95]. The authors suggested that this organism can cause asymptomatic cholangitis[95]. The organism was found only in patients who also had confirmed gastric infection with *H. pylori*. In another study a microorganism closely resembling *H. pylori*, by PCR of the urease B gene and immunohistochemical staining, was found in the resected gallbladder mucosa of a 41-year-old woman admitted to the hospital with fever and right upper quadrant pain[94]. The *in-vitro* susceptibility to bile and the specific tissue tropism of *H. pylori*, however, argues against colonization of the biliary system by this gastric helicobacter[96]. Another report has noted that gastric helicobacter infection increases following cholecystectomy[97]. Surgery for peptic ulcers resulting in high reflux scores, hypochlorhydria and increased bile acid concentration can eliminate *H. pylori*, suggesting that bile acids inhibit *H. pylori* colonization *in vivo*[98].

SUMMARY

Clearly, though EHS are well-established pathogens in experimental animals, further studies are needed to define what role, if any, EHS and/or *H. pylori* play in hepatic and biliary disease in humans. Additional studies should concentrate not only in identifying by culture, *in-vitro* immunocytochemistry, and PCR, *Helicobacter* spp. in diseased hepatobiliary tissue, but also confirm their absence in healthy tissue. Serological assays should also be developed in order to conduct epidemiological studies to ascertain association and possible causality of EHS with liver disease. Finally, continued investigations of EHS in animal models to understand pathogenetic mechanisms of this important group of pathogens should remain a priority.

References

1. Ward JM, Fox JG, Anver MR et al. Chronic active hepatitis and associated liver tumors in mice caused by a persistent bacterial infection with a novel *Helicobacter* species. J Natl Cancer Inst. 1994;86:1222–7.
2. Fox JG, Dewhirst FE, Tully JG et al. *Helicobacter hepaticus* sp. nov., a microaerophilic bacterium isolated from livers and intestinal mucosal scrapings from mice. J Clin Microbiol. 1994;32:1238–45.
3. Shames B, Fox JG, Dewhirst FE, Yan L, Shen Z, Taylor NS. Identification of widespread *Helicobacter hepaticus* infection in feces in commercial mouse colonies by culture and PCR assay. J Clin Microbiol. 1995;33:2968–72.
4. Fox JG, Li X, Yan L et al. Chronic proliferative hepatitis in A/JCr mice associated with persistent *Helicobacter hepaticus* infection: a model of *Helicobacter*-induced carcinogenesis. Infect Immun. 1996;64:1548–58.
5. Cahill RJ, Foltz CJ, Fox JG, Dangler CA, Powrie F, Schauer DB. Inflammatory bowel disease: an immune mediated condition triggered by bacterial infection with *Helicobacter hepaticus*. Infect Immun. 1997;65:3126–31.
6. Foltz CJ, Fox JG, Cahill RJ et al. Spontaneous inflammatory bowel disease in multiple mutant mouse lines: association with colonization by *Helicobacter hepaticus*. Helicobacter. 1998;3:69–78.
7. Whary MT, Morgan TJ, Dangler CA, Gaudes KJ, Taylor NS, Fox JG. Chronic active hepatitis induced by *Helicobacter hepaticus* in the A/JCr mouse is associated with a Th1 cell-mediated immune response. Infect Immun. 1998;66:3142–8.
8. Kullberg MC, Ward JM, Gorelick PL et al. *Helicobacter hepaticus* triggers colitis in specific pathogen free interleukin-10 (IL-10) deficient mice through an IL-12 and gamma interferon-dependent mechanism. Infect Immun. 1998;66:5157–66.
9. von Freeden-Jeffry U, Davidson N, Wiler R, Fort M, Burdach S, Murray R. IL-7 deficiency prevents development of a non-T cell non-B cell-mediated colitis. J Immunol. 1998;15:5673–80.
10. Fox JG, Yan L, Shames B, Campbell J, Murphy JC, Li X. Persistent hepatitis and enterocolitis in germfree mice infected with *Helicobacter hepaticus*. Infect Immun. 1996;64:3673–81.
11. Fox JG, MacGregor J, Shen Z, Li X, Lewis R, Dangler CA. Comparison of methods to identify *Helicobacter hepaticus* in $B6C3F_1$ used in a carcinogenesis bioassay. J Clin Microbiol. 1998;36:1382–7.
12. Hailey JR, Haseman JK, Bucher JR et al. Impact of *Helicobacter hepaticus* infection in B6C3F1 mice from 12 NTP two year carcinogenesis studies. Toxicol Pathol. 1998;26:602–11.
13. Foley JE, Marks S, Munson L et al. Isolation of *Helicobacter canis* from a colony of Bengal cats with endemic diarrhea. J Clin Microbiol. 1999;37:3271–5.

14. Sutton P, Wilson J, Genta R et al. A genetic basis for atrophy: dominant non-responsiveness and *Helicobacter* induced gastritis in F(1) hybrid mice. Gut. 1999;45:335–40.
15. Malkinson AM, Nesbitt MN, Skamene E. Susceptibility to urethane-induced pulmonary adenomas between A/J and C57B1/J mice: use of AXB and BXA recombinant inbred lines indicating a three-locus genetic model. J Natl Cancer Inst. 1985;75:971–4.
16. Malo D, Vidal SM, Hu J, Skamene E, Gros P. High resolution linkage map in the vicinity of the host resistance locus. Genomics. 1993;16:655–63.
17. Skamene E, Gros A, Forget PA, Kongshavn SCC, Taylor BA. Genetic regulation of resistance to intra-cellular pathogens. Nature. 1982;297:506–9.
18. Ihrig M, Schrenzel M, Fox JG. Differential susceptibility to hepatic inflammation and proliferation in AXB recombinant inbred mice chronically infected with *Helicobacter hepaticus*. Am J Pathol. 1999;155:571–82.
19. Dindzans VJ, Skamene E, Levy GA. Susceptibility/resistance to mouse hepatitis virus strain 3 and macrophage procoagulant activity are genetically linked and controlled by two non-H-2-linked genes. J Immunol. 1986; 137:2355–60.
20. Kongshavn PA. Genetic control of resistance to *Listeria* infection. Curr Top Microbiol Immunol. 124:67–85.
21. Manly KF, Cudmore RH Jr, Kohler G. Map Manager QT: a program for genetic mapping of mendelian and quantitative trait loci. 1997.
22. Ye YL, Suen JL, Chen YY, Chiang BL. Phenotypic and functional analysis of activated B cells of autoimmune NZB X NZW F1 mice. Scand J Immunol. 1998;47:122–6.
23. Steinberg P, Steinbrecher R, Radaeva S et al. Oval cell lines OC/CDE 6 and OC/CDE 22 give rise to cholangio-cellular and undifferentiated carcinomas after transformation. Lab Invest. 1994;71:700–9.
24. Isfort RJ, Cody DB, Richards WG, Yoder BK, Wilkinson JE, Woychik RP. Characterization of growth factor responsiveness and alteration in growth factor homeostatis involved in the tumorigenic conversion of mouse oval cells. Growth Factors. 1998;15:81–94.
25. Spencer J, Wotherspoon AC. Gastric MALT lymphoma and *Helicobacter pylori*. Cancer Surv. 1997;30:213–31.
26. Yumoto N, Furukawa M, Kurosu K, Mikata A. A particular characteristic of IgH complementarity-determining region 3 suggests autoreactive B-cell origin of primary gastric B-cell lymphomas. Lab Invest. 1998;78:261–8.
27. Nyska A, Maronpot R, Eldridge S, Haseman J, Hailey J. Alteration in cell kinetics in control B6C3F1 mice infected with *Helicobacter hepaticus*. Toxicol Pathol. 1997;25:591–6.
28. Diwan BA, Rice JM, Oshima M, Ward JM. Interstain differences in susceptibility to liver carcinogenesis initiated by N-nitrosodiethylamine and its promotion by phenobarbital in C57BL/6NCr, C3H/HeNCr^{MTV-} and DBA/2NCr mice. Carcinogenesis. 1986;7:215–20.
29. Weghorst CM, Pereira MA, Klaunig JE. Strain differences in hepatic tumor promotion by phenobarbital in diethylnitrosamine- and dimethylnitrosamine-initiated infant male mice. Carcinogenesis. 1989;10:1409–12.
30. Canella KA, Diwan BA, Gorelick PL et al. Liver tumorigenesis by *Helicobacter hepaticus*: considerations of mechanism. In Vivo. 1996;10:285–92.
31. Diwan BA, Ward JM, Ramljak D, Anderson LM. Promotion by *Helicobacter hepaticus*-induced hepatitis of hepatic tumors initiated by N-nitrosodimethylamine in male A/JCr mice. Toxicol Pathol. 1997; 25:597–605.
32. Sipowicz MA, Weghorst CM, Shiao YH et al. Lack of *p53* and *ras* mutations in *Helicobacter hepaticus*-induced liver tumors in A/JCr mice. Carcinogenesis. 1997;18:233–6.
33. Fox JG, Wishnok JS, Murphy JC, Tannenbaum SR, Correa P. MNNG-induced gastric carcinoma in ferrets infected with *Helicobacter mustelae*. Carcinogenesis. 1993;14:1957–61.
34. Flavell DJ, Lucas SB. Promotion of N-nitrosodimethylamine-initiated bile duct carcinogenesis in the hamster by the human liver fluke, *Opisthorchis viverrini*. Carcinogenesis. 1983;7:927–30.
35. Franklin CL, Beckwith CS, Livingston RS et al. Isolation of a novel *Helicobacter* species, *Helicobacter cholecystus* sp. nov., from the gallbladders of Syrian hamsters with cholangiofibrosis and centrilobular pancreatitis. J Clin Microbiol. 1996;34:2952–8.
36. Sipowicz MA, Chomarat P, Diwan BA et al. Increase oxidative DNA damage and hepatocyte overexpression of specific cytochrome P450 isoforms in hepatitis of mice infected with *Helicobacter hepaticus*. Am J Pathol. 1997;151:933–41.

37. Cahill RJ, Kilgallen C, Beattie S, Hamilton H, O'Morain C. Gastric epithelial kinetics in the progression from normal mucosa to gastric carcinoma. Gut. 1996;38:177–81.
38. Hall PA, Coates PJ, Ansari A, Hopwood D. Regulation of cell number in mammalian gastrointestinal tract:the importance of apoptosis. J Cell Sci. 1994;107:3569–77.
39. Moss SF, Calam J, Agarwal B, Wang S, Holt PR. Induction of gastric epithelial apoptosis by *Helicobacter pylori*. Gut. 1996;38:498–501.
40. Fan XJ, Gunasena H, Gonzales M. et al. *Helicobacter pylori* urease binds to class II MHC molecules on gastric epithelial cells to initiate apoptosis. Gastroenterology. 1998;114:G0485.
41. Wagner S, Beil W, Westermann J et al. Regulation of gastric epithelial cell growth by *Helicobacter pylori*: evidence for a major role of apoptosis. Gastroenterology. 1997;113:1836–47.
42. Crabtree JE, Shallcross TM, Heatley RV, Wyatt JI. Mucosal tumor necrosis factor x and interleukin-6 in patients with *Helicobacter pylori* associated gastritis. Gut. 1991;32:1473–7.
43. Karttunen R, Karttunen T, Ekre HP, MacDonald TT. Interferon gamma and interleukin 4 secreting cells in the gastric antrum in *Helicobacter pylori* positive and negative gastritis. Gut. 1995;36:341–45.
44. Noach LA, Bosma NB, Jansen J, Hoek FJ, van Deventer SJ, Tygat GN. Mucosal tumor necrosis factor-alpha, interleukin-1 beta and interleukin-8 production in patients with *Helicobacter pylori*. Scand J Gastroenterol. 1994;29:425–9.
45. Davies GR, Banatvala N, Collins CE et al. Relationship between infection load of *Helicobacter pylori* and reactive oxygen metabolite production in antral mucosa. Scand J Gastroenterol. 1994;29:419–24.
46. Mannick EE, Bravo LE, Zarama G et al. Inducible nitric oxide synthase, nitrotyrosine, and apoptosis in *Helicobacter pylori* gastritis: effect of antibiotics and antioxidants. Cancer Res. 1996;56:3238–43.
47. Assreuy J, Cunha FQ, Epperlein MM et al. Production of nitric oxide and superoxide by activated macrophages and killing of *Leishmania major*. Eur J Immunol. 1994;24:672–6.
48. Floyd RA. The role of 8-hydroxyguanine in carcinogenesis. Carcinogenesis. 1990;11:1447–50.
49. Luperchio S, Tamir S, Tannenbaum SR. NO-induced oxidative stress and glutathione metabolism in rodent and human cells. Free Radical Biol Med. 1996;21:513–19.
50. Schulte-Hermann R, Timmermann-Trosiener I, Schuppler SJ. Promotion of spontaneous pre-neoplastic cells in rat liver as a possible explanation of tumor production by non-mutagenic compounds. Cancer Res. 1983;43:839–44.
51. Drinkwater N, Ginsler JJ. Genetic control of hepatocarcinogenesis in C57BL/6J and C3H/HeJ inbred mice. Carcinogenesis. 1986;7:1701–7.
52. Drinkwater NR. Genetic control of hepatocarcinogenesis in C3H mice. Drug Metab. 1994;26:201–8.
53. Li X, Fox JG, Whary MT, Yan L, Shames B, Zhao Z. Scid/NCr mice naturally infected with *Helicobacter hepaticus* develop progressive hepatitis, proliferative typhlitis and colitis. Infect Immun. 1998;66:5477–84.
54. Ward JM, Benveniste RE, Fox CH, Battles JK, Gonda MA, Tully JG. Autoimmunity in chronic active *Helicobacter hepatitis* of mice: serum antibodies and expression of heat shock protein 70 in liver. Am J Pathol. 1996;148:509–17.
55. Foltz C, Fox JG, Yan L, Shames B. Evaluation of antibiotic therapies for the eradication of *Helicobacter hepaticus*. Antimicrob Agents Chemother. 1995;36:1292–4.
56. Foltz CJ, Fox JG, Yan L, Shames B. Evaulation of various oral antimicrobial formulations for eradication of *Helicobacter hepaticus*. Lab Anim Sci. 1996;46:193–7.
57. Fox JG, Yan LL, Dewhirst FE et al. *Helicobacter bilis* sp. nov., a novel *Helicobacter* isolated from bile, livers, and intestines of aged, inbred mice. J Clin Microbiol. 1995;33:445–54.
58. Haines DC, Gorelick PL, Battles JK et al. Inflammatory large bowel disease in immuno-deficient rats naturally and experimentally infected with *Helicobacter bilis*. Vet Pathol. 1998;35:202–8.
59. Shomer NH, Dangler CA, Fox JG. *Helicobacter bilis* induced inflammatory bowel disease (IBD) in defined flora SCID mice. Infect Immun. 1997;65:4858–64.
60. Franklin CL, Riley LK, Livingston RS, Beckwith CS, Besch-Williford C, Hook J. Enterohepatic lesions in SCID mice infected with *Helicobacter bilis*. Lab Anim Sci. 1998;48:334–9.

61. Fox, JG, Dewhirst FE, Shen Z et al. Hepatic *Helicobacter* species identified in bile and gallbladder tissue from Chileans with chronic cholecystitis. Gastroenterology. 1998;114:755–63.
62. Fox JG, Shen Z, Feng Y, Dufour JF, Kaplan MM, Dewhirst F. Enterohepatic *Helicobacter* spp. identified from humans with primary sclerosing cholangitis. Gut. 1998;43:A3 (abstract).
63. Gebhart CJ, Fennell CL, Murtaugh MP, Stamm WE. *Campylobacter cinaedi* is normal intestinal flora in hamsters. J Clin Microbiol. 1989;27:1692–4.
64. Kiehlbauch JA, Tauxe RV, Baker CN, Wachsmuth IK. *Helicobacter cinaedi*-associated bacteremia and cellulitis in immunocompromised patients. Ann Intern Med. 1994;121:90–3.
65. Fox JG, Xu S, Shen Z, Dangler CA, Cullen JM. A novel *Helicobacter* sp. isolated from woodchuck livers infected with woodchuck hepatitis virus (WHV). Gastroenterology. 1999;116:A718 (abstract).
66. Kirkbride CA, Gates CE, Collins JE. Ovine abortion associated with an anaerobic bacterium. J Am Vet Med Assoc. 1985;186:789–91.
67. On SL, Holmes B. Classification and identification of *Campylobacters* and *Helicobacters* and allied taxa numerical analysis of phenotypic characters. Syst Appl Microbiol. 1995;18:374–90.
68. Bryner JH, Ritchie AE, Pollet L, Kirkbride CA, Collins JE. Experimental infection and abortion of pregnant guinea pigs with a unique spirillum-like bacterium isolated from aborted ovine fetuses. Am J Vet Res. 1987;48:91–9.
69. Archer JR, Romero S, Ritchie AE et al. Characterization of an unclassified microaerophilic bacterium associated with gastroenteritis. J Clin Microbiol. 1988;26:101–5.
70. Eaton KA, Dewhirst FE, Paster BJ et al. Prevalence and varieties of *Helicobacter* species in dogs from random sources and pet dogs: animal and public health implications. J Clin Microbiol. 1996;34:3165–70.
71. Lockard VG, Boler RK. Ultrastructure of a spiraled microorganism in the gastric mucosa of dogs. Am J Vet Res. 1970;31:1453–62.
72. Schauer DB, Ghori N, Falkow S. Isolation and characterization of '*Flexispira rappini*' from laboratory mice. J Clin Microbiol. 1993;31:2709–14.
73. Dewhirst FE, Fox JG, Mendes EN et al. *Flexispira rappini* strains represent at least ten *Helicobacter* taxa. Int J Syst Bacteriol. 2000 (In press).
74. Romero S, Archer JR, Hamacher ME, Bologna SM, Schell RF. Case report of an unclassified microaerophilic bacterium associated with gastroenteritis. J Clin Microbiol. 1988;26:142–3.
75. Sorlin P, Vandamme P, Nortier J et al. Recurrent '*Flexispira rappini*' bacteremia in an adult patient undergoing hemodialysis: case report. J Clin Microbiol. 1999;37:1319–23.
76. Tee W, Leder K, Karroum E, Dyall-Smith M. '*Flexispira rappini*' bacteremia in a child with pneumonia. J Clin Microbiol. 1998;36:1679–82.
77. Weir SC, Gibert CL, Gordin FM, Fischer SH, Gill VJ. An uncommon *Helicobacter* isolate from blood: evidence of a group of *Helicobacter* spp. pathogenic in AIDS patients. J Clin Microbiol. 1999;37:2729–33.
78. Burnens AP, Stanley J, Schaad UB, Nicolet J. Novel *Campylobacter*-like organism resembling *Helicobacter fennelliae* isolated from a boy with gastroenteritis and from dogs. J Clin Microbiol. 1993;31:1916–17.
79. Stanley J, Linton D, Burens AP et al. *Helicobacter canis* sp. nov., a new species from dogs: an integrated study of phenotype and genotype. J Gen Microbiol. 1993;139:2495–504.
80. Fox JG, Drolet R, Higgins R et al. *Helicobacter canis* isolated from a dog liver with multifocal necrotizing hepatitis. J Clin Microbiol. 1996;34:2479–82.
81. Stanley J, Linton D, Burens AP et al. *Helicobacter pullorum* sp. nov. – genotype and phenotype of a new species isolated from poultry and from human patients with gastroenteritis. Microbiology. 1994;140:3441–9.
82. Burnens, AP, Stanley J, Nicolet J. Possible association of *Helicobacter pullorum* with lesions of vibrionic hepatitis in poultry. In: Newell DG, Ketley JM, Feldman RA, editors. Campylobacters, Helicobacters, and Related Organisms. New York: Plenum Press; 1996.
83. Gibson JR, Ferrus MA, Woodward D, Xerry J, Owen RJ. Genetic diversity in *Helicobacter pullorum* from human and poultry sources identified by an amplified fragment length polymorphism technique and pulsed-field gel electrophoresis. J Appl Microbiol. 1999;87:602–10.
84. Fox JG, Chien CC, Dewhirst FE et al. *Helicobacter canadensis* sp. nov. isolated from humans with diarrheas: an example of an emerging pathogen. J Clin Microbiol. 2000;38:2546–9.

85. Eaton KA, Krakowka S. Effect of gastric pH on urease-dependent colonization of gnotobiotic piglets by *Helicobacter pylori*. Infect Immun. 1994;62:3604–7.
86. Andrutis KA, Fox JG, Schauer DB et al. Inability of an isogenic urease-negative mutant strain of *Helicobacter mustelae* to colonize the ferret stomach. Infect Immun. 1995;63:3722–5.
87. Shen Z, Schauer DB, Mobley HLT, Fox JG. Development of an PCR-RFLP assay using the nucleotide sequence of the *Helicobacter hepaticus* urease structural genes ureAB. J Clin Microbiol. 1998;36:2447–53.
88. Eaton K, Suerbaum S, Josenhans C, Krakowka S. Colonization of gnotobiotic piglets by *H pylori* deficient in two flagellin genes. Infect Immun. 1996;64:2445–8.
89. Andrutis KA, Fox JG, Schauer DB et al. Infection of the ferret stomach by isogenic flagellar mutant strains of *Helicobacter mustelae*. Infect Immun. 1997; 65:1962–66.
90. Taylor NS, Fox JG, Yan L. *In-vitro* hepatotoxic factor in *Helicobacter hepaticus*, *H. pylori* and other *Helicobacter* species. J Med Microbiol. 1995;42:48–52.
91. Young VB, Knox KA, Schauer DB. Cytolethal distending toxin sequence and activity in the enterohepatic pathogen *Helicobacter hepaticus*. Infect Immun. 2000;68:184–91.
92. Chien CC, Taylor NS, Ge Z, Schauer DB, Young VB, Fox JG. Identification of *cdt*B homologues and cytolethal distending toxin activity in enterohepatic *Helicobacter* spp. J Med Microbiol. 2000;49:525–34.
93. Nilsson HO, Taneera J, Castedal M, Glatz E, Olsson R, Wadstrom T. Identification of *Helicobacter pylori* and other *Helicobacter* species by PCR, hybridization, and partial DNA sequencing in human liver samples from patients with primary sclerosing cholangitis or primary biliary cirrhosis. J Clin Microbiol. 2000;38:1072–6.
94. Kawaguchi M, Saito T, Ohno H et al. Bacteria closely resembling *Helicobacter pylori* detected immunohistologically and genetically in resected gallbladder mucosa. J Gastroenterol. 1996;31:294–8.
95. Lin TT, Yeh CT, Wu CS, Liaw YF. Detection and partial sequence analysis of *Helicobacter pylori* DNA in the bile samples. Dig Dis Sci. 1995;40:2214–19.
96. Hanninen ML. Sensitivity of *Helicobacter pylori* to different bile salts. Eur J Clin Microbiol Infect Dis. 1991;10:515–18.
97. Caldwell MTP, McDermott M, Jazrawi S et al. *Helicobacter pylori* infection increases following cholecystectomy. Irish J Med Sci. 1995;164:52–5.
98. O'Connor HJ, Wyatt JI, Dixon MF, Axon ATR. *Campylobacter*-like organisms and reflux gastritis. J Clin Pathol. 1986;39:531–4.
99. Stills HF, Hook RR, Kinden DA. Isolation of a *Campylobacter*-like organism from healthy Syrian hamsters (*Mesocricetus auratus*). J Clin Microbiol. 1989;27:2497–501.
100. Fennell CL, Totten PA, Quinn TC, Patton DL, Holmes KK, Stamm WE. Characterization of *Campylobacter*-like organisms isolated from homosexual men. J Infect Dis. 1984;149:58–66.
101. Lee A, Phillips MW, O'Rourke JL et al. *Helicobacter muridarum* sp. nov., a microaerophilic helical bacterium with a novel ultrastructure isolated from the intestinal mucosa of rodents. Int J Syst Bacteriol. 1992;42:27–36.
102. Mendes EN, Queiroz DMM, Dewhirst FE, Paster BJ, Moura SB, Fox JG. *Helicobacter trogontum* sp. nov., isolated from the rat intestine. Int J Syst Bacteriol. 1996;46:916–21.
102. Phillips MW, Lee A. Isolation and characterization of a spiral bacterium from the crypts of rodent gastrointestinal tracts. Appl Environ Microbiol. 1983;45:675–83.
103. Dewhirst FE, Seymour C, Fraser GJ, Paster BJ, Fox JG. Phylogeny of *Helicobacter* isolates from bird and swine feces and description of *Helicobacter pametensis* sp. nov. Int J Syst Bacteriol. 1994; 44:553–60.
104. Seymour C, Lewis RJ, Kim M et al. Isolation of *Helicobacter* strains from wild bird and swine feces. Appl Environ Microbiol. 1994;60:1025–8.
105. Weir S, Cuccherini B, Whitney AM et al. Recurrent bacteremia caused by a '*Flexispira*'-like organism in a patient with X-linked (Bruton's) agammaglobulinemia. J Clin Microbiol. 1999;37:2439–45.
106. Shen Z, Fox JG, Dewhirst FE et al. *Helicobacter rodentium* sp. nov., a urease negative *Helicobacter* species isolated from laboratory mice. Int J Syst Bacteriol. 1997;47:627–34.
108. Fox JG, Gorelick PL, Kullberg MC, Ge Z, Dewhirst FE, Ward JM. A novel urease-negative *Helicobacter* species associated with colitis and typhlitis in IL-10-deficient mice. Infect Immun. 1999;67:1757–62.

109. Franklin CL, Riley LK, Livingston RS *et al*. Enteric lesions in SCID mice infected with '*Helicobacter typhlonicus*', a novel urease-negative *Helicobacter* species. Lab Anim Sci. 1999;49:496–505.
110. Trivett-Moore NL, Rawlinson WD, Yuen M, Gilbert GL. *Helicobacter westmeadii* sp. nov., a new species isolated from blood cultures of two AIDS patients. J Clin Microbiol. 1997;35:1144–50.

11
Novel *Helicobacter* species in the intestine

A. LEE

THE ECOLOGICAL NICHE OF INTESTINAL MUCUS

The intestinal tract must have been one of the original microbial ecosystems. Primitive bacteria ingested by early animals would have rapidly evolved to inhabit the many ecological niches provided by the intestine. The niche of particular interest is intestinal mucus. Due to the viscous nature of mucus, successful colonizers acquired a spiral/helical morphology and very active motility; this gave them a selective advantage over other bacteria as they were able to swim down and inhabit the intestinal crypts. The surfaces of the large bowel of most animal species are colonized with large numbers of these bacteria. Different morphological types of these organisms can been seen in different locations, e.g. caecum compared to colon. A collage of these bacteria in the intestinal mucus of a mouse is seen in Figure 1.

We now know that many of these spiral bacteria are *Helicobacter* species; for example in the mouse, the animal that has been most studied, *H. muridarum*, *H. rodentium*, *H. bilis*, *H. hepaticus* and *H. trogontum* have all been isolated.

The discovery of these lower bowel *Helicobacters* has led to be an explosion of the Genus. The current list of *Helicobacter* species isolated is shown in Table 1. It is likely that over the next few years many more will be isolated, as there could be hundreds of species that have evolved to inhabit the intestines of every animal species. The question that needs to asked is how does the gastroenterologist respond to this proliferation of *Helicobacters*?

FRIEND OR FOE

The major issue is whether we consider these bacteria to be normal flora or pathogenic. Logic would suggest that these are the normal flora of intestinal mucus as they have been found to inhabit this niche in all animal species, because of their specialized adaptation. One could also imagine a symbiotic

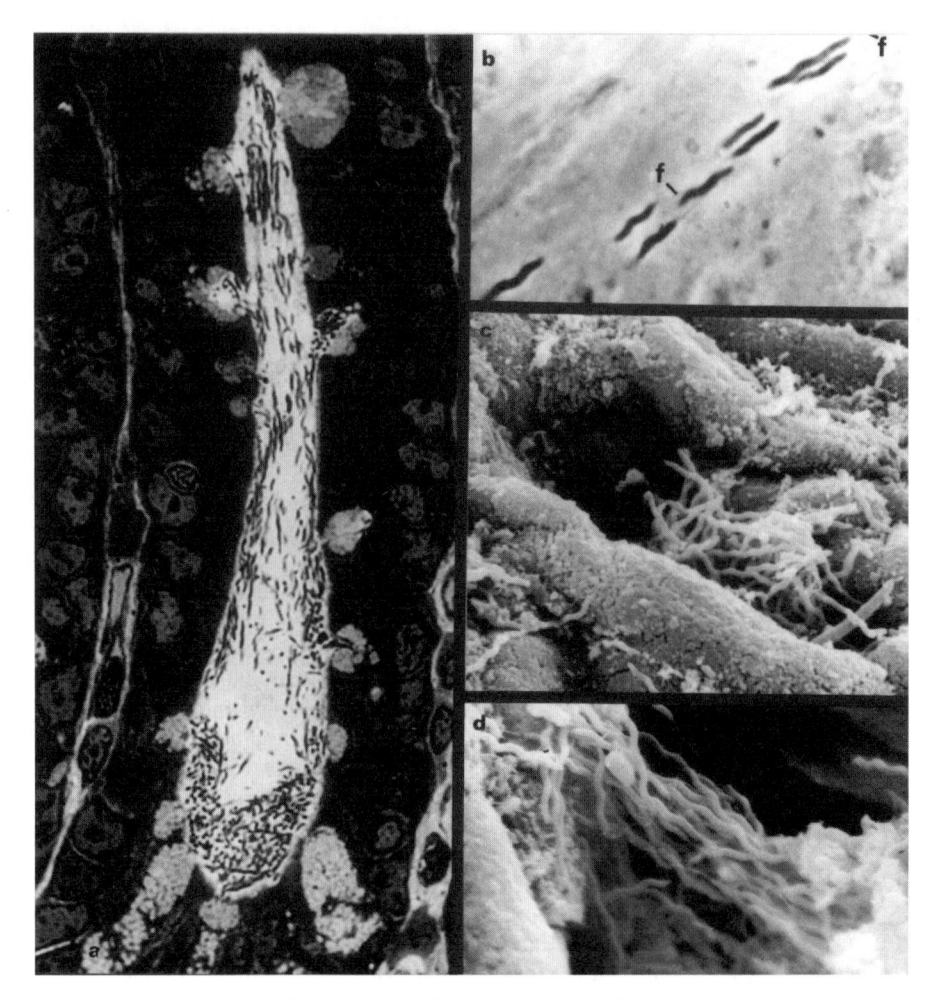

Figure 1. Bacteria in mouse intestinal mucus.

relationship, as is seen with the lumenal lower bowel flora, i.e. colonization of the mucus niche by these evolved normal flora prevents colonization of this niche by potentially pathogenic bacteria. It is interesting that the two well-established pathogens with a spiral, curved morphology that suggests they are also adapted for mucus colonization, *Vibrio cholerae* and *Campylobacter jejuni*, infect the small bowel mucus where there is no resident spiral normal flora.

THE INTESTINAL *HELICOBACTERS* AS PATHOGENS IN ANIMALS

If these bacteria translocate from the gut, they can become opportunistic pathogens in animals, as has been well described in Chapter 10 on the

Table 1. The intestinal *Helicobacter* species and the animals from which they were first isolated

Helicobacter species	Animal of origin	Reference
H. muridarum	Mouse	Lee et al., 1992[1]
H. rodentium	Mouse	Shen et al., 1997[2]
H. hepaticus	Mouse	Fox et al., 1994[3]
H. bilis	Mouse	Fox et al., 1995[4]
H. canis	Dog	Stanley et al., 1993[5]
H. trongontum	Rat	Mendes et al., 1996[6]
H. cholecystus	Syrian Hamster	Franklin et al., 1996[7]
H. pametensis	Birds	Dewhirst et al., 1994[8]
H. cineadi	Human, Hamster	Totten et al., 1985[9]
H. fennelliae	Human, Hamster	Totten et al., 1985[9]
H. pullorum	Chickens, Human	Stanley et al., 1994[10]
'H. typhylonicus'	Mouse	Franklin et al., 1999[11]
'H. colifelis'	Cat	Foley et al., 1998[12]
'H. rappini'	Mice	Schauer et al., 1993[12]
'H. sp.-cottontop'	Cotton top Tamarin	Saunders et al., 1999[14]

hepatic *Helicobacters*. What about causing disease in their normal intestinal niche? There is no doubt that these bacteria do indeed induce significant pathology in the lower intestine of immunocompromised animals. The early demonstrations in mice[15] with *H. hepaticus* have recently been repeated such that Koch's postulates have been fulfilled. Shomer et al. inoculated pure cultures of *H. bilis* by intraperitoneal injection into Tac:Icr:Ha(ICR)-scidfDF mice[16]. The bacteria colonized the mucosa of the caecum and colon and induced varying degrees of inflammatory bowel disease including typhocolitis, crypt hyperplasia, loss of goblet cells and focal mucosal necrosis and suppuration. The number of lower bowel *Helicobacter* species shown to induce changes in the large bowel is increasing, as is the range of immunocompromised mouse strains tested. Thus, a novel urease-negative species was shown to induce colitis and typhilitis in IL-10-deficient mice as well as SCID/NCR and A/JNCR mice[17]. This organism has been provisionally named '*Helicobacter typhlonicus*'[11]. The same may soon be demonstrated in other animal species.

The cottontop tamarin has proved to be an excellent model of human ulcerative colitis. The disease develops spontaneously in approximately 50% of colony-maintained animals. Approximately 25–40% of those with colitis progress to colonic adenocarinoma. In both humans and the primate, clinical features include chronic wasting, bloody diarrhoea and weight loss. The disease in both species responds to sulphadiazine and steroid therapy. Therefore, it is of great interest that a novel *Helicobacter* species has been isolated from tamarins with chronic colitis[14]. The parallels with the mouse models are striking. Similar inoculation studies to the IL-10 mouse experiment in *Helicobacter*-free tamarins are awaited with interest.

Other associations of *Helicobacter* species with disease have been described in cats. In two recent studies, *H. canis* was isolated from a colony of Bengal cats with endemic diarrhoea. A novel *Helicobacter* species was isolated from a kitten, also with severe diarrohea[12,18].

Distinction of these bacteria as pathogen or normal flora remains controversial. Parallels to arguments made in the debate with respect to *H. pylori* are seen here. Rodent inflammatory bowel disease (IBD) is only seen when the host has changed, i.e. become immunodeficient. The cottontop IBD is seen only when the environment changes; i.e. apparently this condition is not seen in tamarins in the wild.

THE LOWER BOWEL *HELICOBACTERS* – DO WE HAVE THEM?

A key question with respect to these new *Helicobacter* species is 'Are they present in the human gut?' Logic would suggest they are. In a study, published the same year as the discovery of *H. pylori*, Croucher examined the surface of the lower bowel of four road accident victims[19]. In the mucus of one of these presumably normal intestines, lightly spiralled bacteria with the typical morphology of *Helicobacter* species were seen. Comparison with similar preparations of mouse intestinal mucus known to be colonized with *Helicobacter rappini* highlights this similarity[13] (Figure 2).

H. fenneliae and *H. cinaedi* have been isolated from the stools of, usually homosexual, patients with proctitis and proctocolitis[9,20,21]. *H. pullorum* has been isolated from humans with gastroenteritis[10,22–24]. As blood culture techniques improve there have been many reports of *Helicobacter* bacteraemia with *H. fenneliae* and *H. cinaedi*, *H. rappini*, *H. westmeadii* and others[20,21,25–36].

Just as with some of the animal studies, causality in these diseases is not proven but often assumed by the authors. One of our very early animal studies, published 10 years before the publication of the Marshall and Warren letters, is relevant here[37]. Spiral bacteria, now known to be *Helicobacter* species, were observed in sections of gut tissue or mucus scrapings. However, these bacteria were rarely seen in specimens of stool. Yet if we induced severe diarrhoea with magnesium sulphate, the luminal bacteria were flushed out and spiral bacteria were the only organisms seen in the diarrhoea stool. We suggested that this experiment challenged the evidence of canine spirochaetosis, a disease for which evidence of aetiology was based solely on observation of spiral organisms in stool. We reasoned that the diarrhoea could be of another cause and the spirals were simply flushed out normal flora. In the kitten study described above, diarrhoea was not induced when faeces from the diarrhoeal kitten was inoculated in pure culture to other kittens. In short, isolation of a *Helicobacter* species from human specimens does not prove causality. Much more rigorous proof is required.

HELICOBACTERS AND CIVILIZATION

Lack of isolation of lower bowel *Helicobacter* species consistently from human specimens could be simply due to a lack of use of the fastidious methods needed for culture of these bacteria. An alternative explanation could be a similar situation found with *H. pylori*. That is, as humans become more civilized so they lose their gastric *Helicobacters*. Could the developed

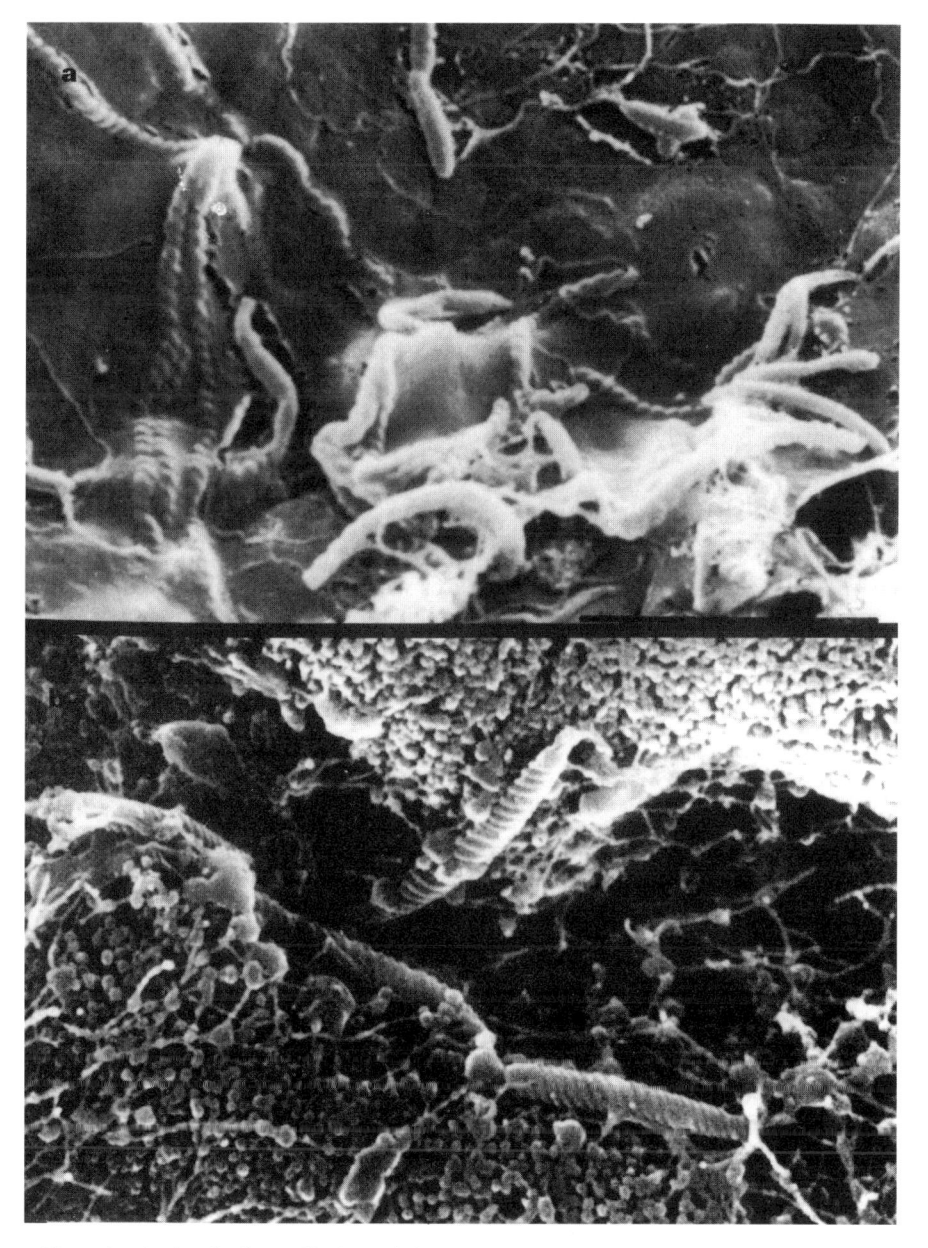

Figure 2. (*top*) *Helicobacter*-like bacteria in the mucus of the human large bowel (from ref. 19). (*bottom*) Helicobacter species on the large bowel mucosa of mice (from ref. 13).

world also have lost their lower bowel *Helicobacter* species? I predict that, in the future, these bacteria will be found to be normal flora of the intestine of many humans in the developing world. It is even possible that as a consequence of evolution they play a beneficial role either by protecting the intestinal mucus from colonization by potential pathogens or protecting the mucosa by exerting an immunomodulating role. Should this bacterial balance change, could not the disease potential of bacteria in the mucus change? This is the niche closest to the mucosa and the most likely to induce damage should conditions change from 'normal'. Could this be why IBD is always seen in the developed world? The lower bowel *Helicobacters* probably do not cause IBD in humans as they do in the animal models. However, these models will tell us much about the role of mucus-associated bacteria and large bowel inflammation. The observation that the intestinal mucus layers from human patients with IBD contain higher numbers of bacteria compared to controls is clearly relevant to these speculations[38].

CONCLUSION

The next few years will see a continuation of the explosion of the genus *Helicobacter*. Many new intestinal species will be discovered in humans and experimental animals. The challenge remains to demonstrate disease causation in humans and to understand mechanisms of pathogenesis in other animals.

References

1. Lee A, Phillips MW, O'Rourke JL et al. *Helicobacter muridarum* sp. nov., a microaerophilic helical bacterium with a novel ultrastructure isolated from the intestinal mucosa of rodents. Int J Syst Bacteriol. 1992;42:27–36.
2. Shen Z, Fox JG, Dewhirst FE et al. *Helicobacter rodentium* sp. nov., a urease-negative *Helicobacter* species isolated from laboratory mice. Int J Syst Bacteriol. 1997;47:627–34.
3. Fox JG, Dewhirst FE, Tully JG et al. *Helicobacter hepaticus* sp. nov., a microaerophilic bacterium isolated from livers and intestinal mucosal scrapings from mice. J Clin Microbiol. 1994;32:1238–45.
4. Fox JG, Yan LL, Dewhirst FE et al. *Helicobacter bilis* sp. nov., a novel *Helicobacter* species isolated from bile, livers, and intestines of aged, inbred mice. J Clin Microbiol. 1995; 33:445–54.
5. Stanley J, Linton D, Burnens AP et al. *Helicobacter canis* sp. nov., a new species from dogs – an integrated study of phenotype and genotype. J Gen Microbiol. 1993;139:2495–504.
6. Mendes EN, Queiroz DMM, Dewhirst FE, Paster BJ, Moura SB, Fox JG. *Helicobacter trogontum* sp. nov., isolated from the rat intestine. Int J Syst Bacteriol. 1996;46:916–21.
7. Franklin CL, Beckwith CS, Livingston RS et al. Isolation of a novel *Helicobacter* species, *Helicobacter cholecystus* sp. nov., from the gallbladders of syrian hamsters with cholangiofibrosis and centrilobular pancreatitis. J Clin Microbiol. 1996;34:2952–8.
8. Dewhirst FE, Seymour C, Fraser GJ, Paster BJ, Fox JG. Phylogeny of *Helicobacter* isolates from bird and swine feces and description of *Helicobacter pametensis* sp. nov. Int J Syst Bact. 1994;44:553–60.
9. Totten PA, Fennell CL, Tenover FC et al. *Campylobacter cinaedi* (sp. nov.) and *Campylobacter fennelliae* (sp. nov.): two new *Campylobacter* species associated with enteric disease in homosexual men. J Infect Dis. 1985;151:131–9.
10. Stanley J, Linton D, Burnens AP et al. *Helicobacter pullorum* sp. nov. – genotype and phenotype of a new species isolated from poultry and from human patients with gastroenteritis. Microbiology-UK. 1994;140:3441–9.

11. Franklin CL, Riley LK, Livingston RS et al. Enteric lesions in SCID mice infected with 'Helicobacter typhlonicus', a novel urease-negative Helicobacter species. Lab Anim Sci. 1999;49:496-505.
12. Foley JE, Solnick JV, Lapointe JM, Jang S, Pedersen NC. Identification of a novel enteric Helicobacter species in a kitten with severe diarrhea. J Clin Microbiol. 1998;36:908-12.
13. Schauer DB, Ghori N, Falkow S. Isolation and characterisation of 'Flexispira rappini' from laboratory mice. J Clin Microbiol. 1993;31:2709-14.
14. Saunders KE, Shen ZL, Dewhirst FE, Paster BJ, Dangler CA, Fox JG. Novel intestinal Helicobacter species isolated from cotton-top tamarins (Saguinus oedipus) with chronic colitis. J Clin Microbiol. 1999;37:146-51.
15. Cahill RJ, Foltz CJ, Fox JG, Dangler CA, Powrie F, Schauer DB. Inflammatory bowel disease – an immunity-mediated condition triggered by bacterial infection with Helicobacter hepaticus. Infect Immun. 1997;65:3126-31.
16. Shomer NH, Dangler CA, Schrenzel MD, Fox JG. Helicobacter bilis-induced inflammatory bowel disease in scid mice with defined flora. Infect Immun. 1997;65:4858-64.
17. Fox JG, Gorelick PL, Kullberg MC, Ge ZM, Dewhirst FE, Ward JM. Novel urease-negative Helicobacter species associated with colitis and typhlitis in IL-10-deficient mice. Infect Immun. 1999;67:1757-62.
18. Foley JE, Marks SL, Munson L et al. Isolation of Helicobacter canis from a colony of Bengal cats with endemic diarrhea. J Clin Microbiol. 1999;37:3271-5.
19. Croucher S, Houston A, Bayliss C, Turner R. Bacterial populations associated with different regions of the human colon wall. Appl Environ Microbiol. 1983;45:1025-33.
20. Tee W, Street AC, Spelman D, Munckhof W, Mijch A. Helicobacter cinaedi bacteraemia – varied clinical manifestations in three homosexual males. Scand J Infect Dis. 1996;28:199-203.
21. Orlicek SL, Welch DF, Kuhls TL. Septicemia and meningitis caused by Helicobacter cinaedi in a neonate. J Clin Microbiol. 1993;31:569-71.
22. Burnens AP, Stanley J, Morgenstern R, Nicolet J. Gastroenteritis associated with Helicobacter pullorum. Lancet. 1994;344:1569-70.
23. Steinbrueckner B, Haerter G, Pelz K et al. Isolation of Helicobacter pullorum from patients with enteritis. Scand J Infect Dis. 1997;29:315-18.
24. Atabay HI, Corry JEL, On SLW. Identification of unusual Campylobacter-like isolates from poultry products as Helicobacter pullorum. J Appl Microbiol. 1998;84:1017-24.
25. Kemper CA, Mickelsen P, Morton A, Walton B, Deresinski SC. Helicobacter-(Campylobacter) fennelliae-like organisms as an important but occult cause of bacteraemia in a patient with AIDS. J Infect. 1993;26:97-101.
26. Kiehlbauch JA, Tauxe RV, Baker CN, Wachsmuth IK. Helicobacter cinaedi-associated bacteremia and cellulitis in immunocompromised patients. Ann Intern Med. 1994;121:90-93.
27. Burman WJ, Cohn DL, Reves RR, Wilson ML. Multifocal cellulitis and monoarticular arthritis as manifestations of Helicobacter cinaedi bacteremia. Clin Infect Dis. 1995;20:564-70.
28. Mammen MP, Aronson NE, Edenfield WJ, Endy TP. Recurrent Helicobacter cinaedi bacteremia in a patient infected with human immunodeficiency virus – case report. Clin Infect Dis. 1995;21:
29. Vanderven A, Kullberg BJ, Vandamme P, Meis J. Helicobacter cinaedi bacteremia associated with localized pain but not with cellulitis. Clin Infect Dis. 1996;22:710-12.
30. Sullivan AK, Nelson MR, Walsh J, Gazzard BG. Recurrent Helicobacter cinaedi cellulitis and bacteraemia in a patient with HIV infection. Int J STD AIDS. 1997;8:59-60.
31. Trivett-Moore NL, Rawlinson WD, Yuen M, Gilbert GL. Helicobacter westmeadii sp. nov., a new species isolated from blood cultures of two AIDS patients. J Clin Microbiol. 1997;35:1144-50.
32. Hung CC, Hsueh PR, Chen MY et al. Bacteremia caused by Helicobacter cinaedi in an AIDS patient. J Formosan Med Assoc. 1997;96:558-60.
33. Tee W, Leder K, Karroum E, Dyallsmith M. Flexispira rappini bacteremia in a child with pneumonia. J Clin Microbiol. 1998;36:1679-82.
34. Sorlin P, Vandamme P, Nortier J et al. Recurrent 'Flexispira rappini' bacteremia in an adult patient undergoing hemodialysis: Case report. J Clin Microbiol. 1999;37:1319-23.
35. Weir S, Cuccherini B, Whiney AM et al. Recurrent bacteremia caused by a 'Flexispira'-like organism in a patient with X-linked (Bruton's) agammaglobulinemia. J Clin Microbiol. 1999;37:2439-45.

36. Weir SC, Gibert CL, Gordin FM, Fischer SH, Gill VJ. An uncommon *Helicobacter* isolate from blood: evidence of a group of *Helicobacter* spp. pathogenic in AIDS patients. J Clin Microbiol. 1999;37:2729–33.
37. Leach WD, Lee A, Stubbs RP. Localization of bacteria in the gastrointestinal tract: a possible explanation of intestinal spirochaetosis. Infect Immun. 1973;7:961–72.
38. Schultsz C, Van Den Berg F, Ten Kate F, Tytgat G, Dankert J. The intestinal mucus layer from patients with inflammatory bowel disease harbors high numbers of bacteria compared with controls. Gastroenterology. 1999;117:1089–7.

Section IV
Diagnosis of *Helicobacter pylori* infection

12
Diagnosis of *Helicobacter pylori* infection: faecal antigen determination

D. VAIRA, C. RICCI, M. MENEGATTI, C. ACCIARDI,
L. GATTA, A. GEMINIANI and M. MIGLIOLI

INTRODUCTION

Helicobacter pylori is a human pathogen that causes chronic gastritis, has a role in gastric and duodenal ulcer, is involved in gastric carcinogenesis and the bacteria have been classified as a class I or definite gastric carcinogen to humans[1]. *H. pylori* is also regarded as a possible important factor in at least a subset of patients with functional dyspepsia. Beside its definite role as a gastroduodenal pathogen, *H. pylori* is now being actively investigated for possible involvement in various non-gastrointestinal conditions such as impaired growth, coronary heart disease, migraine headache, Reynaud's phenomenon, diabetes and gallstone disease[2].

H. pylori causes a chronic gastric infection, which is usually life-long, and many epidemiological studies have shown that this is probably one of the most common bacterial infections throughout the world, involving 50% of the population in developed countries and up to 80–90% of the population in developing regions[3]. It is, therefore, clear that the diagnosis of *H. pylori* infection represents at the least a key step in the management of many of the patients referred to the gastroenterologist. However, due to the wide range and relevance of pathologies possibly related to infection, including malignancies, there is the potential for *H. pylori* to be a major health problem.

H. pylori infection can be diagnosed by both endoscopy, and non-endoscopic techniques, which do not require endoscopy with biopsy sampling[4]. Each of the available diagnostic techniques has advantages as well as disadvantages, and it is now clear that the discussion over the different diagnostic methods cannot be oversimplified by thinking just in terms of 'which is the best diagnostic tool?' The problem should be more directly addressed by asking 'what is the best diagnostic tool in each definitive situation'. This means that the choice has to take into account different factors such as whether we dealing with normal subjects screened for epidemiological purposes or with a patient referred to a gastroenterologist. If a patient is already following a failed eradication attempt are we are looking for susceptibility to antibodies? Are we aiming at diagnosing the infection in a clinical setting or are we interested in other possibly relevant factors? These might include putative markers of increased virulence/pathogenicity of the strain such as *cagA* or *vacA* which are more commonly sought in a research setting. Eventually we should also ask when the cost of the diagnostic technique is relevant. We must take into account all the factors involved, such as the need for the endoscopy, for a technician/nurse to assist the patient, the need for a dedicated laboratory, instrumentation/material to evaluate breath sample, etc. or the use of facilities already widely available even in a small hospital or in developing countries, as is usually the case for serology.

Bearing in mind these and other similar questions, we will discuss the possibility of testing stool samples, to non-invasively diagnose *H. pylori* infection.

Until now there have been only two widely available non-invasive methods (1) ^{13}C or ^{14}C labelled urea breath test (UBT – which is based on the detection of ^{13}C or ^{14}C labelled CO_2 expired air as result of *H. pylori* urease activity)[4,5] and (2) serology, which is based on the detection of a specific anti-*H. pylori* immune response, mostly by IgG antibodies, in a patient's serum[4–6]. Being non-invasive these tests, most often serology due to simplicity and lower cost, have been widely employed in epidemiological studies to assess the prevalence of *H. pylori* infection in different populations. Apart from epidemiological research, non-invasive *H. pylori* testing can be successfully employed in two other settings: (1) pre-endoscopic screening of patients to refer to a gastroenterology service for investigation of dyspepsia and (2) therapeutic monitoring following eradication therapy to confirm cure of infection. The widespread availability of endoscopy means that this technique has become the mainstay for investigation of dyspepsia, and this has led to increased waiting lists and medical costs. In an attempt to obviate the need for endoscopy, without affecting the safety of the patients, several pre-endoscopic screening procedures have been proposed. It has been shown that young *H. pylori*-negative patients, as determined via non-invasive tests, without alarm symptoms or taking NSAIDs, could safely avoid endoscopy and be treated with a trial of medical therapy. Endoscopy could be reserved for those whose symptoms do not improve, or who relapse shortly after discontinuing therapy[7].

On the other hand, apart from patients with gastric ulcer, who probably are best managed with endoscopy due to the possibility of underlying gastric malignancy, two approaches have been advocated for patients treated with *H. pylori* eradication regimens: (1) wait and see (i.e. not testing to confirm eradication, assuming that if patients experience prolonged symptom relief this could be taken as an indirect sign of successful eradication). This approach may not be accepted by some patients for whom fear of the consequences of *H. pylori* infection requires a positive confirmation of eradication. Moreover, such a strategy is based on the unproven assumption of a clear relationship between *H. pylori* infection and symptoms; and (2) test and confirm eradication, which is probably best accomplished with non-invasive testing, bearing in mind that the UBT can be used 4 weeks after treatment, whilst serology requires waiting for a longer period to permit a fall in the antibody titre.

THE *H. PYLORI* STOOL ASSAYS

Over the past few years it has become possible to culture *H. pylori* from stool, but viable organisms are present in only a small percentage of cases[8]. Despite the difficulties encountered in stool culture the fact that the organism was sometimes present raised the possibility of developing a non-invasive diagnostic test based on the detection of bacterial antigen in stool. Over the past 2 years, an enzymatic immunoassay (EIA), which detects the presence of *H. pylori* antigen in stool, has become available (HpSA^{TM} – *H. pylori* Stool Antigen, Meridian Diagnostics Inc., Cincinnati, USA). This has now been tested in clinical practice to evaluate its performance compared to that of the other available diagnostic tests.

The HpSA test has recently been approved by the United States Food and Drugs Administration (FDA) for two indications: diagnosis of *H. pylori* infection in symptomatic adult patients and monitoring response to therapy in adult patients. The test utilizes polyclonal anti-*H. pylori* antibody absorbed to microwells. The stool specimen can be stored at 2–8°C for up to 3 days or indefinitely at −20°C before the test. This makes it possible to collect multiple samples over several days or weeks, which is valuable in a small hospital with a low number of patients, to be tested in one session, thus reducing the cost. Moreover, this allows the storage of samples, which could be employed in future analysis. A small portion of the specimen is diluted and no further manipulation is needed.

Diluted faecal samples and a peroxidase conjugated polyclonal antibody are added to the wells and incubated for 1 h at room temperature, followed by washing to remove unbound material. Substrate is then added and incubated for 10 min at room temperature. In the presence of bound *H. pylori* antigens, a colour change develops. Finally, a stop solution is added and the results are read spectrophotometrically (450 nm). According to the manufacturer's instruction, the cut off values are as follows: <0.140 negative (i.e. no *H. pylori* antigens in the stool sample, patients not infected); 0.140 to 0.159 equivocal/indeterminate. According to the manufacturer's instruction, indeterminate results should be repeated. If the repeat result is equivocal, a new specimen should be obtained. If the result is ≥0.160 it is positive and *H. pylori* antigens are present in the stool samples, indicating that the patient is infected.

It is clear that such a test, which detects bacterial antigen in an actual ongoing infection, is theoretically useful not only for screening, but also as an early predictor of successful treatment. In this section we will briefly consider the currently available evidence supporting a possible role for a non-invasive diagnostic test.

Table 1. Prospective European multicentre study: sensitivity and specificity of HpSA compared to ^{13}C UBT before and after treatment (percentages)

	Before therapy (n = 501 patients)		After therapy (n = 133 patients)	
	HpSA	^{13}C UBT	HpSA	^{13}C UBT
Sensitivity	94.3	95.3	92.3	88.5
Specificity	91.8	97.7	96.2	99.4

As this test has become available only recently, it is understandable that there are only a few studies, most of which are on limited populations, assessing the diagnostic accuracy in terms of sensitivity and specificity compared to standardized techniques. This is particularly true in studies assessing patients post-eradication. A remarkable exception to these points comes from a European multicentre study carried out in 11 endoscopic units with a specific interest in *H. pylori* infection[9]. The first part of this prospective study was planned to assess the accuracy of HpSA compared to standardized techniques. The authors enrolled 501 consecutive patients, not previously treated for *H. pylori* infection, who underwent endoscopy with multiple biopsies, for histology in both antrum and corpus, rapid urease test and culture and ^{13}C UBT. A stool sample was collected from all patients. According to the recently published guidelines for clinical trials[10] in *H. pylori* infection, patients were considered *H. pylori*-positive if at least two tests were positive. If culture alone was positive, in view of its absolute specificity the patients were also considered positive. Using this gold standard, the overall sensitivity and specificity for the two tests were 94% (CI 90.6–96.6) and 91.8% (CI 87.3–95.1) versus 95.3% (CI 94.8–99.3) for HpSA and ^{13}C UBT respectively (Table 1). It is also important to emphasize that, in this study, clear-cut results were obtained for most of the patients, with only 10/501 tests (2%) giving equivocal results.

There appears to be agreement that HpSA is very accurate in untreated patients (Table 2)[9,11–21]. The issue, however, concerns its value as a test of successful bacterial eradication after treatment (Table 3)[12,13,15,17,22]. Controversial results were reported by two authors. The first study[13], by Makristathis *et al.*, reports a specificity of 68.3% for HpSA in 55 patients tested 4 weeks following treatment. Surprisingly, in this study, PCR had a lower specificity of 48.8%. The authors found 21 and 13 positive results for PCR and HpSA respectively in 41 patients successfully treated as assessed by histology and culture. These findings cast some doubt on the validity of the histology and culture results obtained. In contrast to the above report, a recent study by Trevisani *et al.*[12] reported a sensitivity and specificity of 93% and 82% respectively in 116 patients after treatment. They obtained 12 false-positive results by HpSA but used a fixed cut-off without grey zone. In fact, most of the false-positive cases in their study were borderline. A key point in our study is that we recognized a grey zone from 0.140 to 0.159. We undertook a multicentre study, involving dedicated centres. In the 501 patients the sensitivity and the specificity of UBT were performed independently in each centre, as well as the HpSA, giving values of 95.3% and

Table 2. Pretreatment diagnostic accuracy of HpSA: papers ($n = 1793$ patients)

Reference	Patients ($n = 1793$)	Sensitivity (%)	Specificity (%)
11, Italy	107	92.6	96
12, Italy	146	94	90
13, Austria	100	93.7	88.9
9, Europe	501	94.1	91.8
14, Italy	84	98.2	96.4
15, Italy	45	91	100
16, Greece	43	89	100
17, Germany	90	92.2	97.4
18, Italy	203	98	99
19, Austria	72	80	98
20, Switzerland	102	96	93
21, Italy	300	96.8	89.7
Weighted mean		93	95

Table 3. Post-treatment diagnostic accuracy of HpSA: papers ($n = 566$)

Reference	Patients ($n = 566$)	Sensitivity (%)	Specificity (%)
13, Austria	55	85.7	68.3
12, Italy	116	93	82
15, Italy	45	73	93
17, Germany	115	91.3	94.6
22, Europe	235	93.8	96.9

97.7% respectively with 13 false-positive and five false-negative results for UBT.

We have recently presented our post-therapy follow-up study[22] conducted in 10 of the 11 European centres, involved in the first paper. We were able to confirm the sensitivity and specificity of the HpSA and UBT of 93.8% and 96.9%, and 90.6% and 99.2% respectively. These results were assessed against endoscopy-based tests for *H. pylori* status. In 162 re-endoscoped patients 4 weeks after stopping treatment there were in the HpSA results: four false-positive, one indeterminate, two false-negative; and in the ^{13}C UBT results: one false-positive; three false-negative. Two other papers support our findings. The first, from Germany, reports a sensitivity and specificity of 91.3% and 94.6% in 115 patients assessed 4 weeks after treatment[17]. The second, in children with a mean age of 7 years, reports a sensitivity and specificity of 100% and 97.2% respectively[18].

Apart from evaluating the accuracy of the HpSA compared to other tests, several interesting issues are being addressed by investigators around the world. Up to now these are largely in abstract form and include the possible influence of concomitant use of proton-pump inhibitors (PPI)[23]; the kinetics of stool antigen during and after therapy[24,25]; the possibility of cross-reaction with antigen from bacteria other than *H. pylori*[26]; the possibility that HpSA may detect CLO and histology-negative *H. pylori*-infected patients[27] and finally the cost-effectiveness of the test[28].

Taylor et al.[26] evaluated the HpSA for possible cross-reactivity with *Helicobacter* species other than *H. pylori*, including *H. canis*, *H. rodentium*, *H. felis*, *H. pullorum*, *H. cineady*, *H. fenneliae*, *H. bilis*, *H. hepaticus*, *H. rappini* and *H. bizzozzeroni*. The study was carried out in animal models using faeces from *Helicobacter*-infected animals: mice, ferrets and cats. The authors found that other *Helicobacter* species, some of which have been reported in human disease, react with the *H. pylori* antigen capture assay. They concluded that these data require confirmation in a human study to determine the relevance of these findings in a clinical setting.

Hsu and colleagues[27] investigated four *H. pylori*-positive patients undergoing eradication treatment. In these patients stool samples were collected every other day during antibiotic treatment and at 4 weeks after treatment. Eradication was confirmed by ^{13}C-UBT, biopsies from the antrum and corpus for culture, CLO test and histology. The authors found that, at 4 weeks, incomplete eradication in two patients resulted in a positive UBT and HpSA, but negative endoscopy tests, and they concluded that larger-scale studies will be needed to verify the cost-effectiveness of HpSA as a non-invasive test for eradication.

The topic of the cost-effectiveness of HpSA was addressed by Vakil[28]. He established a model based on the cost-effectiveness of stool testing, UBT, office serology, ELISA serology and whole blood testing in the initial diagnosis of the *H. pylori* infection and the cost-effectiveness of UBT and stool studies in patients given eradication therapy. In this US model, Vakil found that, before therapy, the stool test compared favourably to the other techniques assuming a prevalence of *H. pylori* infection of 30% in dyspeptic patients. When the prevalence of infection dropped to 19% the stool test was the most cost-effective because of the higher specificity than office-based blood/serum tests. In post-therapy testing the stool test was cost-effective compared to ^{14}C and ^{13}C-UBT with an average cost of \$183/197 versus 213/99 versus 369/105 respectively. He concluded that: (1) stool tests are a cost-effective alternative to office based serology testing and that (2) their most promising role is in post-treatment assessment.

CONCLUSION

From the data available, it seems that the *H. pylori* stool antigen assay represents a very accurate diagnostic tool to detect *H. pylori* infection both before and shortly after therapy. As a test which is non-invasive, accurate, simple and cost-effective, it has the potential to become the preferred diagnostic tool in many different clinical settings from epidemiological studies to paediatric investigation, from pre-endoscopic screening strategies to post-therapy monitoring.

References

1. International Agency for Research on Cancer, World Health Organisation. Infection with *Helicobacter pylori*. In: Schistosomes, Liver Flukes and *Helicobacter pylori*. Lyon: IARC; 1994:177–202.

2. Gasbarrini A, Franceschi F, Gasbarrini G, Pola P. Extraintestinal pathology associated with *Helicobacter* infection. Eur J Gastroenterol Hepatol. 1997;9:231–3.
3. Vaira D, Miglioli M, Mulè P et al. Prevalence of peptic ulcer in *Helicobacter pylori* positive blood donors. Gut. 1994;35:309–12.
4. Mégraud F. How should *Helicobacter pylori* infection be diagnosed? Gastroenterology. 1997;112:S93–8.
5. Logan RPH. The ^{13}C urea breath test. In: Lee A, Mégraud F, editors. *Helicobacter pylori*: Technique for Clinical Diagnosis and Basic Research. Philadelphia: Saunders; 1996:74–81.
6. Vaira D, Stanghellini V, Menegatti M, Miglioli M, Corinaldesi R and The Italian *Helicobacter* Study Group. IgG ELISA antibodies and detection of *Helicobacter pylori* in elderly patients. Lancet. 1996;1:269–70.
7. Vaira D, Stanghellini V, Menegatti M, Palli D, Corinaldesi R, Miglioli M. Prospective screening of dyspeptic patients by *Helicobacter pylori* serology: a safe policy? Endoscopy. 1997;29:595–601.
8. Thomas JE, Gibson GR, Darboe MK, Dale A, Weaver LT. Isolation of *Helicobacter pylori* from human faeces. Lancet. 1992;340:1194–5.
9. Vaira D, Malfertheiner P, Mégraud F et al. and the European *Helicobacter pylori* HPSA Study Group. Diagnosis of *Helicobacter pylori* infection using a novel, noninvasive antigen based assay in a European multicentre study. Lancet. 1999;354:30–3.
10. Working party of the European *Helicobacter pylori* Study Group. Technical annex: tests used to assess *Helicobacter pylori* infection. In: Guidelines for Clinical Trials in *Helicobacter* Infection. Gut. 1997;41(Suppl. 2):S10–18.
11. Trevisani L, Sartori S, Galvani F et al. Detection of *Helicobacter pylori* in faeces with a new enzyme immunoassay method: preliminary results. Scand J Gastroenterol. 1998;33:893.
12. Trevisani L, Sartori S, Galvani F et al. Evaluation of a new enzyme immunoassay for detecting *Helicobacter pylori* in faeces; a prospective pilot study. Am J Gastroenterol. 1999;94:1831–3.
13. Makristathis A, Pasching E, Schùtze K et al. Detection of *Helicobacter pylori* in stool specimens by PCR and antigen enzyme immunoassay. J Clin Microbiol. 1998;36:2772–4.
14. Fanti L, Mezzi G, Cavallero A, Gesu G, Bonato C, Masci E. A new simple immunoassay for detecting *Helicobacter pylori* infection: antigen in stool specimens. Digestion. 1999;60:456–60.
15. Plebani M, Basso D. Diagnosis of *Helicobacter pylori* infection by HpSA test. Lancet. 1999;354:1210.
16. Archimandritis A, Giontzis A, Smilakon S, Tzivras M, Davaris P. Diagnosis of *Helicobacter pylori* infection by HpSA test. Lancet. 1999;2:1210–11.
17. Braden B, Teuber G, Dietrich CF et al. Stool test may defeat breath test: new faecal antigen detects *Helicobacter pylori* infection and eradication. Br Med J. 2000;320:148.
18. Oderda G, Rapa A, Ronchi B et al. High accuracy of the *Helicobacter pylori* stool antigen test for detection of the infection in children. A multicentre Italian study. Br Med J. 2000;320:347–8.
19. Puspok A, Bakos S, Oberhuber G. A new non-invasive method for detection of *Helicobacter*: validity in the routine clinical setting. Eur J Gastroenterol Hepatol. 1999;11:1139–42.
20. Lehmann F, Drewe J, Terraciano L, Stuber R, Frei R, Beglinger C. Comparison of stool immunoassay with standard methods for detecting *Helicobacter pylori* infection. Br Med J. 1999; 319:1409.
21. Trevisani L, Sartori S, Ruina M, Caselli M et al. *Helicobacter pylori* stool antigen test. Clinical evaluation and cost analysis of a new enzyme immunoassay. Dig Dis Sci. 1999;44:2303–6.
22. Vaira D, Malfertheiner P, Mégraud F et al. and the European *Helicobacter pylori* HPSA Study Group. Non-invasive antigen based assay for assessing *Helicobacter pylori* eradication. A European multicenter study. Am J Gastroenterol. 2000 (In press).
23. Vakil N, Affi A, Sundaram M, Robinson J, Dunn B, Phadnis S. Prospective blinded evaluation of the accuracy of a stool test for the detection of *H. pylori*. Gastroenterology. 1999;116:A342.
24. van't Hoff B, Vaira D, Vakil N et al. Early diagnosis of failed *Helicobacter pylori* (HP) eradication using a stool antigen test. Gastroenterology. 2000 (In press).
25. Petersen JR, Adesoji B, Okorodudu A, Mohammed A, Sifuentes D, Soloway RD. Using the *Helicobacter pylori* stool antigen (HpSA) in monitoring antibiotic treatment response of *Helicobacter pylori*. Gastroenterology. 1999;116:A281.

26. Taylor NS, Esteves M, Fox JG. Cross reactivity with *Helicobacter species* assayed with a *Helicobacter pylori* antigen capture assay. Gastroenterology. 1999;116:A830.
27. Hsu RK, Solnick J, Ruebner B. Premier HpSA *Helicobacter pylori* stool antigen may detect CLO and histology negative infection after antibiotic therapy. A prospective study. Gastroenterology. 1999;116:A191.
28. Vakil N. Cost effectiveness of non-invasive testing methods for *H. pylori* before in dyspeptic patients. Am J Gastroenterol. 2000 (In press).

13
Pitfalls in *Helicobacter pylori* diagnosis

P. MALFERTHEINER, A. LEODOLTER and C. GERARDS

INTRODUCTION

Tests for the detection of *Helicobacter pylori* infection embrace a large battery of methods based on varying principles, and represent a model situation with no comparative analogy in infectious diseases. They range from direct visualization in culture and on biopsy samples to measurement of specific bacterial metabolic products, as well as the systemic immune response. The biological samples on which these measurements can be performed include gastric mucosal specimens, gastric juice, breath samples, blood, stool and urine. Some general aspects require consideration for avoiding pitfalls but, in addition, each individual test needs specific attention.

In this chapter general aspects of biopsy-based tests will be touched on briefly. The main consideration will be given to serology and urea breath tests since the faceal antigen test is dealt with elsewhere in this book.

Significant progress has been made in recent years with the introduction of new tests and by learning what factors interfere with test accuracy and influence the interpretation of the test result. Some of the pitfalls have been known for a long time while others have been learned recently.

GENERAL ASPECTS

With the premise that all tests are carefully and properly performed according to the individual directions, there remain some general aspects to be taken into account for the correct interpretation of the results:

(a) The *H. pylori* prevalence in the population studied.
(b) Type of medication taken by the patient prior to and at the time of testing.
(c) Selection of the test best suited for the clinical question.

(a) The sensitivity and specificity of diagnostic tests for the detection of *H. pylori* infection vary from satisfactory to very good, but their usefulness for clinical decision-making also depends on other factors, such as the *H. pylori* prevalence in differing populations. To obtain useful positive or negative predictive values for *H. pylori* infection in a given population, knowledge of the prevalence of *H. pylori* in that population is crucial. To illustrate this we can consider the example from a recent meta-analysis on the value of commercial serological kits, which reported an overall sensitivity of 85% and a specificity of 79%[1]. The authors provided predictive values for the absence or presence of *H. pylori* infection when the *H. pylori* prevalence theoretically changed from 10% to 90% in a given population. In a population with a 10% prevalence of *H. pylori* a negative result almost completely (98%) excludes infection. The chance of infection with the same negative test result in a population with a 90% prevalence of *H. pylori* infection remains at 63%. The opposite occurs with the positive predictive value, which is very high (97%) in the presence of a 90% prevalence, but drops dramatically if the *H. pylori* prevalence is 10%.

For clinical decision-making the physician has to rely on tests with a sufficiently high diagnostic accuracy which, in respect of the local prevalence of infection, provide reliable positive and negative predictive values.

With the commercial serological kits presently available, patients with a duodenal ulcer would probably be correctly diagnosed as *H. pylori*-positive. In contrast, patients with non-ulcer dyspepsia, in which the prevalence of infection ranges between 20% and 40%, would be at risk of a false positive or negative result and inappropriate clinical management.

(b) Several drugs (proton pump inhibitors (PPIs)), bismuth and several antibiotics) are either bactericidal or suppress the growth of *H. pylori in vitro*, or may interfere with urease activity, which may be used as a marker for *H. pylori* detection. Thus, these medications need to be stopped for a sufficient time before testing. However, the time for optimizing the test accuracy needs to take into consideration the class and dose of the drug, as well as the duration of treatment. Different tests are influenced in different ways by these variables.

When testing for eradication of *H. pylori* infection after treatment in clinical trials a 4-week interval is recommended before testing, as experience has confirmed that any test is more likely to result in a false-negative result within that time. After treatment with PPI alone, a period of 5–10 days of drug withdrawal is suggested, but there are many uncertainties in this regard.

With PPI therapy the urea breath test, as well as the stool antigen test, may provide false-negative results, depending on the dose and duration of treatment. This will be discussed in detail in the section on urea breath testing (UBT) and on the stool antigen test. However, endoscopy-based tests, including histology, allow accurate diagnosis even during PPI treatment, if the sites of biopsies are correctly chosen, and take into account the possible disappearance of *H. pylori* from the antrum and the increased bacterial density in the fundus and proximal body of the stomach[2,3].

(c) The selection of proper testing in relation to the clinical problem becomes more important as new strategies for the management of this infection are established. In young patients with dyspepsia, and without alarm symptoms or a family history of malignancy, some guidelines now recommend to test and treat[4]. For this purpose, non-invasive testing such as serology, UBT and stool antigen tests provide the options. In areas with a high prevalence of gastric cancer, endoscopy is required for primary diagnosis. In all other conditions, and in patients > 45 years of age, an endoscopy-based diagnosis is better, because of the ability to detect the degree and type of mucosal damage, especially with respect to premalignant and malignant conditions.

In general, for each specific clinical question the diagnostic tests require careful choice to avoid pitfalls and to optimize management.

I. BIOPSY-BASED TESTS

Biopsy-based tests include the rapid urease test, histology and culture. All rely on biopsies obtained during endoscopy and are prone to sampling error. To reduce the impact of sampling error it is recommended that four or five biopsies are taken for histology, two for the rapid urease test and two for culture taken from defined sites in the stomach in the antrum and body. The tests may also be influenced by different treatments, which interfere with *H. pylori* growth and metabolism. All tests yield the best sensitivity in untreated patients if biopsies are taken from the antrum. During or following PPI treatment the sensitivity is better when biopsies are taken from the proximal stomach[2,3].

Rapid urease tests were widely available and distributed as well-presented test kits, which are accurate and reliable[5]. Reading of any colour change should be done no later than 24 h after biopsy, otherwise the specificity is inappropriately low. Moreover, the colour change is induced by rise in pH, which can be artificially induced in several ways, such as by xylocaine, blood, etc. False-positives also may occur by contamination with urease-producing bacteria from the oral cavity.

For histology, an appropriate stain, such as the modified Giemsa or Warthin–Starry stains, should be used. Appropriate stains lower the inter-observer variation among pathologists, which is still surprisingly high. A well-known pitfall for the pathologist is an area of intestinal metaplasia, which is not colonized by *H. pylori*, and organisms should be diligently sought in different areas of the biopsy specimen.

For culture, the essential requirements include optimal conditions of isolation, transportation and culture media and a close working relationship between the gastroenterologist and microbiologist. Pitfalls are many and beyond the remit of this chapter. The time of transportation, the duration of culture and, in our opinion, dedication of specialized and involved microbiology staff and microbiologist avoid most of these pitfalls.

II. SEROLOGY

Since the appearance of the first serological tests for the detection of *H. pylori* infection in the mid-1980s, these tests have become more attractive because of their precision and the ability to obtain rapid results, their lower costs in comparison to UBT and stool antigen tests and their wide availability[6,7].

Table 1. Pitfalls in *H. pylori* diagnosis: serology

Method-related pitfalls	Cross-reactivity of the antigen
	Lack of antibody production
	Antibody group (IgA, IgM, IgG)
	Titre dynamics of specific antigens
	Rapid blood tests: accurate reading time, observer experience
	Manufacturers' instructions
Clinical application-related pitfalls	Age
	Prevalence of *H. pylori*
	Ethnicity/geographical difference
	Other diseases than *H. pylori*
	Medication (e.g. NSAID)
	Post-eradication
Pitfalls in interpretation of results	Inter-laboratory variability
	Definition of the reference method
	Definition of grey zone, cut-off point, reading point

Based on progress in the development of *H. pylori* serology the European *H. pylori* Study Group recommends non-invasive tests using serology or the UBT at the primary-care level in dyspeptic patients younger than 45 years, who do not present with alarm symptoms[4]. The stool antigen test deserves to be added to these two tests in a new edition of these recommendations. Based on these results clinical management can be directed by the result, provided that local validation of the serological test has been performed. Serology seems more convenient than the UBT or the stool antigen test for the primary diagnosis of *H. pylori* infection in the general practice setting. The follow-up testing after eradication needs separate consideration[7,8] and will be discussed later.

A multitude of different serological tests have been introduced for routine use during the past few years. The most common are conventional ELISA tests, rapid whole-blood/serum tests and immunoblot methods. While conventional ELISA tests can give quantitative results, most of the rapid blood tests only provide a qualitative result. There are still several pitfalls which require caution in the serological assessment of *H. pylori* infection (Table 1).

Serological tests allow the detection of chronic infection but may indicate a pre-existing infection. Acute infections are rare in adults and might be missed due to a delay in antibody production, which could lead to a false-negative result[9].

The detection of IgM antibodies is reported in only 8–10% of infected subjects, mainly in children. IgA titres are not useful because only in 60% or so of infected patients can IgA be detected. The sensitivity of ELISA based on IgA ranges between 65% and 85%. No further improvement in sensitivity or specificity can be achieved by a combination of ELISA IgA + IgG versus IgG alone. Moreover, the combination may even lower the specificity of IgG[10–12].

Immunoblot assays for the detection of *H. pylori* antibodies were originally developed for 'in-house' testing to answer specific scientific questions, particularly concerning the antibody response to specific antigens in relation to disease expression. Recently, immunoblot assays have become commercially available.

These immunoblot kits have a defined antigen preparation and are ready for incubation. This shortens the performance time and reduces the need for special equipment. Studies with these immunoblot kits are more comparable because of the defined antigen spectrum and comparable assay conditions; but, like all other serological tests they need local validation.

Although they have some advantages, immunoblot assays are still not recommended for routine serology for the following reasons:

1. They are much more expensive than ELISA tests and no more accurate.
2. For routine serology, where often only *H. pylori* positivity or negativity is important, time and costs are disproportionate to outcome.
3. Interpretation of results is tricky because, in contrast to ELISA tests, no cut-off is defined. Therefore, sera with few antibodies against specific antigens would result in a positive immunoblot response, even when testing is negative with an ELISA test.
4. There may be a positive antibody reaction against individual specific *H. pylori* antigens such as CagA or VacA without a reaction against other specific *H. pylori* antigens. This is likely to represent a false-positive test result[13].

Furthermore, it has been suggested that the antibody response against specific antigens such as CagA or VacA may be disease-specific and indicate a higher pathogenicity of bacterial strains, but this needs to be evaluated with respect to individual populations[14].

Consequently, immunoblot assays for *H. pylori* are recommended at this time only for scientific studies or as second-line assays for results after first-line testing with ELISA.

II.1. Rapid whole-blood/serum test and other serological tests

In addition to the conventional ELISA test, rapid blood tests offer the advantage of very quick results and can be performed by general practitioners without any special equipment. In the past the problem of rapid blood tests was the limited accuracy, but recent data from the US suggest an accuracy which is comparable with ELISA tests[15-17]; nevertheless the overall accuracy of these tests is still limited. When using these tests as a sole means of testing *H. pylori*, clinicians should be particularly aware of these limitations.

Several aspects must be considered: first the reading time of rapid blood tests is critical. A time of 10 min[18] to 3 h[19,20] using different kits has been reported. Increasing the reading time increases sensitivity. On the other hand the false-negative rate decreases with longer time periods[19]. Second, subjectivity in the interpretation of the tests is a problem; 10% of rapid blood tests were difficult to read in a study reported by Stone *et al*[18]. Third, a very weak colour change in a rapid blood test should be regarded with caution[18]. Increasing the grey zone in order to increase the accuracy of the test is at the expense of less certain results. Enroth *et al.* suggested that the higher the antibody in the sample observed by serology, the stronger and more reliable the visual scoring of the rapid test would be[21]. Inter-observer errors may also occur even when the test is considered readable[18].

Saliva antibody tests show a low sensitivity and specificity and have the same problems as conventional serological tests in the definition of cut-off points[22,23]. Even the combination of two different serological tests does not always result in detection of *H. pylori* infection with a high sensitivity or specificity (sensitivity 60–95%, specificity 79–95%)[9].

II.2. Pitfalls related to clinical application

The consistency of a test must be established in different geographical and regional settings[23]. Sometimes there is a need to modify the manufacturers' instructions in order to improve the performance of a test[24].

The result of a serological test must be considered in relation to the clinical application. Serological results might be influenced by the patient sample, the size of the group, age and ethnic background, prevalence of *H. pylori* infection in the test population, underlying diseases of the test group and their medical treatment, and the titre in the individual patient after eradication.

There is a special relationship between serological *H. pylori* positivity and gastric cancer; and in many studies blood samples for *H. pylori* testing were obtained long before the disease was diagnosed. Serology in samples taken at the time of disease manifestation, however, indicates a lower prevalence of *H. pylori*, because at this stage the ecological environment for *H. pylori* colonization may have been lost through gastric atrophy as well as the declining antibodies.

However, once gastric cancer is established serological results are still more frequently positive than histology[13,21,25]. The antibody spectrum has been reported to be different between *H. pylori*-positive controls and cancer patients. A higher seropositivity against low-molecular-weight bands (< 28 kDa) and in the 33–66 kDa region was observed in control individuals compared with *H. pylori*-positive gastric cancer patients. In patients with gastric cancer the antibody recognition of high-molecular antigens such as to CagA or VacA is better preserved[13].

NSAIDs may influence the specificity of some serological tests for *H. pylori* infection[24]. Proton-pump inhibitors or antibiotics may influence the specificity of serological tests because these substances influence reference methods based on the direct detection of *H. pylori* or its urease activity[24].

II.3. Age/prevalence of *H. pylori* infection

Using serology in the elderly, one study reported that 32% may be serologically positive but do not have an active infection. On the other hand 21% of serologically negative patients were infected as detected by histology[26]. Several other studies confirmed a decline in specificity, sensitivity, and positive and negative predictive value of ELISA in older patients[18,22,27]. The reason for a high rate of negative histology with positive serology might be due to the higher prevalence of mucosal atrophy and intestinal metaplasia in elderly patients[28–30]. An increase in prevalence of *H. pylori* infection with higher age is well recognized, and the influence of *H. pylori* prevalence on the positive and negative predictive value has been mentioned.

II.4. Ethnicity/geographical differences

Another important factor resulting from the geographical variability of *H. pylori* antigens is the ethnic origin of the population tested. The influence of geographical differences on test results has been shown in South Asia[18], Chinese[31] and Belgians in comparison to those from Mediterranean areas[32]. These results emphasize that serological tests must be standardized for individual regions and populations.

II.5. *H. pylori* assessment following eradication

In several studies, serological tests have been evaluated for their use to determine successful eradication after treatment. The criterion is a significant titre reduction within a definite time interval after eradication, rather than seronegativity itself. For monitoring successful treatment serological tests can only be employed over a long time period, using paired sera. This approach has been suggested to be useful in adult patients free of complaints, with the aim of detecting rare reinfection[33]. Several authors found, in more than 90% of cases, a decline in titre within 6 months[8,32,34,35]. Cutler and Prasad described a 20% decline in IgG concentration 12–21 months after successful eradication with a sensitivity of 93%. Seronegativity was seldom detected; 65% were still seropositive 1 year after eradication[36]. Kosunen found that the decrease in titres continues, and most patients have normal titres within 2 years, depending on the original titre concentration[34]. If results are needed before 6 months, conventional serological tests are of no value. One exception is a new approach combining an IgG-capture method with a streptavidin–biotin technique for the detection of bound *H. pylori* antigens. In a first report, a higher reliability for the assessment of *H. pylori* eradication was shown using paired sera[37]. Nevertheless the UBT and, more recently with rather inconsistent results in different trials, the stool antigen test are the methods of choice, providing reliable results within 4–6 weeks after treatment[8,38–40].

II.6. Pitfalls in interpretation of results

A meta-analysis of 11 ELISA and one latex-agglutination test did not show significant differences in sensitivity and specificity[1]. The inter-laboratory comparison for eight commercially available ELISA kits reported by Feldman *et al.* clearly demonstrated a high variability in sensitivity and specificity even for the same kits[23]. Handling problems in some laboratories using certain kits have been identified, and the need for local validation of each kit has to be stressed.

A major issue is the choice of the reference method[21,23,41]. As shown in Tables 2 and 3 there is a high variability in the 'gold standards' used. Some define the *H. pylori* status by just one method, whereas others rely on three out of four methods with positive results. Even using the same reference method, such as histology, differences in biopsy sampling can influence the

Table 2. Validity of IgG-ELISA for the detection of *H. pylori*

Author/ref.	Test	Reference	n	Sensitivity (%)	Specificity (%)	PPV (%)	NPV (%)
Loy et al.[1]	Meta-analysis, 11 × ELISA, 1 × latex agglutination			85	79		
van der Wouw et al.[27]	Pyloriset IgG (ELISA)	H, C, direct urease test	154	81	89	97	51
Feldman et al.[23]	Interlaboratory: 8 × ELISA, 17 laboratories	C	59	80–99	86–99		
van der Wouw et al.[12]	Pyloriset E-IAG	C and/or H$^+$ direct urease testing	154	100	79	95	100

H = histology, C = culture.

Table 3. Validity of rapid blood tests for the detection of *H. pylori*

Author/ref.	Test	Reference	n	Sensitivity (%)	Specificity (%)	PPV (%)	NPV (%)
Jones et al.[67]	Helisal rapid blood test	2 × ELISA	123	83	78	83	78
Graham et al.[68]	Flexure *H. pylori*	UBT	551	94	87	89	93
Borody et al.[41]	Helisal rapid blood test	H, C, RUT	203	82	91		
Reilly et al.[22]	Helisal rapid blood test	H, UBT or RUT	303	85	80		
Enroth et al.[21]	BM-test *H. pylori*	ELISA, C, H	192	88–96	44–95	57–94	77–96
Stone et al.[18]	Cortecs Helisal rapid blood test	Antral H, RUT C, ELISA	200	91–92	56–62	55	89–92
Laine et al.[15]	Stat Simple	H, RUT	201	90	79		
Faigel et al.[16]	FlexSure HP Serum	Antral H, RUT, UBT	97	90	94		
	FlexSure HP			87	90		
	QuickView			83	96		
	Accustat			76	96		
	StatSimple			90	98		
Chey et al.[17]	FlexPack HP	H, RUT	131	76	79		
	QuikVue			78	90		
	Accumeter			84	90		

H = histology, C = culture, RUT = rapid urease test, UBT = urea breath test.

Table 4. Pitfalls in *H. pylori* diagnosis: UBT

Pitfall	Results
Hydrolysis of urea by other bacteris from the oral cavity	False-positive results
Medication (PPI, antibiotics, bismuth salts)	False-negative results
Bacterial overgrowth of the upper gastrointestinal tract	False-positive results
Insufficient quantity of substrate (min. 75 mg [^{13}C]urea	False-negative results
Insufficient test meal	False-negative/positive results
Performance of UBT without test meal	False-negative results
Insufficient breath collection	False-negative/positive results

outcome. In some studies only antral, but in most studies antral and corpus, biopsies have been taken. Due to the patchy distribution *H. pylori* might be missed by histology performed only on one biopsy specimen. As a consequence a weak gold standard reduces the specificity of a serological test.

In summary, the definition of the cut-off point is a common problem with ELISA tests. By lowering the cut-off values, sensitivity is increased but specificity is decreased[27]. In the elderly it may be recommended to reduce the cut-off due to a decreased immunoreactivity[19,42]. In other populations the definition of a larger grey zone leads to 'better' sensitivity and specificity of the method[23]. The definition of the cut-off by the manufacturer sometimes needs adaptation to the local conditions[27]. An increase in sensitivity by extending the reading time has been shown by Duggan et al.[20]. On the other hand the false-positive rate increased. Clear instructions by the manufacturers of rapid blood tests may improve reading of tests in cases of weak colour changes. Finally, sufficient training of those performing the tests increases their diagnostic accuracy.

III. UREA BREATH TEST (UBT)

The UBT is a non-invasive test of choice for detecting *H. pylori* infection with the greatest accuracy under pre- and post-treatment conditions[43-45]. Recent data indicate that the stool antigen test is comparable in accuracy with the UBT[39]. In post-treatment conditions, however, reports are conflicting about the accuracy of the stool test[39,40,46].

The interpretation of the UBT results needs to take into consideration (a) modifications of the test procedure, (b) gastric physiology and (c) the influence of drugs (see Table 4). In this way more pitfalls can be avoided.

Role of test procedure

The correct performance of the urea breath test is essential and should guarantee the collection of breath samples before and at a definite time point following administration of the [^{13}C] urea. The preparation of the test meal and [^{13}C]urea (commonly dissolved in a liquid) should be meticulous to avoid mistakes such as forgetting to mix the [^{13}C]urea substrate with the test drink. Patients need to be carefully instructed in how to perform and collect breath samples. Changing the dose of [^{13}C]urea, or the timing for taking the second breath sample, leads to different cut-off values[47], and this needs to be taken into account.

The UBT is commonly based on a test meal or test drink given before the substrate [^{13}C]urea, but the substrate can also be dissolved in the test drink and administered simultaneously[48]. The composition of the test meal has an important impact on the diagnostic accuracy of the UBT. Various options, such as gavage-like test meals with low lipid content (i.e. Ensure), gavage with high lipid content (i.e. combination of Ensure and Calogen) and citric acid[49], all yield high diagnostic accuracy. In conditions of low urease activity and borderline results the use of citric acid appears to provide a better sensitivity than other test meals[49,50]. The use of orange juice, in our hands, is less effective than citric acid, probably due to a greater delay in gastric emptying induced by citric acid than by orange juice, or by better exposure of bacterial urease activity[51]. Another group reported recently that the acidity of the test drink with a lowered intragastric pH is responsible for the increased effectiveness of citric acid[52].

The aim of the test meal or drink is to provide a prolonged reaction time for [^{13}C]urea and *H. pylori* urease[50,51,53]. Using scintigraphy, it has been shown that a test meal is crucial for the delivery of the urea solution to the gastric body and fundus. Without a test meal the UBT results may reflect only the urease activity of bacteria colonizing the antrum[53], and because of the lower density of *H. pylori* in the antrum after therapy with antisecretory drugs the test may give a false-negative result. For omeprazole, it has been well established that after 4 weeks of treatment the colonization density of *H. pylori* in antrum and distal body was significantly reduced, while it was increased in the fundus[2,3]. The test meal promotes an equal distribution of the substrate, and measurement of global urease activity in the stomach becomes more predictable.

Before a new UBT test meal can be recommended proper validation should be provided. It is important to consider also the population in which the test will be used during validation. An example is apple juice, which apparently works in children[54], but seems unsuitable for the UBT in adults[55]. In contrast to serology, once a UBT test is validated there is no need for further local validation.

Impact of gastric physiology on UBT results

The UBT is influenced by the gastric physiology. Rapid gastric emptying with only a short contact time of [^{13}C]urea with *H. pylori* leads to false-negative results[53]. Rapid gastric emptying is seen after gastric surgery, and this may lead to negative results. However, false-positive results may also occur with intestinal colonization by other urease-producing bacteria[56]. Urease-producing bacteria are also detectable in the oropharynx, and the activity measured in breath samples collected within the first 10 min after ingestion of the [^{13}C]urea may be confounded with *H. pylori* infection[57]. A full stomach following ingestion of a normal meal decreases the contact of the substrate with *H. pylori* and lowers the individual test results, but seems to have no influence on diagnostic accuracy[58]. The latter was only shown in pre-treatment conditions and not after eradication therapy, where bacterial load is reduced in those patients who have not been successfully eradicated[38].

Use of antibiotics, bismuth salts and proton-pump inhibitors

False-negative results with the UBT will occur if patients are on treatment with antibiotics, bismuth salts, or with high doses of proton-pump inhibitors (PPI) in short-term or long-term treatment.

With short-term treatment the dose of omeprazole seems to play an important role. We found a significant decrease of urease activity after 5 days with 80 mg/day of omeprazole, whereas 20 or 40 mg/day over 5 days did not influence urease activity[59]. Perri et al. performed studies to evaluate the influence of a short course of sucralfate (5 g), colloidal bismuth (600 mg), amoxycillin (2.5 g) or omeprazole (40 mg), and confirmed that a false-negative UBT can occur even after 1 day of therapy[58].

Long-term treatment leads to an increase of false-negative results even with lower doses of the PPI. As an example, patients after 14 days treatment with lansoprazole, 30 mg/day, had an equivocal or false-negative [^{14}C]UBT in 61%, with omeprazole 20 mg/day in 38.5% and with ranitidine in 18%. This effect lasted up to 5 days after stopping treatment[60,61]. The increase in false-negative results with long-term treatment also seems to depend on the PPI dose, but the dose is lower than for short-term treatment. For example Weill et al. described 25% versus 50% false-negative results measured by [^{14}C]UBT in patients after 28 days of treatment with omeprazole 20 versus 40 mg/day[62].

Recent studies indicate that the stool antigen test is affected in a similar way by PPI treatment. Bravo et al. found a significant proportion of false-negative stools after 7 days of lansoprazole treatment (45 mg/day, 15% negative) and of bismuth treatment (bismuth subsalicylate 780 mg/day, 10% negative), but the simultaneously performed UBT was more affected by PPI/bismuth treatment (30% and 45%)[63]. Controversially, Manes et al. reported that after 7 days treatment with omeprazole 20 mg/day only 13% false-negative UBTs occurred, but 57% of stool antigen tests were false-negative[64].

Caution is needed when interpreting studies of the UBT in patients on PPIs depending on the choice of reference methods. For example, treatment with a PPI decreases H. pylori density in the antrum and leads to a shift of H. pylori to proximal parts of the stomach. This leads to a decrease in the sensitivity of antral and corpus biopsies for detecting H. pylori both by urease testing and histological examination[65]. Therefore, studies of the effect of omeprazole on the UBT using histology or/and rapid urease tests as a reference need a sufficient number of biopsies from the corpus as well as from the antrum in addition to another reference method such as serology.

The effect of a 4-week treatment with tripotassium-dicitrato-bismuthate (DeNol®) has been studied by Dill et al.[66]. Immediately after treatment, five patients out of 55 had a false-negative UBT compared with histology and the rapid urease test. In these patients the H. pylori load was appreciably decreased. Four weeks after the end of treatment in four of these patients the UBT was positive again[66].

For practical purposes, when using the UBT, it is necessary to know the class, dose and duration of drug intake in order to interpret negative results. Treatment with a drug influencing the UBT should be stopped as soon as possible before performing the UBT. In clinical practice a standard recommendation to wait 4 weeks after the end of eradication treatment is still valid. With other drugs potentially influencing the urease activity, but not given for *H. pylori* eradication, the time may be shortened to 5 days. Exact data are not yet available to make definitive recommendations.

CONCLUSIONS

Testing for *H. pylori* infection encompasses all kinds of invasive and non-invasive approaches. The accuracy of different methods is influenced by factors such as the background prevalence of *H. pylori* infection, as well as specific individual technical or methodological factors. In addition, drugs impacting on the *H. pylori* infection (i.e. PPI influence the bacterial distribution within the stomach and inhibits the urease activity) exert an important influence on test accuracy and interpretation. Important studies have been made to identify factors that cause method-interest error or lead to wrong interpretation of correct results, but there is still more to learn about pitfalls in *H. pylori* diagnosis.

References

1. Loy CT, Irwig LM, Katelaris PH, Talley NJ. Do commercial serological kits for *Helicobacter pylori* infection differ in accuracy? A meta-analysis. Am J Gastroenterol. 2000;91:1138–44.
2. Logan RP, Walker MM, Misiewicz JJ, Gummett PA, Karim QN, Baron JH. Changes in the intragastric distribution of *Helicobacter pylori* during treatment with omeprazole. Gut. 1995;36:12–16.
3. Stolte M, Bethke B. Elimination of *Helicobacter pylori* under treatment with omeprazole. Z Gastroenterol. 1990;28:271–4.
4. Current European concepts in the management of *Helicobacter pylori* infection. The Maastricht Consensus Report. European *Helicobacter pylori* Study Group. Gut. 1997;41:8–13.
5. Malfertheiner P, Enrique Dominguez-Munoz J, Heckenmuller H, Neubrand M, Fischer HP, Sauerbruch T. Modified rapid urease test for detection of *Helicobacter pylori* infection. Eur J Gastroenterol Hepatol. 1996;8:53–6.
6. Megraud F. How should *Helicobacter pylori* infection be diagnosed? Gastroenterology. 1997;113(Suppl. 6):S93–8.
7. Megraud F. The most important diagnostic modalities for *Helicobacter pylori*, now and in the future. Eur J Gastroenterol Hepatol. 1997;9(Suppl. 1):S13–15.
8. Atherton JC. Non-endoscopic tests in the diagnosis of *Helicobacter pylori* infection. Aliment Pharmacol Ther. 1997;11(Suppl. 1):11–20.
9. Allerberger F, Oberhumer G, Wrba F, Puspok A, Dejaco C, Dierich MP. Detection of *Helicobacter pylori* infection using single serum specimens: comparison of five commercial serological tests. Hepatogastroenterology. 1996;43:1656–9.
10. Jaskowski TD, Martins TB, Hill HR, Litwin CM. Immunoglobulin A antibodies to *Helicobacter pylori*. J Clin Microbiol. 1997;35:2999–3000.
11. Karvar S, Karch H, Frosch M, Burghardt W, Gross U. Use of serum-specific immunoglobulins A and G for detection of *Helicobacter pylori* infection in patients with chronic gastritis by immunoblot analysis. J Clin Microbiol. 1997;35:3058–61.
12. van de Wouw BA, de Boer WA, Jansz AR, Roymans RT, Staals AP. Comparison of three commercially available enzyme-linked immunosorbent assays and biopsy-dependent diagnosis for detecting *Helicobacter pylori* infection. J Clin Microbiol. 1996;34:94–7.

13. Klaamas K, Held M, Wadstrom T, Lipping A, Kurtenkov O. IgG immune response to *Helicobacter pylori* antigens in patients with gastric cancer as defined by ELISA and immunoblotting. Int J Cancer. 1996;67:1–5.
14. Mitchell HM, Hazell SL, Li YY, Hu PJ. Serological response to specific *Helicobacter pylori* antigens: antibody against CagA antigen is not predictive of gastric cancer in a developing country. Am J Gastroenterol. 2000;91:1785–8.
15. Laine L, Knigge K, Faigel D et al. Fingerstick *Helicobacter pylori* antibody test: better than laboratory serological testing? Am J Gastroenterol. 1999;94:3464–7.
16. Faigel DO, Magaret N, Corless C, Lieberman DA, Fennerty MB. Evaluation of rapid antibody tests for the diagnosis of *Helicobacter pylori* infection. Am J Gastroenterol. 2000;95:72–7.
17. Chey WD, Murthy U, Shaw S et al. A comparison of three fingerstick, whole blood antibody tests for *Helicobacter pylori* infection: a United States, multicenter trial. Am J Gastroenterol. 1999;94:1512–16.
18. Stone MA, Mayberry JF, Wicks AC et al. Near patient testing for *Helicobacter pylori*: a detailed evaluation of the Cortecs Helisal Rapid Blood test. Eur J Gastroenterol Hepatol. 1997;9:257–60.
19. Wilcox MH, Dent TH, Hunter JO et al. Accuracy of serology for the diagnosis of *Helicobacter pylori* infection – a comparison of eight kits. J Clin Pathol. 1996;49:373–6.
20. Duggan A, Logan R, Knifton A. Accuracy of near-patient blood tests for *Helicobacter pylori*. Lancet. 1996;348:617.
21. Enroth H, Rigo R, Hulten K, Engstrand L. Diagnostic accuracy of a rapid whole-blood test for detection of *Helicobacter pylori*. J Clin Microbiol. 1997;35:2695–7.
22. Reilly TG, Poxon V, Sanders DS, Elliott TS, Walt RP. Comparison of serum, salivary, and rapid whole blood diagnostic tests for *Helicobacter pylori* and their validation against endoscopy based tests. Gut. 1997;40:454–8.
23. Feldman RA, Deeks JJ, Evans SJ. Multi-laboratory comparison of eight commercially available *Helicobacter pylori* serology kits. *Helicobacter pylori* Serology Study Group. Eur J Clin Microbiol Infect Dis. 1995;14:428–33.
24. Taha AS, Reid J, Boothmann P et al. Serological diagnosis of *Helicobacter pylori* – evaluation of four tests in the presence or absence of non-steroidal anti-inflammatory drugs. Gut. 1993;34:461–5.
25. Menegatti M, Vaira D, Miglioli M et al. *Helicobacter pylori* in patients with gastric and nongastric cancer. Am J Gastroenterol. 1995;90:1278–81.
26. Liston R, Pitt MA, Banerjee AK. IgG ELISA antibodies and detection of *Helicobacter pylori* in elderly patients. Lancet. 1996;347:269.
27. van de Wouw BA, de Boer WA, Jansz AR, Staals AP, Roymans RT. Serodiagnosis of *Helicobacter pylori* infection: an evaluation of a commercially available ELISA-IgG. Neth J Med. 1995;47:272–7.
28. Testoni PA, Colombo E, Cattani L et al. *Helicobacter pylori* serology in chronic gastritis with antral atrophy and negative histology for *Helicobacter*-like organisms. J Clin Gastroenterol. 1996;22:182–5.
29. Osawa H, Inoue F, Yoshida Y. Inverse relation of serum *Helicobacter pylori* antibody titres and extent of intestinal metaplasia. J Clin Pathol. 1996;49:112–15.
30. Kokkola A, Rauteliln H, Puolakkainen P et al. Diagnosis of *Helicobacter pylori* infection in patients with atrophic gastritis: comparison of histology, ^{13}C-urea breath test, and serology. Scand J Gastroenterol 2000;35:138–41.
31. Wong BC, Wong W, Tang VS et al. An evaluation of whole blood testing for *Helicobacter pylori* infection in the Chinese population. Aliment Pharmacol Ther. 2000;14:331–5.
32. Goossens H, Blupczynski Y, Burette A et al. Evaluation of a commercially available complement fixation test for diagnosis of *Helicobacter pylori* infection and for follow-up after antimicrobial therapy. J Clin Microbiol. 1992;30:3230–3.
33. Hirschl AM, Rotter ML. Serological tests for monitoring *Helicobacter pylori* eradication treatment. J Gastroenterol. 1996;31(Suppl. 9):33–6.
34. Kosunen TU. Antibody titres in *Helicobacter pylori* infection: implications in the follow-up of antimicrobial therapy. Ann Med. 1995;27:605–7.
35. Wang WM, Chen CY, Jan CM et al. Long-term follow-up and serological study after triple therapy of *Helicobacter pylori*-associated duodenal ulcer. Am J Gastroenterol. 1994;89:1793–6.

36. Cutler AF, Prasad VM. Long-term follow-up of *Helicobacter pylori* serology after successful eradication. Am J Gastroenterol. 2000;91:85–8.
37. Savio A, Buffoli F, Landi F et al. The value of a new capture ELISA system for the diagnosis and the follow-up of *Helicobacter pylori* infection. Gut. 1999;45(Suppl. 3):128 (abstract).
38. Leodolter A, Dominguez-Munoz JE, Von Arnim U, Kahl S, Peitz U, Malfertheiner P. Validity of a modified ^{13}C-urea breath test for pre- and posttreatment diagnosis of *Helicobacter pylori* infection in the routine clinical setting. Am J Gastroenterol. 1999;94:2100–4.
39. Vaira D, Malfertheiner P, Megraud F et al. Diagnosis of *Helicobacter pylori* infection with a new non-invasive antigen-based assay. HpSA European Study Group. Lancet. 1999; 354:30–3.
40. Makristathis A, Pasching E, Schutze K, Wimmer M, Rotter ML, Hirschl AM. Detection of *Helicobacter pylori* in stool specimens by PCR and antigen enzyme immunoassay. J Clin Microbiol. 1998;36:2772–4.
41. Borody TJ, Andrews P, Shortis NP. Evaluation of whole blood antibody kit to detect active *Helicobacter pylori* infection. Am J Gastroenterol. 2000;91:2509–12.
42. Rollan A, Giancaspero R, Arrese M et al. Accuracy of invasive and noninvasive tests to diagnose *Helicobacter pylori* infection after antibiotic treatment. Am J Gastroenterol. 1997;92:1268–74.
43. Bazzoli F, Zagari M, Fossi S et al. Urea breath tests for the detection of *Helicobacter pylori* infection. Helicobacter. 1997;2(Suppl. 1):S34–7.
44. Logan RP. Urea breath tests in the management of *Helicobacter pylori* infection. Gut. 1998;43(Suppl. 1):S47–50.
45. Metz DC, Furth EE, Faigel DO et al. Realities of diagnosing *Helicobacter pylori* infection in clinical practice: a case for non-invasive indirect methodologies. Yale J Biol Med. 1998; 71:81–90.
46. Trevisani L, Sartori S, Galvani F et al. Evaluation of a new enzyme immunoassay for detecting *Helicobacter pylori* in feces: a prospective pilot study. Am J Gastroenterol. 1999;94:1830–3.
47. Klein PD, Malaty HM, Martin RF, Graham KS, Genta RM, Graham DY. Noninvasive detection of *Helicobacter pylori* infection in clinical practice: the ^{13}C urea breath test. Am J Gastroenterol. 1996;91:690–4.
48. Leodolter A, Dominguez-Munoz JE, Von Arnim U, Manes G, Malfertheiner P. ^{13}C-urea breath test for the diagnosis of *Helicobacter pylori* infection. A further simplification for clinical practice. Scand J Gastroenterol. 1998;33:267–70.
49. Dominguez-Monoz JE, Leodolter A, Sauerbruch T, Malfertheiner P. A citric acid solution is an optimal test drink in the ^{13}C-urea breath test for the diagnosis of *Helicobacter pylori* infection. Gut. 1997;40:459–62.
50. Graham DY, Runke D, Anderson SY, Malaty HM, Klein PD. Citric acid as the test meal for the ^{13}C-urea breath test. Am J Gastroenterol. 1999;94:1214–17.
51. Leodolter A, Dominguez-Munoz JE, Von Arnim U, Malfertheiner P. Citric acid or orange juice for the ^{13}C-urea breath test: the impact of pH and gastric emptying. Aliment Pharmacol Ther. 1999;13:1057–62.
52. Pantoflickowa D, Lew E, Dorta G et al. Intragastric pH affects the results of the ^{13}C-urea breath test (UBT) in the diagnosis of *H. pylori* (Hp). Gastroenterology. 2000;118:4 (abstract).
53. Atherton JC, Washington N, Blackshaw PE et al. Effect of a test meal on the intragastric distribution of urea in the ^{13}C-urea breath test for *Helicobacter pylori*. Gut. 1995;36:337–40.
54. Kindermann A, Demmelmair H, Koletzko B, Krauss-Etschmann S, Wiebecke B, Koletzko S. Influence of age on ^{13}C-urea breath test results in children. J Pediatr Gastroenterol Nutr. 2000;30:85–91.
55. Ellenrieder V, Glasbrenner B, Stoffels C et al. Qualitative and semi-quantitative value of a modified ^{13}C-urea breath test for identification of *Helicobacter pylori* infection. Eur J Gastroenterol Hepatol. 1997;9:1085–9.
56. Lotterer E, Ludtke FE, Tegeler R, Lepsien G, Bauer FE. The ^{13}C-urea breath test – detection of *Helicobacter pylori* infection in patients with partial gastroectomy. Z Gastroenterol. 1993;31:115–19.
57. Logan R, Rousseau M. The ^{13}C-urea breath test. In: Lee A, Megraud F, editors. *Helicobacter pylori*: Techniques for Clinical Diagnosis and Basic Research. London: W. B. Saunders; 1996:74–81.

58. Perri F, Maes B, Geypens B, Ghoos Y, Hiele M, Rutgeerts P. The influence of isolated doses of drugs, feeding and colonic bacterial ureolysis on urea breath test results. Aliment Pharmacol Ther. 1995;9:705–9.
59. Stoschus B, Dominguez-Munoz JE, Kalhori N, Sauerbruch T, Malfertheiner P. Effect of omeprazole on *Helicobacter pylori* urease activity *in vivo*. Eur J Gastroenterol Hepatol. 1996;8:811–13.
60. Chey WD, Woods M, Scheiman JM, Nostrant TT, DelValle J. Lansoprazole and ranitidine affect the accuracy of the ^{14}C-urea breath test by a pH-dependent mechanism. Am J Gastroenterol. 1997;92:446–50.
61. Chey WD, Spybrook M, Carpenter S, Nostrant TT, Elta GH, Scheiman JM. Prolonged effect of omeprazole on the ^{14}C-urea breath test. Am J Gastroenterol. 1996;91:89–92.
62. Weil J, Bell GD, Powell K *et al.* Omeprazole and *Helicobacter pylori*: temporary suppression rather than true eradication. Aliment Pharmacol Ther. 1991;5:309–13.
63. Bravo LE, Realpe JL, Campo C, Mera R, Correa P. Effects of acid suppression and bismuth medications on the performance of diagnostic tests for *Helicobacter pylori* infection. Am J Gastroenterol. 1999;94:2380–3.
64. Manes G, Lioniello M, Piccirillo MM, Reccia L, Balzano A. Omeprazole markedly impairs the accuracy of the new *H. pylori* stool antigen (HpSA) test. Gut. 1999;45(Suppl. 3):111 (abstract).
65. Dickey W, Kenny BD, McConnell JB. Effect of proton pump inhibitors on the detection of *Helicobacter pylori* in gastric biopsies. Aliment Pharmacol Ther. 1996;10:289–93.
66. Dill S, Payne-James JJ, Misiewicz JJ *et al.* Evaluation of ^{13}C-urea breath test in the detection of *Helicobacter pylori* and in monitoring the effect of tripotassium dicitratobismuthate in non-ulcer dyspepsia. Gut. 1990;31:1237–41.
67. Jones R, Phillips I, Felix G, Tait C. An evaluation of near-patient testing for *Helicobacter pylori* in general practice. Aliment Pharmacol Ther. 1997;11:101–5.
68. Graham DY, Evans DJJ, Peacock J, Baker JT, Schrier WH. Comparison of rapid serological tests (FlexSure HP and QuickVue) with conventional ELISA for detection of *Helicobacter pylori* infection Am J Gastroenterol. 2000;91:942–8.

Section V
Inflammation and the Immune Response to *Helicobacter pylori* Infection

14
Overview of immune and inflammatory changes due to *Helicobacter* infection

A. HAMLET and K. CROITORU

INTRODUCTION

Helicobacter pylori infection causes gastric inflammation and is linked to the development of duodenal and gastric ulceration, gastric atrophy and gastric cancer. The high prevalence of *Helicobacter pylori* infection in the world, and its link to these diseases, makes this one of the world's leading health problems[1]. Eradication of *H. pylori* infection prevents ulcer recurrence and treatment of *H. pylori* infection is indicated in all patients with peptic ulcer disease as well as MALT lymphoma. On the other hand, the benefits of treating all *H. pylori*-infected patients remains controversial given the cost of treatment, the concerns regarding the side-effects of antibiotics and the increasing incidence of antibiotic-resistant *H. pylori* strains[2,3]. Nonetheless, as the strength of the evidence for an association between *H. pylori* and dyspepsia and, more importantly, gastric cancer increases, the arguments in favour of treating all *H. pylori*-infected patients become more convincing. Therefore, there is a need for new treatment strategies that can be applied to large populations[2,4].

Natural infection with *H. pylori* in humans and animal models is associated with a measurable immune response; nevertheless the gastric infection remains chronic[5]. On the other hand, once *H. pylori* infection is eradicated in adults re-infection is uncommon[6,7], suggesting that immune mechanisms can prevent re-infection. Animal studies show that oral vaccines co-administered with mucosal adjuvants such as cholera toxin (CTx), prevent and even lead to elimination of established *Helicobacter* infection[8-12]. Therefore, effective immunity can be achieved in *Helicobacter* infection. Our ability to design new vaccines or therapeutic approaches that will generate effective immunity will rely on understanding the mucosal inflammatory and immune response in the stomach.

MUCOSAL IMMUNE RESPONSE

The mucosa associated lymphoid tissue or MALT comprises the organized lymphoid structures, e.g. Peyer's pathches, lymphoid follicles and mesenteric lymph nodes (MLN) and the immune cells in the epithelium and lamina propria in the small intestine[13]. Overlying the Peyer's patches are specialized epithelial cells referred to as 'M cells', which serve as points of antigen uptake[14]. Within the Peyer's patches B cells switch from IgM to IgA production[15]. Antigen-stimulated cells leave the Peyer's patches and recirculate selectively to other mucosal sites[16]. Hence, immunization at one mucosal surface confers immunity at other mucosal surfaces[17].

The normal stomach is devoid of organized lymphoid elements; in fact few immune cells are found in the normal lamina propria of the stomach. *Helicobacter pylori* infection leads to gastric inflammation characterized by neutrophils, lymphocyte and plasma cell infiltrates in the lamina propria and epithelium[18-21]. With time the lymphoid cells become organized into follicular structures: however, M cells have not been identified in the stomach and there is no direct evidence for antigen uptake in the stomach. On the other hand, epithelial cells in the inflamed gastric mucosa express MHC class II[22] and B7-1 and B7-2 antigens[23], permitting antigen-presenting function. It remains that local mucosal lymphoid cells participate in the effector arm of the immune response, producing antibodies and cytokines. The ability of these cells to recirculate to the gastric mucosa has not been formally demonstrated. In spite of the progress in understanding the immune response to *Helicobacter* infection, the innate and adaptive immune response in the stomach remains poorly understood.

T CELLS AND CYTOKINES

In the mouse the cytokine-secreting profile of helper T cells distinguishes between Th1 cells producing IL-2 and IFN-γ (contribute to delayed-type hypersensitivity) and Th2 cells producing IL-4, IL-5, IL-6 and IL-10 (contribute to antibody responses, e.g. IgA and IgE, and stimulate eosinophilia and mast cell hyperplasia)[24]. Il-12 is a strong inducer of IFN-γ and along with IFN-γ promotes Th1 responses and inhibits Th2 responses. Conversely, IL-4 and IL-10 stimulate Th2 and inhibit Th1 responses[25-27]. Although this is an oversimplified analysis of both mouse and human T cell differentiation and function, it provides a framework for the study of cytokine responses in infections and chronic inflammatory diseases. For example, primary infection with *Leishmania major* in Balb/c mice leads to a progressive disease associated with a Th2 response. In contrast, mice strains responding with a Th1-type response, i.e. IFN-γ, are protected from lethal infection[28]. Recently, new subsets of T cells including a regulatory T cell, Tr1, that produces IL-10 and little IL-4, have been identified. These Tr1 cells appear to be vital for the regulation of a controlled response to normal gut flora in the intestine[29,30]. Presumably similar T cell subsets are present in the gastric mucosa. More work is required to establish how these T cell subsets and their cytokines influence the immune response to *Helicobacter* infection.

THE INFLAMMATORY/IMMUNE RESPONSE TO *HELICOBACTER* INFECTION IN HUMANS

Antigen-specific and non-specific arms of the immune system contribute to gastric inflammation and to the immune response induced by *Helicobacter*. These responses may participate in the control of the infection but may also contribute to mucosal damange. For example, IL-4 administration to humans, and IFN-γ to mice, leads to mucosal damage[31,32]. Increases in iNOS and Cox-2 enzymes, seen in *H. pylori* gastritis, can lead to increases in NO and prostanoids respectively. *H. pylori* infection is also associated with increases in epithelial-derived IL-6, IL-8 and other C-X-C and C-C chemokines such as GROα, RANTES, and MIP-1α[33–35]. These molecules contribute to the early influx of neutrophils and mononuclear cells long before the T cell response has developed. Urease and genes in the *Cag* pathogenicity island contribute to this response[36,37].

In humans, *H. pylori*-specific IgG and IgA antibody are found in gastric secretions, supporting the belief that the gastric mucosa participates in the effector arm of the immune response[38]. The cellular response to *H. pylori* in humans is less well defined. *H. pylori* resides in the mucous layer overlying gastric epthelial cells, and immune/inflammatory cells are not seen in direct contact with *H. pylori* in these sites. Therefore, it is unclear how cellular responses would influence *H. pylori* colonization. Nonetheless, increases in CD4 and CD8 T cells in the lamina propria and CD8 T cells in the gastric epithelium during *H. pylori* infection have been defined[39,40]. Isolated gastric lymphocytes proliferate and secrete IFN-γ *in vitro* in response to *H. pylori* antigen; however, *H. pylori*-negative patients with gastritis also produce IFN-γ[41,42]. It appears that *H. pylori* stimulates elements of the innate immune system, e.g. non-antigen-specific NK cells[43] and mucosal macrophages[37], leading to production of pro-inflammatory cytokines such as IL-1β, IL-6, IL-8, TNF-α and IFN-γ[44–46]. *H. pylori*-specific T cells and clones have also been identified in the peripheral blood and in the gastric mucosa of patients infected with *H. pylori*[47].

During chronic *H. pylori* infection in humans, and acute infections in rhesus macaques, the T cell production of cytokines is skewed towards a Th1 response[40,48], with very few Th2 cytokines such as IL-4 detectable. Activation of the cellular immune response during *H. pylori* infection may release soluble mediators that contribute to mucosal damage as well as aid in controlling the infection. It should be noted that patients with AIDS due to HIV infection have a decrease in incidence in *Helicobacter* gastritis, leading to the speculation that an intact immune system may prevent *H. pylori* elimination. Studying the role of the immune response to natural infection in humans is difficult. Elimination of *H. pylori* infection in rhesus monkeys does not leave protective immunity, suggesting that in primates it may be difficult to elicit an effective immune response. It should be noted that these primates failed to develop a measurable IgA response[49].

IMMUNE RESPONSES TO *HELICOBACTER* IN THE MOUSE

H. felis infection causes inflammation of the gastric antrum and fundus in the mouse[40]. In this model the influence of T cells on the inflammatory response is not clear. One study of *H. felis* gastritis in SCID mice showed no difference in inflammation when compared to immunocompetent Balb/c mice[51]. A more recent study showed that the degree of inflammation was actually decreased in RAG-1 and T cell receptor-deficient mice[52]. Furthermore, *H. pylori*-infected SCID mice adoptively transferred with splenocytes from *H. pylori*-infected B/6 mice developed an increase in gastritis that was correlated with the development of DTH responses. Thus, it would appear that T cells contribute to mucosal inflammation.

The specific cytokine response also influences the development of mucosal inflammation, as shown by comparing *H. felis* gastritis in Balb/c and C57BL/6 (B6) mice[53]. Balb/c mice tend to produce a more Th2-type response, while B6 mice produce a Th1 response[54], and this correlated with a greater degree of gastritis in the latter strain. Furthermore, treatment of *H. felis*-infected B6 mice with anti-IFN-γ decreased mucosal inflammation[55], and mice lacking IFN-γ developed less inflammation[56]. Therefore, it would appear that Th1 cytokines contribute to the development of mucosal injury. On the other hand, mice lacking the Th2 cytokine, IL-10, developed more severe hyperplastic gastritis[57], and another study of *H. felis* infection in Balb/c mice showed an increase in colonization[58]. Therefore, the contribution of defined cytokine responses to gastric inflammation is more complex that simply a Th1/Th2 dichotomy.

Antigen-specific responses to *Helicobacter* infection are reflected by increases in serum anti-*H. felis* IgM and IgG antibody[59–61], and both serum and gut IgA[61]. Although IgG and IgA antibody confer protection in passive immunization experiments[62,63], oral vaccines are not dependent on antibody[64].

Cellular responses to *Helicobacter* described in the mouse include *Helicobacter*-independent responses against urease and heat shock proteins, and *H. felis*-specific responses characterized by cellular proliferation and IFN-γ production[32,55]. As mentioned, the response to natural *Helicobacter* infection in both humans and mice is predominantly Th1. Adoptive transfer of *H. felis*-specific Th2 cell lines decreases *H. felis* colonization in the mouse, suggesting that Th2 responses are required for protection against or elimination of *H. felis*[55]. This does not rule out the possibility that Th1 cytokines can influence colonization. The method by which either of these immune responses controls *Helicobacter* infection in the mouse remains to be defined.

IMMUNIZATION

Oral immunization with a protein antigen leads to Th1 responses with IL-12 and IFN-γ release, followed by anergy and apoptosis of specific T cells and/or induction of suppressor type T cells[65–67]. This is referred to as oral tolerance. Other studies have shown that immunization at mucosal sites delivers the best local immunity, e.g. vaginal or nasal mucosa[68]. Oral vaccines of *H. felis* given with a mucosal adjuvant such as cholera toxin (Ctx) or *E. coli* heat-labile enterotoxin (LT), confers long-lasting protection against infection in mice[8,9,50,69,70]. Oral immunization with urease B plus CTx also eliminates established *H. felis* infection in mice and ferrets[10,12]. CTx can break oral tolerance to protein antigens presented to the mucosal immune system[71–73]. CTx also shifts T cell cytokine responses from Th1 to Th2 responses[74–76]. Given that Th2 cytokines stimulate local IgA responses, it has been argued that this is the mechanism responsible for the effect of mucosal adjuvants on *Helicobacter* infection; however, as mentioned previously these vaccines are effective in antibody-deficient mice[64,77].

The role of Th1/Th2 cytokines in protective immunity is not straightforward. For example, IL-4 knockout mice and IL-4 transgenic mice are colonized to a similar degree as normal mice, suggesting that IL-4 is not a major contributor to resistance to *H. pylori* infection[78]. On the other hand, CTx confers protective immunity in the presence or absence of IFN-γ and IFN-γ-deficient mice are more susceptible to *H. pylori* infection. This suggests that IFN-γ may also play a role in protective immunity[56].

The effect of CTx on Th1/Th2 cytokine balance is controversial in that CTx can induce a mixed Th1/Th2 response, and in some instances stimulates IFN-γ responses[73,79,80]. It also appears that the protection conferred by oral immunization is not absolute in that small numbers of residual bacteria persist after oral challenge and lead to the persistence of the gastritis[50,55,81]. Therefore, it is possible that oral vaccines reduce colonization to a low level, and do not completely prevent or totally eliminate *Helicobacter* infection. Our current understanding of the mechanism of action of adjuvant-based oral vaccines has not fully explained the mechanisms required for effective immunity[72,73]. The potential toxicity associated with the use of mucosal adjuvants such as CTx in humans may limit its clinical use[82], and initial results of clinical studies using oral urease B subunit vaccines with *E. coli* heat-labile enterotoxin have been disappointing[83,84].

IMMUNOMODULATION

Since an *H. pylori*-specific immune response develops during *H. pylori* infection, appropriate modulation of that response may lead to an effective immune response. Therefore, as an alternative to antigen-specific adjuvant-based immunization, we explored modulating the immune response in a non-specific manner. Previous work showed that injection of replication defective adenovirus (RDA) carrying cytokine genes modulates the response in a number of models of infectious agents and allergens[85–88]. The vector used was adenovirus-5, in which the foreign cytokine gene is inserted into the E1 and/or E3 region of the viral genome, rendering the virus replication defective[89,90]. A single injection of Ad-IL-12 can protect Balb/c mice against *Leishmania major* infection, while Ad-IL-4 had the opposite effect[91]. Ad-IL-12 also prevented death due to *Klebsiella pneumoniae* infection[92]. Therefore, cytokine delivery via this vector can modulate the host response.

We examined the effect of the RDA vector itself on *H. felis* colonization and the associated inflammatory response. Our study showed that RDA significantly decreased *H. felis* colonizaton in the C57BL/6 (B6) mouse, and this was dependent on the Th1 cytokines, IFN-γ and IL-12[61]. Therefore, stimulation of Th1 cytokines without specific antigen successfully modulated *H. felis* infection. These findings are in keeping with a recent report that systemic vaccination with complete Freund's adjuvant (CFA), a Th1-type adjuvant, was protective against *H. pylori* infection in the mouse[77]. In addition, Fox et al. have examined the ability of a helminth infection to modulate *H. pylori* infection through stimulating Th2 responses. In their study *H. pylori* infected mice co-infected with *Heligmosomoides polygyrus* developed a decrease in gastric inflammation that was associated with a decrease in gastric mucosal Th1 cytokines and an increase in Th2 cytokines. Interestingly, in spite of these changes in gastritis and Th1/Th2 responses, the degree of colonization at 16 weeks was increased in mice co-infected with *H. polygyrus*[93].

CONCLUSION

Helicobacter infection induces inflammation and stimulates an ineffective immune response. The ability of the organism to evade the immune system and maintain chronic colonization may relate to the unique environmental niche occupied by the organism, or to the selective induction of an immune response that interferes with effective elimination. Defining the mechanisms that determine an ineffective immune response vs. an immune response that eliminates the infection is critical to the design of appropriate novel treatment strategies. Immunomodulation may be an important and practical means of eliminating infection in large populations. Understanding the cellular and molecular elements involved in the response to *Helicobacter* is a prerequisite to such an undertaking. Insight into the mucosal response to normal gut flora will also help our understanding of the pathophysiology of inflammatory disease of the gastrointestinal tract in general.

Acknowledgements

K.C. holds an Ontario Ministry of Health Career Scientist Award; A.H. holds a Canadian Association of Gastroenterology/AstraZeneca Medical Research Council Fellowship. The work described has received support from the Hamilton Health Sciences Corporation Research Foundation, the Canadian Association of Gastroenterology, AstraZenica, the Medical Research Council of Canada and the Swedish MRC.

References

1. Parsonnet J. *Helicobacter pylori*: the size of the problem. Gut. 1998;43:S6–9.
2. Graham DY. Can therapy ever be denied for *Helicobacter pylori* infection? Gastroenterology. 1997;113:S113–17.
3. Hopkins RJ. Current FDA-approved treatments for *Helicobacter pylori* and the FDA approval process. Gastroenterology. 1997;113:S126–30.
4. Michetti P. Vaccine against *Helicobacter pylori*: fact or fiction? Gut. 1997;41:728–30.
5. Croitoru K, Snider DP. What determines the vigor of the immune response to *Helicobacter pylori*? In: Hunt RH, Tytgat GNJ, editors. *Helicobacter pylori*: Basic Mechanisms to Clinical Cure, 1996. Dordrecht: Kluwer; 1996:158–67.
6. Mitchell HM, Hu P, Chi Y, Chen MH, Li YY, Hazell SL. A low rate of reinfection following effective therapy against *Helicobacter pylori* in a developing nation (China). Gastroenterology. 1998;114:256–61.

7. Gisbert JP, Pajares JM, García-Valriberas R et al. Recurrence of *Helicobacter pylori* infection after eradication: incidence and variables influencing it. Scand J Gastroenterol. 1998; 33:1144–51.
8. Czinn SJ, Nedrud JG. Oral immunization against *Helicobacter pylori*. Infect Immun. 1991;59:2359–63.
9. Chen M, Lee A, Hazell S. Immunization against gastric *Helicobacter* infection in a mouse/*Helicobacter felis* model (letter). Lancet. 1992;339:1120–1.
10. Corthésy-Theulaz I, Porta N, Glauser M et al. Oral immunization with *Helicobacter pylori* urease B subunit as a treatment against *Helicobacter* infection. Lancet. 1995;109:115–21.
11. Doidge C, Gust I, Lee A, Buck F, Hazell S, Manne U. Therapeutic immunization against *Helicobacter* infection. Lancet. 1994;343:914–15.
12. Cuenca R, Blanchard TG, Czinn SJ et al. Therapeutic immunization against *Helicobacter mustelae* in naturally infected ferrets (See comments). Gastroenterology. 1996;110:1770–5.
13. Croitoru K, Bienenstock J. Characteristics and functions of mucosa-associated lymphoid tissue. In: Ogra PL, Strober W, Mestecky J, McGhee JR, Lamm ME, Bienenstock J, editors. Handbook of Mucosal Immunology. San Diego: Academic Press; 1994:141–9.
14. Neutra MR, Kraehenbuhl J-P. The role of transepithelial transport by M cells in microbial invasion and host defense. J Cell Sci. 1993;106(Suppl. 17):209–15.
15. Weinstein PD, Cebra JJ. The preference for switching to IgA expression by Peyer's patch germinal center B cells is likely due to the intrinsic influence of their microenvironment. J Immunol. 1991;147:4126–35.
16. Reynolds JD, Kennedy L, Peppard J, Pabst R. Ileal Peyer's patch emigrants are predominantly B cells and travel to all lymphoid tissues in sheep. Eur J Immunol. 1991;21:283–9.
17. McDermott MR, Bienenstock J. Evidence for a common mucosal immunologic system. I. Migration of B immunoblasts into intestinal, respiratory, and genital tissues. J Immunol. 1979;122:1892–8.
18. Crabtree JE. Immune and inflammatory responses to *Helicobacter pylori* infection. Scand J Gastroenterol. 1996;31:3–10.
19. Genta RM, Wentzell Hamner H, Graham DY. Gastric lymphoid follicles in *Helicobacter pylori* infection: frequency, distribution, and response to triple therapy. Hum Pathol. 1993;24:577–83.
20. Stolte M, Eidt S. Lymphoid follicles in antral mucosa: immune response to *Campylobacter pylori*? J Clin Pathol. 1989;42:1269–71.
21. Hood CJ, Lesna M. Immunocytochemical quantitation of inflammatory cells associated with *Helicobacter pylori* infection. Br J Biomed Sci. 1993;50:82–8.
22. Papadimitrou CS, Ioachim-Velogianni EE, Tsianos EB, Moutsopoulos HM. Epithelial HLA-DR expression and lymphocyte subsets in gastric muocsa in type B chronic gastritis. Virchows Arch (A). 1988;413:197–204.
23. Ye G, Barrera C, Fan X et al. Expression of B7-1 and B7-2 costimulatory molecules by human gastric epithelial cells: potential role in CD4+ T cell activation during *Helicobacter pylori* infection. J Clin Invest. 1997;99:1628–36.
24. Mosmann TR, Coffman RL. Heterogeneity of cytokine secretion patterns and functions of helper T cells. Adv Immunol. 1989;46:111–48.
25. Thompson-Snipes L, Dhar V, Bond MW, Mosmann TR, Moore KW, Rennick DM. Interleukin 10: a novel stimulatory factor for mast cells and their progenitors. J Exp Med. 1991;173:507–10.
26. Trinchieri G. Interleukin-12: a proinflammatory cytokine with immunoregulatory functions that bridge innate resistance and antigen-specific adaptive immunity. Annu Rev Immunol. 1995;13:251–76.
27. Carter LL, Dutton RW. Type 1 and type 2: a fundamental dichotomy for all T-cell subsets. Curr Opin Immunol. 1996;8:336–42.
28. Locksley RM, Scott P. Helper T-cell subsets in mouse leishmaniasis: induction, expansion and effector function. Immunol Today. 1991;12:A58–61.
29. Groux H, O'Garra A, Bigler M et al. A CD4$^+$ T-cell subset inhibits antigen-specific T-cell responses and prevents colitis. Nature. 1997;389:737–42.
30. Mason D, Powrie F. Control of immune pathology by regulatory T cells. Curr Opin Immunol. 1998;10:649–55.
31. Rubin JT, Lotze MT. Acute gastric mucosal injury associated with the systemic administration of interleukin-4 Surgery. 1992;111:274–80.

32. Mohammadi M, Nedrud J, Redline R, Lycke N, Czinn SJ. Murine CD4 T-cell response to *Helicobacter* infection: TH1 cells enhance gastritis and TH2 cells reduce bacterial load. Gastroenterology. 1997;113:1848–57.
33. Crowe SE, Alvarez L, Dytoc M et al. Expression of interleukin 8 and CD54 by human gastric epithelium after *Helicobacter pylori* infection *in vitro*. Gastroenterology. 1995;108:65–74.
34. Shimoyama T, Everett SM, Dixon MF, Axon ATR, Crabtree JE. Chemokine mRNA expression in gastric mucosa is associated with *Helicobacter pylori* cagA positivity and severity of gastritis. J Clin Pathol. 1998;51:765–70.
35. Yamaoka Y, Kita M, Kodama T et al. Chemokines in the gastric mucosa in *Helicobacter pylori* infection. Gut. 1998;42:609–17.
36. Crabtree JE, Kersulyte D, Li SD, Lindley IJ, Berg DE. Modulation of *Helicobacter pylori* induced interleukin-8 synthesis in gastric epithelial cells mediated by cag PAI encoded VirD4 homologue. J Clin Pathol. 1999;52:653–7.
37. Harris PR, Ernst PB, Kawabata S, Kiyono H, Graham MF, Smith DP. Recombinant *Helicobacter pylori* urease activates primary mucosal macrophages. J Infect Dis. 1998; 178:1516–20.
38. Perez-Perez GI, Dworkin BM, Chodos JE, Blaser MJ. *Campylobacter pylori* antibodies in humans. Ann Intern Med. 1998;109:11–17.
39. Jaskiewicz K, Louw JA, Marks IN. Local cellular and immune response by antral mucosa in patients undergoing treatment for eradication of *Helicobacter pylori*. Dig Dis Sci. 1993; 38:937–43.
40. Bamford KB, Fan XJ, Crowe SE et al. Lymphocytes in the human gastric mucosa during *Helicobacter pylori* have a T helper cell 1 phenotype. Gastroenterology. 1998;114:482–92.
41. Karttunen R. Blood lymphocyte proliferation, cytokine secretion and appearance of T cells with activation surface markers in cultures with *Helicobacter pylori*. Comparison of the responses of subjects with and without antibodies to *H. pylori*. Clin Exp Immunol. 1991;83:396–400.
42. Fan XJ, Chua A, Shahi CN, McDevitt J, Keeling PW, Kelleher D. Gastric T lymphocyte responses to *Helicobacter pylori* in patients with *H. pylori* colonisation. Gut. 1994;35:1379–84.
43. Tarkkanen J, Kosunen TU, Saksela E. Contact of lymphocytes with *Helicobacter pylori* augments natural killer cell activity and induces production of gamma interferon. Infect Immun. 1993;61:3012–16.
44. Haberle H, Kubin M, Trinchieri G et al. Activated Th cells are recruited to the gastric epithelium and lamina propria during *H. pylori* infection. Clin Immunol Immunopathol. 1995;76:S8.
45. Sommer F, Faller G, Konturek P et al. Antrum- and corpus mucosa-infiltrating CD4[+] lymphocytes in *Helicobacter pylori* gastritis display a Th1 phenotype. Infect Immun. 1998; 66:5543–6.
46. Vanderlaan M, Thomas CB. Characterization of monoclonal antibodies to bromodeoxyuridine. Cytometry. 1985;6:501–5.
47. Di Tommaso A, Xiang Z, Bugnoli M et al. *Helicobacter pylori*-specific CD4 + T-cell clones from peripheral blood and gastric biopsies. Infect Immun. 1995;63:1102–6.
48. Mattapallil JJ, Dandekar S, Canfield DR, Solnick JV. A predominant Th1 type of immune response is induced early during acute *Helicobacter pylori* infection in rhesus macaques. Gastroenterology. 2000;118:307–15.
49. Dubois A, Berg DE, Incecik ET et al. Host specificity of *Helicobacter pylori* strains and host responses in experimentally challenged nonhuman primates. Gastroenterology. 1999; 116:90–6.
50. Michetti P, Corthésy-Theulaz I, Davin C et al. Immunization of BALB/c mice against *Helicobacter felis* infection with *Helicobacter pylori* urease. Gastroenterology. 1994; 107:1002–11.
51. Blanchard TG, Czinn SJ, Nedrud JG, Redline RW. *Helicobacter*-associated gastritis in SCID mice. Infect Immun. 1995;63:1113–15.
52. Roth KA, Kapadia SB, Martin SM, Lorenz RG. Cellular immune responses are essential for the development of *Helicobacter felis*-associated gastric pathology. J Immunol. 1999; 163: 1490–7.

53. Mohammadi M, Redline R, Nedrud J, Czinn S. Role of the host in pathogenesis of *Helicobacter*-associated gastritis: *H. felis* infection of inbred and congenic mouse strains. Infect Immun. 1996;64:238–45.
54. Finkelman FD, Pearce DJ, Urban JF, Sher A. Regulation and biological function of helminth-induced cytokine response. Immunol Today. 1991;12:A62–6.
55. Mohammadi M, Czinn S, Redline R, Nedrud J. *Helicobacter*-specific cell-mediated immune responses display a predominant Th1 phenotype and promote a delayed-type hypersensitivity response in the stomachs of mice. J Immunol. 1996;156:4729–38.
56. Sawai N, Kita M, Kodama T et al. Role of gamma interferon in *Helicobacter pylori*-induced gastric inflammatory responses in a mouse model. Infect Immun. 1999;67:279–85.
57. Berg DJ, Lynch NA, Lynch RG, Lauricella DM. Rapid development of severe hyperplastic gastritis with gastric epithelial dedifferentiation in *Helicobacter felis*-infected IL-10(−/−) mice. Am J Pathol. 1998;152:1377–86.
58. Sakagami T, Dixon M, O'Rourke J et al. Atrophic gastric changes in both *Helicobacter felis* and *Helicobacter pylori* infected mice are host dependent and separate from antral gastritis. Gut. 1996;39:639–48.
59. Lee A, Fox JG, Otto G, Murphy J. A small animal model of human *Helicobacter pylori* active chronic gastritis. Gastroenterology. 1990;99:1315.
60. Fox JG, Blanco M, Murphy JC et al. Local and systemic immune responses in murine *Helicobacter felis* active chronic gastritis. Infect Immun. 1993;61:2309–15.
61. Bo J, Jordana M, Xing Z et al. Replication defective adenovirus infection reduces *Helicobacter felis* colonization in the mouse in an interferon- and IL-12 dependent manner. Infect Immun. 1999 (In press).
62. Czinn SJ, Cai A, Nedrud JG. Protection of germ-free mice from infection by *Helicobacter felis* after active oral or passive IgA immunization. Vaccine. 1993;11:637–42.
63. Ferrero RL, Thiberge JM, Labigne A. Local immunoglobulin G antibodies in the stomach may contribute to immunity against *Helicobacter* infection in mice. Gastroenterology. 1997;113:185–94.
64. Ermak TH, Giannasca PJ, Nichols R et al. Immunization of mice with urease vaccine affords protection against *Helicobacter pylori* infection in the absence of antibodies and is mediated by MHC class II-restricted responses. J Exp Med. 1998;188:2277–88.
65. Neurath M, Fuss I, Kelsall BL, Presky DH, Waegell W, Strober W. Experimental granulomatous colitis in mice is abrogated by induction of TGF-β mediated oral tolerance. J Exp Med. 1996;183:2605.
66. Chen Y, Kuchroo VK, Inobe J, Hafler DA, Weiner HL. Regulatory T cell clones induced by oral tolerance: suppression of autoimmune encephalomyelitis. Science. 1994;265:1237–40.
67. Fowler E, Weiner HL. Oral tolerance: elucidation of mechanisms and application to treatment of autoimmune diseases. Biopolymers. 1997;43:323–35.
68. Gallichan WS, Rosenthal KL. Long-lived cytotoxic T lymphocyte memory in mucosal tissues after mucosal but not systemic immunization. J Exp Med. 1996;184:1879–90.
69. Lee CK, Weltzin R, Thomas WD et al. Oral immunization with recombinant *Helicobacter pylori* urease induces secretory IgA antibodies and protects mice from challenge with *Helicobacter felis*. J Infect Dis. 1995;172:161–72.
70. Marchetti M, Arico B, Burroni D, Figura N, Rappuoli R, Ghiara P. Development of a mouse model of *Helicobacter pylori* infection that mimics human disease. Science. 1995;267:1655–8.
71. Elson CO, Ealding W. Generalized systemic and mucosal immunity in mice after mucosal stimulation with cholera toxin. J Immunol. 1984;132:2736–41.
72. Holmgren J, Lycke N, Czerkinsky C. Cholera toxin and cholera B subunit as oral–mucosal adjuvant and antigen vector systems. Vaccine. 1993;11:1179–84.
73. Snider DP. The mucosal adjuvant activities of ADP-ribosylating bacterial enterotoxins. Crit Rev Immunol. 1995;15:317–48.
74. Clements JD, Hartzog NM, Lyon FL. Adjuvant activity of *Escherichia coli* heat labile enterotoxin and effect on the induction of oral tolerance in mice to unrelated protein antigens. Vaccine. 1998;6:269–77.
75. Xu-Amano J, Jackson RJ, Fujihashi K, Kiyono H, Staats HF, McGhee JR. Helper Th1 and Th2 cell responses following mucosal or systemic immunization with cholera toxin. Vaccine. 1994;12:903–11.

76. Xu-Amano J, Kiyono H, Jackson RJ et al. Helper T cell subsets for immunoglobulin A responses: oral immunization with tetanus toxoid and cholera toxin as adjuvant selectively induces Th2 cells in mucosa associated tissues. J Exp Med. 1993;178:1309–20.
77. Blanchard TG, Gottwein JM, Targoni et al. Systemic vaccination inducing either Th1 or Th2 immunity protects mice from challenge with *H. pylori*. Gastroenterology. 1999;116:A695.
78. Chen W, Shu D, Chadwick VS. *Helicobacter pylori* infection in interleukin-4-deficient and transgenic mice. Scand J Gastroenterol. 1999;34:987–92.
79. Hörnquis E, Grdic KD, Mak T, Lycke N. CD8-deficient mice exhibit augmented mucosal immune response and intact adjuvant effects to cholera toxin. Immunology. 1996;87:220–9.
80. Snider DP, Marshall JS, Perdue MH, Liang H. Production of IgE antibody and allergic sensitization of intestinal and peripheral tissues after oral immunization with protein Ag and cholera toxin. J Immunol. 1994;153:647–57.
81. Ermak TH, Ding R, Ekstein B et al. Gastritis in urease-immunized mice after *Helicobacter felis* challenge may be due to residual bacteria. Gastroenterology. 1997;113:1118–28.
82. Czinn SJ. What is the role for vaccination in *Helicobacter pylori*? Gastroenterology. 1997;113:S149–53.
83. Saldinger PF, Blum AL, Corthesy-Theulaz IE. Perspectives of anti-*H. pylori* vaccination. J Physiol Pharmacol. 1997;48(Suppl. 4):59–65.
84. Michetti P, Kreiss C, Kotloff KL et al. Oral immunization with urease and *Escherichia coli* heat-labile exterotoxin is safe and immunogenic in *Helicobacter pylori*-infected adults. Gastroenterology. 1999;116:804–12.
85. Papp Z, Middleton DM, Mittal SK, Babiuk LA, Baca-Estrada ME. Mucosal immunization with recombinant adenoviruses: induction of immunity and protection of cotton rats against respiratory bovine herpes virus type 1 infection. J Gen Virol. 1997;78:2933–43.
86. Wilson ME, Young BM, Davidson BL, Mente KA, McGowan SE. The importance of TGF-beta in murine visceral leishmaniasis. J Immunol. 1998;161:6148–55.
87. Stampfli MR, Ritz SA, Neigh GS et al. Adenoviral infection inhibits allergic airways inflammation in mice. Clin Exp Allergy. 1998;28:1581–90.
88. Xing Z, Ohkawara Y, Jordana M, Graham FL, Gauldie J. Adenoviral vector-mediated interleukin-10 expression *in vivo*: intramuscular gene transfer inhibits cytokine responses in endotoxemia. Gene Ther. 1997;4:140–9.
89. Bett AJ, Hadara W, Prevec L, Graham FL. An efficient and flexible system for construction of adenovirus vectors with insertions or deletions in early regions 1 and 3. Proc Natl Acad Sci USA. 1994;91:8802–6.
90. Xing Z, Braciak TA, Jordana M, Croitoru K, Graham FL, Gauldie J. Adenovirus-mediated cytokine gene transfer at tissue sites. Overexpression of IL-6 induces lymphocytic hyperplasia in the lung. J Immunol. 1994;153:4059–69.
91. Gabaglia CR, Pedersen B, Hitt M et al. A single intramuscular injection with an adenovirus-expressing IL-12 protects BALB/c mice against *Leishmania major* infection, while treatment with an IL-4-expressing vector increases disease susceptibility in B10.D2 mice. J Immunol. 1999;162:753–60.
92. Greenberger MJ, Kenkel SL, Strieter RM et al. IL-12 gene therapy protects mice in lethal *Klebsiella pneumonia*. J Immunol. 1996;157:3006–12.
93. Fox JG, Beck P, Dangler CA et al. Concurrent enteric helminth infection modulates inflammation and gastric immune responses and reduces *Helicobacter*-induced gastric atrophy. Nature Med. 2000 (In press).

15
Interaction of *Helicobacter pylori* with gastric epithelium

E. SOLCIA, V. RICCI, P. SOMMI, V. NECCHI, M. CANDUSSO and R. FIOCCA

RELEASE OF VacA AND OUTER MEMBRANE VESICLES

Many *Helicobacter pylori* organisms colonizing the human stomach are free-floating in the mucous layer covering the gastric epithelium. Only a fraction of these bacteria are found to adhere to the luminal surface of the epithelium either with close contact, apparent fusion or juxtaposition of the bacterial outer membrane with the luminal membrane or with a number of thin filaments radiating from the bacterial surface and joining the two membranes[1,2]. It has been shown that bacterial adhesion causes rearrangement of the underlying cell cytoskeleton and a number of other morphological and biochemical changes. It is postulated that at the site of adhesion Cag proteins of the bacterial membrane, encoded by genes of the so-called pathogenicity island, may form secretory channels allowing direct delivery of bacterial constituents from the bacterial body into the cell cytoplasm[3]. Other bacterial products, such as the vacuolating cytotoxin, VacA, are believed to be actively secreted, probably by a type II mechanism. This implies transport of the VacA protoxin across the inner bacterial membrane, via a sec-mediated pathway, followed by transport across the outer membrane via a channel formed by the C-terminus of VacA itself[4-6]. In support of this concept, we localized VacA immunoreactivity by the immunogold test in the periplasm and outer membrane of intact bacteria, either cultured *in vitro* or colonizing the gastric mucosa *in vivo*. In addition, we detected free VacA in the peribacterial space, within culture medium or gastric mucus, a likely result of active toxin secretion. During these investigations outer membrane vesicles (OMVs), 50–250 nm in size, have been found to be released by the bacteria, both in culture and in the gastric lumen, through budding of outer membrane blebs enveloping periplasmic expansions, which later detach from the bacterium to form free-floating vesicles carrying VacA immunoreactivity[6]. Thus, OMVs were found free in bacterial culture medium, during both growth and stationary phases. They were easily separated from the bacteria by centrifugation, while largely passing through a 0.22-μm cellulose acetate filter, so that they were partly retained in the broth culture filtrates used in tests on gastric MKN28 cell cultures[7]. In these conditions OMVs were found to adhere in part to the cell membrane at sites of luminal-type differentiation, similar to the behaviour of intact H. pylori organisms. Both free VacA and OMVs contacting the cell membrane can be taken up by the cell, apparently by endocytosis, to be concentrated in cytoplasmic vesicles of an endosomal nature, where they may persist for more than 3 days while retaining VacA biological activity[6,7]. A similar behaviour of free VacA and VacA-immunoreactive OMVs in respect to colonized gastric epithelium has been observed in gastric biopsies.

ENDOSOMAL VESICLES AND CYTOPLASMIC VACUOLES

A consistent finding of the colonized gastric epithelium with adhering H. pylori bacteria is the appearance of a number of small (100–500 nm) clear vesicles in the juxtaluminal cytoplasm[2,8,9]. The endocytic–endosomal nature of such vesicles is supported by their occasional content of OMVs and by their storage of immunoreactive VacA as well as cathepsin E[6,8,9]. In normal, non-colonized gastric epithelium only a very few endocytic vesicles were found, usually small and flattened. This dramatic expansion of endocytic–endosomal vesicles seems to be elicited by bacterial adhesion and may reflect H. pylori activation of epithelial endocytosis resulting in a substantial uptake of bacterial antigens and toxins (as well as other luminal contents).

Cytoplasmic vesicles are easily formed by expansion, dilation, and reciprocal fusion of endosomal vesicles in MKN28 cells incubated with VacA and ammonia[10]. MKN28 cells, derived from a human gastric carcinoma, show gastric-type luminal differentiation in the apparent absence of mucous secretion, thus allowing easy interaction of bacteria and their broth culture filtrates with cell membranes, without interposition of the mucous layer shown by the gastric epithelium *in vivo*. Cytoplasmic vacuolization is much less prominent in biopsies of gastric epithelium, despite extensive H. pylori colonization. The *in-vivo* situation can better be compared to the behaviour of VacA incubated, confluent MNK28 cell cultures, where only scanty vacuoles were observed and few cells showed expanded endosomes with VacA content. It seems likely that the subconfluent cell cultures usually employed in vacuolization experiments represent a highly sensitive but rather unphysiological model for investigation of H. pylori toxins, to be compared only to a gastric epithelium with disrupted or highly permeable tight junctions.

ANTIGEN TRANSPORT AND POSSIBLE PROCESSING/PRESENTATION

Colonized human gastric epithelium undergoes several histochemical changes, among which enhanced expression of cathepsin E and interleukin 8 and *de-novo* expression of HLA-DR are most prominent. Cathepsin E has been shown to be crucial for processing of antigens to be presented in the context of class II HLA molecules[11]. In colonized gastric epithelium the cathepsin E content was dramatically increased and extended from the basal endoplasmic reticulum, where normally it is likely to be retained in an inactive proenzyme form, to the supranuclear cytoplasm, inclusive of the endosomal vesicles where it may interact with bacterial antigens internalized by the cell[8,9,12]. Endosomal localization of cathepsin E has also been reported in other cell types known to be active in antigen sampling, transport and processing, such as Langerhans cells[13] and intestinal M cells of follicle-associated epithelium[14]. The concomitant expression of HLA-DR and B7 costimulatory molecules[15] may be important for antigen presentation to immunocompetent cells of the lamina propria immediately underlying the epithelium. On the other hand, interleukin-8 epithelial overexpression, which is secondary to interaction with viable *H. pylori* bacteria carrying the *cag* pathogenicity island, seems crucial to elicit an active inflammatory process in the underlying mucosa[16].

In conclusion, it seems likely that the gastric epithelium, activated by colonizing bacteria, has an important role in the modulation of the type and severity of the mucosal immune-inflammatory response. However, the precise link between modified epithelial function and mucosal response remains largely to be clarified.

References

1. Tricottet V, Bruneval P, Vire O et al. *Campylobacter*-like organisms and surface epithelium abnormalities in active, chronic gastritis in humans: an ultrastructural study. Ultrastruct Pathol. 1986;10:113–22.
2. Fiocca R, Villani L, Turpini F, Solcia E. High incidence of *Campylobacter*-like organisms in endoscopic biopsies from patients with gastritis, with or without peptic ulcer. Digestion. 1987;38:234–44.
3. Censini S, Lange C, Xiang Z et al. Cag, a pathogenicity island of *Helicobacter pylori*, encodes type I-specific and disease-associated virulence factors. Proc Natl Acad Sci USA. 1996;93:14648–53.
4. Cover TL, Tummuru MKR, Thompson SA, Blaser MJ. Divergence of genetic sequences for the vacuolating cytotoxin among *Helicobacter pylori* strains. J Biol Chem. 1994;269:10566–73.
5. Telford JL, Ghiara P, dell'Orco M et al. Gene structure of the *Helicobacter pylori* cytotoxin and evidence of its key role in gastric disease. J Exp Med. 1994;179:1653–8.
6. Fiocca R, Necchi V, Sommi P et al. Release of *Helicobacter pylori* vacuolating cytotoxin by both a specific secretion pathway and budding of outer membrane vesicles. Uptake of released toxin and vesicles by gastric epithelium. J Pathol. 1999;188:220–6.
7. Sommi P, Ricci V, Fiocca R et al. Persistence of *Helicobacter pylori* VacA toxin and vacuolating potential in cultured gastric epithelial cells. Am J Physiol. 1998;275:G681–8.
8. Fiocca R, Luinetti O, Villani L et al. Epithelial cytotoxicity, immune responses, and inflammatory components of *Helicobacter pylori* gastritis. Scand J Gastroenterol. 1994;29(Suppl. 205):11–21.
9. Solcia E, Villani L, Luinetti O, Trespi E, Fiocca R. The mucosal response to *Helicobacter pylori* infection and its contribution to gastric pathology. Microecol Ther. 1995;25:121–32.
10. Ricci V, Sommi P, Fiocca R et al. Cytotoxicity of *Helicobacter pylori* on human gastric epithelial cells in vitro: role of cytotoxin(s) and ammonia. Eur J Gastroenterol Hepatol. 1993;5:687–94.
11. Bennett K, Levine T, Ellis JS et al. Antigen processing for presentation by class II major histocompatibility complex requires cleavage by cathepsin E. Eur J Immunol. 1992;22:1519–24.

12. Fiocca R, Villani L, Tenti P et al. The foveolar cell component of gastric cancer. Hum Pathol. 1990;21:260–70.
13. Solcia E, Paulli M, Fiocca R et al. Cathepsin E in antigen presenting cells: Langerhans cells of the epidermis and interdigitating reticulum cells of lymphoid tissues. Eur J Histochem. 1993;37:19–26.
14. Finzi G, Cornaggia M, Capella C et al. Cathepsin E in follicle associated epithelium of intestine and tonsils: localization to M cells and possible role in antigen processing. Histochemistry. 1993;99:201–11.
15. Ye G, Barrera C, Fan X et al. Expression of B7–1 and B7–2 costimulatory molecules by human gastric epithelial cells. J Clin Invest. 1997;99:1628–36.
16. Crabtree JE, Covacci A, Farmery SM et al. *Helicobacter pylori* induced interleukin-8 expression in gastric epithelial cells is associated with cagA positive phenotype. J Clin Pathol. 1995;48:41–5.

16
Helicobacter pylori and the epithelial barrier: role of oxidative injury

S.-Z. DING and S. E. CROWE

INTRODUCTION

During *Helicobacter pylori* infection the gastric mucosa is subjected to potentially injurious factors of bacterial and host origin that alter barrier function and the regulation of epithelial cell growth. Disruption of barrier function may be due to direct bacterial actions or occur secondarily as a consequence of activation of an inflammatory response. Although *H. pylori* infection is normally restricted to the mucosal surface, increased gastric permeability permits further damage from bacteria and their products that gain access into the mucosa. Our research focuses on altered epithelial cell growth and death that occurs during *H. pylori* infection and the role that reactive oxygen species (ROS) play in these events. ROS are released by *H. pylori*, as well as from immune cells, and accumulate in gastric epithelial cells in response to infection, exogenous oxidative metabolites, and inflammatory cytokines. Epithelial cell apoptosis is increased in *H. pylori* infection and there is some evidence that antioxidants reduce ROS accumulation and programmed cell death in the epithelium during infection. During *H. pylori* infection both bacterial factors and the host inflammatory response serve as sources of oxidative stress, a factor that plays a role in determining the net effect on the health of the gastric epithelium. As the epithelial response is an important determinant of the outcome of infection, an understanding of the factors that disturb the epithelial barrier is relevant.

THE GASTRIC MUCOSAL BARRIER

The mucosal layer of the gastrointestinal tract forms an important interface between the host and the microenvironment of the lumen of the gut. This layer functions as a barrier to infection by various pathogenic microorganisms, the uptake of foreign material including food and microbial antigens, and injury from material secreted into the lumen such as bile and acid, or ingested toxins, including ethanol and non-steroidal anti-inflammatory drugs (NSAIDs). At the same time, the mucosa performs key functions that include acid secretion, maintenance of fluid and electrolyte balance, and digestion and absorption of nutrients. Injury to the mucosa results in an interruption of these normal functions of the gut.

The gastric barrier consists of three main components when considered in physiological terms. The pre-epithelial layer includes mucus and bicarbonate secretion[1]; the epithelial component comprises phospholipid expression, cell restitution and proliferation; and the post-epithelial aspect involves the microcirculation[2]. It is increasingly recognized that mesenchymal cells such as myofibroblasts and immune cells, as well as neural elements in the sub-epithelial compartment, may play a role in mucosal barrier function. Relatively fewer studies have focused on these aspects in the stomach compared to the intestine, however.

A large number of factors are considered as protective and aid in maintaining the mucosal barrier. These include prostaglandins, nitric oxide, epidermal growth factor (EGF), transforming growth factor-alpha (TGF-α), and trefoil peptides. So-called 'aggressive factors' interfere with the health of the gastric mucosal barrier. Stress, non-selective NSAIDs, *H. pylori* infection, acid/pepsin, bile, and ischaemia represent some of the most-studied factors that can impair the gastric barrier[2]. The mechanisms by which barrier function is altered have been well established for some of these factors but, as will be discussed, the processes involved in *H. pylori* infection remain less defined.

There are several methods available to evaluate gastrointestinal barrier function. Since the gut epithelium forms a polarized monolayer, measurement of transepithelial resistance can be used as a means to evaluate mucosal integrity. Fluxes in the transport of macromolecules such as horseradish peroxidase, or of labelled ions, represent other *in-vitro* measures of gut permeability. Human studies of gut barrier function have relied upon the absorption and subsequent urinary excretion of macromolecules including disaccharides and labelled compounds. Recently, sucrose absorption has been shown to reflect enhanced gastric permeability since any uptake of this sugar, which is readily degraded into glucose and fructose in the proximal duodenum, must take place in the stomach[3,4]. Enhanced gastric uptake of macromolecules, reflecting altered epithelial permeability, has been reported in allergic reactions, NSAID gastropathy, corticosteroid administration, and lymphocytic gastritis[3-9].

Enhanced permeability can result from loss of epithelial cells from necrosis or apoptosis, failure of normal cell restitution and repair mechanisms, alterations of the tight junction, and increased transepithelial transfer of macromolecules. *In-vitro* studies employing polarized intestinal epithelial cell lines have greatly enhanced our understanding of the mechanisms regulating the intestinal epithelial barrier[10,11]. The lack of polarized gastric cell models has precluded parallel advancements of knowledge concerning the stomach, although it is likely that similar regulatory factors are involved. Specialized epithelial cells, M cells, are a major site of antigen uptake in the intestinal tract, but as M cells are not present in the gastric mucosa, this represents one difference in the mucosal barrier of the stomach compared to the small and large intestine. As will be discussed, polarized intestinal epithelial cell lines have been used to examine *H. pylori*-mediated changes.

H. PYLORI INFECTION AND MUCOSAL BARRIER FUNCTION

Several studies have used the sucrose permeability test to evaluate gastric permeability in *H. pylori*-infected human subjects. A study from Graham and colleagues demonstrated normal sucrose permeability test results in *H. pylori*-infected subjects while aspirin ingestion was associated with a marked increase in gastric sucrose permeability[7]. Another report from this group described a small but statistically significant reduction of sucrose excretion after *H. pylori* eradication, suggesting that *H. pylori* may have an effect on gastric permeability[12]. Sucrose permeability was found to be increased in Peruvian children with *H. pylori* infection and endoscopic 'gastritis', but not in infected subjects with endoscopically normal mucosa[13]. Sucrose permeability was also shown to be increased in Swedish adults with asymptomatic *H. pylori* infection, and correlated with the degree of neutrophil infiltration in the mucosa, but not atrophy or intestinal metaplasia[14]. Together, these *in vivo* studies suggest that infection may alter gastric permeability, but the mechanisms by which this occurs cannot be proved by such studies.

In order to examine alterations of gastric permeability on a more mechanistic basis, a number of investigators have performed *in-vitro* studies using gastric mucosa and cultured epithelial cells. IL-8-stimulated transmigration of neutrophils across primary rabbit gastric epithelial cells cultured on membranes with 3 µm pores was associated with increased back-diffusion of sodium ion, suggesting some impairment of gastric epithelial barrier function[15]. This finding is not unexpected, as earlier studies using T84 intestinal epithelial cells showed similar results[16]. *H. pylori* infection of HT-29-19A polarized intestinal epithelial cells was accompanied by an increase in transcellular macromolecular transport without an effect on paracellular transport[17]. In contrast, *H. pylori* sonicates decreased transepithelial resistance of T84 intestinal epithelial cell monolayers and increased paracellular permeability of a marker macromolecule, mannitol[18]. This study also demonstrated that *H. pylori* sonicates increased permeability to mannitol in rat gastric mucosa studied in Ussing chambers. As protein kinase C (PKC) is known to regulate tight junctions, and since sonicate-induced increases in T84 resistance were inhibited by a PKC activator, the authors concluded that *H. pylori* stimulates intracellular signalling to counteract the effects of PKC. In another study, vacuolating cytotoxin (VacA) was shown to increase paracellular permeability for small molecules, including nutrient ions, in T84, canine kidney MDCK I, and murine mammary gland epH4 epithelial cell lines[19]. Increased permeability to macromolecules was measured *in vitro* in gastric mucosa from *H. pylori* infected mice as well as mucosa from mice in which inflammation persisted after eradication of infection[19b]. A number of studies have previously shown increased intestinal epithelial permeability induced by cytokines, including IL-4, IFN-γ and

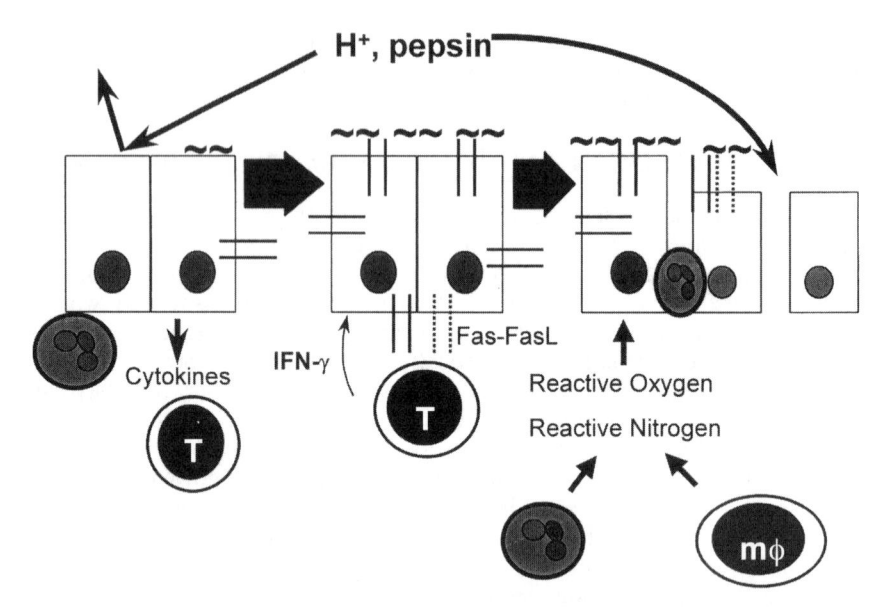

Figure 1. The gastric epithelial barrier during *Helicobacter pylori* infection. Attachment of *H. pylori* to receptors on gastric epithelial cells initiates intracellular signalling that leads to the secretion of chemoattractant cytokines that recruit and activate various immune cells. Cytokines from activated T cells, such as interferon (IFN)-γ, affect barrier function through direct effects on the epithelium including modulation of tight junction and transporter function, and induction of apoptosis. IFN-γ also up-regulates the expression of class II MHC molecules that act as receptors for *H. pylori*, and by enhancing Fas–FasL interactions that lead to cell death. Tumour necrosis factor (TNF)-α, released from macrophages and other cells, can also induce cell death. Activated phagocytic cells release reactive oxygen species (ROS) and reactive nitrogen species (RNS) which can lead to apoptosis or necrosis of epithelial cells. Accelerated loss of epithelium, impaired epithelial restitution, and transepithelial migration of neutrophils induced by *H. pylori* infection and the associated inflammatory response, lead to alterations of gastric epithelial barrier function. This, in turn, allows increased exposure to acid and pepsin, as well as enhanced uptake of potentially antigenic and inflammatory bacterial products from the gastric lumen, leading to further inflammation and mucosal injury.

TNF-α, and by the transmigration of neutrophils or eosinophils[16,20–23]. While these *in-vitro* studies have certain limitations, together they provide some evidence that bacteria, inflammatory cytokines, and neutrophil migration can alter epithelial barrier function during *H. pylori* infection (Figure 1).

MECHANISMS OF ALTERED GASTRIC BARRIER FUNCTION IN *H. PYLORI* INFECTION

Bacterial and host factors can damage the gastric mucosal barrier and lead to alterations of epithelial cell growth and differentiation (Table 1). *H. pylori* infection is associated with increased proliferation *in vivo*[24,25] although most *in-vitro* studies demonstrate bacterial inhibition of cell growth[26], suggesting that other factors regulate cell growth in the complex milieu of the infected gastric mucosa. Increased numbers of apoptotic cells are found in the gastric

Table 1. Factors affecting gastric mucosal barrier function in *H. pylori* infection

Bacterial factors	Host factors
Phosphatases	Cytokines
Phospholipases	Growth factors
Proteases	Eicosanoids
Ammonia generation	Reactive oxygen species
Lipopolysaccharide	Reactive nitrogen species
Platelet-activating factor	Complement
Reactive oxygen species	Proteolytic enzymes

epithelium of infected patients[27–30] with similar findings in cultured gastric epithelial cells[26,31]. Proliferative rates[24,25] and apoptotic rates[27,30] have both been shown to return to control levels after eradication of infection. Potential stimulatory factors include certain cytokines and growth factors, although others may reduce growth. One can speculate that the balance of inhibitory or stimulatory influences on epithelial growth may mediate epithelial outcomes that include ulceration, intestinal metaplasia, and gastric neoplasia.

Cell death represents one mechanism whereby epithelial growth can be regulated. In contrast to necrosis, apoptosis is a programmed form of cell death in which accumulation of DNA fragments consisting of multiples of 180 base pairs forms the basis of several assays to detect apoptosis[32]. Apoptosis is rarely detected in normal intestinal epithelium but is increased in melanosis coli, graft-versus-host disease, NSAID-induced enteropathy, HIV infection, and with chemotherapy or radiation[33,34]. Defective apoptosis is thought to play a role in carcinogenesis, since certain genes that are associated with the development of colorectal cancer (*c-myc*, *p53*, and *bcl-2*) regulate apoptosis[35]. It is also proposed that increased apoptosis stimulates a compensatory increase in proliferation that then increases the chances of mutations that can lead to malignancy[27]. A number of studies in human gastric mucosa and in gastric epithelial cell lines have shown that *H. pylori* infection increases programmed cell death.

GASTRIC EPITHELIAL CELL APOPTOSIS IN *H. PYLORI* INFECTION

Moss and colleagues were the first to publish that, while apoptotic cells were rare and located superficially in gastric glands of uninfected tissue samples, apoptotic cells were present in increased numbers and located throughout the depth of the gastric glands in samples from patients with *H. pylori* infection[27]. Eradication of *H. pylori* infection reduced apoptotic rates to those of uninfected samples. Increased epithelial apoptosis in gastric biopsies from *H. pylori*-infected patients, and its decrease after successful eradication therapy, was confirmed in two other studies[28,30]. The frequency of epithelial apoptosis was found to be significantly lower in other forms of gastritis or non-inflamed mucosa in one study[30]. Immunohistochemical staining for inducible nitric oxide synthase expression and for a marker of peroxynitrite formation was increased in infected tissues[28]. Together these studies demonstrate that *H. pylori* infection is associated with increased epithelial apoptosis. One report suggested that the effect on apoptosis was due to cagA status since their data showed increased apoptosis in biopsies from patients infected with cagA$^-$ strains while cagA$^+$ strains were associated with increased epithelial proliferation but apoptosis was not different from that of uninfected controls[29]. Other studies have not confirmed an association of strain with apoptosis, however[36].

Studies from our laboratory[31] and from Wagner *et al.*[26] show that *H. pylori* induces apoptosis in gastric epithelial cell lines. IFN-γ or TNF-α also induces apoptosis, and when combined with bacteria, IFN-γ has a synergistic effect. Other inflammatory factors including NH_2Cl and nitric oxide induce apoptosis. Recent work indicates that various mutations of different *H. pylori* genes modulate the gastric cell cycle in various ways[37]. Together, these studies imply that bacterial and host factors act, together, to regulate epithelial cell growth and programmed cell death (Figure 1).

OXIDATIVE INJURY

Reactive oxygen species (ROS) including superoxide ($O_2^{-\cdot}$), hydroxyl radical (OH$^\cdot$), and hydrogen peroxide (H_2O_2) can be produced endogenously in at least four general ways; by: (1) metabolic cellular processes, mainly oxidative phosphorylation (OXPHOS); (2) cytokines or growth factors; (3) nitric oxide (NO) second messenger; and (4) neutrophil or macrophage stimulation at sites of injury[38,39].

Within the mitochondria, leakage of electrons from the electron transport chain (primarily complexes I and III) generates reactive oxygen. It has been estimated that 1–4% of all the oxygen consumed by mitochondria is released as superoxide or hydrogen peroxide. Manganese superoxide dismutase (SOD), the mitochondrial form of SOD, converts superoxide to hydrogen peroxide, and is induced by several oxidants. Several other biochemical reactions within the cell can produce ROS. For example, xanthine oxidase (XO) generates uric acid and superoxide from oxygen and xanthine. Another potential source of mitochondrial-generated hydrogen peroxide is monoamine oxidase (MAO), which is located in the outer mitochondrial membrane.

Several recent reports have suggested that growth factors such as platelet-derived growth factor and TNF-α, as well as other cytokines, induce a transient surge of H_2O_2, which is essential for the action of these agents[40-42]. A variety of cells including neutrophils and macrophages express NO$^\cdot$ synthase (NOS) and produce NO$^\cdot$. NO$^\cdot$ has been shown to inhibit mitochondrial enzymes such as aconitase and inhibit the electron transport chain. Thus, NO$^\cdot$ toxicity may be caused directly by the inhibition of normal mitochondrial function, and the leakage of reactive oxygen. NO$^\cdot$ can react with superoxide to form peroxynitrite (ONOO$^-$). This can spontaneously break down to form hydroxyl radical or singlet oxygen, both of which are highly reactive with DNA.

ROS are generated during the respiratory burst in phagocytic cells through mitochondrial and microsomal electron transport chains and by oxidant enzymes including xanthine oxidase (described above), cyclooxygenase and lipoxygenase. In the presence of neutrophil myeloperoxidase, H_2O_2 combines with free chloride to form hypochlorous acid (HOCl). HOCl is $\sim$ 100 times more reactive than H_2O_2, can react with primary amines to form N-chloramines and monochloramine, and eventually leads to lipid damage[38]. Hydroxyl radicals are extremely reactive and very short-lived. If free Fe^{2+} is available it may participate directly in the production of OH˙ radicals via the Fenton reaction. Hydroxyl radicals can also be generated by superoxide in the Haber–Weiss reaction. These processes can act together to yield large quantities of OH˙ radicals, which are very reactive with macromolecules. Activated macrophages also produce TNF-α, which can exert a wide range of cellular effects including the direct production of mitochondrial ROS and cell death.

A number of endogenous systems help regulate the production of ROS. In addition to the mitochondrial MnSOD (SOD2) discussed above, extracellular (EcSOD, SOD3) and copper–zinc cytoplasmic (CuZnSOD, SOD1) isozymes also exist. These enzymes work in concert with catalase and glutathione peroxidase (GSX) to break down SOD-generated H_2O_2 in water. It has been suggested that GSX reactions are more important than catalase for the breakdown of hydrogen peroxide, since (with the exception of muscle) mitochondria lack catalase. Besides enzymatic breakdown of ROS, tissues contain several antioxidant scavengers, including tocopherol (vitamin E), β-carotene, and vitamin C, the latter being decreased in *H. pylori* infection[43,44].

The three major types of cellular damage resulting from ROS are lipid peroxidation (discussed above), protein oxidation and oxidation of DNA[45,46]. ROS, such as OH˙, are thought to play a causal role in malignant transformation through the induction of DNA damage, which is composed of single-strand breaks (SSB), alkali-labile sites in DNA (such as abasic sites) as well as many forms of base damage. A critical cell cycle control protein, p53, which is induced after DNA damage and is important for DNA damage-induced apoptosis, directs cellular arrest in G1 by the induction of several proteins, such as p21/WAF-1[47]. This delay in cell cycle progression allows the cell to repair the damaged DNA. However, if the damage is severe the cell will undergo a p53-dependent programmed cell death. There are many other genes (e.g. *c-myc*, *bcl-2* and its homologues) that are being recognized to regulate gastrointestinal epithelial cell growth and apoptosis and the development of cancer.

Many different cell types have been shown to undergo a paradoxical response of either mitogenesis or cell death by ROS[38]. For example, low amounts of reactive oxygen can result in the induction of immediate early response genes such as *c-fos* and *c-jun*[48]. In addition, the transcription factor nuclear factor κB (NFκB) is activated by a variety of stimuli include oxidative stress, UV light, or ionizing radiation, and has recently been linked to ageing tissues. NFκB is known to regulate the expression of several acute-phase response genes involved in inflammation and cellular proliferation. However, higher levels or prolonged exposure to ROS can lead to pro-

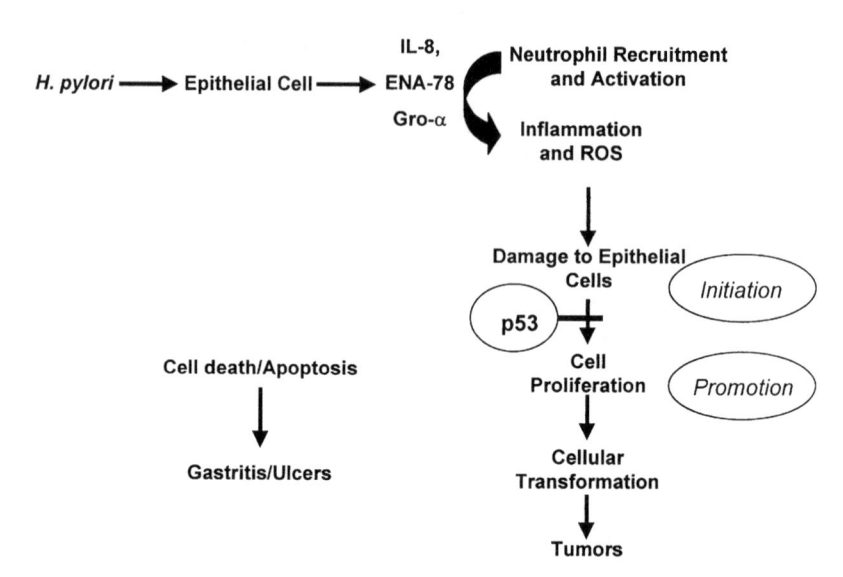

Figure 2. *H. pylori*, epithelial cell injury and reactive oxygen species. Schematic diagram illustrating proposed key events in the initiation of inflammation, epithelial injury, and development of gastric cancer in *H. pylori* infection. Gastric epithelial cell lines secrete chemokines in response to infection with non-invasive *H. pylori*. Neutrophils are recruited into the gastric mucosa and activated to release ROS, which can damage the gastric epithelium. *H. pylori* can also release ROS and induce accumulation of ROS in epithelial cells. The result of ROS-mediated injury depends on the expression of various genes such as p53, the extent and type of the injury, the existence of DNA repair mechanisms, and the contribution of growth-regulating factors. These events regulate the balance between cell death and cell proliferation and the subsequent progression of cellular transformation and the development of gastric cancer. (Modified with permission from ref. 39.)

grammed cell death[49]. ROS have been shown to contribute to p53[47], Fas–Fas ligand[50,51], ceramide[52], and TNF-mediated killing (Figure 2). It is known that mammalian cells respond to oxidative stress with the initial generation of ROS and the subsequent activation of reduction–oxidation (redox) sensitive signalling pathways which control the transcription of genes that may regulate cell growth, repair the death processes[38]. A number of studies including work from our laboratory indicate that ROS are involved in the pathogenesis of *H. pylori* infection.

H. PYLORI INFECTION AND OXIDATIVE STRESS

There is increasing evidence that microbial pathogens induce oxidative stress in infected host cells[53-55] and this may represent an important mechanism leading to epithelial injury in *H. pylori* infection. It is known from other cell systems that oxidative stress regulates cell cycle events in multiple ways with net responses that include aberrant proliferation, adaptation cytotoxicity and cell death[38]. Oxidative stress could well play a role in the altered epithelial proliferation, increased apoptosis and increased oxidative DNA damage[56,57] associated with *H. pylori* infection (Figure 2). Increased levels of ROS have been measured in the mucosa of infected patients[58,59]. While activated phagocytic leucocytes recruited to the gastric mucosa during infection that release ROS represent one obvious source of oxidative stress[58,60], recent studies demonstrate that *H. pylori* also generates ROS[61,62]. The decreased levels of ascorbic acid that are associated with *H. pylori* infection[44,63] also contribute to a pro-oxidative environment.

Mycobacterium avium-intracellulare complex, bovine viral diarrhoea virus and human immunodeficiency virus, have been shown to exert their effects on host cells via ROS generation[54,55]. Another species of *Helicobacter*, *H. hepaticus*, has been shown to induce oxidative DNA damage in hepatocytes of infected mice[53]. We have shown that *H. pylori* infection stimulates the accumulation of intracellular ROS in different gastric epithelial cell lines[64], confirming the findings of a previous report describing the accumulation of ROS in another human gastric epithelial cell line, CRL 1739, after infection with *H. pylori*[61]. Superoxide anion was also detected in epithelial cell preparations isolated from guinea pig gastric mucosa after experimental *H. pylori* infection[62]. A preliminary report demonstrating decreased levels of glutathione in *H. pylori*-infected HMO2 human gastric epithelial cells[65] provides additional evidence that *H. pylori* serves as a stimulus for the accumulation of ROS within gastric epithelial cells. We have shown that ROS levels are higher in gastric epithelial cells isolated from infected subjects, compared to those from uninfected subjects, demonstrating that *H. pylori*-induced oxidative stress is not an artifact of cultured cells or animal models and does occur in naturally infected native human epithelial cells. Further evidence that oxidative stress may be involved in the alterations of epithelial cell growth in *H. pylori* infection is found in a study in which decreased epithelial cell apoptosis was observed in gastric tissues for *H. pylori*-infected patients treated with antioxidant therapy only[28]. Although ROS have not been previously shown to play a role in programmed cell death of gastric epithelial cells, they have been implicated in apoptosis in other cell types resulting from various stimuli[49].

Host factors also contribute to oxidative stress during *H. pylori* infection. Activated neutrophils or macrophages are potent sources of ROS[66], including H_2O_2, which lead to an accumulation of intracellular ROS and apoptosis of gastric epithelial cells. Cytokines that are increased in the gastric mucosa of infected subjects, including TNF-α, IFN-γ and IL-1β[67], also induce oxidative stress and apoptosis. This is consistent with other cell types in which cytokines have been reported to induce ROS[40–42].

The role of bacterial genotype has been a focus of recent investigations into *H. pylori* pathogenesis. Strains that are *cagA*$^+$ have been shown to be associated with increased gastric inflammation, increased bacterial load and both peptic ulcer disease and gastric cancer[68,69]. Strains bearing the pathogenicity island (PAI) induce higher levels of IL-870 and activate transcription factors, NFκB[71,72] and activator protein (AP)-1[73]. *cag* PAI status may also influence the ability of *H. pylori* to induce intracellular ROS in gastric epithelial cells, providing further insight into how bacterial genetic factors

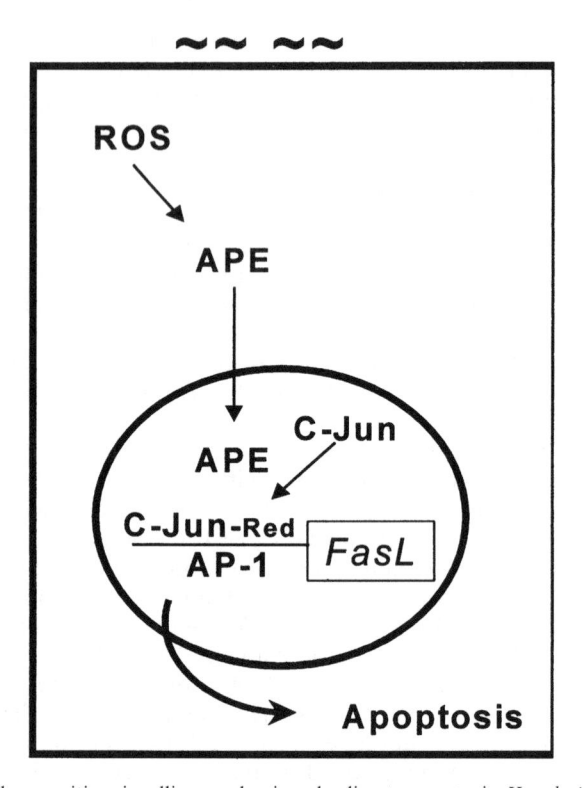

Figure 3. Redox-sensitive signalling mechanisms leading to apoptosis. *H. pylori*, or the associated inflammatory response, leads to apoptosis and the accumulation of intracellular ROS. ROS damage cellular proteins, lipids, and DNA as well as regulating the activation of transcription factors that induce the expression of redox-sensitive genes encoding DNA repair enzymes, antioxidant proteins, cytokines, and factors regulating cell growth and apoptosis. AP endonuclease, also known as redox factor-1 (ref. 1), has been shown to be necessary for the reduction of cysteine residue 252 in the DNA binding portion of c-Jun and c-Fos[76]. *H. pylori* increases the expression of AP endonuclease (APE), a multifunctional protein that acts as a DNA repair enzyme which also acts to reductively activate transcription factors such as p53 or c-Jun. This permits DNA binding of the reduced transcription factor, in this case c-Jun (c-Jun-Red), to the binding site (activator protein (AP)-1) upstream of several pro-apoptotic genes including *fasL* or in the case of p53, *bax*. As such, the expression of genes regulated by AP endonuclease is 'redox-sensitive'. Interestingly, many of the genes regulating apoptosis are redox-sensitive, as are signalling pathways such as JNK/SAPK. The net effect of *H. pylori* infection or ROS on gastric epithelial cell signalling is complex, but an understanding of these events may provide insight into disease pathogenesis.

play a role in disease pathogenesis. Moreover, since *cag* PAI-positive strains are associated with greater inflammation, the host response may also contribute to enhanced oxidative stress associated with these strains. Differential induction of ROS may be relevant to the reported associations of the *cag* PAI and the activation of epithelial cell signalling pathways[70,73]. With the identification of *H. pylori* genome sequences the opportunity exists to identify more specific bacterial genes that regulate ROS generation[74,75].

CONCLUSIONS

Helicobacter pylori infection is an aetiological factor in various disorders of the gastric epithelium including ulceration, metaplasia, dysplasia, and carcinoma. Alterations of epithelial cell growth and enhanced programmed cell death play a role in *H. pylori* disease manifestations, as failure of mucosal adaptation can lead to ulceration and abnormal repair may predispose to malignancy. There is reasonable evidence that *H. pylori* infection affects gastric mucosal barrier function and that the effects on epithelial growth and repair mechanisms, as well as cell death, contribute to the reported changes in gastric permeability. Recent studies indicate that oxidative stress may play a role in the increased programmed cell death that occurs in the epithelium during infection. Further investigation is necessary to explore the cellular and molecular mechanisms by which oxidative stress regulates epithelial responses to *H. pylori* infection (Figure 3), as this will provide new insight into the pathogenesis of *H. pylori*-associated conditions.

Acknowledgements

Support from the National Institute of Health (RO1 DK51677 and RO1 DK50669), the John Sealy Memorial Endowment Fund (Development Grant), and a UTMB President's Cabinet Award is acknowledged.

References

1. Engel E, Guth PH, Nishikazi Y, Kaunitz JD. Barrier function of the gastric mucus gel. Am J Physiol Gastrointest Liver Physiol. 1995;269:G994–9.
2. Konturek PC. Physiological, immunohistochemical, and molecular aspects of gastric adaptation to stress, aspirin, and to *H. pylori*-derived gastrotoxins. J Physiol Pharmacol. 1997;48:3–42.
3. Meddings JB, Sutherland LR, Byles NI, Wallace JL. Sucrose: a novel permeability marker for gastroduodenal disease. Gastroenterology. 1993;104:1619–26.
4. Sutherland LR, Verhoef M, Wallace JL, Van Rosendaal G, Crutcher R, Meddings JB. A simple, non-invasive marker of gastric damage: sucrose permeability. Lancet. 1994;343:998–1000.
5. Hatz RA, Bloch KJ, Harmatez PR *et al*. Divalent hapten-induced intestinal anaphylaxis in the mouse enhances macromolecular uptake from the stomach. Gastroenterology. 1990;98:894–900.
6. Curtis GH, Gall DG. Macromolecular transport by rat gastric mucosa. Am J Physiol Gastrointest Liver Physiol. 1992;1262:G1033–40.
7. Rabassa AA, Goodgame R, Sutton FM, Ou CN, Rognerud C, Graham DY. Effects of aspirin and *Helicobacter pylori* on the gastroduodenal mucosal permeability to sucrose. Gut. 1996;39:159–63.
8. Vogelsang H, Oberhuber G, Wyatt J. Lymphocytic gastritis and gastric permeability in patients with celiac disease. Gastroenterology. 1996;111:73–7.
9. Catto-Smith AG, Patrick MK, Scott RB, Davison JS, Gall DG. Gastric response to mucosal IgE-mediated reactions. Am J Physiol. 1989;257:G704–8.
10. Madara JL. Loosening tight junctions: lessons from the intestine. J Clin Invest. 1989;83:1089–94.
11. Madara JL. Pathobiology of the intestinal epithelial barrier. Am J Pathol. 1990;137:1273–81.
12. Graham DY, Malaty HM, Goodgame R, Ou CN. Effect of cure of *H. pylori* infection on the gastric mucosal permeability. Gastroenterology. 1996;110:A122 (abstract).

13. Vera JF, Gotteland M, Chavez E, Vial MT, Kakarieka E, Brunser O. Sucrose permeability in children with gastric damage and *Helicobacter pylori* infection. J Pediatr Gastroenterol Nutr. 1997;24:506–11.
14. Borch K, Sjostedt C, Hannestad U, Soderholm JD, Franzen L, Mardh S. Asymptomatic *Helicobacter pylori* gastritis is associated with increased sucrose permeability. Dig Dis Sci. 1998;43:749–53.
15. Fujiwara Y, Arakawa T, Fukuda T et al. Interleukin-8 stimulates leukocyte migration across a monolayer of cultured rabbit gastric epithelial cells. Effect associated with the impairment of gastric epithelial barrier function. Dig Dis Sci. 1997;42:1210–15.
16. Nash S, Stafford J, Madara JL. Effects of polymorphonuclear leukocyte transmigration on the barrier function of cultured intestinal epithelial monlayers. J Clin Invest. 1987; 80:1104–13.
17. Matysiak-Budnik T, Terpend K, Alain S et al. *Helicobacter pylori* alters exogenous antigen absorption and processing in a digestive tract epithelial cell line model. Infect Immun. 1998;66:5786–91.
18. Terres AM, Pajares JM, Hopkins AM et al. *Helicobacter pylori* disrupts epithelial barrier function in a process inhibited by protein kinase C activators. Infect Immun. 1998; 66:2943–50.
19. Papini E, Satin B, Norais N et al. Selective increase of the permeability of polarized epithelial cell monolayers by *Helicobacter pylori* vacuolating toxin. J Clin Invest. 1998;102:813–20.
19b. Matysiak-Budnik T, Hashimoto K, Heyman M, de Mascarel A, Desjeux JF, Megraud F. Antral gastric permeability to antigens in mice is altered by infection with *Helicobacter felis*. Eur J Gastroenterol Hepatol. 1999;11:1371–7.
20. Madara JL, Stafford J. Interferon-γ directly affects barrier function of cultured intestinal epithelial monolayers. J Clin Invest. 1989;83:724–7.
21. Colgan SP, Resnick MB, Parkos CA et al. IL-4 directly modulates function of a model human intestinal epithelium. J Immunol. 1994;153:2122–9.
22. Parkos CA, Colgan SP, Delp C, Arnaout MA, Madara JL. Neutrophil migration across a cultured epithelial monolayer elicits a biphasic resistance response representing sequential effects on transcellular and paracellular pathways. J Cell Biol. 1992;117:757–64.
23. Resnick MB, Colgan SP, Patapoff TW et al. Activated eosinophils evoke chloride secretion in model intestinal epithelia primarily via regulated release of 5′-AMP. J Immunol. 1993;151:5716–23.
24. Cahill RJ, Xia H, Kilgallen C, Beattie S, Hamilton H, O'Morain C. Effect of eradication of *Helicobacter pylori* infection on gastric epithelial cell proliferation. Dig Dis Sci. 1995; 40:1627–31.
25. Lynch DAF, Mapstone NP, Clarke AMT et al. Cell proliferation in *Helicobacter pylori* associated gastritis and the effect of eradication therapy. Gut. 1995;36:346–50.
26. Wagner S, Beil W, Westermann J et al. Regulation of gastric epithelial cell growth by *Helicobacter pylori*: evidence for a major role of apoptosis. Gastroenterology. 1997; 113:1836–47.
27. Moss SF, Calam J, Agarwal B, Wang S, Holt PG. Induction of gastric epithelial apoptosis by *Helicobacter pylori*. Gut. 1996;38:498–501.
28. Mannick EE, Bravo LE, Zarama G et al. Inducible nitric oxide synthase, nitrotyrosine, and apoptosis in *Helicobacter pylori* gastritis: effect of antibiotics and antioxidants. Cancer Res. 1996;56:3238–43.
29. Peek Jr RM, Moss SF, Tham KY et al. *Helicobacter pylori* cagA$^+$ strains and dissociation of gastric epithelial cell proliferation from apoptosis. J Natl Cancer Inst. 1997;89:863–8.
30. Jones NL, Shannon PT, Cutz E, Yeger H, Sherman PM. Increase in proliferation and apoptosis of gastric epithelial cells early in the natural history of *Helicobacter pylori* infection. Am J Pathol. 1997;151:1695–703.
31. Fan X, Crowe SE, Behar S et al. The effect of class II major histocompatibility complex expression on adherence of *Helicobacter pylori* and induction of apoptosis in gastric epithelial cells: a mechanism for T helper cell type 1-mediated damage. J Exp Med. 1998;187:1659–69.
32. Hetts SW. To die or not to die. An overview of apoptosis and its role in disease. J Am Med Assoc. 1998;279:300–7.
33. Watson AJM. Necrosis and apoptosis in the gastrointestinal tract. Gut. 1995;37:165–7.

34. Que FG, Gores G. Cell death by apoptosis: basic concepts and disease relevance for the gastroenterologist. Gastroenterology. 1996;110:1238–43.
35. Wyllie AH. Apoptosis and carcinogenesis. Eur J Cell Biol. 1997;73:189–97.
36. Zhu H, Yang XL, Lai KC et al. Nonsteroidal antiinflammatory drugs could reverse *Helicobacter pylori*-induced apoptosis and proliferation in gastric epithelial cells. Dig Dis Sci. 1998;43:1957–63.
37. Peek Jr RM, Blaser MJ, Mays DJ et al. *Helicobacter pylori* strain-specific genotypes and modulation of the gastric epithelial cell cycle. Cancer Res. 1999;59:6124–31.
38. Janssen YMW, Van Houten B, Borm PJA, Mossman BT. Biology of disease. Cell and tissue responses to oxidative damage. Lab Invest. 1993;69:261–74.
39. Van Houten B, Crowe SE. The role of the host response in oxidative damage and malignant transformation. Mucosal Immunol Update. 1997;5:64–75.
40. Matsubara T, Ziff M. Increased superoxide anion release from human endothelial cells in response to cytokines. J Immunol. 1986;137:3295–8.
41. Meier B, Radeke HH, Selle S et al. Human fibroblasts release reactive oxygen species in response to interleukin-1 or tumour necrosis factor-α. Biochem J. 1989;263:539–45.
42. Radeke HH, Meier B, Topley N, Floge J, Habermehl GG, Resch K. Interleukin 1-α and tumor necrosis factor-α induce oxygen radical production in mesangial cells. Kidney Int. 1990;37:767–75.
43. Sobala GM, Crabtree JE, Dixon MF et al. Acute *Helicobacter pylori* infection: clinical features, local and systemic immune response, gastric mucosal histology, and gastric juice ascorbic acid concentrations. Gut. 1991;32:1415–18.
44. Ruiz B, Carlton Rood J, Fontham ETH et al. Vitamin C concentration in gastric juice before and after anti-*Helicobacter pylori* treatment. Am J Gastroenterol. 1994;89:533–9.
45. Wiseman H, Halliwell B. Damage to DNA by reactive oxygen and nitrogen species: role in inflammatory disease and progression to cancer. Biochem J. 1996;313–17–29.
46. Cross CE, Halliwell B, Borish ET et al. Oxygen radicals and human disease [clinical conference]. Ann Intern Med. 1987;107:526–45.
47. Polyak K, Xia Y, Zweier JL, Kinzler KW, Vogelstein B. A model of p53-induced apoptosis. Nature. 1997;389:300–5.
48. Muller JM, Rupec RA, Baeuerle PA. Study of gene regulation by NF-κB and AP-1 in response to reactive oxygen intermediates. Methods Enzymol. 1997;11:301–12.
49. Buttke TM, Sandstrom PA. Oxidative stress as a mediator of apoptosis. Immunol Today. 1994;15:7–10.
50. Hug H, Strand S, Grambihler A et al. Reactive oxygen intermediates are involved in the induction of CD95 ligand mRNA expression by cytostatic drugs in hepatoma cells. J Biol Chem. 1997;272:28191–3.
51. Bauer MKA, Vogt M, Los M, Siegel J, Weselborg S, Schulze-Osthoff K. Role of reactive oxygen intermediates in activation-induced CD95 (APO-1/Fas) ligand expression. J Biol Chem. 1998;273:8084–55.
52. Quillet-Mary A, Jaffrezou JP, Mansat V, Bordier C, Naval J, Laurent G. Implication of mitochondrial hydrogen peroxide generation in ceramide-induced apoptosis. J Biol Chem. 1997;272:21388–95.
53. Sipowicz MA, Chomarat P, Diwan BA et al. Increased oxidative DNA damage and hepatocyte overexpression of specific cytochrome p450 isoforms in hepatitis of mice infected with *Helicobacter hepaticus*. Am J Pathol. 1997;151:933–41.
54. Schweizer M, Peterhans E. Oxidative stress in cells infected with bovine viral diarrhoea virus: a crucial step in the induction of apoptosis. J Gen Virol. 1999;80:1147–55.
55. Giri DK, Mehta RT, Kansal RG, Aggarwal BB. *Mycobacterium avium-intracellulare* complex activates nuclear transcription factor-κB in different cell types through reactive oxygen intermediates. J Immunol. 1998;161:4834–41.
56. Baik S-C, You H-S, Chung M-H et al. Increased oxidative DNA damage in *Helicobacter pylori*-infected human gastric mucosa. Cancer Res. 1996;56:1279–82.
57. Farinati F, Cardin R, Degan P et al. Oxidative DNA damage accumulation in gastric carcinogenesis. Gut. 1998;42:351–6.
58. Davies GR, Simmonds NJ, Stevens TRJ et al. *Helicobacter pylori* stimulates antral mucosal reactive oxygen metabolite production *in vivo*. Gut. 1994;35:179–85.
59. Drake IM, Mapstone NP, Schorah CJ et al. Reactive oxygen species activity and lipid peroxidation in *Helicobacter pylori* associated gastritis: relation to gastric mucosal ascorbic acid concentrations and effect of *H. pylori* eradication. Gut. 1998;42:768–71.

60. Zhang QB, Dawodu JB, Husain A, Etolhi G, Gemmell CG, Russell RI. Association of antral mucosal levels of interleukin 8 and reactive oxygen radicals in patients infected with *Helicobacter pylori*. Clin Sci. 1998;92:69–73.
61. Bagchi D, Bhattacharya G, Stohs SJ. Production of reactive oxygen species by gastric cells in association with *Helicobacter pylori*. Free Rad Res. 1996;24:439–50.
62. Teshima S, Rokutan K, Nikawa T, Kishi K. Guinea pig gastric mucosal cells produce abundant superoxide anion through an NADPH oxidase-like system. Gastroenterology. 1998;115:1186–96.
63. Sobalo GM, Schorah CJ, Shires S et al. Effect of eradication of *Helicobacter pylori* on gastric juice ascorbic acid concentrations. Gut. 1993;34:1038–41.
64. Boldogh I, Ding SZ, Fan XJ, Patel J, Minohara Y, Crowe SE. Oxidative stress in gastric epithelial cells during *Helicobacter pylori* infection. Gastroenterology. 1999;116:A141 (abstract).
65. Beil W, Wagner S, Obst B, Kirchner G, Sewing K-F. *Helicobacter pylori* attenuates sulfhydryl levels in the gastric cell line HM02. Gastroenterology. 114:A71 (abstract).
66. Thelen M, Dewald B, Baggiolini M. Neutrophil signal transduction and activation of the respiratory burst. Physiol Rev. 1993:73:797–821.
67. Noach LA, Bosma NB, Jansen J, Hoek FJ, van-Deventer SJ, Tytgat GN. Mucosal tumor necrosis factor-alpha, interleukin-1 beta and interleukin-8 production in patients with *Helicobacter pylori*. Scand J Gastroenterol. 1994;29:425–9.
68. Blaser MJ, Perez-Perez GI, Kleanthous H et al. Infection with *Helicobacter pylori* strains possessing cagA is associated with an increased risk of developing adenocarcinoma of the stomach. Cancer Res. 1995;55:2111–15.
69. Peek Jr RM, Miller GG, Tham KT et al. Heightened inflammatory response and cytokine expression *in vivo* to $cagA^+$ *Helicobacter pylori* strains. Lab Invest. 1995;71:760–70.
70. Li SD, Kersulyte D, Lindley IJD, Neelam B, Berg DE, Crabtree JE. Multiple genes in the left half of the *cag* pathogenicity island of *Helicobacter pylori* are required for tyrosine kinase-dependent transcription of interleukin-8 in gastric epithelial cells. Infect Immun. 1999;67:3893–9.
71. Keates S, Youssef SH, Upton M, Kelly CP. *Helicobacter pylori* infection activates NF-kB in gastric epithelial cells. Gastroenterology. 1997;113:1099–109.
72. Sharma SA, Tummuru MK, Blaser MJ, Kerr LD. Activation of IL-8 gene expression by *Helicobacter pylori* is regulated by transcription factor nuclear factor-kappa B in gsatric epithelial cells. J Immunol. 1998;160:2401–7.
73. Naumann M, Wessler S, Bartsch C et al. Activation of activator protein 1 and stress response kinases in epithelial cells colonized by *Helicobacter pylori* encoding the *cag* pathogenicity island. J Biol Chem. 1999;274:31655–62.
74. Tomb J-F, White O, Kerlavage AR et al. The complete genome sequence of the gastric pathogen *Helicobacter pylori*. Nature. 1997;388:539–47.
75. Marais A, Mendz GL, Hazell SL, Megraud F. Metabolism and genetics of *Helicobacter pylori*: the genome era. Microbiol Mol Biol Rev. 1999;63:642–74.
76. Abate C, Patel L, Rauscher III FJ, Curran T. Redox regulation of Fos and Jun DNA-binding activity *in vitro*. Science. 1990;249:1157–61.

17
Immuno-inflammatory response to *Helicobacter pylori* in children

S. J. CZINN, J. C. EISENBERG, J. G. NEDRUD and
T. G. BLANCHARD

INTRODUCTION

Since the isolation and culture of *Helicobacter pylori* less than 20 years ago, the terms diffuse chronic active gastritis and multifocal atrophic gastritis have been introduced in an effort to explain the fundamental role this organism plays in the development of gastroduodenal disease[1]. A number of epidemiological studies have also demonstrated that once this infection is acquired it is rarely cleared, and persists for the life of the individual[2]. In addition to gastritis and peptic ulcer disease, chronic long-lasting *H. pylori* infection, particularly when acquired in childhood, can significantly increase the risk of developing gastric cancer[3]. These studies were so compelling that in 1994 the World Health Organization classified *H. pylori* as a human carcinogen[4]. Unfortunately, most epidemiological studies of *H. pylori* infection have been performed in adults, who were probably infected for decades prior to the diagnosis. Therefore, very little information is available regarding the natural history of the acute phase of the infection.

ACQUISITION AND TRANSMISSION OF *H. PYLORI* INFECTION

Studies from all continents have now established that the overwhelming majority of individuals in developing countries are infected with *H. pylori* during childhood[5,6]. Data to support the early acquisition of *H. pylori* infection come from retrospective studies, which estimate the incidence of new *H. pylori* infections in adults to be 0.4% per patient-year. At the present time there are also data suggesting that *H. pylori* infection clusters within families, and that the acquisition of this infection is strongly linked to conditions associated with lower socioeconomic status during childhood, such as residential crowding[7-9]. A recent study by Goodman and Correa suggests that transmission occurs from older siblings to their younger siblings rather than from the parents[10]. Close contact does not in itself always result in transmission of infection. A prospective study investigating the evolution of *H. pylori* infection in infants born to *H. pylori*-positive mothers was unable to demonstrate transmission of infection. At 1 year of age, 67 children underwent a C-13 urea breath test which demonstrated that only one of these children had become infected with *H. pylori*. This study demonstrates that, despite close personal contact with their mothers, children born to *H. pylori*-positive mothers do not appear to have an increased risk of becoming infected with *H. pylori* during the first year of life. Since most of these mothers were breastfeeding, it is possible that protective factors in the mothers' milk were responsible for the low rate of *H. pylori* acquisition[11]. We can speculate that the rate of transmission would have been higher if the mothers were not breastfeeding. Support for the hypothesis of person-to-person transmission of *H. pylori*, either via the oral–oral route or the fecal–oral route, comes from a number of recent reports. Parsonnet and colleagues confirmed the presence of live *H. pylori* bacteria in numbers as high as 30,000 bacteria/ml of vomitus, as well as in the ambient air following emetic-induced vomiting in *H. pylori*-positive patients[12]. In addition, this as well as other reports have also confirmed the presence of viable *H. pylori* organisms recovered from human faeces[13,14]. Although water and pets have also been suggested as an environmental source of *H. pylori* infection, to date the only known reservoir for *H. pylori* continues to be the human stomach.

ANTIBODY RESPONSES IN CHILDREN INFECTED WITH *H. PYLORI*

Although there appears to be a consensus of opinion that the majority of individuals become infected with *H. pylori* during childhood, a number of additional epidemiological differences do exist between children and adults with regard to *H. pylori* infection. In addition to the acquisition of *H. pylori* during childhood, young children also appear to be at increased risk of reinfection following antimicrobial eradication of the organism[15]. A number of investigators have suggested that transient *H. pylori* infection is a common phenomenon in children during the first few years of life. It is unclear whether this is strictly due to socioeconomic factors or whether other factors such as the host immune response to *H. pylori* infection is significantly different in children from that of adults.

Immunoglobulin A is the primary immunoglobulin of the mucosal immune system and is thought to play a major role in preventing enteric infections. Ingested by the infant in colostrum and milk, IgA acts at the epithelial surface to exclude foreign microbial and food-borne antigens. Thomas and colleagues studied Gambian mother–infant pairs during the first year of life, and demonstrated that higher maternal anti-*H. pylori* IgA antibody titres resulted in delay of acquisition of *H. pylori* infection. The same authors also demonstrated that breast milk IgA antibody levels in mothers or infants who remained free of infection were 2–4 times higher than those of mothers of infants who acquired *H. pylori* infection before the age of 1 year. Studies such as these suggest that human milk may also prevent *H. pylori* infection through antibody-dependent mechanisms[7,16].

Older children infected with *H. pylori* develop serum and gastric anti-*H. pylori* antibody responses which were initially thought to be quite similar to those of adults. However, the mean serological antibody titre among infected paediatric patients is lower than the mean titres in infected adult patients[17–19]. Interestingly, anti-*H. pylori* IgG but not IgA antibody levels are significantly increased in paediatric patients infected with *H. pylori*. The lower IgA antibody titres may be a factor in promoting the acquisition of *H. pylori* in children[20]. Additionally there may also be a difference in the quality of the serum antibody response between adults and children. Western blot analysis has shown that the immunodominant *Helicobacter* proteins recognized in children may differ from those recognized in adults[21]. Additional studies will be required to determine the exact route of *H. pylori* acquisition, so that adequate preventive strategies for this extremely common infection can be developed.

Based on epidemiological studies, a number of investigators have suggested that transient *H. pylori* infection is a common phenomenon in children. Is there a role for the host immune response in explaining the ability of a child to spontaneously clear this infection? We have recently been able to study a paediatric patient who spontaneously cleared his *H. pylori* infection[22]. In this case report a 10-year old boy with a documented duodenal bulb ulcer and chronic *H. pylori*-associated gastric inflammation spontaneously cleared his *Helicobacter* infection. The Western blot analysis from this patient demonstrated numerous bands during chronic infection but only one prominent band with a molecular weight of 76 kDa following spontaneous clearance of infection. Subsequent Western blot analysis using purified recombinant *H. pylori ureB* showed that this convalescent serum recognized urease. These data suggest that qualitative as well as quantitative differences in antibody responses may explain not only why children are more susceptible to *H. pylori* infection, but also why a subset of the paediatric population acutely infected with *H. pylori* can then clear the infection.

BACTERIAL PATHOGENESIS OF *H. PYLORI*

Several virulence factors of *H. pylori* have now been identified and either play a direct role in the ability of the bacteria to colonize the gastric mucosa or may contribute to the pathogenesis of disease. The most notable virulence factors include VacA and the CagA pathogenicity island. It is likely that genotypic differences among bacteria are important in the progression of disease. In studies performed in adults, there is evidence that strains of *H. pylori* which express the VacA and the CagA pathogenicity island are more likely to result in the development of duodenal ulcer or gastric cancer. Although upwards of 50% of all *H. pylori* strains fall into the virulent designation, only a small minority of adults infected with such strains develop such serious disease. Little information is available regarding the relationship of such bacterial virulence factors and clinical outcomes in paediatric patients. Data from an ongoing collaborative pediatric *H. pylori* study in

North America have been unable to confirm a relationship between the putative virulence factors VacA and CagA and the development of peptic ulcer disease. Seventy-five per cent of the children with ulcers, and 60% of the children with only histological gastritis, had *H. pylori* strains that were $CagA+$ genotype (manuscript in preparation).

The degree of histological gastritis did, however, appear to correlate with the serum antibody response. In a study of children with *H. pylori* gastritis, the mean serum anti-*H. pylori* antibody titres were 0.274 ± 0.126 in the presence of mild gastritis, 0.778 ± 0.55 in the presence of moderate gastritis, and finally when severe gastritis was present the serum antibody titre was 1.32 ± 0.6. Thus, in children, the serum IgG immune response appears to correlate with the degree of histological gastritis[23]. Currently, it is unclear whether the humoral immune response promotes the inflammatory response or whether the decreased serum antibody response seen in children as compared to adults may, primarily, be due to an initial milder inflammatory response.

CELLULAR IMMUNE RESPONSE TO *H. PYLORI* INFECTION

Because there are studies linking the early acquisition of *H. pylori* to childhood diarrhoea, malnutrition, short stature, and the potential for developing gastric cancer, there may be a need to develop effective methods to prevent this infection. A number of laboratories have confirmed that oral and systemic immunization strategies are capable of preventing *H. pylori* infection.

Early studies suggested that immunization by either the oral or intranasal route, in combination with a suitable mucosal adjuvant or carrier system, was necessary for the induction of protective immunity at the gastric mucosa[24-26]. However, several recent studies by us and others indicate that protective immunity appears to be an antibody-independent phenomenon and can be achieved in adult animal models by traditional systemic immunizations when a suitable adjuvant is employed[27,28]. Since infection is believed to occur primarily in early life, such a vaccination would have to be effective when administered in early childhood. Immunization of neonatal mice by both the subcutaneous and intraperitoneal routes resulted in a pronounced immune response, as demonstrated by the production of *H. pylori*-specific antibodies and the ability of spleen T cells to secrete significant amounts of cytokine following stimulation with antigen *in vitro*. Mice immunized subcutaneously or intraperitoneally as neonates, like their adult counterparts, had a significant reduction in bacterial load ($p < 0.0001$) compared to mice immunized with an irrelevant protein antigen. Recently weaned mice (4 weeks old) also showed a marked reduction in bacterial load when immunized with *H. pylori* antigen and IFA intraperitoneally. These mice had a five-fold reduction in *H. pylori* cfu per mg of stomach. These experiments demonstrate that protective immunity against *H. pylori* infection can be induced by prophylactic immunization of newborn and recently weaned mice. These immunizations can be administered by systemic injection and can be accomplished with a TH2 biased adjuvant, similar in its immune induction properties to aluminium hydroxide, a commonly used systemic adjuvant in humans. These results suggest that systemic immunization may be a practical approach for the prevention of *H. pylori* infection in developing countries where prevalence is significant and associated with potentially serious physical manifestations.

References

1. Dixon MF, Genta RM, Yardley JH, Correa P. Participants in the international workshop on the histopathology of Gastritis in Houston in 1994. Classification and grading of gastritis. The updated Sydney System. Am J Surg Pathol. 1996;20:1161–81.
2. NIH Consensus Conference. *Helicobacter pylori* in peptic ulcer disease. NIH Consensus Development Panel on *Helicobacter pylori* in peptic ulcer disease. J Am Med Assoc. 1994;272:65–9.
3. Forman D, Webb P, Parsonnet J. *H. pylori* and gastric cancer. Lancet. 1994;343:243–4.
4. World Health Organization. Infection with *Helicobacter pylori*. Schistosomes, Liver Flukes and *Helicobacter pylori*, vol. 61. Lyon: International Agency for Research on Cancer; 1994:177–241.
5. Valle J, Kekki M, Sipponen P, Ihamaki T, Siurla M. Long-term course and consequences of *Helicobacter pylori* gastritis. Scand J Gastroenterol. 1996;31:546–50.
6. Kilbridge PM, Dahms BBV, Czinn SJ. *Campylobacter pylori* associated gastritis and peptic ulcer disease in children. Am J Dis Child. 1988;142:1149–52.
7. Thomas JE, Whatmore AM, Barer MR, Eastham EJ, Kehoe ME. Serodiagnosis of *Helicobacter* infection in childhood. J Clin Microbiol. 1990;28A:2641–6.
8. Perez-Perez GI, Witkin SS, Decker MD, Blaser MJ. Seroprevalence of *Helicobacter pylori* infection in couples. J Clin Microbiol. 1991;29:642–4.
9. Malaty HM, Graham DY. Importance of childhood socioeconomic status on the current prevalence of *Helicobacter pylori* infection. Gut. 1994;35:742–5.
10. Goodman KJ, Correa P. Transmission of *Helicobacter pylori* among siblings. Lancet. 2000;355:358–62.
11. Blecker U, Lanciers S, Keppens E, Vandenplas Y. Evolution of *Helicobacter pylori* positivity in infants born from positive mothers. J Pediatr Gastroenterol Nutr. 1994;87–90.
12. Parsonnet J, Shmuely H, Haggerty T. Fecal and oral shedding of *Helicobacter pylori* from healthy infected adults. J Am Med Assoc. 1999;282:2240–1.
13. Megraud F. Transmission of *Helicobacter pylori*: fecal–oral versus oral–oral. Aliment Pharmacol Ther. 1995;9 (Suppl. 2):85–92.
14. Kelly SM, Pitcher MC, Farmery SM, Gibson GR. Isolation of *Helicobacter pylori* from feces of patients with dyspepsia in the United Kingdom. Gastroenterology. 1994;107:1671–4.
15. Rowland M, Dumar D, Daly L, O'Connor P, Vaughan D, Drumm B. Low rates of *Helicobacter pylori* reinfection in children. Gastroenterology. 1999;117:336–41.
16. Thomas JE, Austin S, Dale A et al. Specific human mild IgA antibody protects against *Helicobacter pylori* infection in infancy. Lancet. 1993;392:121.
17. Westblom TU, Lagging LM, Midkiff BR, Czinn SJ. Evaluation of QuickVue, a rapid enzyme immunoassay test for the detection of serum antibodies to *Helicobacter pylori*. Diagn Microbiol Infect Dis. 1993;16:317–20.
18. Westblom TU, Lagging LM, Milligan TW, Midkiff BR, Czinn SJ. Differences in antigenic recognition between adult and pediatric patients infected with *Helicobacter pylori*: analysis using Western blot technique. Acta Gastroenterol Belg. 1993;56:84.
19. Khanna B, Cutler A, Israel N et al. Use caution with serologic testing for *Helicobacter pylori* infection in children. J Infect Dis. 1998;178:460–5.
20. Czinn SJ, Carr HS, Speck WT. Diagnosis of gastritis caused by *Helicobacter pylori* in children by means of ELISA. Rev Infect Dis. 1991;13 (Suppl. 8): S700–3.
21. Czinn S, Carr H, Sheffler L, Aronoff S. Serum IgG antibody to the outer membrane proteins of *Campylobacter pylori* in children with gastroduodenal disease. J Infect Dis. 1989;159:596–9.
22. Blanchard TG, Nedrud JG, Czinn SH. Local and systemic antibody responses in humans with *Helicobacter pylori* infection. Can J Gastroenterol. 1999;13:591–4.

23. Czinn SJ. *Helicobacter pylori* induced gastritis in childhood. In: Malfertheiner P, Ditschuneit H, editors. *Helicobacter pylori*, Gastritis and Peptic Ulcer. Springer Verlag: Berlin, Heidelberg: 1990;180–7.
24. Chen M, Lee A, Hazell S, Hu P, Li Y. Immunization against gastric infection with *Helicobacter pylori* species: first step in the prophylaxis of gastric cancer? Zentralblatt Bakteriol. 1993;280:155–65.
25. Czinn SJ, Cai A, Nedrud JG. Protection of germ-free mice from infection by *Helicobacter felis* after active oral or passive IgA immunization. Vaccine. 1993;11:637–42.
26. Weltzin R, Kleanthous H, Guirdkhoo F, Monath TP, Lee CK. Novel intranasal immunization techniques for antibody induction and protection of mice against gastric *Helicobacter felis* infection. Vaccine. 1997;15:370–6.
27. Ermak TH, Giannasca PJ, Nichols R *et al.* Immunization of mice with urease vaccine affords protection against *Helicobacter pylori* infection in the absence of antibodies and is mediated by MHC class II-restricted responses. J Exp Med. 1998;188:2277–88.
28. Guy B, Hessler C, Fourage S *et al.* Systemic immunization with urease protects mice against *Helicobacter pylori* infection. Vaccine. 1998;16:850–6.

18
Severity and reversibility of mucosal inflammation in children and adolescents infected with *Helicobacter pylori*

P. M. SHERMAN

INTRODUCTION

Helicobacter pylori infects at least half of the world's human population. Increasing evidence points to acquisition of the gastric infection during the childhood years[1]. Intrafamilial clustering suggests person-to-person transmission of the infection which could occur by the faecal-to-oral route, an oral-to-oral route, or via vomitus[2,3]. Recent reports of successful culture of viable bacteria from emesis provide additional support for the latter method of transmission[4]. However, precisely how this route of transmission would explain transfer of infection from infected parents to their uninfected young children remains enigmatic.

Alternatively, acquisition of infection among family members could point to exposure to a common environmental reservoir. Some studies report the successful culture of *H. pylori* from sources of drinking water[5]. Reports of domestic cats as a source of infection have not been confirmed. The concept of a zoonotic infection acquired from farm animals and their products also has not been confirmed experimentally.

Whatever the source of the initial exposure to *H. pylori*, it is clear that this generally occurs early during the childhood years. There is some evidence to suggest that breast feeding can protect infants from the gastric infection, particularly if the mother is herself colonized[6]. This finding could indicate a role for *H. pylori*-specific immunoglobulin A antibodies present in mothers' milk. However, recent studies indicate that non-immune constituents of human breast milk and bovine colostrum also have anti-*Helicobacter* activity[7].

CONSEQUENCES OF INITIAL *H. PYLORI* INFECTION IN CHILDREN

The natural history of gastric infection in the childhood years has not been studied extensively. Current evidence indicates that the overwhelming majority of *H. pylori*-infected children and adolescents develop a chronic-active, antral predominant gastritis. There is a single report suggesting the potential for *H. pylori* colonization of the stomach of children in the absence of documented mucosal inflammation in the antrum[8]. On the other hand, the overwhelming majority of studies indicate that mucosal inflammation in the antrum is an invariable feature of *H. pylori* infection in children and adolescents.

Whether there is a pangastritis with inflammation extending to involve the body of the stomach, and if *H. pylori* infection is always associated with carditis, are important issues that require additional evaluation in a variety of paediatric populations. Initial evidence suggests that there is a pangastritis in children infected with *H. pylori*[9,10]. However, a formal mapping study to delineate the extent and severity of bacterial colonization of the stomach, as well as the accompanying host cell mucosal inflammatory response to infection, has yet to be carried out. A prospective study in preschool-aged children would be of particular interest in this regard.

NODULAR GASTRITIS AND LYMPHOID FOLLICLES

A prominent endoscopic feature of *H. pylori* infection in children is the presence of nodularity in the antrum of the stomach (Figure 1). The antral nodularity is more prominent after taking an endoscopic biopsy because the associated bleeding provides a contrast with the gastric mucosa. Nodularity of the antrum is a highly specific feature of *H. pylori* infection in children. It is rarely seen in uninfected children with normal mucosal histology. For example, Mitchell *et al.*[1] found a nodular antrum at endoscopy in only one of 195 (0.5%) children without evidence of *H. pylori* infection. Rosh *et al.*[11] detected antral nodularity only in the five cases of *H. pylori* infection among a series of 500 consecutive paediatric diagnostic upper gastrointestinal endoscopies. Antral nodularity is not observed endoscopically in other non-infectious conditions that cause inflammation in the antrum of the stomach in children (for example, eosinophilic gastritis and gastric Crohn's disease).

Although antral nodularity is a specific feature of paediatric *H. pylori* infection[12], the endoscopic finding is seen in only approximately half of infected children and adolescents[9,13]. Therefore, antral nodularity is not a sensitive marker of gastric infection, and a normal-appearing antrum at the time of upper gastrointestinal endoscopy does not exclude the presence of *H. pylori*. Therefore, biopsies of the antrum should be taken in all children undergoing elective diagnostic oesophagogastroduodenoscopy.

It remains uncertain whether the endoscopic nodules are a visual feature that mirrors microscopic evidence of lymphoid follicles (Figure 2). Lymphoid follicles are a highly specific histological feature of *H. pylori* infection because they are rarely observed in the gastric mucosa in the absence of mucosal

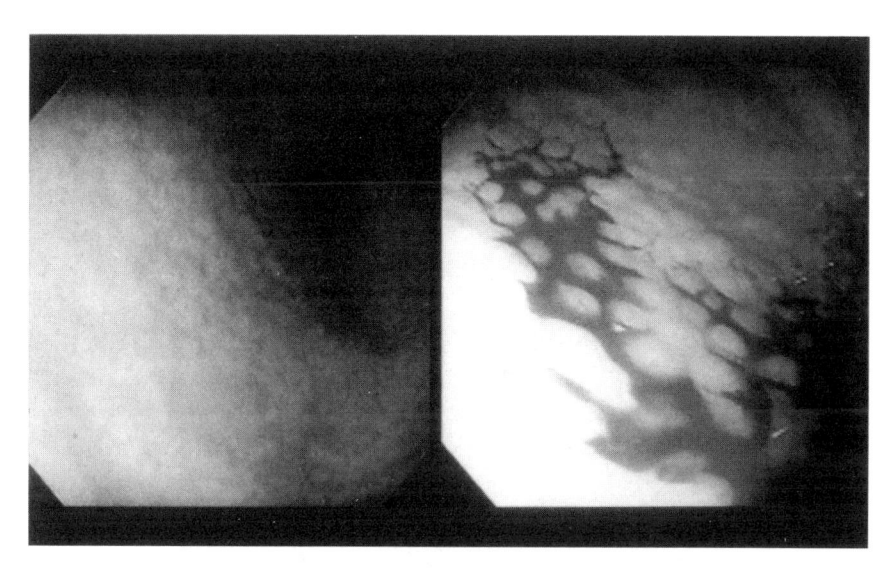

Figure 1. Photograph of the antral mucosa taken at the time of diagnostic upper endoscopy in a child with *H. pylori*-induced gastritis. The left panel shows a pattern of nodules on the surface of the gastric antrum. The nodules are more prominent in the right panel after a per-endoscopic forceps biopsy has been taken from the antrum resulting in a small amount of haemorrhage.

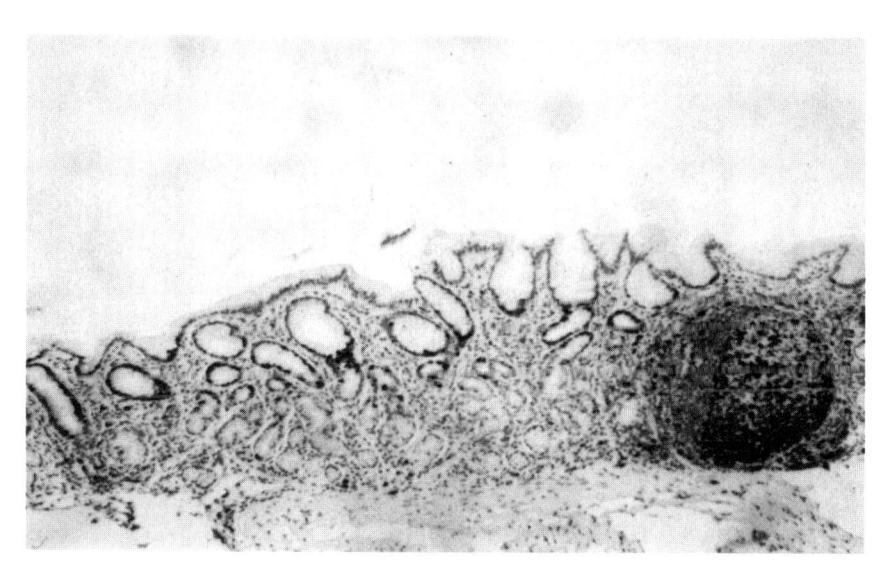

Figure 2. Bright-field microscopy of antral mucosa obtained from a child with *H. pylori*-induced gastritis. A prominent lymphoid follicle is evident on the right-hand side of the photograph (MIB-1 immunohistochemical staining, original approximate magnification, ×40).

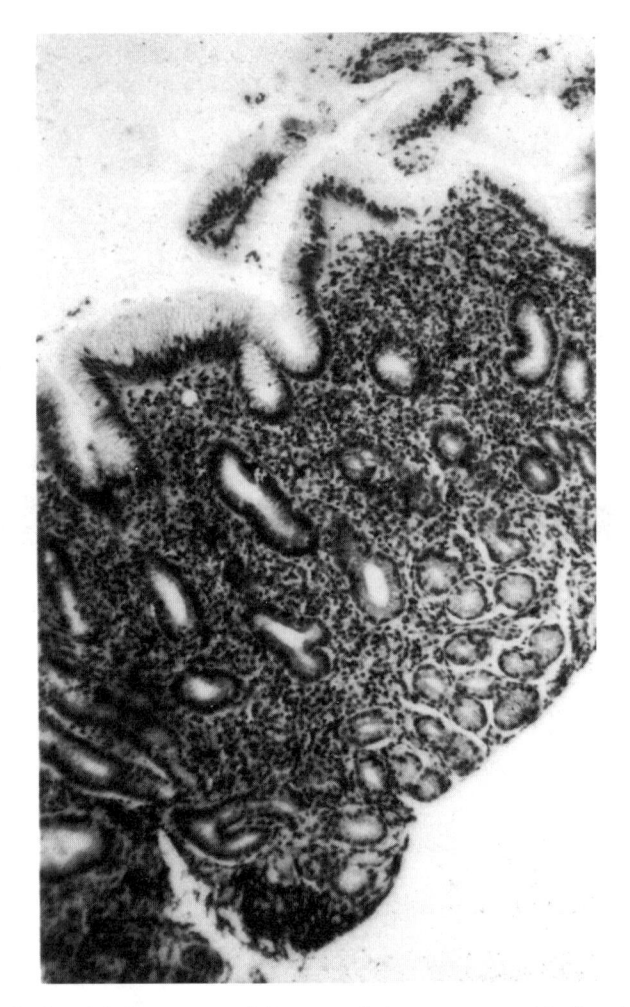

Figure 3. Histology of the antrum of the stomach in a teenager with *H. pylori* infection documented by both culture and staining with silver of gastric mucosa. There is evidence of a moderate gastritis with a mixed acute and chronic inflammatory cell infiltrate without disruption or destruction of glands. The overlying surface mucosa is intact (haematoxylin and eosin staining, original approximate magnification, ×40).

inflammation or in the setting of gastric inflammation arising due to causes other than *H. pylori*[14]. Evidence that lymphoid follicles in the gastric mucosa are a specific marker of infection with *H. pylori* in adults also has been reported[15,16].

PATHOLOGICAL RESPONSES IN THE STOMACH TO *H. PYLORI*

In *H. pylori*-infected children the neutrophil infiltrate in the gastric mucosa tends to be less prominent compared to that observed in adults[17,18]. The

Table 1. Demographic summary and frequency of gastric metaplasia and duodenitis in three study groups

	Gastritis H. pylori-*positive*	Gastritis H. pylori-*negative*	Normal antral mucosa
Number	31	33	33
Age (years)	13.4 ± 3.4	13.8 ± 4.8	13.1 ± 4.1
Sex (female/male)	10/21	11/22	11/22
Metaplasia positive (%)	13* (42)	2 (6)	1 (3)
Duodenitis positive (%)	24* (77)	4 (12)	2 (6)

* Percentage positive is significantly higher than in the two comparison groups, $p < 0.01$. Taken from ref. 24, with permission.

reasons for these apparent differences are not defined, and are worthy of future study, as they could provide important clues as to the nature of the host response to infection. The superficial gastritis that is present in children is primarily composed of lymphocytes (both T cells and B cells) as well as plasma cells, eosinophils, mast cells and, to a lesser extent, basophils infiltrating into the mucosa[19] (Figure 5).

Gastric atrophy and intestinal metaplasia in the stomach of *H. pylori*-infected children are extremely uncommon histopathological findings in the paediatric population[9]. This may simply reflect the duration of infection rather than differing host responses related to chronological age.

H. pylori infection in children causes enhanced epithelial cell proliferation in gastric crypts that is associated with the expression of p53 protein and increased apoptosis of cells lining the surface epithelium[20]. Apoptosis of host epithelial cells is due to both direct effects of the bacterium and indirect immune responses mediated by Fas ligand on T lymphocytes and Fas receptor on gastric epithelial cells[21]. Nevertheless, the development of gastric cancers including adenocarcinoma, lymphoma, or MALToma presenting in children and adolescents is an exceedingly uncommon consequence of *H. pylori* infection[22]. This has generally been attributed to the length of bacterial colonization rather than any biological features unique to the developing and maturing host.

INFLAMMATION AND GASTRIC METAPLASIA IN THE DUODENUM

As in adults, *H. pylori* infection is accompanied by changes in the proximal duodenum, including both mucosal inflammation and the presence of ectopic gastric mucosa that will serve as a site for bacterial colonization. It is clear that the gastric mucosa present in the duodenum occurs as a consequence of *H. pylori* infection and accompanying inflammation[23]. As shown in Table 1, in comparison with *H. pylori*-infected children, duodenitis occurs with a much lower frequency and gastric metaplasia is less extensive in children without bacterial colonization of the stomach[24].

A prospective study not only confirmed these findings, but suggested that the ectopic gastric mucosa is a potential risk factor for developing complications from *H. pylori* infection[25]. Peptic ulceration was identified more frequently in those children with *H. pylori* infection and gastric metaplasia compared to infected children without ectopic gastric mucosa in the proximal duodenum.

NATURAL HISTORY OF *H. PYLORI* INFECTION

In older children, adolescents and adults it appears that *H. pylori* infection and the accompanying gastritis are life-long unless specific eradication therapies are employed. By contrast, several epidemiological studies, using either serology[26-28] or urea breath testing[29,30] as indirect markers of gastric infection, report that spontaneous clearance might occur in pre-school-aged children. If confirmed by other investigators this would provide a subgroup worthy of study to determine novel mechanisms to eradicate infection in other age groups of the human population. However, it should be noted that there are concerns about the accuracy of the indirect methodologies employed to determine the presence or absence of *H. pylori* infection in children under 5 years of age.

Ganga-Zandzou et al.[31] prospectively monitored, over a period of 2 years, the consequences of untreated *H. pylori* infection in a group of 18 asymptomatic children in Lille, France. Even though the density of bacterial colonization was not changed, there was both more marked antral nodularity and more severe mucosal inflammation in the antrum over the period of follow-up (Figure 4). Comparable studies in other paediatric populations (for example, among those residing in a developing nation) and for even longer periods of follow-up would be required to more clearly define the histopathological consequences of childhood *H. pylori* infection. However, such studies will probably prove to be exceedingly difficult to undertake. The requirement for repeated endoscopic evaluations is not an insignificant ethical issue when considering the potential benefits for those children who would be entered into such a protocol. It is more likely that such information will have to be derived from cross-sectional studies entering children of a variety of ages who reside in a relatively homogeneous community.

BACTERIAL FACTORS CONTRIBUTING TO MUCOSAL INFLAMMATORY RESPONSES

Recent studies have focused on the potential role of a vacuolating cytotoxin (VacA) or a cytotoxin-associated outer membrane protein (CagA) encoded on a segment of chromosomal DNA of lower $G+C$ content than the remainder of the bacterial genome (referred to as the cag pathogenicity island). Extrachromosomal elements, such as plasmids, that frequently encode virulence genes in other bacterial pathogens, do not appear to be involved in the pathogenicity of *H. pylori* strains.

An association between VacA and the presence of disease outcome (that is, peptic ulceration compared to gastritis alone) has been reported in some

PATHOLOGY OF *H. PYLORI* INFECTION IN CHILDREN

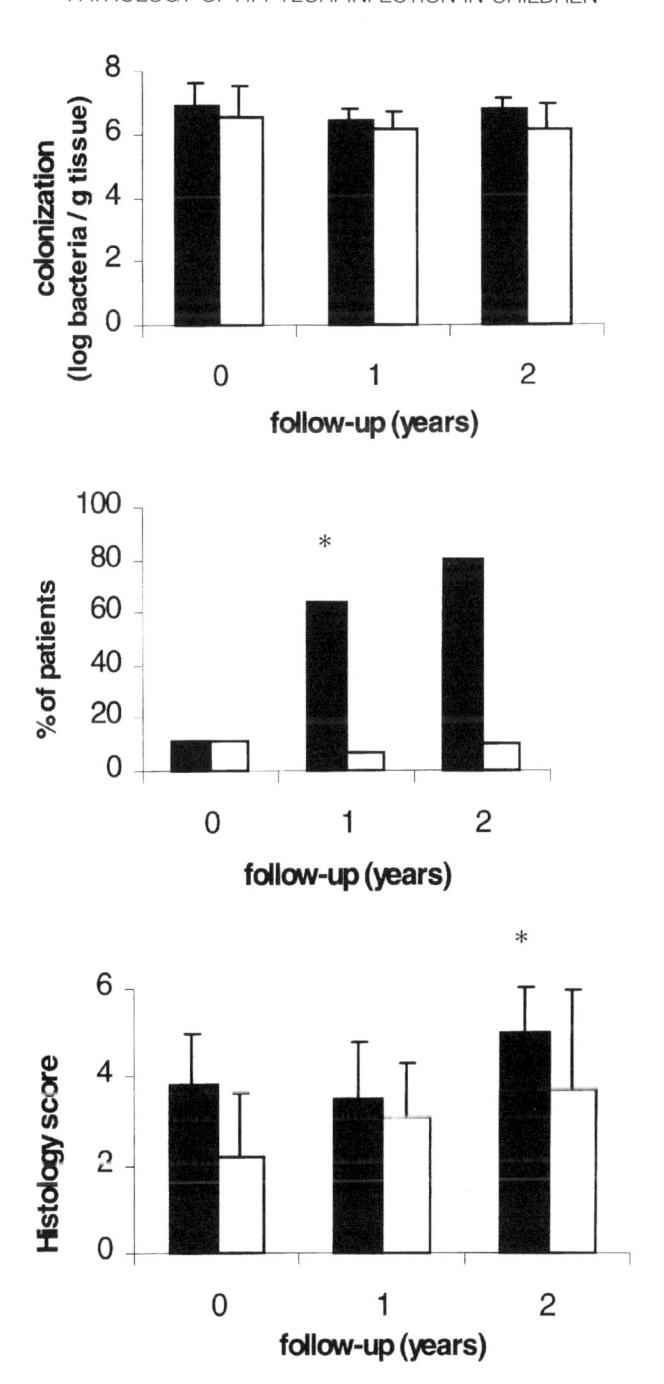

Figure 4. Bacterial colonization (panel A), antral nodularity at endoscopy (panel B), and antral gastritis evident on histopathology (panel C) in untreated *H. pylori*-infected children at diagnosis ($n = 18$), after 12 months ($n = 14$), and after 24 month ($n = 10$) of follow-up. Adapted from ref. 31, with permission.

studies evaluating infected adults. The results of studies undertaken to date in children are less convincing. For example, the VacA phenotype of *H. pylori* isolated from children and adolescents in Toronto, Canada, did not correlate with either the presence of peptic ulceration or with any of the pathological criteria examined, including the presence and severity of gastritis, duodenitis and gastric metaplasia in the duodenum[32]. However, an initial report from researchers in Brazil indicates that an evaluation of the *vac*A genotype might serve as a better predictor of disease outcome in children. The s1m1 allele was identified in 87% of 16 children with endoscopic evidence of duodenal ulceration, whereas the s1m2 and s2m2 alleles were more common among children with gastritis alone (26 of 37, 70%; $p = 0.01$)[33]. Additional studies testing *vac*A alleles in *H. pylori* strains isolated from children residing in disparate geographic settings are warranted to confirm the observations in South America.

At least three reports indicate that the frequency of antral nodularity and the severity of mucosal inflammation is greater in children infected with CagA-positive *H. pylori* strains compared to those infected with CagA-negative isolates[34-36]. However, the correlation of CagA status with peptic ulceration reported in some adult populations has been difficult to reproduce in the paediatric setting. For example, in a study from Japan more than 80% of children infected with *H. pylori* had anti-CagA antibodies present in the serum[37]. The high frequency of circulating antibodies was present in children with gastric ulcer (80%), duodenal ulcer (95%), nodular gastritis (93%), and gastritis alone (82%, ANOVA $p > 0.05$). Amongst Canadian children, when tested by polymerase chain reaction, more than 80% of the *H. pylori* strains isolated from children were *cag*A-positive[38]. *cag*A status was independent of the child's country of origin. In addition, *cag*A status did not correlate with the presence of endoscopic evidence of peptic ulceration or with histological evidence of the severity of gastritis, presence and severity of duodenitis, or gastric mucosa present ectopically in the proximal duodenum. In a study undertaken in Spain, the frequency of infection with *cag*A *H. pylori* strains increased with advancing chronological age[39]. In children the *cag*A genotype was more frequent among those with peptic ulcer disease (three of five, 60%) compared to subjects with gastritis alone (12 of 38, 32%). In Brazilian children the presence of the *cag*A gene, identified by polymerase chain reaction, is also identified in *H. pylori* strains more frequently in patients with duodenal ulceration (27 of 27) compared to those with gastritis alone (33 of 53, 62%; $p < 0.001$)[40].

Other factors encoded on the *cag* pathogenicity island of the bacterial genome might also serve to determine host response to infection. In contrast to targeted disruptions of the *cag*A gene, which do not affect the ability of a *H. pylori* strain to induce chemokine production by gastric epithelial cells, mutations in the *cag*E gene (also referred to by some investigators as *pic*B) impair interleukin-8 transcription and secretion from infected host cells[41]. Therefore, we have tested *cag*E as a potential virulence marker in infected children. In contrast to VacA and *cag*A which did not distinguish infection complicated by duodenal ulcer from gastritis alone, *cag*E was present more commonly in *H. pylori* isolates from Toronto children with endoscopic evidence of mucosal ulceration (12 of 13, 92%) compared to those with gastritis alone (five of 16, 31%; $p < 0.01$). This provides initial evidence that bacterial virulence factors do, indeed, affect disease outcome in the paediatric setting[38]. Additional studies are now required to confirm this observation, and to determine whether additional virulence factors contained either within the pathogenicity island or on the rest of the bacterial genome modulate host responses to infection and thereby impact upon disease outcome[42,43].

REVERSIBILITY OF PAEDIATRIC H. PYLORI INFECTION

Unfortunately, to date there have been no randomized controlled trials evaluating the efficacy of anti-*Helicobacter* eradication therapy in the paediatric setting. Nevertheless, small case series reported in the literature suggest that the efficacy of triple therapy and quadruple therapy regimens is comparable to that achieved in adults[44].

The rapidity of healing of mucosal inflammation following successful eradication of the gastric infection is not known. However, at least one study provides indirect evidence to suggest that resolution of the inflammatory response may well occur faster in children compared to what has been reported in adults. Kato *et al.*[45] showed that there is a relatively rapid reduction in *H. pylori*-specific IgG and IgA titres in the serum of children following successful treatment (Figure 5). Among 34 treated children, a 30% drop in IgA antibody titre at 6 months provided evidence of successful eradication with a sensitivity of 91% and a specificity of 100%. From the completion of eradication therapy the mean time to seroreversion was 11.2 ± 7.0 months for IgG and 11.6 ± 7.8 months for *H. pylori*-specific IgA.

CONCLUSIONS

H. pylori infection generally first occurs during the childhood years. In a critical editorial a number of years ago, McKinlay and colleagues[46] stated: 'Children represent a particularly important population group who may help to clarify our understanding of *H. pylori* infection.' As detailed in this review, the developing human does not respond in precisely the same manner to the gastric infection as that reported in the mature and ageing host. Research aimed at modulating the inflammatory and immune responses during development should provide additional insights into the intricacies of the interactions between this unique microbe and its host. Such information could provide new strategies aimed at resolving bacterial colonization of the stomach, and thereby prevent disease complications in future generations.

Acknowledgement

Work in the author's laboratory is supported by the Medical Research Council of Canada.

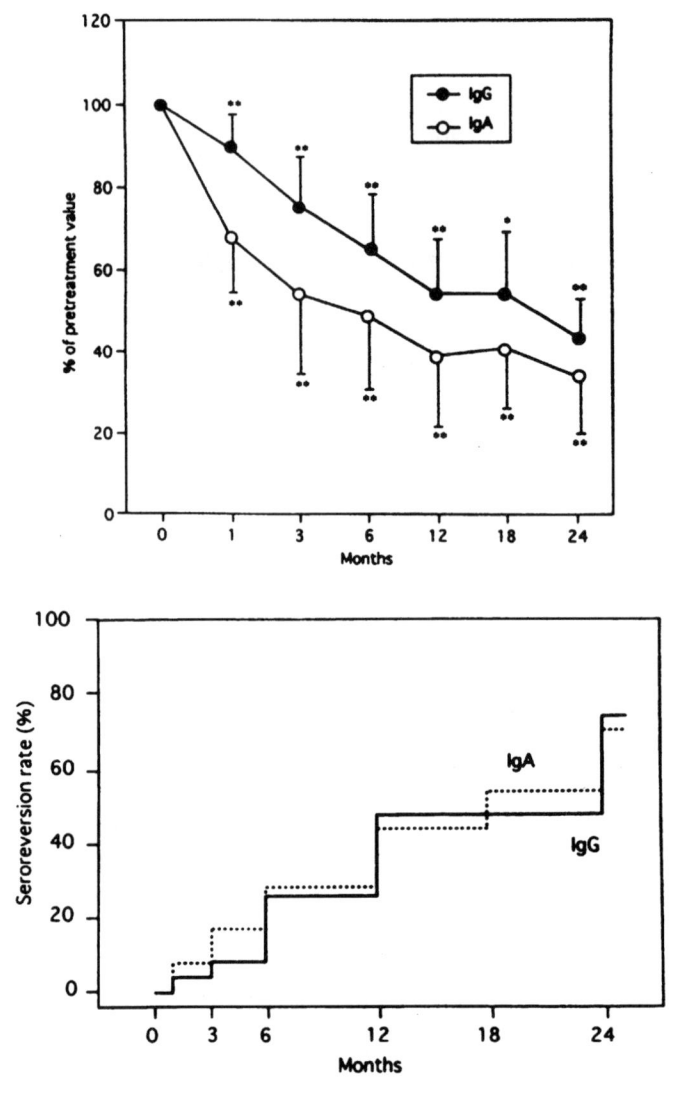

Figure 5. Anti-*Helicobacter* humoral immune responses following eradication therapy in children. Panel A: serum anti-*H. pylori* IgG and IgA antibody titres in patients with successful eradication of the gastric infection. Post-treatment titres are expressed as percentages of pretreatment titres. Panel B: cumulative seroreversion rates of serum *H. pylori*-specific IgG (solid line) and IgA (broken line) antibodies in children with successful eradication therapy. Adapted from ref. 45, with permission.

References

1. Mitchell HM, Li YY, Hu PJ *et al.* Epidemiology of *Helicobacter pylori* in southern China: identification of early childhood as the critical period for acquisition. J Infect Dis. 1992;166:149–53.

2. Drumm B, Perez-Perez GI, Blaser MJ, Sherman PM. Intrafamilial clustering of *Helicobacter pylori* infection. N Engl J Med. 1990;322:359–63.
3. Dominici P, Bellentani S, Di Biase AR et al. Familial clustering of *Helicobacter pylori* infection: population based study. Br Med J. 1999;319:537–41.
4. Parsonet J, Shmuely H, Haggerty T. Fecal and oral shedding of *Helicobacter pylori* from healthy infected adults. J Am Med Assoc. 1999;282:2240–5.
5. Goodman KJ, Correa P. The transmission of *Helicobacter pylori*: a critical review of the evidence. Int J Epidemiol. 1995;24:875–87.
6. Thomas JE, Austin S, Dale A et al. Protection by human milk IgA against *Helicobacter pylori* infection in infancy. Lancet 1993;342:121.
7. Bitzan MM, Gold BD, Philpott DJ et al. Inhibition of *Helicobacter pylori* and *Helicobacter mustelae* binding to lipid receptors by bovine colostrum. J Infect Dis. 1998;177:955–61.
8. Gottrand F, Cullu F, Turck D et al. Normal gastric histology in *Helicobacter pylori*-infected children. J Pediatr Gastroenterol Nutr. 1997;25:74–8.
9. Queiroz DMM, Rocha GA, Mendes EN et al. Differences in distribution and severity of *Helicobacter pylori* gastritis in children and adults with duodenal ulcer disease. J Pediatr Gastroenterol Nutr. 1991;12:178–81.
10. Dohil R, Hassall E, Jevon G, Dimmick J. Gastritis and gastropathy of childhood. J Pediatr Gastroenterol Nutr. 1999;29:378–94.
11. Rosh JR, Kurfist LA, Benkov KJ, Toor AH, Bottone EJ, LeLeiko NS. *Helicobacter pylori* and gastric lymphonodular hyperplasia in children. Am J Gastroenterol. 1992;87:135–9.
12. Hassall E, Dimmick JE. Unique features of *Helicobacter pylori* disease in children. Dig Dis Sci. 1991;36:417–23.
13. Mitchell HM, Bohane TD, Tobias V et al. *Helicobacter pylori* infection in children: potential clues to pathogenesis. J Pediatr Gastroenterol Nutr. 1993;16:120–5.
14. Genta RM, Hamner HW. The significance of lymphoid follicles in the interpretation of gastric biopsy specimens. Arch Pathol Lab Med. 1994;118:740–3.
15. Genta RM, Hamner HW, Graham DY. Gastric lymphoid follicles in *Helicobacter pylori* infection: frequency, distribution, and response to triple therapy. Hum Pathol. 1993;24:577–83.
16. Sbeih F, Abdullah A, Sullivan S, Merenkov Z. Antral nodularity, gastric lymphoid hyperplasia, and *Helicobacter pylori* in adults. J Clin Gastroenterol. 1996;22:227–30.
17. Ashorn M. What are the specific features of *Helicobacter pylori* gastritis in children? Ann Med. 1995;27:617–20.
18. Whitney AE, Guarner F, Hutwagner L, Gold BD. Histopathological differences between *Helicobacter pylori* gastritis of children and adults. Gastroenterology. 1998;114:G1351 (abstract).
19. Jones NL, Sherman PM, Croitoru K. Immunobiology of the stomach: the *Helicobacter* model. Can J Allerg Clin Immunol. 1998;3:58–63.
20. Jones NL, Shannon PT, Cutz E, Yeger H, Sherman PM. Increase in proliferation and apoptosis of gastric epithelial cells early in the natural history of *Helicobacter pylori* infection. Am J Pathol. 1997;151:1695–703.
21. Jones NL, Day AS, Jennings HA, Sherman PM. *Helicobacter pylori* induces gastric epithelial cell apoptosis in association with increased Fas receptor expression. Infect Immun. 1999;67:4237–42.
22. Riddell RH. Pathobiology of *Helicobacter pylori* infection in children. Can J Gastroenterol. 1999;13:599–603.
23. Elitsur Y, Triest WE. Is duodenal gastric metaplasia a consequence of *Helicobacter pylori* infection in children? Am J Gastroenterol. 1997;92:2216–19.
24. Shahib S, Cutz E, Drumm B, Sherman PM. Association of gastric metaplasia and duodenitis with *Helicobacter pylori* infection in children. Am J Clin Pathol. 1994;102:188–91.
25. Gormally SM, Kierce BM, Daly LE et al. Gastric metaplasia and duodenal ulcer disease in children infected by *Helicobacter pylori*. Gut. 1996;38:513–17.
26. Malaty HM, Graham DY, Wattigney WA, Srinivasan SR, Osato M, Berenson GS. Natural history of *Helicobacter pylori* infection in childhood:12-year follow-up cohort study in a biracial community. Clin Infect Dis. 1999;28:279–82.
27. Tindberg Y, Blennow M, Granstrom M. Clinical symptoms and social factors in a cohort of children spontaneously clearing *Helicobacter pylori* infection. Acta Paediatr. 1999;88:631–5.

28. Lindkvist P, Enquselassie F, Asrat D, Nilsson I, Muhe L, Giesecke J. *Helicobacter pylori* infection in Ethiopian children: a cohort study. Scand J Infect Dis. 1999;31:475–80.
29. Perri F, Pastore M, Clemente R et al. *Helicobacter pylori* infection may undergo spontaneous eradication in children: a 2-year follow-up study. J Pediatr Gastroenterol Nutr. 1998;27:181–3.
30. Thomas JE, Dale A, Harding M, Coward WA, Cole TJ, Weaver LT. *Helicobacter pylori* colonization in early life. Pediatr Res. 1999;45:218–23.
31. Ganga-Zandzou PS, Michaud L, Vincent P et al. Natural outcome of *Helicobacter pylori* infection in asymptomatic children: a two-year follow-up study. Pediatrics. 1999;104:216–21.
32. Loeb M, Jayaratne P, Jones N, Sihoe A, Sherman P. Lack of correlation between vacuolating cytotoxin activity, *cag*A gene, and peptic ulcer disease in *Helicobacter pylori* in children. Eur J Clin Microbiol Infect Dis. 1998;17:653–6.
33. Rocha GA, Mendes EN, Gusmao VR et al. *vac*A genotypes in *Helicobacter pylori* strains isolated from children. Gut, 1998;43(Suppl. 2):A72 (abstract).
34. Luzza F, Contaldo A, Imeneo M et al. Testing for serum IgG antibodies to *Helicobacter pylori* cytotoxin-associated protein detects children with higher grades of gastric inflammation. J Pediatr Gastroenterol Nutr. 1999;29:302–7.
35. Kolho K-L, Karttunen R, Heikkila P, Lindahl H, Rautelin H. Gastric inflammation is enhanced in children with CagA-positive *Helicobacter pylori* infection. Pediatr Infect Dis J. 1999;18:337–41.
36. Elitsur Y, Neace C, Werthammer MC, Triest WE. Prevalence of CagA and VacA antibodies in symptomatic and asymptomatic children with *Helicobacter pylori* infection. Helicobacter. 1999;4:100–5.
37. Kato S, Sugiyama T, Kudo M et al. CagA antibodies in Japanese children with nodular gastritis or peptic ulcer disease. J Clin Microbiol. 2000;38:68–70.
38. Day AS, Jones NL, Lynett JT, Jennings HA, Fallone CA, Beech R, Sherman PM. *cag*E is a virulence factor associated with *Helicobacter pylori*-induced duodenal ulceration in children. J Infect Dis. 2000;181:1370–5.
39. Alarcon T, Domingo D, Martinez MJ, Lopez-Brea M. *cag*A gene and *vac*A alleles in Spanish *Helicobacter pylori* clinical isolates from patients of different ages. FEMS Immunol Med Microbiol. 1999;24:215–19.
40. Queiroz DMM, Mendes EN, Carvalho AST et al. Factors associated with *Helicobacter pylori* infection by a *cag*A-positive strain in children. J Infect Dis. 2000;181:626–30.
41. Atherton JC. *Helicobacter pylori* virulence factors. Br Med Bull. 1998;54:105–20.
42. Ge Z, Taylor DE. Contributions of genome sequencing to understanding the biology of *Helicobacter pylori*. Annu Rev Microbiol. 1999;53:353–87.
43. Marias A, Mendz GL, Hazell SL, Megraud F. Metabolism and genetics of *Helicobacter pylori*: the genome era. Microbiol Mol Biol Rev. 1999;63:642–74.
44. Gold BD. Current therapy for *Helicobacter pylori* infection in children and adolescents. Can J Gastroenterol. 1999;13:571–9.
45. Kato S, Furuyama N, Ozawa K, Ohnuma K, Iinuma K. Long-term follow-up study of serum immunoglobulin G and immunoglobulin A antibodies after *Helicobacter pylori* eradication. Pediatrics. 1999;104:e22–6.
46. McKinlay AW, Upadhyay R, Gemmell CG, Russell RI. *Helicobacter pylori*; bridging the credibility gap. Gut. 1990;31:940–5.

19
Elimination of *Helicobacter pylori* is dependent on a Th2 response

A. LEE

QUALIFICATIONS

The views of this chapter represent the arguments to support the debate. The value of debate is that it forces a polarization of views, which may be useful in putting the issue in perspective.

WHY Th2?

The most important function of the immune response is to protect the host against infectious diseases. As microorganisms can live on human cells or within them, this immune response evolved by different effector mechanisms. Extracellular pathogens require an antibody response to eliminate them, either by preventing colonization, facilitating phagocytosis or destroying them via antibody-mediated lysis. In contrast, to cope with intracellular pathogens the response is cell-mediated with macrophages acquiring an increased capacity to destroy the ingested organism. Evolution resulted in an efficient system, whereby both arms of the response arise from precursor T cells, which develop following contact with cells presenting antigen from the particular pathogen, and under the influence of the local cytokine environment, into either Th1 or Th2 cells. Th1 cells acquire the ability to synthesize the cytokines TNF-β and IFN-γ which activate macrophages such that they can destroy the intracellular pathogen. In contrast, Th2 cells produce IL-10, IL-4 and IL-5, resulting in maturation of plasma cells and production of various immunoglobulin classes of antibody.

HELICOBACTER PYLORI – AN EVOLVED PARASITE

H. pylori has infected humans for centuries. Over this time the parasite has evolved to survive the very substantial host responses mounted against it.

Indeed, *H. pylori* has been so successful in this endeavour that it can inhabit the gastric mucosa for life. The chosen niche for the bacterium is the surface mucus or the surface epithelium. Thus, *H. pylori* is an *extracellular pathogen* and the logical immune response to remove the organism would be a Th2 response. However, numerous studies on cells and cytokines in the gastric mucosa of infected individuals show production of IFN-γ and a Th1 phenotype. No Th2 cells or IL-4 are observed[1-8]. So the immune response against *H. pylori* is Th1. This may be important in the inability of the host to eliminate host infection. Note that a Th2 response would be able to *eliminate*. Given this, is it not logical that, over the ages of evolution, *H. pylori* has indeed selected for hosts or manipulated the response towards Th1, a response that not only would not harm but may even benefit it due to nutrients produced by inflammation[9]? Certainly the bacterium seems to have benefited by acquisition of the Cag pathogenicity island which makes it more inflammatory, a project that would normally be against the organism's survival[10].

THE ANIMAL EVIDENCE FOR Th2 AND ELIMINATION

The evidence that a Th2 response can indeed eliminate *H. pylori* comes from mouse studies on vaccination. Using either whole cell sonicate or recombinant protein antigens such as urease, a number of workers have shown that both *H. pylori* and its close relative, *H. felis*, can be cleared from the stomach following multiple immunizing doses[11,12]. Two statements taken from one such paper add strong support to the thesis of this chapter:

> Immunization induced a proliferative response of splenic CD4(+) cells, a progressive decrease in interferon gamma secretion and a concomitant increase in interleukin 4 secretion after each immunization[13].
>
> Conclusions: In BALB/C mice, therapeutic immunization with rUreB induces progressively a Th2 CD4(+) T cell response resulting in the elimination of the pathogen[13].

Previous work on the adjuvant action of cholera toxin with other antigens is consistent with this conclusion. Thus, immunization of mice with tetanus toxoid as the antigen resulted in significant levels of T cell messenger RNA coding for IL-4 in Peyer's patch preparations from immunized animals while more were seen in control mice[14].

The conclusive proof of the importance of the role of Th2 cells in elimination of *Helicobacter* species was a series of elegant adoptive transfer experiments, where T cells cloned from immunized mice were injected intraperitoneally into mice and the effect on *H. felis* infection was measured[15]. Both Th1 and Th2 clones resulted in an exacerbation of inflammation caused by the organism. However, it was only the Th2 clone that led to a reduction in colonization.

THE FLAWED EVIDENCE OF THE KNOCKOUT MICE

The following chapter tries to use conflicting evidence from genetically manipulated mice to challenge the Th2 hypothesis. Consistent with a role for Th2, orally immunized IL-4 knockout mice show no protection against both *H. pylori* or *H. felis* infections[16]. However, orally immunized IFN-γ knockouts, also show reduced protection[17]. Even more confusing is the evidence from three groups who orally immunized μMT mice that are unable to produce antibody. They are still protected against infection against both *Helicobacter* species[18–20]. It will be argued that this is conclusive evidence against the simple Th2 concept. I argue: discount the knockout mice studies; they are artifactual! Two quotes from authoritative sources on the worldwide web highlight the dangers of putting too much reliance on knockout mice studies as there is just too much gene redundancy in these highly artificial animals.

> What to do if you develop a new mouse? Expect the unexpected! (http://www.ncifcrf.gov/vetpath/gam.html).

> The choice of strain may have significant impact on the phenotype as unlinked genes contained in the strain background can have a dramatic effect on the disease phenotype (http://www.csh.org/genes/dev/supplement/x8.htm).

THE HUMAN EVIDENCE

Having discredited the major arguments against my thesis, the final evidence for a Th2 response is the human response. There are accumulating data suggesting that, in contrast to the adult, children can lose their *H. pylori* infection. Thus, in studies in Gambian children the prevalence of a positive urea breath test indicative of *H. pylori* infection increased from 19% at 3 months of age to 84% by 30 months[21]. Reversion to a negative breath test, in association with declining specific antibody levels, occurred in 48/248, i.e. 20% of the children. Experiments in mice have shown that the direction of lymphocyte development can be influenced in the neonatal period[22]. Could it be that Th2 responses are more pronounced in early childhood, and so the *H. pylori* is more easily eliminated. Certainly the product of a Th2 response, IgA, can give rise to protection in the human. In the Gambian children human breast milk IgA was shown to protect against *H. pylori* infection in infancy[23].

CONCLUSION

Based on logic and sound animal data the evidence is overwhelming that elimination of *Helicobacter pylori* is dependent on a Th2 response. The reader is asked to keep these arguments in mind while reading the alternative view.

COMMENT

In reality, the animal studies have shown that the simple Th2 story does not hold up. Yet many points above are relevant. Immunization against *H. pylori* is possible, but our simple concept of removal by local IgA is wrong. Novel, probably cellular, mechanisms are involved. Understand this process and not only will we produce a vaccine that will save millions of lives, but we will have learnt new fundamental lessons about mucosal immunology.

References

1. Hida N, Shimoyama T, Neville P, Dixon MF, Axon ATR, Crabtree JE. Increased expression of IL-10 and IL-12 (p40) mRNA in *Helicobacter pylori* infected gastric mucosa: relation to bacterial cag status and peptic ulceration. J Clin Pathol. 1999;52:658–64.
2. Sommer F, Faller G, Konturek P et al. Antrum- and corpus mucosa-infiltrating CD4(+) lymphocytes in *Helicobacter pylori* gastritis display a TH1 phenotype. Infect Immun. 1998;66:5543–6.
3. Bamford KB, Fan XJ, Crowe SE et al. Lymphocytes in the human gastric mucosa during *Helicobacter pylori* have a T helper cell 1 phenotype. Gastroenterology. 1998;114:482–92.
4. Del Prete G, D'Elios MM, Manghetti M, Romagnani S, Telford J. *H. pylori*-specific Th1 effector cells in the gastric antrum of patients with peptic ulcer disease. Gut. 1996; 39(Suppl. 2):A42.
5. Delios MM, Manghetti M, Decarli M et al. T helper 1 effector cells specific for *Helicobacter pylori* in the gastric antrum of patients with peptic ulcer disease. J Immunol. 1997;158:962–7.
6. Karttunen R, Karttunen T, Ekre HPT, MacDonald TT. Interferon gamma and interleukin 4 secreting cells in the gastric antrum in *Helicobacter pylori* positive and negative gastritis. Gut. 1995;36:341–5.
7. Haeberle HA, Kubin M, Bamford KB et al. Differential stimulation of interleukin-12 (IL-12) and IL-10 by live and killed *Helicobacter pylori in vitro* and association of IL-12 production with gamma interferon-producing T cells in the human gastric mucosa. Infect Immun. 1997;65:4229–35.
8. Yamaoka Y, Kita M, Kodama T, Sawai N, Kashima K, Imanishi J. Expression of cytokine mrna in gastric mucosa with *Helicobacter pylori* infection. Scand J Gastroenterol. 1995;30:1153–9.
9. Ernst PB, Reves VE, Gourley WH, Haberle H, Bamford KB. Is the Th1/Th2 lymphocyte balance upset by *Helicobacter pylori* infection? In: Hunt RH, Tytgat GNJ, editors. *Helicobacter pylori*: Basic Mechanisms to Clinical Cure 1996. Dordrecht: Kluwer; 1996:150–7.
10. Covacci A, Telford JL, Del Giudice G, Parsonnet J, Rappuoli R. *Helicobacter pylori* virulence and genetic geography. Science. 1999;284:1328–33.
11. Doidge C, Gust I, Lee A, Buck F, Hazell S, Manne U. Therapeutic immunisation against *Helicobacter* infection. Lancet. 1994;343:914–15.
12. Corthesy Theulaz I, Porta N, Glauser M et al. Oral immunization with *Helicobacter pylori* urease B subunit as a treatment against *Helicobacter* infection in mice. Gastroenterology. 1995;109:115–21.
13. Saldinger PF, Porta N, Launois P et al. Immunization of BALB/c mice with *Helicobacter* urease B induces a T helper 2 response absent in *Helicobacter* infection. Gastroenterology. 1998;115:891–7.
14. Marinaro M, Staats HF, Hiroi T et al. Mucosal adjuvant effect of cholera toxin in mice results from induction of T helper 2 (Th2) cells and IL-4. J Immunol. 1995;155:4621–9.
15. Mohammadi M, Nedrud J, Redline R, Lycke N, Czinn SJ. Murine CD4 T-cell response to *Helicobacter* infection – TH1 cells enhance gastritis and TH2 cells reduce bacterial load. Gastroenterology. 1997;113:1848–57.
16. Radcliff F, Ramsay AJ, Lee A. Failure of immunisation against *Helicobacter* infection in IL-4 mice: evidence for the TH2 immune response as the basis for protective immunity. Gastroenterology. 1996;110:A997.
17. Radcliff FJ, Ramsey AJ, Lee A. A mixed Th1/Th2 response may be necessary for effective immunity against *Helicobacter*. Immunol Cell Biol. 1997;75:A90.
18. Ermak TH, Giannasca PJ, Nichols R et al. Immunization of mice with urease vaccine affords protection against *Helicobacter pylori* infection in the absence of antibodies and is mediated by MHC class II-restricted responses. J Exp Med. 1998;188:2277–88.

19. Nedrud JR, Blanchard TG, Redline R, Sigmund N, Czinn SJ. Orally immunized μMT antibody-deficient mice are protected against *H. felis* infection. Gastroenterology. 1998; 114:A1049.
20. Sutton P, Wilson J, Kosaka T, Wolowczuk I, Lee A. Therapeutic immunization against *Helicobacter pylori* infection in the absence of antibodies. Immunol Cell Biol. 2000;78:28–30.
21. Thomas JE, Dale A, Harding M, Coward WA, Cole TJ, Weaver LT. *Helicobacter pylori* colonization in early life. Ped Res. 1999;45:218–23.
22. Forsthuber T, Yip H, Lehmann P. Induction of TH1 and TH2 immunity in neonatal mice. Science. 1996;271:1728–30.
23. Thomas JE, Austin S, Dale A *et al.* Protection by human milk IgA against *Helicobacter pylori* infection in infancy. Lancet. 1993;342:121.

20
Elimination of *Helicobacter pylori* is not dependent on a Th2 cytokine response

K. CROITORU

INTRODUCTION

The following evidence argues in support of the resolution that elimination of *Helicobacter pylori* is not dependent on a Th2 response:
1. Th1/Th2 dichotomy is an oversimplification of T cell responses to *H. pylori* infection.
2. Immunization in the absence of IL-4 (Th2) is protective.
3. Viral-induced elimination of *H. pylori* is dependent on IFN-γ and IL-12.
4. Immunization in the absence of IFN-γ is not protective.
5. Systemic immunization without Th2 adjuvants leads to a decrease in colonization.

Th1/Th2 PARADIGM

Helper T cell responses can be polarized, based on the profile of cytokines produced. The initial division of T cells into Th1 and Th2 subsets helped address many of the observations made in studies of immune responses to infections[1]. Therefore, it is reasonable to see the many studies that attempt to classify the T cell/cytokine response to *Helicobacter* infection into either a Th1 or Th2 type response. A number of studies have shown that natural *Helicobacter* infection leads to a Th1-type response[2,3]. Clearly this is an oversimplification of what happens in humans or in rodent models of the infection. In addition to the frequent finding that elements of both Th1 and Th2 responses can be found in any immune responses, other T cell responses can be demonstrated, e.g. Th3 responses where TGF-β is the major cytokine produced[4]. In addition, recent studies have identified regulatory Tr1 cells, which produce IL-10 with little IL-4[5]. The balance between all of these T cells, and others yet to be identified, defines the true nature of the response to *Helicobacter*.

EFFECT OF ABSENCE OF IL-4 ON *HELICOBACTER* INFECTION

In the absence of one of the prototypic Th2 cytokines, IL-4 *H. pylori* (SS1) infection induces gastritis and colonization that is not significantly different from that seen in normal mice. On the other hand, another study showed that *H. felis* infection was slightly increased in IL-4 knockout mice[6]. In addition, the proposed mechanisms by which cholera toxin-based vaccine led to an effective immune response is through promoting Th2 immune responses, which help promote antibody responses, in particular IgA. Although IgA responses can be measured during *Helicobacter* infection, a number of studies have now shown that adjuvant-based vaccines are equally effective in protection or in eliminating established infection in mice lacking B cells[7,8].

On the other hand, *Helicobacter* infection in B/6 and IFN-γ-deficient mice resulted in gastritis that was no different, but the degree of bacterial colonization was increased in the IFN-γ-deficient mice[9]. This would argue against the contention that Th2 responses alone are required for effective immunity.

VIRAL-INDUCED ELIMINATION OF *H. FELIS* IS DEPENDENT ON IFN-γ AND IL-12

Our study showed that *H. pylori* adenovirus-induced elimination of *H. felis* infection was dependent on Th1 cytokines, IFN-γ and IL-12[10]. This implies that Th1 cytokines can be involved in the control or even the elimination of *Helicobacter* infection. On the other hand, in a recent study Fox *et al.* showed that helminth co-infection of *H. pylori*-infected mice leads to a decrease in Th1[11]. Therefore, in addition to viral-induced elimination of *Helicobacter*, helminth modulation increased *Helicobacter* colonization in spite of increasing Th2 cytokines.

IMMUNIZATION IN THE ABSENCE OF IFN-γ IS NOT PROTECTIVE

The inability to induce effective immunization in the absence of IFN-γ (i.e. in a mouse with predominantly Th2 cytokines present) would be very strong evidence that Th2 cytokines are not required. However, the studies examining this issue suggest that vaccination of IFN-γ-deficient mice does lead to effective immunity[9]. Although this does not argue in support of the proposal that elimination of *H. pylori* is not dependent on a Th2 cytokine response, transgenic mice which over express IL-4 remain susceptible to *Helicobacter* infection[6].

SYSTEMIC IMMUNIZATION WITHOUT Th2 ADJUVANTS LEADS TO A DECREASE IN COLONIZATION

In a recent study, systemic immunization of mice with complete Freund's adjuvant, a Th1-stimulating adjuvant, led to protective immunity against

Helicobacter infection[8]. We have examined the effect of systemic immunization with incomplete Freund's adjuvant in mice with established *H. pylori*-infection. In these mice there was a decrease in colonization that was correlated with an increase in DTH responses, suggesting that, without specifically stimulating Th2 response, we could induce an immune response effective in eliminating an established infection.

CONCLUSION

These data support the idea that elimination of *H. pylori* is not dependent on a Th2 response. The significant finding in favour of this proposal is that the design of vaccines is not limited to the stimulation of a Th2 response. Furthermore, it is also possible that modulating the immune response without specific defined antigen would also lead to an effective treatment of *Helicobacter* infection.

Acknowledgements

K.C. holds an Ontario Ministry of Health Career Scientist Award. The work described has received support from the Hamilton Health Sciences Corporation Research Foundation, the Canadian Association of Gastroenterology, AstraZenica and the Medical Research Council of Canada.

References

1. Mosmann TR, Coffman RL. Heterogeneity of cytokine secretion patterns and functions of helper T cells. Adv Immunol. 1989;46:111–48.
2. Bamford KB, Fan XJ, Crowe SE *et al.* Lymphocytes in the human gastric mucosa during *Helicobacter pylori* have a T helper cell 1 phenotype. Gastroenterology. 1998;114:482–92.
3. Mohammadi M, Czinn S, Redline R, Nedrud J. *Helicobacter*-specific cell-mediated immune responses display a predominant Th1 phenotype and promote a delayed-type hypersensitivity response in the stomachs of mice. J Immunol. 1996;156:4729–38.
4. Neurath M, Fuss I, Kelsall BL, Presky DH, Waegell W, Strober W. Experimental granulomatous colitis in mice is abrogated by induction of TGF-β mediated oral tolerance. J Exp Med. 1996;183:2605.
5. Groux H, O'Garra A, Bigler M *et al.* A $CD4^+$ T-cell subset inhibits antigen-specific T-cell responses and prevents colitis. Nature. 1997;389:737–42.
6. Chen W, Shu D, Chadwick VS. *Helicobacter pylori* infection in interleukin-4-deficient and transgenic mice. Scand J Gastroenterol. 1999;34:987–92.
7. Ermak TH, Giannasca PJ, Nichols R *et al.* Immunization of mice with urease vaccine affords protection against *Helicobacter pylori* infection in the absence of antibodies and is mediated by MHC class II restricted responses. J Exp Med. 1998;188:2277–88.
8. Blanchard TG, Gottwein JM, Targoni OS *et al.* Systemic vaccination inducing either Th1 or Th2 immunity protects mice from challenge with *H. pylori*. Gastroenterology. 1999;116:A695 (abstract).
9. Sawai N, Kita M, Kodama T *et al.* Role of gamma interferon in *Helicobacter pylori*-induced gastric inflammatory responses in a mouse model. Infect Immun. 1999;67:279–85.
10. Jiang B, Jordana M, Xing Z *et al.* Replication-defective adenovirus infection reduces *Helicobacter felis* colonization in the mouse in a gamma interferon- and interleukin-12-dependent manner. Infect Immun. 1999;67:4539–44.
11. Fox JG, Beck P, Dangler CA *et al.* Concurrent enteric helminth infection modulates inflammation and gastric immune responses and reduces *Helicobacter*-induced gastric atrophy. Nature Med. 2000 (In press).

21
The inflamatory activity in *Helicobacter pylori* infection is predominantly organism related

P. MICHETTI

INTRODUCTION

Helicobacter pylori is remarkably adapted to survival in its niche on the surface of the human gastric mucosa. It persists for decades with minimal damage in the majority of those infected. Nevertheless, infection is almost invariably associated with some degree of chronic active gastritis. The intensity of this inflammation of the gastric mucosa has been correlated with the risk of developing complications of the infection such as peptic ulcer, and the inflammation invariably abates after successful elimination of the infection. To modulate the host response, *H. pylori* has evolved a complex set of genes. Recent genetic studies contributed to defining the function of some of these genes. In addition, these studies, as well as the analysis of the two complete genomes of *H. pylori*, have provided important information regarding the mechanisms by which *H. pylori* modulates gene expression. Gene regulation allows the pathogen to further adapt to its environment and to further modulate its relationship to its host, including inflammation.

STRAIN-SPECIFIC GENE PRODUCTS OF *H. PYLORI* CAN MODULATE GASTRIC INFLAMMATION

Adhesins

Adhesion of the bacteria may not be required for persistence of the infection, but *H. pylori* selectively binds to gastric epithelial cells, and its colonization of the digestive tract is limited to areas lined by gastric-type epithelial cells. On adhesion, tyrosine phosphorylation and cytoskeletal rearrangement occur, leading to a remodelling of the apical surface of the epithelial cells[1]. Adhesion is necessary for the initiation of the inflammation cascade. In particular adhesion is a prerequisite for interleukin 8 (IL-8) secretion by gastric epithelial cells[2]. Evidence also accumulates that adherence may promote the development of more severe disease. Transgenic mice that expressed the Lewis b blood group antigen, the receptor for the BabA adhesin[3] developed autoreactive antibodies, and had more severe chronic gastritis and parietal cell loss than animals without the transgene[4]. More recently, BabA was associated with duodenal ulcer, distal gastric cancer, and more severe gastritis[5]. Furthermore, ablation of parietal cells in transgenic mice by genetic engineering caused expansion of epithelial progenitor cells that expressed another species of receptor molecules for *H. pylori* (terminal NeuAcα2,3Galβ1,4). *H. pylori* was found to bind to these progenitor cells, resulting in an increased immune response and more severe gastritis, confirming that adhesion plays a role in inflammation[6]. Other factors may also participate in *H. pylori* adhesion, such as the two highly related proteins AlpA and AlpB. Like the Le^b binding adhesin BabA, AlpA and AlpB are members of the large family of related outer membrane proteins (Hop proteins). Both AlpA and AlpB are required for adhesion to Kato III cells and to human gastric tissue sections[7]. BabA and the Alp proteins are not present in all strains of *H. pylori*, and thus may represent means by which the pathogen gains control of the host response.

Lipopolysaccharide

Lipopolysaccharides (LPS), also known as endotoxins, comprise an important group of bacterial surface carbohydrates that have been implicated in a variety of biological interactions between Gram-negative bacteria and their hosts. *H. pylori* LPS has unusually low endotoxic and immunostimulating activities compared to the LPS of other Gram-negative bacteria. Recent evidence indicates that the low endotoxin potency of *H. pylori* LPS is due to a slow transfer of *H. pylori* LPS from LPS-binding protein to CD14, the final cellular receptor for endotoxin[8,9]. Although this mechanism of action of LPS is analogous to other bacterial LPS, this slower transfer could account for the lower pro-inflammatory effect of *H. pylori* LPS as compared to *E. coli* or *S. typhimurium* LPS[10]. Studies in mice naturally unresponsive to LPS showed that these mice had decreased macrophage infiltration of the gastric mucosa and slower progression towards gastric mucosal atrophy than wild-type congenic animals[11]. Finally, *H. pylori* adapts its pattern of Lewis antigen expression to mimic that of its host, indicating that the pathogen is able to regulate this virulence factor[12].

The vacuolating cytotoxin A (VacA)

The association of VacA with peptic ulcer disease, MALT lymphoma, and gastric cancer is well validated, at least in Europe where the background population has a low incidence of type I strains (defined as CagA and VacA positive)[13–15]. *H. pylori vacA s1* strains have been associated with high cytotoxin activity, high VacA expression or the occurrence of peptic ulcer disease[15,16]. *vacA s1* may even be a surrogate marker for the presence of the *cag* PAI[17]. The *vacA m2* allele is also associated with peptic ulcer disease and gastric cancer[18]. The mechanism of action of VacA has recently been further described. Binding of free or membrane-bound VacA to epithelial cells is receptor-mediated[19,20], and receptor usage may differ for VacA m1 and VacA m2[18]. VacA forms pores in lysosomal membranes, increasing anion permeability and generating vacuoles, in a process that may require cellular proteins[21,22]. In addition, VacA may increase paracellular permeability to small molecules[23]. Finally, VacA inhibits *de-novo* antigen binding by MHC class II receptor, a mechanism that can contribute to a down-regulation of the host immune response[24], which has been correlated in mice with increased gastritis and atrophy[25].

CagA and the *cag*-associated pathogenicity island (*cag*-PAI)

There is evidence that CagA$^+$ strains are more infectious[26], achieve higher bacterial density on the gastric mucosa, and cause more inflammation than CagA$^-$ strains[27]. These findings suggest that the *cag*-PAI contains genes involved in colonization and host response. Among them, six membrane proteins, including the one encoded by the *picB* gene, have been shown to be required for the up-regulation of NF-κB and associated with increased gastric IL-8 expression[2,28]. The *cag*-PAI is composed of two parts, split by a transposable element IS605[29]. In the second part of the PAI, named *cagII*, Akopyants *et al.*[29] identified four proteins homologous to components of multiprotein complexes of *Bordetella pertussis*, *Agrobacterium tumefaciens* and of bacterial plasmids that deliver pertussis toxin, tumour-inducing DNA, and conjugated genes to their respective targets. These proteins may assemble in a membrane complex used to signal gastric epithelial cells, and induce IL-8 secretion. One of the *cagII* genes, named *virD4*, has been shown to decrease IL-8 production by gastric epithelial cells, suggesting that *cag*-PAI genes may have a bimodal role in the control of the host response[30]. The CagA protein, which was long considered merely a marker for the *cag*-PAI, has recently been shown to be the signal transmitted by PAI-encoded proteins. Upon binding of the bacteria, CagA is translocated into the host epithelial cells and tyrosine-phosphorylated. In addition, several host proteins are dephosphorylated[31,32].

IceA

Two alleles of a novel *H. pylori* gene, *iceA* (induced by contact with epithelium) were recently characterized. In contrast to its homologue *iceA2*, the *iceA1* allele is associated with peptic ulcer and increased mucosal concentration of IL-8[33]. A recent study in Japan showed that the *iceA1* allele is associated with increased gastric inflammation[34]. Another study in Europe associated *iceA1* with an increased risk of duodenal ulcer disease[35].

GENE REGULATION MECHANISMS OF *H. PYLORI*

The analysis of the two complete genome sequences of *H. pylori* showed that approximately 7% of the sequences present in one strain were lacking in the other. Subtractive hybridization techniques demonstrated further strain-specific genes[36]. The function of these strain-specific genes is as yet unknown, but they may participate in the adaptation of *H. pylori* to individual hosts, ethnic groups, or may affect the clinical course of the infection. Although the genetic variability of *H. pylori* has been described earlier, the mechanisms underlying this diversity remained largely unclear. Population genetic studies[37,38], as well as careful analyses of multiple strains isolated from a single patient, provide novel insights into these mechanisms[39]. These studies indicate that strain diversity in *H. pylori* has been created by recombination between strains, and that new recombinant genotypes continue to be generated in patients infected with multiple strains. Frequent recombination may be one mechanism that permits *H. pylori* to adapt to individual host organisms. In addition, this form of genetic exchange could facilitate global spread of chromosomal mutations such as those that confer resistance against some antibiotics.

Specific promoters

Gene regulation in *H. pylori* may also represent an important pathogenic function. The genome analyses showed that *H. pylori* lacks some of the known bacterial master regulatory features. However, the analysis of intergenic sequences in the *cag*-PAI revealed three overlapping functional promoters between the two divergently transcribed *cagA* and *cagB* genes[40]. These putative promoter sequences showed high homology to the *E. coli* $\sigma 70$–10 promoter consensus sequences, suggesting that promoters are active in the regulation of the *cag* genes.

Sequence repeats

The genome of *H. pylori* contains numerous short repetitive nucleotide sequences, located mainly within genes encoding surface-exposed molecules. Recent experimental evidence showed that length variation in these repeat sequences provides a means of switching genes on and off. A fucosyltransferase (*fucT2*) of *H. pylori* can be switched off by a change of repeat length within the coding region that causes a frame-shift and a premature stop codon[41]. The resulting inactivation of *fucT2* affects the expression of Lewis^Y antigen in the LPS molecule. This mechanism of antigenic variation may be relevant for molecular mimicry and avoidance of the host immune system.

Environment-dependent gene expression

The slow growth and the complex media requirement of *H. pylori* impair the identification of the conditions that activate the *H. pylori* virulence programme. Using subtractive RNA hybridization of bacteria incubated at pH 4 and 7, McGowan and co-workers[42] have recently identified an acid-induced gene that is involved in LPS biosynthesis and adaptation to acid stress. The *iceA* gene, which is a putative restriction endonuclease, was identified by a similar approach. This gene is induced by contact of the bacteria with epithelial cells[33].

CONCLUSIONS

The genome of *H. pylori* contains numerous genes encoding for factors involved in the control of gastric inflammation. These genes can be exchanged between strains, and their expression is controlled by several independent mechanisms. This complex machinery provides H. pylori with the ability to regulate the host response, and thus represents an integral part of its pathogenesis.

Reference

1. Segal ED, Falkow S, Tompkins LS. *Helicobacter pylori* attachment to gastric cells induces cytoskeletal rearrangements and tyrosine phosphorylation of host cell proteins. Proc Natl Acad Sci USA. 1996;93:1259–64.
2. Keates S, Hitti YS, Upton M, Kelly CP. *Helicobacter pylori* infection activates NF-kappa B in gastric epithelial cells. Gastroenterology. 1997;113:1099–109.
3. Ilver D, Arnqvist A, Ogren J et al. *Helicobacter pylori* adhesin binding fucosylated histo-blood group antigens revealed by retagging. Science. 1998;279:373–7.
4. Guruge JL, Falk PG, Lorenz RG et al. Epithelial attachment alters the outcome of *Helicobacter pylori* infection. Proc Natl Acad Sci USA. 1998;95:3925–30.
5. Gerhard M, Lehn N, Neumayer N et al. Clinical relevance of the *Helicobacter pylori* gene for blood-group antigen-binding adhesin. Proc Natl Acad Sci USA. 1999;96:12778–83.
6. Syder AJ, Guruge JL, Li Q et al. *Helicobacter pylori* attaches to NeuAc alpha 2,3Gal beta 1,4 glycoconjugates produced in the stomach of transgenic mice lacking parietal cells. Mol Cell. 1999;3:263–74.
7. Odenbreit S, Till M, Hofreuter D, Faller G, Haas R. Genetic and functional characterization of the alpAB gene locus essential for the adhesion of *Helicobacter pylori* to human gastric tissue. Mol Microbiol. 1999;31:1537–48.
8. Cunningham MD, Seachord C, Ratcliffe K, Bainbridge B, Aruffo A, Darveau RP. *Helicobacter pylori* and *Porphyromonas gingivalis* lipopolysaccharides are poorly transferred to recombinant soluble CD14. Infect Immun. 1996;64:3601–8.
9. Kirkland T, Viriyakosol S, Perez-Perez GI, Blaser MJ. *Helicobacter pylori* lipopolysaccharide can activate 70Z/3 cells via CD14. Infect Immun. 1997;65:604–8.
10. Semeraro N, Montemurro P, Piccoli C et al. Effect of *Helicobacter pylori* lipopolysaccharide (LPS) and LPS derivatives on the production of tissue factor and plasminogen activator inhibitor type 2 by human blood mononuclear cells. J Infect Dis. 1996;174:1255–60.
11. Sakagami T, Vella J, Dixon MF et al. The endotoxin of Helicobacter pylori is a modulator of host-dependent gastritis. Infect Immun. 1997;65:3310–16.
12. Wirth HP, Yang M, Peek RM, Jr, Tham KT, Blaser MJ. *Helicobacter pylori* Lewis expression is related to the host Lewis phenotype. Gastroenterology. 1997;113:1091–8.
13. de Figueiredo Soares T, de Magalhaes Queiroz DM, Mendes EN et al. The interrelationship between *Helicobacter pylori* vacuolating cytotoxin and gastric carcinoma. Am J Gastroenterol. 1998;93:1841–7.
14. Rudi J, Kolb C, Maiwald M et al. Diversity of *Helicobacter pylori* *vacA* and *cagA* genes and relationship to VacA and CagA protein expression, cytotoxin production, and associated diseases (see comments). J Clin Microbiol. 1998;36:944–8.
15. Yang JC, Kuo CH, Wang HJ, Wang TC, Chang CS, Wang WC. Vacuolating toxin gene polymorphism among *Helicobacter pylori* clinical isolates and its association with m1, m2, or chimeric vacA middle types. Scand J Gastroenterol. 1998;33.1152–7.
16. Miehlke S, Meining A, Morgner A et al. Frequency of vacA genotypes and cytotoxin activity in *Helicobacter pylori* associated with low-grade gastric mucosa-associated lymphoid tissue lymphoma. J Clin Microbiol. 1998;36:2369–70.
17. Yamaoka Y, Kodama T, Kita M, Imanishi J, Kashima K, Graham DY. Relationship of *vacA* genotypes of *Helicobacter pylori* to *cagA* status, cytotoxin production, and clinical outcome. Helicobacter. 1998;3:241–3.
18. Pagliaccia C, de Bernard M, Lupetti P et al. The m2 form of the *Helicobacter pylori* cytotoxin has cell type-specific vacuolating activity. Proc Natl Acad Sci USA. 1998;95:10212–17.
19. Massari P, Manetti R, Burroni D et al. Binding of the *Helicobacter pylori* vacuolating cytotoxin to target cells. Infect Immun. 1998;66:3981–84.

20. Sommi P, Ricci V, Fiocca R et al. Persistence of *Helicobacter pylori* VacA toxin and vacuolating potential in cultured gastric epithelial cells. Am J Physiol. 1998;275:G681–8.
21. de Bernard M, Burroni D, Papini E, Rappuoli R, Telford J, Montecucco C. Identification of the *Helicobacter pylori* VacA toxin domain active in the cell cytosol. Infect Immun. 1998;66:6014–16.
22. Pai R, Wyle FA, Cover TL, Itani RM, Domek MJ, Tarnawski AS. *Helicobacter pylori* culture supernatant interferes with epidermal growth factor-activated signal transduction in human gastric KATO III cells. Am J Pathol. 1998;152:1617–24.
23. Papini E, Satin B, Norais N et al. Selective increase of the permeability of polarized epithelial cell monolayers by *Helicobacter pylori* vacuolating toxin. J Clin Invest. 1998;102:813–20.
24. Molinari M, Salio M, Galli C et al. Selective inhibition of Ii-dependent antigen presentation by *Helicobacter pylori* toxin VacA. J Exp Med. 1998;187:135–40.
25. Sutton P, Wilson J, Genta R et al. A genetic basis for atrophy: dominant non-responsiveness and *Helicobacter* induced gastritis in F(1) hybrid mice (See comments). Gut. 1999;45:335–40.
26. Wirth HP, Beins MH, Yang M, Tham KT, Blaser MJ. Experimental infection of Mongolian gerbils with wild-type and mutant *Helicobacter pylori* strains. Infect Immun. 1998;66: 4856–66.
27. Gunn MC, Stephens JC, Stewart JA, Rathbone BJ, West KP. The significance of cagA and vacA subtypes of *Helicobacter pylori* in the pathogenesis of inflammation and peptic ulceration. J Clin Pathol. 1998;51:761–4.
28. Glocker E, Lange C, Covacci A, Bereswill S, Kist M, Pahl HL. Proteins encoded by the *cag* pathogenicity island of *Helicobacter pylori* are required for NF-kappaB activation. Infect Immun. 1998;66:2346–8.
29. Akopyants NS, Clifton SW, Kersulyte D et al. Analyses of the *cag* pathogenicity island of *Helicobacter pylori*. Mol Microbiol. 1998;28:37–53.
30. Crabtree JE, Kersulyte D, Li SD, Lindley IJ, Berg DE. Modulation of *Helicobacter pylori* induced interleukin-8 synthesis in gastric epithelial cells mediated by *cag* PAI encoded VirD4 homologue. J Clin Pathol. 1999;52:653–7.
31. Odenbreit S, Puls J, Sedlmaier B, Gerland E, Fischer W, Haas R. Translocation of *Helicobacter pylori* CagA into gastric epithelial cells by type IV secretion. Science. 2000;287:1497–500.
32. Segal ED, Cha J, Lo J, Falkow S, Tompkins LS. Altered states: involvement of phosphorylated CagA in the induction of host cellular growth changes by *Helicobacter pylori*. Proc Natl Acad Sci USA. 1999;96:14559–64.
33. Peek RM Jr, Thompson SA, Donahue JP et al. Adherence to gastric epithelial cells induces expression of a *Helicobacter pylori* gene, *iceA*, that is associated with clinical outcome. Proc Assoc Am Phys. 1998;110:531–44.
34. Nishiya D, Shimoyama T, Fukuda S, Yoshimura T, Tanaka M, Munakata A. Evaluation of the clinical relevance of the iceA1 gene in patients with *Helicobacter pylori* infection in Japan. Scand J Gastroenterol. 2000;35:36–9.
35. van Doorn LJ, Figueiredo C, Sanna R et al. Clinical relevance of the *cagA*, *vacA*, and *iceA* status of *Helicobacter pylori*. Gastroenterology. 1998;115:58–66.
36. Akopyants NS, Fradkov A, Diatchenko L et al. PCR-based subtractive hybridization and differences in gene content among strains of *Helicobacter pylori*. Proc Natl Acad Sci USA. 1998;95:13108–13.
37. Achtman M, Azuma T, Berg DE et al. Recombination and clonal groupings within *Helicobacter pylori* from different geographical regions. Mol Microbiol. 1999;32:459–70.
38. Suerbaum S, Smith JM, Bapumia K et al. Free recombination within *Helicobacter pylori*. Proc Natl Acad Sci USA. 1998;95:12619–24.
39. Kersulyte D, Chalkauskas H, Berg DE. Emergence of recombinant strains of *Helicobacter pylori* during human infection. Mol Microbiol. 1999;31:31–43.
40. Spohn G, Beier D, Rappuoli R, Scarlato V. Transcriptional analysis of the divergent *cagAB* genes encoded by the pathogenicity island of *Helicobacter pylori*. Mol Microbiol. 1997; 26:361–72.
41. Wang G, Rasko DA, Sherburne R, Taylor DE. Molecular genetic basis for the variable expression of Lewis Y antigen in *Helicobacter pylori*: analysis of the alpha (1,2) fucosyltransferase gene. Mol Microbiol. 1999;31:1265–74.
42. McGowan CC, Necheva A, Thompson SA, Cover TL, Blaser MJ. Acid-induced expression of an LPS-associated gene in Helicobacter pylori. Mol Microbiol. 1998;30:19–31.

22
The inflammatory activity in *Helicobacter pylori* infection is predominantly host-related

P. B. ERNST

THE HOST RESPONSE IS A MAJOR FACTOR THAT DETERMINES PATHOGENICITY

There are several examples that illustrate the principle that the host immune/inflammatory response is necessary for the manifestation of disease caused by infection (Table 1). For example, it is well recognized that some infections trigger autoimmune disease. While the microbe is the trigger, the host response is the bullet that leads to the actual disease. Others have shown that infection with *Clostridium difficile* causes enteritis but administration of antibodies that impair the homing of immune/inflammatory cells to the gut prevents the manifestation of diarrhoea[1]. Even the prototype for a microbial virulence factor, cholera toxin, cannot exert its pathogenic effect without an intact host response. Infection of mice deficient in stem cell factor or its receptor does not induce fluid accumulation in the intestinal lumen after administration of the cholera toxin[2]. Thus, the host response must often be considered an essential element of microbial pathogenicity.

If the host response contributes to pathogenicity, then it is possible to extend the notion such that it can actually define pathogenicity. The digestive tract is colonized with a robust flora including 200–300 different species of bacteria. In fact, the normal intestinal immune response is designed to limit its reactivity to antigenic stimuli that persist in the lumen. However, several

Table 1. Evidence favouring a role for the host response in defining microbial pathogenesis

Enteric infections trigger autoimmune disease[32]
Cholera in SCF-deficient mice does not cause diarrhoea[2]
Antibodies to CD18 block diarrhoea by *C. difficile*[1]
Antibodies to TNF block diarrhoea by *S. typhimurium* (G. Jackson, personal communciation)
Disrupted immune regulation leads to colitis[33]
Gastric disease associated with *H. pylori*

experimental models have shown that disruption of the delicate balance in immune regulation renders the otherwise innocuous luminal flora extremely dangerous[3]. With the advent of genetic engineering in animal models it readily became apparent that targeted manipulations of the immune system result in colitis. For example, deletion of the genes encoding IL-2, IL-10, the T cell receptor alpha chain, class II MHC as well as TGF-β, all resulted in the spontaneous development of colitis in these animal models[4–6]. Subsequently, it was shown that Th1 responses were over-represented in these animals. Based on this, it was predicted that manipulating genes encoding receptors for these cytokines, or disrupting signalling mechanisms that favoured Th1 development, also led to colitis[7,8]. In most of the models tested, disease is completely prevented by housing the animals in germ-free conditions. Therefore, colitis was not due to the introduction of a new pathogen *per se*, but rather the altered immune response rendered some element of the normal flora pathogenic. In essence, the host response defined the pathogenicity of the organisms. The same model can be applied to *H. pylori*-related disease.

PROBLEMS IN THE VIRULENCE FACTOR MODEL

Since gastroduodenal diseases can be attributed to infection with *Helicobacter pylori*, it is natural to assume that pathogenicity will be defined by bacterial factors. Stanley Falkow recently discussed properties of pathogenicity[9] including the important property that a pathogen must breach host cell barriers. This process is facilitated by the ability of the organism to avoid, subvert or otherwise circumvent the host's immune response, thus leading to damage and eventually illness. Based on the discussion above, the host response should not be considered solely as an element of protection, but also as an instrument that translates the bacterial virulence factor into a disease process. It is also important to consider that some bacteria cause disease quite rapidly while others, like *H. pylori*, do so over decades. Thus, the presence and/or potency of virulence factors must vary among different bacterial species. In the case of chronic infections there is no advantage to the bacteria to risk killing the host; therefore, bacteria causing chronic infections would logically evolve to favour colonization and persistence while tending to lose virulence factors that cause significant disease directly.

While *H. pylori* produces products, including urease, that are necessary for colonization, studies have tried to identify virulence factors that cause gastroduodenal disease. *H. pylori* infection is essentially limited to the gastroduodenal lumen, where it colonizes under the mucus layer, adjacent to the epithelium, allowing the bacteria to cause damage to the gastric mucosa. Leunk and colleagues[10] described the ability of *H. pylori* to induce vacuolization in the membrane of epithelial cells. Subsequently, a vacuolating toxin, VacA, was purified, characterized, cloned and used to understand the pathogenesis of these vacuoles[11–13]. The cytotoxin-associated gene, *cagA*, was also identified. While the *cagA* gene does not actually encode the vacuolating toxin, it was often co-expressed with *vacA*[14].

Several studies have examined the association of these genes with the more severe disease manifestations associated with *H. pylori* infection. CagA has been associated with duodenal ulcer as well as gastric cancer[15,16]. Similarly, the examination of the *vacA* locus has undergone extensive scrutiny. VacA is capable of causing epithelial cell damage and is sufficient to cause gastritis in mice[13]. Atherton and colleagues have suggested that virulence and clinical outcome are associated with strains of *H. pylori* that have a particular pattern of nucleotides in the *vacA* gene[11]. Based on their studies, strains of *H. pylori* with the *vacA* signal sequence type s1a were associated with enhanced gastric inflammation and duodenal ulceration. However, the genotype of strains based on these genes varies widely among different geographic regions and does not always associate with disease in different regions of the globe[17].

Using the *cagA* and *vacA* genotypes, investigators have pursued the association of virulence factors and gastroduodenal disease. This led to the description of 'type I' and 'type II' strains, defined by the presence or absence of both the *cagA* and *vacA* genes[14]. The type I strains, which express both factors, have been implicated as a predictor of more adverse disease outcome. On further dissection it became evident that these tools would not significantly help identify individuals at greater risk of peptic ulcer or gastric cancer. To begin with, strains expressing CagA constitute 70–95% of all isolates, depending on the study and the geographic location of the subjects. As peptic ulcer affects approximately 10% of all infected subjects and gastric cancer less than 1%, the presence of CagA does not predict disease. This therefore suggests that this gene product alone does not translate into a 'virulence factor' the way cholera toxin would. Similarly, the association of the variants of the *vacA* gene fail to effectively predict the outcome of infection when one considers that 90% of the strains in Asia bear this genotype, yet disease expression is relatively low.

Other studies have focused on simultaneously following many genes in an effort to identify a stronger correlation between infection and disease outcome. In one such study, cagA, vacAs1 and iceA1 status of *H. pylori* was shown to be associated with peptic ulcer disease[18]. However, patients infected with strains lacking these genetic markers can still develop peptic ulceration[11,18]. Moreover, patients may be infected simultaneously with more than one strain that varies in their genotype, for example, in the *cag* pathogenicity island (PAI) region[19], thus making the studies of disease association difficult. It also should not be forgotten that the overwhelming majority of individuals infected with 'high-risk' strains identified to date do not suffer the more severe clinical consequences (see Figure 1). Thus, no single entity or array of genes has yet been identified that can serve as a marker(s) for predicting the development of gastric disease. This could be attributed to the role of other factors that govern disease expression. In particular, changes in gastric physiology[20] and the host immune/inflammatory response[21] have been implicated in the pathogenesis of gastric disease.

SHAPING THE IMUNE RESPONSE DURING INFECTION

Most infected humans carry strains of *H. pylori* expressing the PAI. The dominance of these strains suggests that they may have a selective advantage,

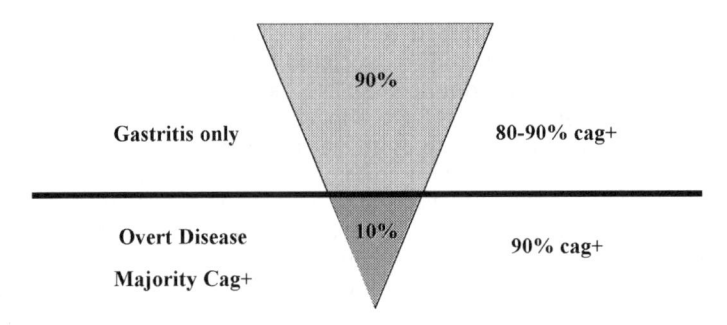

```
                    90%
Gastritis only                    80-90% cag+
─────────────────────────────────────────────
Overt Disease      10%
                                  90% cag+
Majority Cag+
```

Figure 1. Varying perspectives on the role of the *cag* pathogenicity island as a virulence factor. The *cag* PAI provides an interesting model to study bacterial–host interactions. Genes linked to the *cag* PAI have been associated with more severe gastritis, duodenal ulcer and an increased risk of gastric cancer. However, these strains predominate globally and are found in the majority of infected subjects who do not develop the more severe manifestation of *H. pylori* infection. Clearly, the fact that many subjects without significant disease also have strains bearing this or other phenotypes putatively described as being virulence factors makes it difficult to ascribe disease to a virulence factor alone. Thus, other bacterial factors may be important, or the variation in disease manifestation may be regulated by more complex interactions among the bacteria, host and environmental factors. Modified from ref. 34.

perhaps achieved by avoiding a protective immune response. This is consistent with the model described by Falkow, which proposes that a pathogen can usually circumvent the host defence mechanisms[9]. Little direct evidence for this process has been described in the context of *H. pylori* infection. It has been suggested that the bacterium may adapt its immunogenicity by acquiring the ability to express antigens that mimic the host. For example, the Lewis antigen phenotype of *H. pylori* has been reported to mirror that of the host[22]. It could be possible that these antigens activate local T cells that secrete 'anti-inflammatory' cytokines which attenuate the host response via a bystander effect. That is, a small population of T cells that confer tolerance may be activated and impair the immune reactivity to other T cells around them[23]. However, this has not been substantiated based on the cytokine analysis, as it appears that most of the cytokines in the gastric mucosa during infection are inflammatory rather than anti-inflammatory[21]. This in itself may favour chronic infection because the predominant Th1 response observed during infection is unlikely to be effective against a pathogen within the lumen. Indeed, a Th1 response is far more likely to have adverse effects on the host and actually contribute to gastroduodenal disease.

Another possibility is that a natural infection with *H. pylori* may selectively inhibit antigen-specific responses. Recent studies describe the ability of *H. pylori* to induce death in T cells through Fas/FasL interactions (manuscript submitted). Interestingly, the induction of apoptosis was restricted to *H. pylori* bearing the *cag* PAI and not observed with *cag* PAI-deficient strains or *C. jejuni*, suggesting that it is a specific mechanism of immune evasion. Since *cag* PAI strains predominate in humans, it is possible that this ability to induce apoptosis in T cells confers a selective advantage that

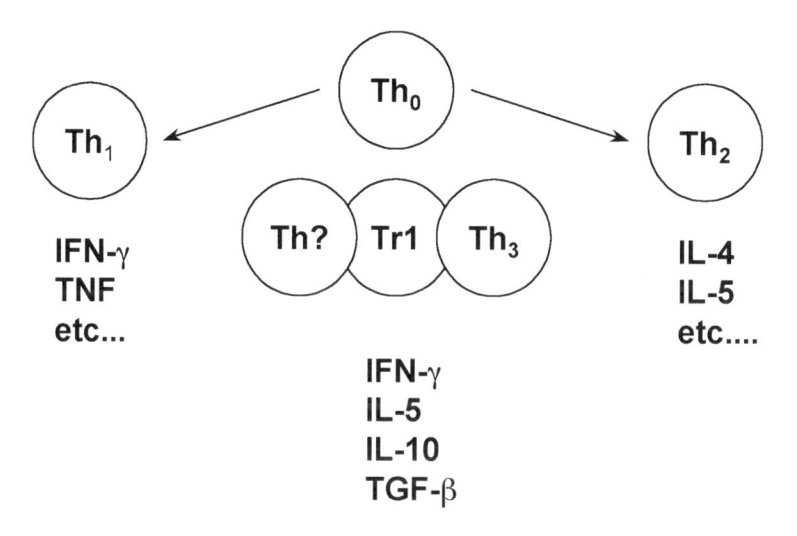

```
        ┌─────┐
        │ Th₀ │
        └─────┘
       ↙       ↘
┌─────┐              ┌─────┐
│ Th₁ │              │ Th₂ │
└─────┘              └─────┘

IFN-γ   ┌────┐┌────┐┌────┐   IL-4
TNF     │Th? ││Tr1 ││Th₃ │   IL-5
etc...  └────┘└────┘└────┘   etc....
              IFN-γ
              IL-5
              IL-10
              TGF-β
```

Dampens Reactivity to Luminal Antigens

Figure 2. Th cell responses controlling inflammation in the digestive tract. As described in the text, helper T cells display a tremendous amount of heterogeneity. Gastric T cell responses during *H. pylori* infection are predominantly of the Th1 type. While Th2 responses have been suggested to control inflammation, the more recently described Th3/Tr1 subsets may predominate in this role. These subsets are sufficient to limit the host response to luminal antigen. For example, intravenous injection of Tr1 cells into mice prevents the development of colitis. The relative absence of these cells in the gastric and duodenal mucosa could exacerbate inflammation and tissue damage favouring the development of gastroduodenal ulcers and the oxidative stress that contributes to gastric cancer.

complements other mechanisms favouring the persistent growth and survival of these strains.

CONTROL OF INFLAMMATION BY THE HOST RESPONSE

While strains of *H. pylori* expressing the *cag* PAI may avoid a protective response, they are still capable of inducing greater levels of inflammation in the gastric mucosa than strains lacking the *cag* PAI[24–26]. Thus, it is possible that any association between strains bearing the *cag* PAI and disease may be governed by the variation in the host response to infection in general, and these strains in particular. While significant advances have been made in our understanding of immune regulation in the gastrointestinal tract, new evidence suggests it is even more complex than previously thought.

Helper T cell responses have been viewed as primarily belonging to one of two major subsets – Th1 or Th2 – based on their cytokine profile (Figure 2). Through the production of IFN-γ, TNF-α and IL-2, Th1 cells select for a rather specific panel of immune responses including cell-mediated immunity, while Th2 cells preferentially regulate mucosal IgA responses through the production of TGF-β, IL-4, IL-5, IL-6 and IL-10[27]. This model is a vast over-simplification of the complex processes regulating multiple genes in Th cells[28] that is now becoming better appreciated. For example, a subset of helper Th cells that produces TGF-β and inhibits the host response to antigens that persist in the lumen has been referred to as Th3 cells[29,30]. More recently, investigators have described a subset of helper T cells that produce copious amounts of IL-10 and are capable of preventing colitis in a model of aberrant immune regulation to luminal flora[31]. What these models suggest is that defining T cell phenotype based on a limited number of cytokines misses important changes in the overall T cell response. Complicated inter- and intracellular signalling mechanisms will dictate the total phenotype based on the expression or repression of dozens of cytokines of immune effector molecules. In the case of controlling the host response to luminal antigens, it appears that a cell that differs from the Th1 or Th2 cell, perhaps a Th3 cell, Tr1 cell or some hybrid, will be important.

This model suggests that the gastric immune responses, which appear to be directed towards a relatively homogeneous Th1 response, may lack sufficient control to prevent immune-mediated damage. For example, Th1 cells not only impart damage to the epithelium directly, but are capable of increasing the recruitment and activation of neutrophils, B cells, mast cells and macrophages that have already been shown to be capable of damaging gastric structure and function. Should this be correct, then the driving factor in many gastric diseases might be linked to environmental factors, genetic predisposition or other, as yet undefined, immune/inflammatory responses that attenuate the anti-inflammatory control conferred by Th3 or Tr1 cells.

References

1. Kelly CP, Becker S, Linevsky JK et al. Neutrophil recruitment in *Clostridium difficile* toxin A enteritis in the rabbit. J Clin Invest. 1994;93:1257–65.
2. Klimpel GR, Chopra AK, Langley KE et al. A role for stem cell factor and c-kit in the murine intestinal tract secretory response to cholera toxin. J Exp Med. 1995;182:1931–42.
3. Powrie F, Leach MW. Genetic and spontaneous models of inflammatory bowel disease in rodents: evidence for abnormalities in mucosal immune regulation. Ther Immunol. 1995; 2:115–23.
4. Kuhn R, Lohler J, Rennick D, Rajewsky K, Muller W. Interleukin-10-deficient mice develop chronic enterocolitis. Cell. 1993;75:263–74.
5. Mombaerts P, Mizoguchi E, Grusby MJ, Glimcher LH, Bhan AK, Tonegawa S. Spontaneous development of inflammatory bowel disease in T cell receptor mutant mice. Cell. 1993;75:275–82.
6. Strober W, Ehrhardt RO. Chronic intestinal inflammation: an unexpected outcome in cytokine or T cell receptor mutant mice. Cell. 1993;75:203–5.
7. Spencer SD, Di Marco F, Hooley J et al. The orphan receptor CRF2-4 is an essential subunit of the interleukin 10 receptor. J Exp Med. 1998;187:571–8.
8. Wirtz S, Finotto S, Kanzler S et al. Chronic intestinal inflammation in STAT-4 transgenic mice: characterization of disease and adoptive transfer by TNF-plus IFN-gamma-producing CD4+ T cells that respond to bacterial antigens. J Immunol. 1999;162:1884–8.
9. Falkow S. What is a pathogen? ASM News. 1997:359–65.
10. Leunk RD, Johnson PT, David BC, Kraft WG, Morgan DR. Cytotoxic activity in broth-culture filtrates of *Campylobacter pylori*. J Med Microbiol. 1988;36:93–9.
11. Atherton JC, Peek RM, Jr, Tham KT, Cover TL, Blaser MJ. Clinical and pathological importance of heterogeneity in vacA, the vacuolating cytotoxin gene of *Helicobacter pylori*. Gastroenterology. 1997;112:92–9.

12. Cover TL, Blaser MJ. Purification and characterization of the vacuolating toxin from *Helicobacter pylori*. J Biol Chem. 1992;267:10570–5.
13. Telford JL, Ghiara P, Dellorco M et al. Gene structure of the *Helicobacter pylori* cytotoxin and evidence of its key role in gastric disease. J Exp Med. 1994;179:1653–8.
14. Xiang Z, Censini S, Bayeli PF et al. Analysis of expression of CagA and VacA virulence factors in 43 strains of *Helicobacter pylori* reveals that clinical isolates can be divided into two major types and that CagA is not necessary for expression of the vacuolating toxin. Infect Immun. 1995;63:9463–98.
15. Blaser MJ, Perez-Perez GI, Kleanthous H et al. Infection with *Helicobacter pylori* strains possessing cagA is associated with an increased risk of developing adenocarcinoma of the stomach. Cancer Res. 1995;55:2111–15.
16. Hamlet A, Thoreson AC, Nilsson O, Svennerholm AM, Olbe L. Duodenal *Helicobacter pylori* infection differs in cagA genotype between asymptomatic subjects and patients with duodenal ulcers. Gastroenterology. 1999;116:259–68.
17. Yamaoka Y, Kodama T, Gutierrez O, Kim JG, Kashima K, Graham DY. Relationship between *Helicobacter pylori* iceA, cagA, and vacA status and clinical outcome: studies in four different countries. J Clin Microbiol. 1999;37:2274–9.
18. Van Doorn L-J, Figueiredo C, Sanna R et al. Clinical relevance of the *cagA*, *vacA* and *iceA* status of *Helicobacter pylori*. Gastroenterology. 1998;115:58–66.
19. Covacci A, Telford JL, Del Giudice G, Parsonnet J, Rappuoli R. *Helicobacter pylori* virulence and genetic geography. Science. 1999;284:1328–33.
20. Graham DY. *Helicobacter pylori* infection in the pathogenesis of duodenal ulcer and gastric cancer: a model. Gastroenterology. 1997;113:1983–91.
21. Ernst PB Michetti P, Smith PD. The Immunobiology of *Helicobacter pylori*. From Pathogenesis to Prevention. Philadelphia: Lippencott-Raven; 1997.
22. Wirth HP, Yang M, Peek RM, Jr, Tham KT, Blaser MJ. *Helicobacter pylori* Lewis expression is related to the host Lewis phenotype. Gastroenterology. 1997;113:1091–8.
23. Ridgway WM, Weiner HL, Fathman CG. Regulation of autoimmune response. Curr Opin Immunol. 1994;6:946–55.
24. Peek RM, Jr, Miller GS, Tham KT et al. Heightened inflammatory response and cytokine expression in vivo to cagA+ *Helicobacter pylori* strains. Lab Invest. 1995;73:760–70.
25. Yamaoka Y, Kita M, Sawai N, Imanishi J. *Helicobacter pylori* cagA gene and expression of cytokine messenger RNA in gastric mucosa. Gastroenterology. 1996;110:1744–52.
26. Yamaoka Y, Kita M, Kodama T, Sawai N, Kashima K, Imanishi J. Induction of various cytokines and development of severe mucosal inflammation by cagA gene positive *Helicobacter pylori* strains. Gut. 1997;41:442–51.
27. Xu-Amano BJ, Kiyono H, Jackson RJ et al. Helper T cell subsets for immunoglobulin A responses: oral immunization with tetanus toxoid and cholera toxin as adjuvant selectively induces Th2 cells in mucosa associated tissues. J Exp Med. 1993;178:1309–20.
28. Kelso A. Th1 and Th2 subsets: paradigms lost? Immunol Today. 1995;16:374–9.
29. Inobe J, Slavin AJ, Komagata Y, Chen Y, Liu L, Weiner HL. IL-4 is a differentiation factor for transforming growth factor-beta secreting Th3 cells and oral administration of IL-4 enhances oral tolerance in experimental allergic encephalomyelitis. Eur J Immunol. 1998;28:2780–90.
30. Fukaura H, Kent SC, Pietrusewicz MJ, Khoury SJ, Weiner HL, Hafler DA. Induction of circulating myelin basic protein and proteolipid protein-specific transforming growth factor-beta1-secreting Th3 T cells by oral administration of myelin in multiple sclerosis patients. J Clin Invest. 1996;98:70–7.
31. Groux H, O'Garra A, Bigler M et al. A CD4+ T-cell subset inhibits antigen-specific T-cell responses and prevents colitis. Nature. 1997;389:737–42.
32. Rath HC, Herfarth HH, Ikeda JS et al. Normal luminal bacteria, especially *Bacteroides* species, mediate chronic colitis, gastritis and arthritis in HLS-B27/human beta2 microglobulin transgenic rats. J Clin Invest. 1996;98:945–53.
33. Strober W. Animal models of inflammatory bowel disease – an overview. Dig Dis Sci. 1985;30:3–10S.
34. Ernst PB, Gold B. The disease spectrum of *H. pylori*: the immunopathogenesis of gastroduodenal ulcer and gastric cancer. Annu Rev Microbiol. 2000. (In press).

Section VI
Helicobactor pylori and Gastritis

23
Helicobacter pylori gastritis – a global view

Y. LIU, C. I. J. PONSIOEN, G. J. WAVERLING, S.-D. XIAO, G. N. J. TYTGAT and F. J. W. TEN KATE

INTRODUCTION

Helicobacter pylori infection is considered the leading cause of gastric mucosal inflammation. Chronic inflammation ultimately leads in some individuals to atrophic changes and intestinal metaplasia[1-3]. The latter condition may predispose to gastric malignancy[4-9]. The processes that govern the development of atrophy and intestinal metaplasia are complex. Duration of chronic active inflammation together with environmental factors may be of major importance in explaining differences in speed of developments between various geographical areas.

Gastric cancer is the most ominous outcome of *H. pylori* infection. Many experts feel that population screening for *H. pylori* infection should be considered if efficacious, *H. pylori*-specific, well tolerated and safe antimicrobial therapy became available. The optimal timing for such theoretical population screening would obviously depend on the onset and speed of worsening of gastric inflammation, atrophy, intestinal metaplasia and dysplasia. Many investigators have studied gastric mucosal morphology as a function of age. However, comparing the results of those studies turns out to be hazardous, if not impossible, because of lack of uniform definitions and criteria for grading gastric atrophy or intestinal metaplasia.

A systematic study of gastric biopsies in *H. pylori*-infected individuals using the latest Houston modification[10] of the Sydney classification system[11] by the same pathologists has not yet been carried out. The aim of this study was therefore to compare gastric mucosa in various age cohorts of *H. pylori*-infected dyspeptic individuals from several geographical areas in the world using a standardized grading system, in order to compare the degrees of atrophy and intestinal metaplasia according to age. In addition, the prevalence of atrophy and intestinal metaplasia was compared to respective gastric cancer incidence.

Table 1. *H. pylori* gastritis – study population

Patient groups	No. of patients	Mean age (years)	Sex ratio M : F
Finland (FI)	104	53 ± 10	0.8 : 1
Netherlands (NL)	269	50 ± 13	1.4 : 1
Guangzhou (GU)	104	42 ± 13	2.8 : 1
New Orleans (NO)	50	45 ± 11	0.5 : 1
Colombia (CA)	35	50 ± 9	0.7 : 1
Shanghai (SH)	342	43 ± 11	1.2 : 1
Thailand (TH)	250	48 ± 15	1 : 1
Germany (GE)	250	54 ± 18	0.9 : 1
Xi-an (XI)	176	50 ± 11	1.6 : 1
Portugal (PO)	221	49 ± 17	1 : 1
Japan (JP)	242	52 ± 13	1.9 : 1

MATERIALS AND METHODS

Study populations

Sequential gastric biopsies were obtained from different geographical areas as summarized in Table 1. Exclusion criteria were age less than 18 or greater than 75 years, history of gastrectomy, active upper gastrointestinal bleeding or perforation and severe gastro-oesophageal reflux disease.

Study protocol

At least two biopsy specimens were taken from the antrum within 2–3 cm from the pylorus in *H. pylori*-positive individuals. Two corpus biopsies were also taken of the lesser and greater curve, some 10 cm from the cardia, except in the Netherlands and Xi-an.

Patients were divided into five different age categories: less than 30 years; between 30 and 40 years; between 40 and 50 years; between 50 and 60 years; over 60 years.

HISTOPATHOLOGICAL ASSESSMENT

A detailed histopathological classification was used in order to allow registration of minor variations in atrophy and intestinal metaplasia. Therefore the categories 'mild', 'moderate' and 'severe' as used in the updated Sydney system were each subdivided into two further subcategories to allow some fine-tuning[12]; therefore a 1–6 scale was applied: 1–2 (mild), 3–4 (moderate), 5–6 (severe), corresponding to the updated Sydney system[13].

Atrophy was defined as the loss of specialized gastric glandular tissue, with or without replacement by intestinal metaplasia. Grade 1 equals focally few gastric glands lost or replaced by intestinal-type epithelium; grade 2 equals small areas of gastric glands disappearing or replaced by intestinal-type epithelium; 3 corresponds to 25% of gastric glands lost or replaced by intestinal-type epithelium, 4 corresponds to 25–50% of gastric glands lost or replaced by intestinal epithelium; 5 corresponds to more than 50% of gastric glands lost or replaced by intestinal epithelium; 6 is diagnosed when only a few areas of gastric glands are remaining.

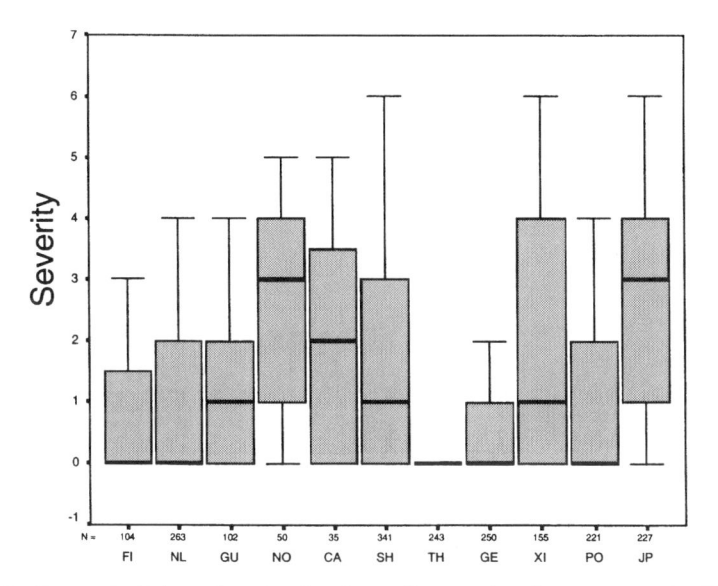

Figure 1. Box and whiskers plots showing the median severity of antrum atrophy. The box extends from the 25th percentile to the 75th percentile with a horizontal line at the median (50th percentile). Whiskers extend down the smallest value and up to the largest.

Intestinal metaplasia was diagnosed when gastric foveolar and glandular epithelium was focally or diffusely replaced by intestinal-type epithelium: grade 1 equals only one focus (one crypt) replaced in intestinal-type epithelium; 2 equals one focal area (one to four crypts) (in one of the biopsies); 3 corresponds to the presence of two separate foci; 4 indicates multiple foci in at least one of the biopsies; 5 corresponds to more than 50% of gastric epithelium diffusely replaced by intestinal metaplasia; 6 is diagnosed when only a few small areas of gastric epithelium, not replaced by intestinal metaplasia, are left.

Because gastric cancer incidence rates may differ markedly between males and females, incidence rates were calculated for populations mimicking the male/female ratios of the respective gastritis study population.

RESULTS

A total of 1991 *H. pylori*-infected subjects, who underwent gastroscopy for upper gastrointestinal complaints, and for whom all data were complete, were analysed.

The overall results of antrum biopsies expressed as 'box and whiskers' plots, showing the 75th percentile and range, both for degrees of atrophy and intestinal metaplasia, are summarized in Figures 1 and 2.

The highest scores for antrum atrophy (Figure 1) were found in Japan (JP) and among New Orleans blacks (NO), and slightly lower scores in Colombia (CA). Lower scores were seen in China, Guangzhou (GU), Shanghai (SH) and Xi-an (XI). The lowest scores were found in Europe:

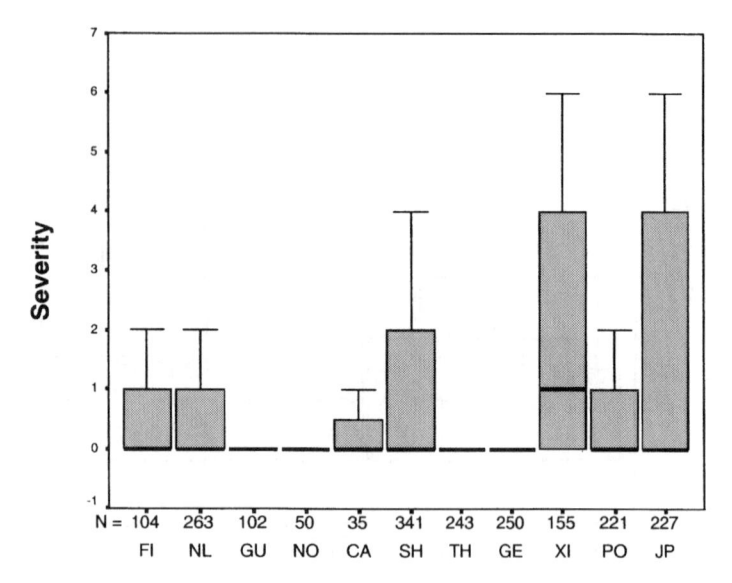

Figure 2. Box and whiskers plot showing the severity of antrum intestinal metaplasia.

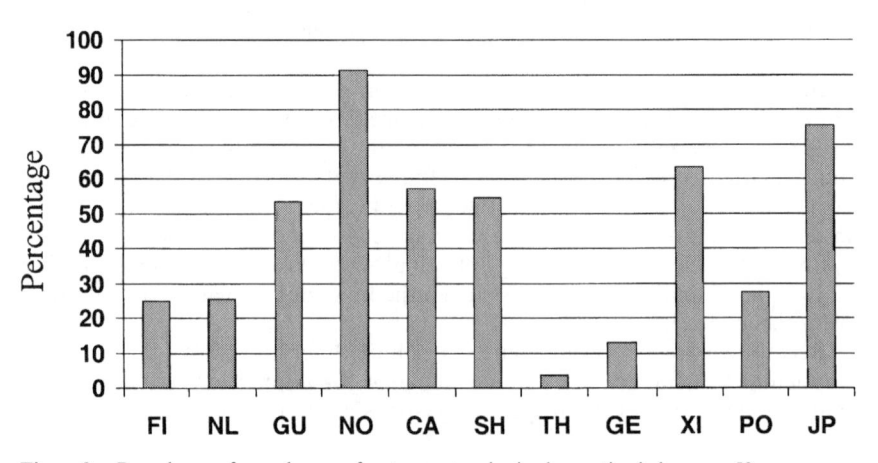

Figure 3. Prevalence of any degree of antrum atrophy in dyspeptics below age 50 years.

Finland (FI), Netherlands (NL), Germany (GE), Portugal (PO) and especially in Thailand (TH). Degrees of atrophy in corpus biopsies were low throughout in all countries and are not shown.

The severity of the intestinal metaplasia scores in the antrum was in general low except for Xi-an, Japan and Shanghai (Figure 2). Intestinal metaplasia in corpus biopsies was negligible throughout.

The overall prevalence of atrophy and intestinal metaplasia in individuals less than 50 years of age is summarized in Figures 3 and 4. The prevalence of antrum atrophy and intestinal metaplasia is compared to gastric cancer incidence in Tables 2 and 3. For antrum atrophy the correlation was 0.527

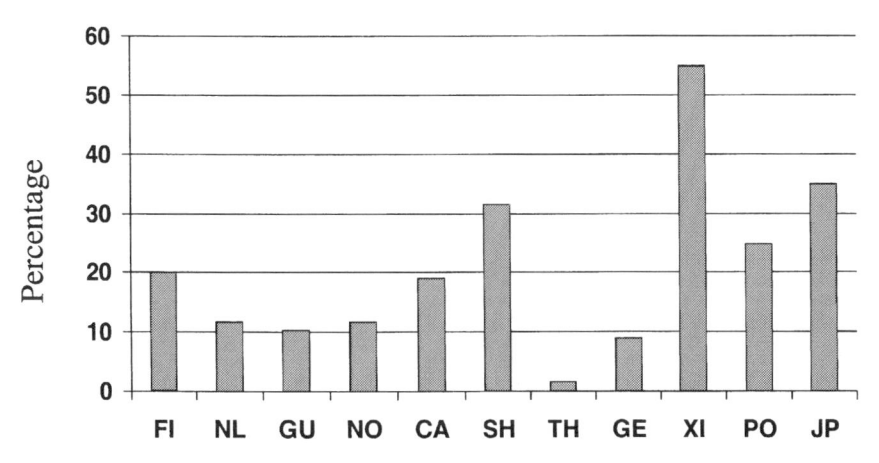

Figure 4. Prevalence of any degree of antrum intestinal metaplasia in dyspeptics below age 50 years.

Table 2. Antrum atrophy (any degree)

	<30 (%)	31–40 (%)	41–50 (%)	51–60 (%)	>60 (%)	Overall (%)	Gastric cancer*
FI		27	21	46	70	44	14
NL	23	23	35	65	60	42	15
GU	48	53	60	60	68	60	32
NO	100	87	93	69	100	86	7
CA	0	71	50	100	80	71	26
SH	45	55	57	66	59	56	38
TH	6	2	4	21	22	12	4
GE	7	8	21	34	44	29	15
XI	60	58	68	57	79	65	55
PO	15	29	38	62	42	38	24
JP	50	71	80	80	90	80	91

*Gastric cancer incidence per 100 000.

($p = 0.096$). For antrum intestinal metaplasia the correlation was 0.708 ($p = 0.015$). The degree of antrum intestinal metaplasia correlated significantly with atrophy (Table 4).

DISCUSSION

Analysis of random biopsies, particularly from the antrum from consecutive *H. pylori*-infected dyspeptic patients with/without ulcer diathesis, reveals substantial geographical differences in age-related degree of atrophy and intestinal metaplasia. The atrophic/metaplastic changes were largely limited to the antrum and much less pronounced in corpus biopsies. The overall prevalence of atrophy and intestinal metaplasia mirrored the respective incidence of gastric cancer. This finding strengthens the hypothesis that chronic *H. pylori*-associated inflammation is a key factor in gastric carcino-

Table 3. Antrum intestinal metaplasia (any degree)

	<30 (%)	31–40 (%)	41–50 (%)	51–60 (%)	>60 (%)	Overall (%)	Gastric cancer*
FI		18	18	27	59	33	14
NL	18	6	19	43	41	26	15
GU	10	8	15	10	20	12	32
NO	0	13	14	15	33	14	7
CA	0	29	14	44	20	26	26
SH	19	32	33	39	33	32	38
TH	0	2	2	13	10	6	4
GE	0	3	22	29	33	22	15
XI	60	42	61	48	66	55	55
PO	13	26	35	57	37	34	24
JP	10	29	40	47	58	44	91

*Gastric cancer incidence per 100 000.

Table 4.

	Atrophy med (interquartile range)	Intestinal metaplasia med (interquartile range)	Correlation coefficient* (Spearman's r)	Regression coefficient[†] (10 years)$^{-1}$
FI	0 (0–1)	0 (0–1)	0.834	0.34
NL	0 (0–2)	0 (0–1)	0.777	0.44
GU	1 (0–2)	0 (0–0)	0.396	0.11
NO	3 (1–4)	0 (0–0)	0.237	0.09
CA	2 (0–4)	0 (0–1)	0.486	0.70
SH	1 (0–3)	0 (0–2)	0.705	0.14
TH	0 (0–0)	0 (0–0)	0.692	0.14
GE	0 (0–1)	0 (0–0)	0.870	0.20
XI	1 (0–4)	1 (0–4)	0.947	0.23
PO	0 (0–2)	0 (0–1)	0.943	0.17
JP	3 (1–4)	0 (0–4)	0.801	0.39

*Spearman's r rank correlation between antrum score for atrophy and for intestinal metaplasia; all values except NO significant.
[†]Increase in antrum atrophy score per 10 years age increase.

genesis[13–15]. The observation that atrophy and intestinal metaplasia appeared at younger ages in populations at high risk for gastric cancer than in populations at low risk supports the results of many other studies. Particularly striking was the very low prevalence of atrophy and intestinal metaplasia in Thailand, corresponding to a very low gastric cancer incidence.

Our study has strengths and weaknesses. Strengths of the study relate to the blind character of the biopsy analysis by the same histopathologists, well trained in the analysis of gastric mucosal biopsies and with an acceptable internal reproducibility. All biopsies were essentially obtained within the same time frame. All biopsies had pathological proof of *H. pylori* infection.

Weaknesses of the study relate to the lack of characterization of the infecting organisms (Cag$^-$, Vac$^-$, IceA$^-$ status unknown); lack of information on percentage with ulcer diathesis; smoking, etc.; lack of further characterization of the type of intestinal metaplasia; lack of correlation of gastric mucosal status with gastric secretory function (pepsinogens, gastrins etc.); and the occasional low number of biopsies in certain age categories. Particularly the cytotoxin-associated gene A (*cag*A) seems highly associated with atrophic gastritis[16–18] and gastric adenocarcinoma[19], at least in certain but not all countries.

Despite these shortcomings our study clearly shows that there are major geographical differences in the overall prevalence of atrophy and intestinal metaplasia. Duration of chronic active inflammation is obviously an important element, and a high infection rate very early in life may largely explain the geographical differences in age-related atrophy and metaplasia. In addition environmental factors may also influence the velocity of development of atrophy and metaplasia. Hu *et al.*[21] came to a similar conclusion when they compared the degree of gastric mucosal atrophy in Lanzhou (high gastric cancer incidence) versus Guangzhou (low gastric cancer incidence). We do not know whether those putative environmental factors require the presence of *H. pylori*, or what those environmental factors are (lack of antioxidants in food? smoking? alimentary nitrosamines?).

We were rather surprised to find that atrophy and metaplasia were largely restricted to the antrum and almost absent from the corpus biopsies, even in countries with high gastric cancer prevalence. We cannot rule out that this is caused by the selection of patients with dyspeptic symptoms or with ulcer diathesis, where inflammation is known to be largely antrum-predominant. Caution should be taken not to extrapolate our findings to the general non-symptomatic population in the various geographical areas. Yet in dyspeptics, atrophy and intestinal metaplasia are more common in the antrum and angular area[20].

Cost calculations have been made in the literature with respect to population screening and antimicrobial therapy[22]. In those studies, screening is projected to start at age 50. It would appear from our study that a substantial proportion of the (dyspeptic) population already has variable degrees of atrophy and intestinal metaplasia, especially in countries with high gastric cancer incidence. If ever population screening became feasible, determination of the most appropriate starting age would need to be determined, and may well be earlier, especially in areas with high gastric cancer risk, in order not to pass the 'point of no return' in the inflammation–atrophy–metaplasia–dysplasia cascade.

References

1. Correa P, Munoz N, Cuello C et al. The role of *Campylobacter pylori* in gastroduodenal disease. In: Fenoglio Preiser C, editor. Progression in Surgical Pathology. Philadelphia: Field & Wood; 1989:191–210.
2. Rugge M, DiMario F, Cassaro M et al. Pathology of the gastric antrum and body associated with *Helicobacter pylori* infection in non-ulcerous patients: is the bacterium a promoter of intestinal metaplasia? Histopathology. 1993;22:9–15.
3. Kuipers EJ, Thijs JC, Festen HPM. The prevalence of *Helicobacter pylori* infection in peptic ulcer disease. Aliment Pharmacol Ther/. 1995;9:59–70.
4. Forman D. The prevalence of *Helicobacter pylori* infection in gastric cancer. Aliment Pharmacol Ther. 1995;9:71–6.

5. EUROGAST Study Group. An international association between *Helicobacter pylori* infection and gastric cancer. Lancet. 1993;341:1359–62.
6. Correa P. *Helicobacter pylori* and gastric carcinogenesis. Am J Surg Pathol. 1995;19 (Suppl. 1):S34–7.
7. Correa P. Human gastric carcinogenesis: a multistep and multifactoral process – first American Cancer Society Award Lecture on Cancer Epidemiology and prevention. Cancer Res. 1992;52:6735–40.
8. Varis K, Taylor PR, Sipponen P et al. Gastric cancer and premalignant lesions in atrophic gastritis: a controlled trial on the effect of supplementation with alpha-tocopherol and beta-carotene. Helsinki Gastritis Study Group. Scand J Gastroenterol. 1998;33:294–300.
9. Parsonnet J, Friedman GD, Vandersteen DP et al. *Helicobacter pylori* infection and the risk of gastric carcinoma. N Engl J Med. 1991;325:1127–31.
10. Dixon MF, Genta RM, Yardley JH et al. Classification and grading of gastritis, the updated Sydney system. Am J Surg Pathol. 1996;20:1161–81.
11. Misiewicz JJ, Tytgat GNJ, Goodwin CS. The Sydney System: a new classification of gastritis. J Hepatol Gastroenterol. 1991;6:209–22.
12. Chen X-Y, Van der Hulst RWM, Bruno MJ et al. Interobserver variation in the histopathological scoring of *Helicobacter pylori* related gastritis. J Clin Pathol. 1999;52:612–15.
13. Forman D. *Helicobacter pylori* infection and cancer. Br Med Bull. 1998;54:71–8.
14. Correa P, Haenszel W, Cuella C et al. Gastric precancerous process in a high risk population: cross-sectional studies. Cancer Res. 1990;50:4731–6.
15. Hansson LE, Engstrand L, Nyrén O et al. *Helicobacter pylori* infection: independent risk indicator of gastric adenocarcinoma. Gastroenterology. 1993;105:1098–103.
16. Shimoyama T, Fukuda S, Tanaka M, Mikami T, Saito Y, Munakata A. High prevalence of the *CagA*-positive *Helicobacter pylori* strains in Japanese asymptomatic patients and gastric cancer patients. Scand J Gastroenterol. 1997;32:465–8.
17. Matsukura N, Onda M, Kato S et al. Cytotoxin genes of *Helicobacter pylori* in chronic gastritis, gastroduodenal ulcer and gastric cancer: an age and gender matched case–control study. Jpn J Cancer Res. 1997;88:532–6.
18. Kuipers EJ, Péréz-Péréz GI, Meuwissen SGM, Blaser MJ. *Helicobacter pylori* and atrophic gastritis: importance of the *cagA* status. J Natl Cancer Inst. 1995;73:742–5.
19. Blaser MJ, Pérez-Pérez GI, Kleanthous H et al. Infection with *Helicobacter pylori* strains possessing *cagA* is associated with an increased risk of developing adenocarcinoma of the stomach. Cancer Res. 1995;55:2111–5.
20. Xia HH-X, Kalantar JS, Talley, NJ et al. Antral-type mucosa in the gastric incisura, body, and fundus (antralization): a link between *Helicobacter pylori* infection and intestinal metaplasia? Am J Gastroenterol. 2000;95:114–21.
21. Hu PJ, Li YY, Lin HL et al. Gastric atrophy and regional variation in upper gastrointestinal disease. Am J Gastroenterol. 1995;90:1102–6.
22. Harris RA, Owens DK, Witherell H, Parsonnet J. *Helicobacter pylori* and gastric cancer: what are the benefits of screening only for the CagA phenotype of *H. pylori*. Helicobacter. 1999;4:69–76.

24
Unusual forms of gastric inflammation and their relationship to *Helicobacter pylori* infection

M. F. DIXON

INTRODUCTION

The usual form of inflammation seen in gastric biopsies is that of an active chronic gastritis associated with *Helicobacter pylori* infection. This can be diffuse (a pangastritis) or be more dominant in the antrum or corpus of the stomach. Occasionally, a mild diffuse inactive chronic gastritis without detectable helicobacters is encountered. This form could follow *H. pylori* infection which has been eradicated, either therapeutically or 'spontaneously', or have a totally different aetiology. A focal pattern of chronic inflammation can be a microscopic feature of Crohn's disease[1]. Unusual forms of *H. pylori* infection are also recognized. For instance, in children, infection frequently produces antral lymphoid hyperplasia giving rise to endoscopic nodularity. Likewise 'giant fold' gastritis is another gross pattern of response to *H. pylori* infection that can mimic Ménétrier's disease[2].

In considering 'unusual' forms of gastritis, there are of course more or less specific inflammatory reactions caused by infections such as cytomegalovirus and histoplasmosis, but these are not relevant to a consideration of inflammation which may be related to *H. pylori* infection. Furthermore, the unusual corpus-predominant form of gastritis attributed to autoimmunity and its relation to *H. pylori* are discussed elsewhere in this book. Thus, the following account will be restricted to a group of idiopathic forms of gastric inflammation which are identified only by their predominant histological appearance, namely *lymphocytic, collagenous, granulomatous* and *eosinophilic* gastritis.

LYMPHOCYTIC GASTRITIS

Lymphocytic gastritis is characterized by an increase in intraepithelial lymphocytes (IELs) in surface and foveolar epithelium together with a variable

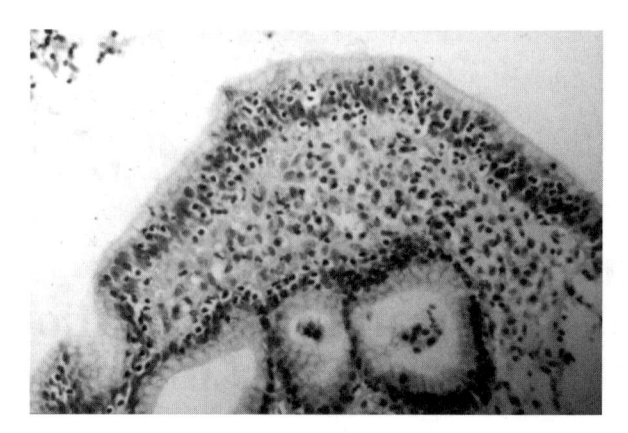

Figure 1. Lymphocytic gastritis. The surface and foveolar epithelium is infiltrated by large numbers of mature small lymphocytes. Many are surrounded by a clear 'halo' characteristic of intraepithelial lymphocytes and on immunostaining the cells are of CD8+ T-cell phenotype.

increase in chronic inflammatory cells in the lamina propria of the gastric mucosa[3,4] (Figure 1). Although the degree of intraepithelial lymphocytosis shows patchy variation, the disorder usually affects the whole stomach. The number of intraepithelial lymphocytes may be increased by 10–15 times that found in *H. pylori* chronic gastritis, and counts above 25 IELs per 100 epithelial cells are considered to be diagnostic. On immunostaining these are exclusively of T cell type, and are of the CD8+ cytotoxic/suppressor phenotype. In the lamina propria CD4+ T lymphocytes are the predominant cell type along with plasma cells, but their numbers are extremely variable[5]. Lymphocytic gastritis is found in 0.83–2.5% of unselected patients undergoing upper gastrointestinal endoscopy[6] and 4.5% of those with histological chronic gastritis[5]. This type of gastritis may be associated with a normal-looking gastric mucosa at endoscopy. However, the classical endoscopic appearances comprise prominent rugal folds bearing small nodular elevations surmounted by small grey-white erosions with hyperaemic margins, maximal in the corpus and fundus, a picture that has been termed 'varioliform' gastritis[4].

An increased density of IELs can also be found in the gastric mucosa of patients with coeliac disease and in a proportion their numbers are sufficient to diagnose lymphocytic gastritis[7–10]. This coeliac disease-associated form of lymphocytic gastritis is usually not associated with the endoscopic picture of varioliform gastritis. Indeed the pattern of gastritis found associated with duodenal villous atrophy is often antral-predominant or a pangastritis in contrast with the classical corpus-predominant pattern of non-coeliac (*isolated*) lymphocytic gastritis[11]. The classical pattern is rarely, if ever, associated with coeliac disease.

The aetiology of lymphocytic gastritis is not known but it has been suggested that it represents an idiosyncratic immune response to *H. pylori*[5,12]. We have shown using multiple tests that many cases of isolated lymphocytic gastritis are associated with *H. pylori* infection, and that eradication of infection brings about a significant reduction in gastric intraepithelial lymphocytic infiltration, corpus inflammation and dyspeptic symptoms[13]. Curiously, in most of these patients, *H. pylori* infection was diagnosed on the basis of positive serology alone, with histology and the carbon-13 urea breath test being negative. We have speculated that in such cases the organism may be present in small numbers and possibly exist in a different (coccoid) form, and that isolated lymphocytic gastritis represents a specific immune response to the infection. This response may be genetically determined, as the majority of these patients with isolated lymphocytic gastritis possess the coeliac-associated HLA DQB1 *0201 allele (unpublished observations).

Lymphocytic gastritis in non-coeliac patients may still be a subtle form of gluten sensitivity. A previous study from our unit demonstrated abnormal intestinal permeability and high duodenal IEL counts in non-coeliac patients with lymphocytic gastritis[14]. It is now recognized that there is a spectrum of gluten-induced intestinal changes, ranging from the classic 'coeliac' lesion of subtotal villous atrophy to more subtle manifestations, such as a high duodenal IEL count in the absence of villous atrophy[15]. Thus, coeliac disease represents a primary small intestinal disorder which can be accompanied by intraepithelial lymphocytosis in the stomach, while lymphocytic gastritis is primarily a gastric disorder accompanied in many cases by intraepithelial lymphocytosis and functional disturbances in the small intestine.

The role of *H. pylori* infection could be to alter the reactivity of the gastric mucosa to foreign antigens in genetically predisposed individuals. Infection and inflammation bring about the acquisition of HLA-DR sites on the gastric epithelium and the cells become capable of antigen presentation. Thus, the initial *H. pylori* gastritis may be followed by suppression or clearance of infection and the acquired capacity of the gastric mucosa to present antigenic material, possibly related to gluten, to which they are peculiarly sensitized. Such an explanation could underlie the link between lymphocytic gastritis and coeliac disease, and explain why both *H. pylori* eradication and gluten withdrawal can achieve a reduction in IELs in gastric mucosa.

COLLAGENOUS GASTRITIS

The entity of collagenous gastritis appears to have been first described in two case reports published in 1989 by Colletti and Trainer[16], and by Borchard and Niedorau[17]. The former reported the finding of a thick band of collagen immediately beneath the surface epithelium in corpus biopsies from a 15-year-old girl who presented with an acute haematemesis and had a history of intermittent epigastric pain. A second paediatric case characterized by severe anaemia was added by Cote *et al*[18]. In both cases histology of the duodenum and colon was normal. However, subsequent reports have documented the coexistence of collagenous gastritis with either lymphocytic colitis[19] or collagenous colitis. In view of the emerging relationship between lymphocytic and collagenous *colitis*,[20] the possibility that collagenous and lymphocytic *gastritis* are linked in some way would provide a fascinating

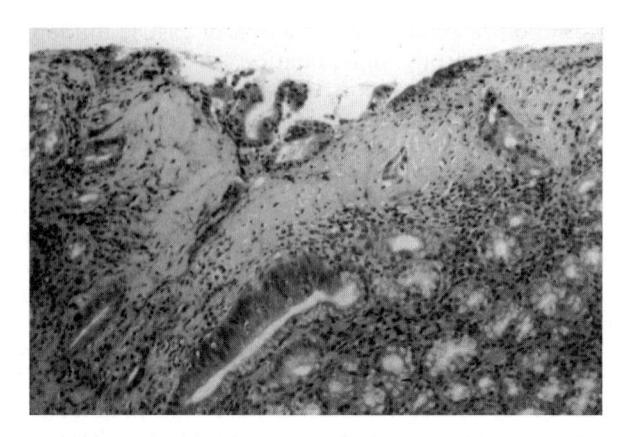

Figure 2. Collagenous gastritis. The gastric mucosa is inflamed and contains a band of hyaline collagen beneath the surface epithelium. The patient presented 3 months before with a markedly active *H. pylori* gastritis, but no eradication therapy was given.

parallel. I have seen a case of collagenous gastritis which followed *H. pylori* gastritis (Figure 2), but as yet this sequence of events has not been reported in the literature. However, it is unlikely to be unique.

GRANULOMATOUS GASTRITIS

Granulomas are circumscribed collections of altered macrophages which have lost much of their phagocytic ability but have an active secretory role. These specialized macrophages, termed epithelioid cells, are usually associated with the finding of multinucleate giant cells formed by cell fusion. Granulomas may be present in the gastric mucosa in Crohn's disease, in sarcoidosis (Figure 3), a variety of infectious diseases, and as a reaction to endogenous and foreign materials. In rare instances, granulomatous gastritis can be part of an immune-mediated vasculitis syndrome[21] or Wegener's disease[22] or accompany a gastric lymphoma[23] or adenocarcinoma[24]. Only after excluding such causes should the diagnosis of *isolated* granulomatous gastritis be made[25].

Symptomatic involvement of the stomach by Crohn's disease, frequently accompanied by contiguous duodenal disease, has been found in 1–2% of patients[26]. However, asymptomatic involvement is such more common and has been found in over 40% of antral biopsies[27]. The finding of granulomas is dependent upon sampling and, where multiple biopsies have been examined, epithelioid granulomas can be found in up to 50%[28]. These are often small, multiple and situated in the deep lamina propria close to the muscularis mucosae[29].

Involvement of the gastrointestinal tract in sarcoidosis is rare, although granulomas were identified in 10% of gastric biopsies from patients with other evidence of systemic sarcoid[30,31].

As regards isolated granulomatous gastritis, a majority of the reported cases show thickening and narrowing of the pre-pyloric region and patients

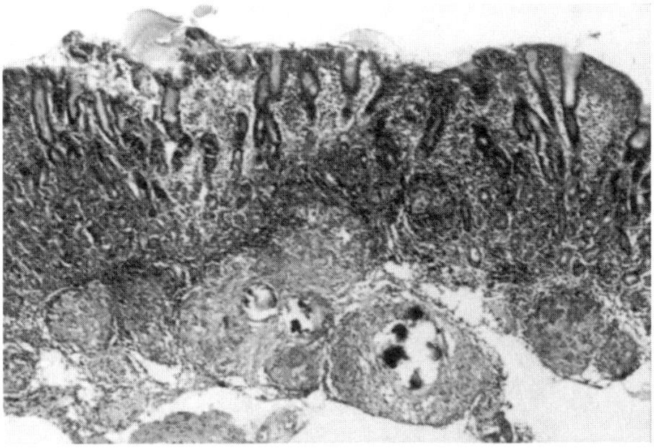

Figure 3. Granulomatous gastritis. The deep mucosa is occupied by large, well-circumscribed granulomas, several of which contain calcified material, so-called conchoidal bodies. The patient had a lung biopsy which confirmed the clinical diagnosis of sarcoidosis 11 years prior to gastric biopsy for dyspeptic symptoms.

have presented with obstructive symptoms[32,33]. In about a third of cases there is a coexistent peptic ulcer[25], but examination of resection specimens has shown that the granulomas are not intimately related to these[34]. The presence of peptic ulceration brings into question the role of *H. pylori* in such cases. Most cases of isolated granulomatous gastritis are *H. pylori*-positive[29], but so are many cases of *specific* granulomatous gastritis. However, granulomas could result from an atypical response to *H. pylori* antigens in the lamina propria. Granulomas were found in 1.1% of cases of *H. pylori* gastritis by Dhillon and Sawyerr[35]. The presence of stainable organisms within the granulomas led the authors to conclude that this infection should be added to the causes of a granulomatous response in the gastric mucosa, but the finding of intramucosal organisms is highly controversial. These observations need to be corroborated using more specific methods of identification, for example *in-situ* hybridization or *in-situ* polymerase chain reaction. The appropriateness of the term *isolated* granulomatous gastritis has already been challenged[36]. If a role for *H. pylori* infection is eventually confirmed, the concept of an isolated or idiopathic form will no doubt disappear.

EOSINOPHILIC GASTRITIS

Eosinophilic gastritis is a rare condition which is thought to be one manifestation of a generalized involvement of the alimentary tract by an allergic reaction – eosinophilic gastroenteritis. The diagnosis should be made with great caution. It is not sufficient to see conspicuous numbers of eosinophils; eosinophils have to be the dominant cell type with little or no increase in other inflammatory cell types. A marked increase in eosinophils can be seen in some cases of Crohn's disease, chronic granulomatous disease of childhood[33], parasitic diseases[37], and accompanying some peptic ulcers and carci-

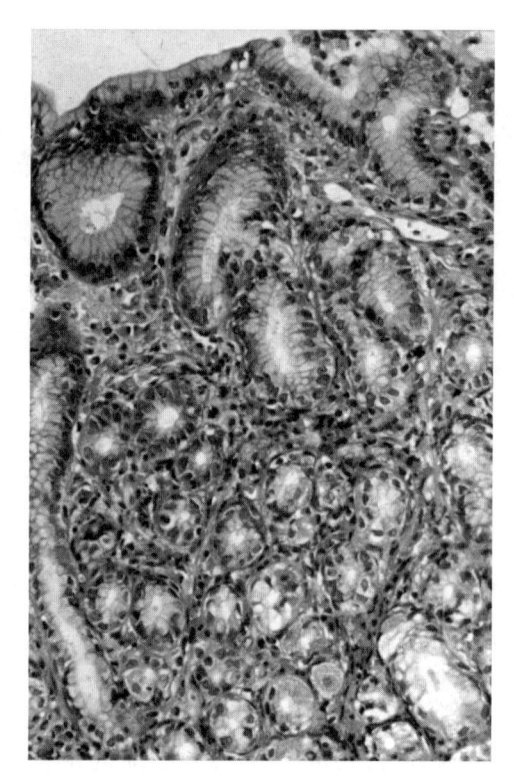

Figure 4. Eosinophilic gastritis. The lamina propria of this antral biopsy contains a dense infiltrate of eosinophil polymorphs. The patient presented with dysphagia and had eosinophilic oesophagitis. She was a long-standing asthmatic and had a raised peripheral blood eosnophil count. She responded rapidly to corticosteroid treatment.

nomas. Eosinophilic gastritis can be diagnosed with greater confidence when there is a history of allergic disease such as asthma (Figure 4), food intolerance and atopic eczema (70% of cases), and there is a peripheral blood eosinophila (40%)[38]. The stomach is the commonest site and eosinophilic infiltration is maximal in the antrum[39], but the oesophagus and small intestine are also frequently involved. However, the diffuse mucosal form of the disease is but one category. A second form primarily affects the muscle layer, while a third involves the subserosa and peritoneum[40].

Mucosal eosinophilic gastroenteritis is the commonest type, accounting for about 65% of the reported cases. The patients present with bleeding and anaemia, malabsorption or a protein-losing state. Gastroscopy reveals reddening of the mucosa with scattered erosions[41], and biopsy reveals intense infiltration of the lamina propria by eosinophils. Muscle layer or 'mural' involvement leads to thickening and deformity of the antrum with narrowing of the pylorus and diminished peristalsis[42], an appearance indistinguishable from infiltrating carcinoma. It may also present as a giant gastric ulcer, which may be refractory to acid suppressive treatment and thus be mistaken for a gastric cancer[43]. Predominantly serosal eosinophilic gastroenteritis gives rise to ascites.

There is no evidence (as yet) to support a role for *H. pylori* in eosinophilic gastroenteritis.

References

1. Oberhuber G, Püspök A, Oesterreicher C et al. Focally enhanced gastritis: a frequent type of gastritis in patients with Crohn's disease. Gastroenterology. 1997;112:698–706.
2. Stolte M, Bätz Ch, Eidt S. Giant fold gastritis – a special form of *Helicobacter pylori* associated gastritis. Z Gastroenterol. 1993:31:289–93.
3. Haot J, Hamichi L, Wallez L, Mainguet P. Lymphocytic gastritis: a newly described entity: a retrospective endoscopic and histological study. Gut. 1988;29:1258–64.
4. Haot J, Jouret A, Willette M, Gossuin A, Mainguet P. Lymphocytic gastritis – prospective study of its relationship with varioliform gastritis. Gut. 1990;31:282–5.
5. Dixon MF, Wyatt JI, Burke DA, Rathbone BJ. Lymphocytic gastritis: relationship to *Campylobacter pylori* infection. J Pathol. 1988;154:125–32.
6. Jaskiewicz K, Price SK, Zak J, Lowrens HD. Lymphocytic gastritis in nonulcer dyspepsia. Dig Dis Sci. 1991;36:1079–83.
7. Wolber R, Owen D, DelBuono L, Appelman H, Freeman H. Lymphocytic gastritis in patients with celiac sprue or spruelike intestinal disease. Gastroenterology. 1990;98:310–15.
8. De Giacomo C, Gianatti A, Negrini R et al. Lymphocytic gastritis: a positive relationship with celiac disease. J Pediatr. 1994;124:57–62.
9. Alsaigh N, Odze R, Goldman H, Antonioli D, Ott MJ, Leichtner A. Gastric and oesophageal intraepithelial lymphocytes in pediatric celiac disease. Am J Surg Pathol. 1996; 20:865–70.
10. Feeley KM, Heneghan MA, Stevens FM, McCarthy CF. Lymphocytic gastritis and coeliac disease: evidence of a positive association. J Clin Pathol. 1998;51:207–10.
11. Hayat M, Arora DS, Wyatt JI, O'Mahony S, Dixon MF. The pattern of involvement of the gastric mucosa in lymphocytic gastritis is predictive of the presence of duodenal pathology. J Clin Pathol. 1999;52:815–19.
12. Niemela S, Karttunen T, Kerola T, Karttunen R. Ten year follow up study of lymphocytic gastritis: further evidence on *Helicobacter pylori* as a cause of lymphocytic gastritis and corpus gastritis. J Clin Pathol. 1995;48:1111–16.
13. Hayat M, Arora DS, Dixon MF, Clark B, O'Mahony S. Effects of *Helicobacter pylori* eradication on the natural history of lymphocytic gastritis. Gut. 1999;45:495–8.
14. Lynch DAF, Sobala GM, Dixon MF et al. Lymphocytic gastritis and associated small bowel disease: a diffuse lymphocytic gastroenteropathy? J Clin Pathol. 1995;48:939–45.
15. Ferguson A, Arranz E, O'Mahony S. Clinical and pathological spectrum of coeliac disease – active, silent, latent, potential. Gut. 1993;34:150–1.
16. Colletti RB, Trainer TD. Collagenous gastritis: a new entity. Gastroenterology. 1989;96:94A (abstract).
17. Borchard F, Niederau C. Kollagene gastroduodenitis. Dtsch Med Wschr. 1989,114.1345.
18. Cote JF, Hankard GF, Faure C et al. Collagenous gastritis revealed by severe anemia in a child. Hum Pathol. 1998;29:883–6.
19. Stolte M, Ritter M, Borchard F et al. Collagenous gastroduodenitis and collagenous colitis. Endoscopy. 1990;22:186–7.
20. Christ AD, Meier R, Bauerfeind P et al. Simultaneous occurrence of lymphocytic gastritis and lymphocytic colitis with transition to collagenous colitis. Schw Med Wochenschr. 1993;123:1487–90.
21. O'Donovan C, Murray J, Staunton H et al. Granulomatous gastritis: part of a vasculitic syndrome. Hum Pathol. 1991;22:1057–9.
22. Temmesfeld-Wollbrueck B, Heinrichs C, Szalay A, Seeger W. Granulomatous gastritis in Wegener's disease: differentiation from Crohn's disease supported by a positive test for antineutrophil antibodies. Gut. 1997;40:550–3.
23. Leach IH, Maclennan KA. Gastric lymphoma associated with mucosal and nodal granulomas: a new differential diagnosis in granulomatous gastritis. Histopathology. 1990;17:87–9.

24. Newton C, Nochomovitz L, Sackier JM. Gastric adenocarcinoma associated with isolated granulomatous gastritis. Ann Surg Oncol. 1998;5:407–10.
25. Fahimi HD, Deren JJ, Gottlieb LS, Zamcheck N. Isolated granulomatous gastritis: its relationship to disseminated sarcoidosis and regional entritis. Gastroenterology. 1963; 45:161–75.
26. Rutgeerts P, Onette E, Vantrappen G et al. Crohn's disease of the stomach and duodenum: a clinical study with emphasis on the value of endoscopy and endoscopic biopsies. Endoscopy. 1980;12:288–94.
27. Oberhuber G, Hirsch M, Stolte M. High incidence of upper gastrointestinal tract involvement in Crohn's disease. Virchows Arch. 1998;432:49–52.
28. Haggitt RC, Meissner WA. Crohn's disease of the upper gastrointestinal tract. Am J Clin Pathol. 1973;59:613–22.
29. Ectors NL, Dixon MF, Geboes KJ et al. Granulomatous gastritis: a morphological and diagnostic approach. Histopathology. 1993;23:55–61.
30. Palmer ED. Note on silent sarcoidosis of the gastric mucosa. J Lab Clin Med. 1958;52:231–4.
31. Moretti AM, Sallustio G, Attimonelli R et al. Gastric localization of sarcoidosis. Rec Progress Med. 1993;84:750–5.
32. Spinzi G, Meucci G, Radaelli F, Sangiovanni A, Terruzzi V, Minoli G. Granulomatous gastritis presenting as gastric outlet obstruction: a case report. Ital J Gastroenterol Hepatol. 1998;30:410–13.
33. Griscom NT, Kirkpatrick JA Jr, Girdany BR et al. Gastric antral narrowing in chronic granulomatous disease of childhood. Pediatrics. 1974;54:456–60.
34. Schinella RA, Ackert J. Isolated granulomatous disease of the stomach. Report of three cases presenting as incidental findings in gastrectomy specimens. Am J Gastroenterol. 1979;72:30–5.
35. Dhillon AP, Sawyerr A. Granulomatous gastritis associated with *Campylobacter pylori*. Acta Pathol Microbiol Immunol Scand. 1989;97:723–7.
36. Shapiro JL, Goldblum JR, Petras RE. A clinicopathologic study of 42 patients with granulomatous gastritis. Is there really an 'idiopathic' granulomatous gastritis? Am J Surg Pathol. 1996;20:462–70.
37. Watt IA, McLean NR, Girdwood RWA et al. Eosinophilic gastroenteritis associated with a larval anisakine nematode. Lancet. 1979;2:893–4.
38. Caldwell JH, Sharma HM, Hurtubise PE, Colwell DL. Eosinophilic gastroenteritis in extreme allergy. Immunopathological comparison with nonallergic gastrointestinal disease. Gastroenterology. 1979;77:560–4.
39. Goldman H, Proujansky R. Allergic proctitis and gastroenteritis in children. Clinical and mucosal biopsy features in 53 cases. Am J Surg Pathol. 1986;10:75–86.
40. Talley NJ, Shorter RG, Phillips SF et al. Eosinophilic gastroenteritis: a clinicopathological study of patients with disease of the mucosa, muscle layers and subserosal tissues. Gut. 1990;31:54–8.
41. Katz AJ, Goldman H, Grand RJ. Gastric mucosal biopsy in eosinophilic (allergic) gastroenteritis. Gastroenterology. 1977;73:705–9.
42. Navab F, Kleinman MS, Algazy K et al. Endoscopic diagnosis of eosinophilic gastritis. Gastrointest Endosc. 1972;19:67–9.
43. Scolapio JS, DeVault K, Wolfe JT. Eosinophilic gastroenteritis presenting as a giant gastric ulcer. Am J Gastroenterol. 1996;91:804–5.

25
Can atrophic gastritis be diagnosed in the presence of *Helicobacter pylori* infection?

R. M. GENTA

INTRODUCTION

No question involving atrophic gastritis can ignore the continuing saga of the consensus agreement or disagreement among pathologists on the recognition and assessment of the histological features that define atrophy. One would expect these apparently tedious debates to have taken their just toll on clinicians' interest. Yet gastroenterologists, whose understanding and management of gastric disorders relies heavily on their pathologists' opinions, continue to follow closely the atrophy debate and to give pathologists space in their journals.

Reports from pathologists' meetings on this subject have been notable for the low kappas (of the infamous κ statistics), dissent on terminology, and even dissent on the very existence of the entity that most – paradoxically, even those who deny its existence – call atrophy. However, after several years of efforts and formal and informal meetings among the members of an international group of gastric pathologists (the 'Atrophy Club'), some tangible progress has been made. The kappas have risen from the depths of discordance, agreements on a definition and on critical histopathological features that characterize atrophy have been reached, and finally solid foundations have been laid on which to build a better understanding of atrophic gastritis. This recently sealed accord will allow us to answer – at least in part – the question asked in the title of this chapter.

GASTRIC ATROPHY AND ATROPHIC GASTRITIS: *NOT* ONE AND THE SAME

In 1983 Cheli and Giacosa published an article entitled 'Chronic atrophic gastritis and gastric mucosal atrophy – one and the same'[1]. The aim of their study was to determine whether the intensity of inflammation in the stomach of patients with fundic gastritis without anaemia ('chronic atrophic gastritis') was different from that in patients with pernicious anaemia ('gastritis mucosal atrophy'). Since no differences were found, the authors concluded that the two entities could not be differentiated histologically.

In recent years we have attempted to resurrect the differentiation between the two terms and to exploit this difference in an effort to improve our ability to diagnose gastritis. 'Gastric atrophy' is defined as the loss of appropriate glands in a given gastric compartment. This is a purely histopathological definition and indicates that in the portion of gastric mucosa under examination the glands expected to be present (for example, oxyntic glands in the mucosa of the corpus) are no longer there, and have been replaced by something else that does not belong to that area. This 'something else' may be extracellular matrix, fibrosis, or other glands that normally are not there (e.g. intestinal-type glands or pseudopyloric glands). In contrast, 'atrophic gastritis' is defined as a type of gastritis characterized by the presence of significant areas of atrophy. The two most common causes of atrophic gastritis are chronic infection with *Helicobacter pylori* and the autoimmune gastritis that may become associated with pernicious anaemia. In the Updated Sydney System[2] the term 'atrophic gastritis' is used in contrast to 'non-atrophic gastritis' or simply 'gastritis', a condition usually more severe in the antrum (hence the term 'antral-predominant') found in most subjects infected with *H. pylori* in the Western industrialized world.

Atrophic gastritis is usually characterized by extensive areas of intestinal metaplasia and has been known for several decades to represent a significant risk factor for gastric adenocarcinoma[3-12]. A diagnosis so loaded with significant prognostic implications ought not to be made lightly but, surprisingly, the histopathological criteria for atrophic gastritis have been and remain vague. This chapter will address three issues: (1) the progress made in the recognition and diagnosis of the histopathological features of atrophy in the gastric mucosa; (2) the possible influence of concurrent *H. pylori* infection on the pathologist's ability to evaluate atrophy; and (3) the need for the establishment of reproducible criteria for the diagnosis of atrophic gastritis.

GASTRIC BIOPSY VERSUS THE STOMACH

In the majority of patients hepatitis and cirrhosis affect the entire liver in a relatively uniform manner. Thus, a specimen obtained through a needle biopsy, even though it may constitute less than one-millionth part of the liver, can be expected to be reasonably representative of the whole organ. In contrast, the changes associated with gastritis (inflammatory infiltrates, lymphoid follicles, atrophy, and metaplasia) are patchily distributed. The topographic distribution and the relative intensity of these lesions in different parts of the stomach are the main determinants used for the classifications of gastritis. Furthermore, different gastric compartments have different functions, and both type and degree of functional damage depend on how each area is affected. Therefore, it is self-evident that, in order to obtain an accurate picture of gastritis in an individual patient, a set of specimens representative of each gastric compartment must be available. Each specimen must be examined according to rigorous criteria, a general impression of the intensity of the features of gastritis must be extrapolated from the various specimens from each compartment, and finally this information must be amalgamated in a topographical diagnosis. These are the principles guiding both the original and the Updated Sydney System.

After the publication of the Sydney Systems there has been little controversy in our understanding of the basic features of gastritis: several studies showed that when pathologists tested their ability to score active and chronic inflammation or bacterial density, the inter-observer variability (most often measured by κ statistics) was within acceptable limits. In contrast, the assessment of atrophy and intestinal metaplasia has been plagued by intellectual disagreement and, more troublesome for clinicians, a low degree of concurrence even among experts[13-16]. The disagreement was magnified when the controversy shifted from 'what is atrophy?' to 'what is atrophic gastritis?' Although the terms have been used interchangeably, I believe that maintaining the distinction between the two is essential to reaching a clinically meaningful understanding of gastric disease.

NATURA ABHORRET VACUUM

When gastric glands are destroyed by any process (inflammatory, chemical, neoplastic) something enters to fill the void. The foundations of our knowledge of the natural progress of *H. pylori* gastritis were laid by studies performed decades before *H. pylori* was known to be the aetiological agent of the condition[9,17-22]. Later, new studies confirmed the validity of this body of knowledge and added the newly acquired information to the initial steps of the process; furthermore, safer and more accessible endoscopic procedures have made it possible to obtain specimens at shorter intervals, providing a clearer picture of the dynamics of chronic gastritis[23-26]. Briefly, the process can be summarized as follows. *H. pylori* infection elicits an inflammatory infiltrate, which, depending on the presence of a variety of yet-unknown cofactors, may progressively destroy the gastric glands. The space liberated by the destroyed glands may be filled by the deposition of extracellular matrix, fibroblasts, and eventually collagen: for the purpose of this discussion this variant of atrophy will be referred to as fibrosis. In another, possibly synchronous or metachronous repair process, the original glands are replaced by an intestinal-type epithelium and glands not normally found in the stomach (intestinal metaplasia), or by glands that are normally not found in that part of the stomach (pseudopyloric metaplasia of the oxyntic mucosa).

H. PYLORI AND FIBROSIS

In the biopsy specimen schematically represented in Figure 1, the lamina propria of the gastric mucosa is almost entirely replaced by fibroblasts and collagen. Only scattered isolated glands are still remaining. *H. pylori* infection is present, and a moderate amount of inflammatory cells (not represented

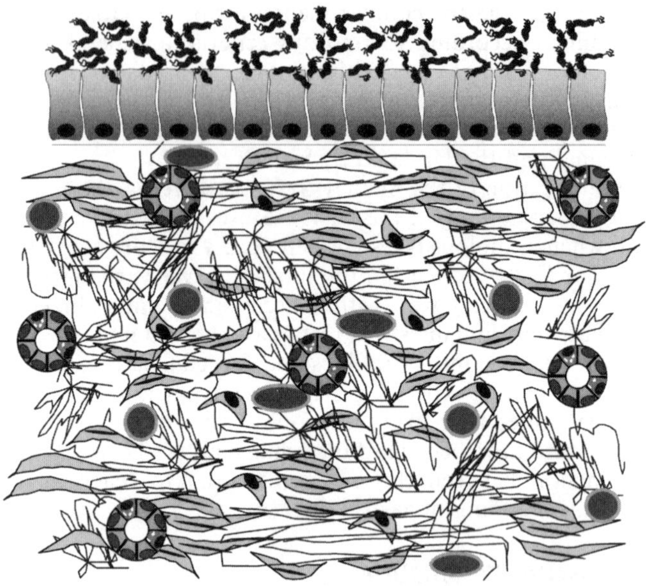

Figure 1. Schematic representation of the gastric epithelium infected with *H. pylori*. There are only rare scattered glands in the lamina propria, which is almost entirely replaced by fibrosis. In such a case the diagnosis of atrophy can be made confidently, irrespective of the presence of *H. pylori*.

in the drawing) may infiltrate epithelium and mucosa. However, the loss of glands is unequivocal; therefore the conditions of the definition of atrophy are fully met. Thus, the diagnosis of atrophy can be made when it is unambiguous that fibrosis has replaced most of the appropriate gastric glands, irrespective of the presence of *H. pylori* infection.

H. PYLORI AND METAPLASIA

When the gastric glands native to a region of the stomach have been destroyed, they may be replaced by other types of glands. Most commonly, an intestinal-type epithelium refurbishes the injured mucosa with intestinal-type crypts. This epithelium may consist of goblet cells, Paneth cells, and absorptive cells similar to those of the small intestine with a brush border and no sulphated mucins (also known as small intestinal type, type I, or complete metaplasia) or of goblet cells mixed with pseudo-absorptive cells with no brush border and variable amounts of sulphated mucins (colonic type, types II and III, or incomplete metaplasia). The metaplastic mucosa, which may consist of a few cells or extend to cover much of the gastric mucosa, is generally inhospitable for *H. pylori* colonization[27], although notable exceptions occur[28,29]. As depicted in Figure 2, when there is intestinal metaplasia the presence of *H. pylori* should have no impact on the evaluation of atrophy: if the native gastric glands have been replaced by metaplastic

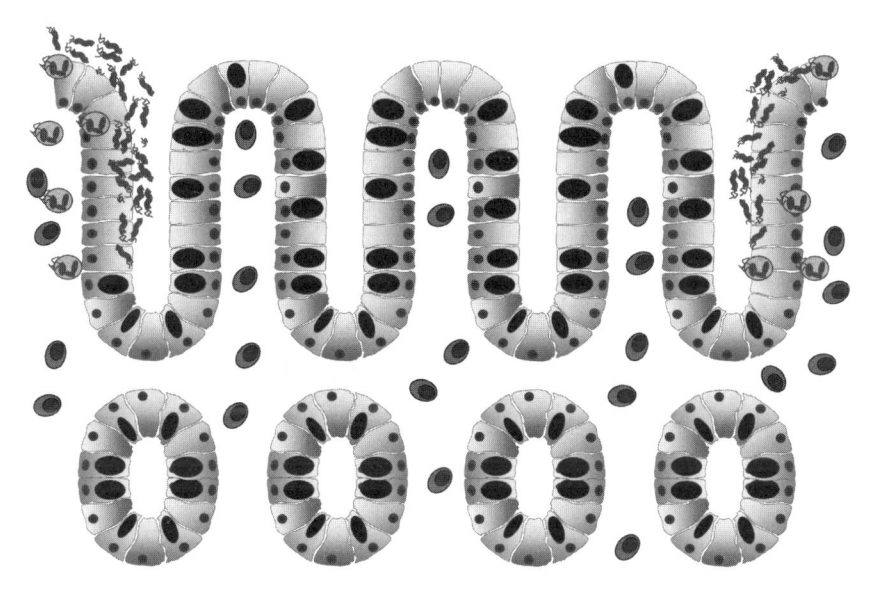

Figure 2. In this portion of gastric mucosa most of the epithelium (surface and glands) has been replaced by intestinal metaplasia. Although the few remnants of gastric epithelium (depicted at each end of the figure) are infected with *H. pylori*, the diagnosis of atrophy is possible, since no appropriate (= native) gastric glands are present in the lamina propria.

epithelium, then the conditions of the definition of atrophy are fully satisfied. Similarly, if antral mucous glands or pyloric glands replace oxyntic glands (phenomena known as antral expansion, pyloric metaplasia, or pseudopyloric metaplasia) atrophy is present because the native glands (the oxyntic glands, in this case) are lost. Again, concurrent *H. pylori* infection would have no effect on the diagnosis of atrophy.

DEFINING THE INDEFINITE

H. pylori infection elicits inflammatory responses in the gastric mucosa of virtually all infected subjects. These responses consist of a mostly polymorphonuclear infiltration in the surface and glandular epithelium, and a mostly mononuclear inflammatory infiltrate accompanied by the formation of lymphoid follicles in the lamina propria (Figure 3). Whereas the presence of neutrophils in the epithelium has a negligible effect on the mucosal architecture, a dense infiltrate in the lamina propria may cause profound alterations in the glandular architecture, in the most extreme cases making the glands completely invisible in histopathological preparations. Under such circumstances *invisibility* is virtually impossible to distinguish from *loss*: the observer does not see the glands, but cannot make an educated guess on whether the unseen glands have disappeared because they have vanished, or because there are so many inflammatory cells around them that they have been displaced and obscured from view.

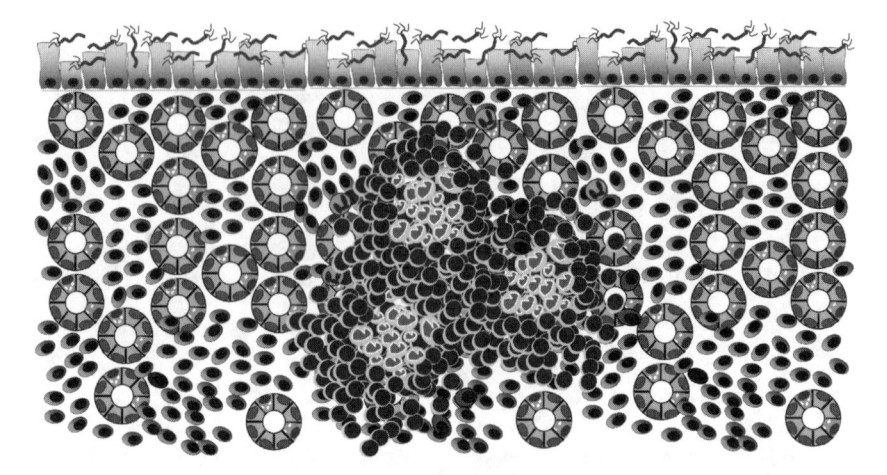

Figure 3. *H. pylori* infection elicits inflammatory responses in the gastric mucosa of virtually all infected subjects. These responses consist of a mostly polymorphonuclear infiltration in the surface and glandular epithelium, and a mostly mononuclear inflammatory infiltrate accompanied by the formation of lymphoid follicles in the lamina propria. When the inflammatory infiltrate is dense, glands may not be seen because they may be truly lost or simply displaced. In such a case the diagnosis of 'indefinite for atrophy' should be made.

At the Atrophy 2000 meeting, which took place in New Orleans in March 2000, the definition of atrophy was modified to *absence of appropriate glands*. This new designation emphasized that: (1) glands must be actually proven to be absent, as opposed to merely obscured or invisible; (2) any replacement of the normal glands in a given compartment of the stomach is equivalent to atrophy.

In many cases, atrophy due to fibrosis can be recognized even in the presence of inflammation; but when the inflammatory infiltrate is particularly dense, histopathologists cannot tell destruction from displacement or obscuration, and the diagnosis of atrophy should not be made. Instead, the term *indefinite for atrophy* ought to be used, postponing the final judgement to 3–6 months after *H. pylori* infection has been cured, and much of the inflammatory infiltrate has receded, unveiling fields of glands or meshes of fibrosis (Figure 4). If this prudent approach were applied, many premature reports hailing the regression of atrophic gastritis would never see the light of publication.

At the risk of being redundant, it must be emphasized that 'indefinite' is not a separate category of atrophy, or even the permanent categorization of an entity. Rather, it is the equivalent of 'indefinite for dysplasia', a term now used for almost two decades in the evaluation of dysplasia associated with ulcerative colitis and Barrett's oesophagus[30,31]. Pathologists use this 'temporary category' when they are unsure whether the epithelial changes in a biopsy specimen are due to reaction to inflammation or true neoplastic changes. When a diagnosis of 'indefinite for dysplasia' is rendered, the clinician's action plan is to attempt to reduce the inflammation (for example,

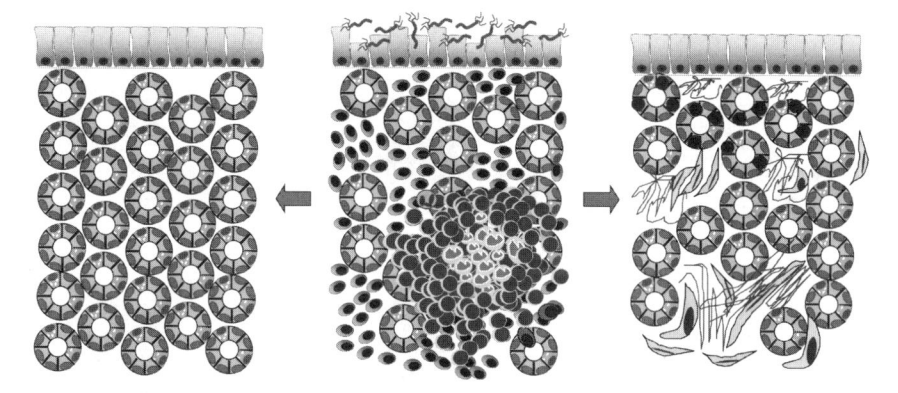

Figure 4. After *H. pylori* infection is cured much of the chronic inflammatory infiltrate resolves within a few months. Thus, an area of mucosa previously deemed to be 'indefinite for atrophy' (centre) may reveal almost intact glands (left) and, therefore, non-atrophic, or may show extensive loss of glands and fibrosis (right), in which case an accurate diagnosis of atrophy will be possible.

by using anti-inflammatory agents in patients with ulcerative colitis or vigorous antisecretory therapy in those with gastro-oesophageal reflux disease) and then obtain a new set of biopsies. Our intent in adding this term to the assessment of atrophy was to elicit a similar response: cure *H. pylori* infection and sample again after a few months, when the chronic inflammatory infiltrate can be expected to have subsided and the structures in the gastric mucosa become more clearly visible.

FUTURE CHALLENGE: THE DEFINITION OF ATROPHIC GASTRITIS

Once the pathologist has acquired the ability to recognize atrophy and assess its extent and severity with a reasonable degree of intra- and interobserver agreement, the next step is to synthesize the information and formulate a useful diagnosis. A useful diagnosis is one that triggers an action plan. The clinician is not interested in learning that there is a small focus of intestinal metaplasia in a specimen from the antrum and a larger area of fibrosis in a biopsy from the corpus. The only use of such descriptive narratives is to enable the pathologist to consolidate the information into a simple but precise diagnostic phrase (e.g. *H. pylori* atrophic pangastritis) that will allow the gastroenterologist to make a management decision.

Too long has the diagnosis of atrophic gastritis been confused with the recognition of atrophy in a single biopsy specimen. Now endoscopy is universally available and reasonably representative gastric bioptic mapping can be performed by any interested gastroenterologist. The challenges remain to define the entity known as atrophic gastritis (Figure 5), determine what is the minimum number of biopsy specimens to diagnose it, and to design clinical studies to provide data on which to base guidelines for treatment and follow-up. This will require the combined efforts of pathologists and

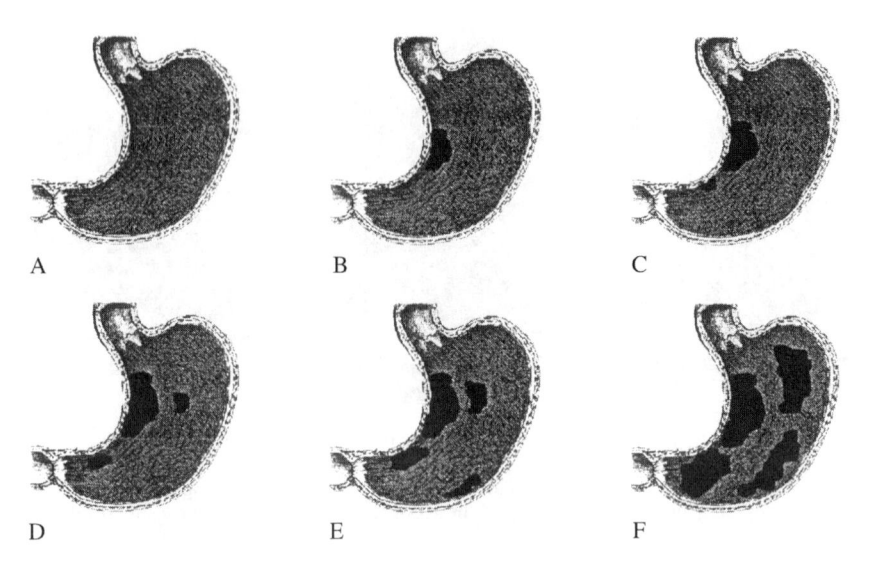

Figure 5. These six schematic representations of the stomach show the possible progression of atrophy, indicated as multifocal patches initiating in the region of the *incisura angularis*. A pathologist with access to representative biopsy samples from these stomachs would probably diagnose 'non-atrophic gastritis' in stomach A and 'atrophic gastritis' in stomachs E and F. However, no guidelines exist, and one could argue that B through E have the disease 'atrophic gastritis'. The next challenge in our understanding of gastric disease is to find reproducible and prognostically accurate criteria for the definition of the still nebulous condition we know as atrophic gastritis.

gastroenterologists as well as the cooperation of several centres in different countries equipped for the performance of large controlled clinical studies. Until this happens our approach to atrophic gastritis will continue to be empirical.

References

1. Cheli R, Giacosa A. Chronic atrophic gastritis and gastric mucosal atrophy – one and the same. Gastrointest Endosc. 1983;29:23–5.
2. Dixon MF, Genta RM, Yardley JH, Correa P. Classification and grading of gastritis. The updated Sydney System. International Workshop on the Histopathology of Gastritis, Houston, 1994. Am J Surg Pathol. 1996;20:1161–81.
3. Correa P. *Helicobacter pylori* and gastric cancer: state of the art. Cancer Epidemiol Biomarkers Prev. 1996;5:477–81.
4. Correa P. Human gastric carcinogenesis: a multistep and multifactorial process – First American Cancer Society Award Lecture on Cancer Epidemiology and Prevention. Cancer Res. 1992;52:6735–40.
5. Kekki M, Villako K, Tamm A, Siurala M. Dynamics of antral and fundal gastritis in an Estonian rural population sample. Scand J Gastroenterol. 1977;12:321–4.
6. Siurala M, Lehtola J, Ihamaki T. Atrophic gastritis and its sequelae. Results of 19–23 years' follow-up examinations. Scand J Gastroenterol. 1974;9:441–6.
7. Siurala M, Kekki M, Varis K, Isokoski M, Ihamaki T. Gastritis and gastric cancer. Br Med J. 1972;3:530–1.
8. Asaka M, Kato M, Kudo M et al. Relationship between *Helicobacter pylori* infection, atrophic gastritis and gastric carcinoma in a Japanese population. Eur J Gastroenterol Hepatol. 1995;7(Suppl. 1):S7–10.

9. Ihamaki T, Sipponen P, Varis K, Kekki M, Siurala M. Characteristics of gastric mucosa which precede occurrence of gastric malignancy: results of long-term follow-up of three family samples. Scand J Gastroenterol Suppl. 1991;186:16–23.
10. Ihamaki T, Saukkonen M, Siurala M. Long-term observation of subjects with normal mucosa and with superficial gastritis: results of 23—27 years' follow-up examinations. Scand J Gastroenterol. 1978;13:771–5.
11. Miehlke S, Hackelsberger A, Meining A *et al.* Severe expression of corpus gastritis is characteristic in gastric cancer patients infected with *Helicobacter pylori*. Br J Cancer. 1998;78:263–6.
12. Walker IR, Strickland RG, Ungar B, Mackay IR. Simple atrophic gastritis and gastric carcinoma. Gut. 1971;12:906–11.
13. El Zimaity HM, Graham DY, Al Assi MT *et al.* Interobserver variation in the histopathological assessment of *Helicobacter pylori* gastritis [see comments]. Hum Pathol. 1996;27:35–41.
14. Andrew A, Wyatt JI, Dixon MF. Observer variation in the assessment of chronic gastritis according to the Sydney system. Histopathology. 1994;25:317–22.
15. Genta RM. Review article: Gastric atrophy and atrophic gastritis–nebulous concepts in search of a definition. Aliment Pharmacol Ther. 1998;12(Suppl. 1):17–23.
16. Tepes B, Ferlan-Marolt V, Jutersek A, Kavcic B, Zaletel-Kragelj L. Interobserver agreement in the assessment of gastritis reversibility after *Helicobacter pylori* eradication. Histopathology. 1999;34:124–33.
17. Cuello C, Correa P, Haenszel W *et al.* Gastric cancer in Colombia. I. Cancer risk and suspect environmental agents. J Natl Cancer Inst. 1976;57:1015–20.
18. Correa P, Cuello C, Duque E *et al.* Gastric cancer in Colombia. III. Natural history of precursor lesions. J Natl Cancer Inst. 1976;57:1027–35.
19. Haenszel W, Correa P, Cuello C *et al.* Gastric cancer in Colombia. II. Case–control epidemiologic study of precursor lesions. J Natl Cancer Inst. 1976;57:1021–6.
20. Kimura K. Chronological transition of the fundic–pyloric border determined by stepwise biopsy of the lesser and greater curvatures of the stomach. Gastroenterology. 1972; 63:584–92.
21. Siurala M, Varis K, Wiljasalo M. Studies of patients with atrophic gastritis: a 10–15-year follow-up. Scand J Gastroenterol. 1966;1:40–8.
22. Villako K, Siurala M. The behaviour of gastritis and related conditions in different population samples. Ann Clin Res. 1981;13:114–18.
23. Fontham ET, Ruiz B, Perez A, Hunter F, Correa P. Determinants of *Helicobacter pylori* infection and chronic gastritis. Am J Gastroenterol. 1995;90:1094–101.
24. Satoh K, Kimura K, Sipponen P. *Helicobacter pylori* infection and chronological extension of atrophic gastritis. Eur J Gastroenterol Hepatol. 1995;7(Suppl. 1):S11–15.
25. Sipponen P, Kimura K. Intestinal metaplasia, atrophic gastritis and stomach cancer: trends over time. Eur J Gastroenterol Hepatol. 1994;6(Suppl. 1):S79–83.
26. Kuipers EJ, Uyterlinde AM, Pena AS *et al.* Long-term sequelae of *Helicobacter pylori* gastritis [see comments]. Lancet. 1995;345:1525–8.
27. Dixon MF. Progress in the pathology of gastritis and duodenitis. Curr Top Pathol. 1990;81:1–40.
28. Genta RM, Gurer IE, Graham DY *et al.* Adherence of *Helicobacter pylori* to areas of incomplete intestinal metaplasia in the gastric mucosa. Gastroenterology. 1996;111:1206–11.
29. Ota H, Katsuyama T, Nakajima S *et al.* Intestinal metaplasia with adherent *Helicobacter pylori*: a hybrid epithelium with both gastric and intestinal features. Hum Pathol. 1998;29:846–50.
30. Reid BJ, Haggitt RC, Rubin CE *et al.* Observer variation in the diagnosis of dysplasia in Barrett's esophagus. Hum Pathol. 1988;19:166–78.
31. Riddell RH, Goldman H, Ransohoff DF *et al.* Dysplasia in inflammatory bowel disease: standardized classification with provisional clinical applications. Hum Pathol. 1983; 14:931–68.

26
Mechanisms involved in gastric atrophy

N. A. WRIGHT

INTRODUCTION

It is usual to start such a discourse with a definition, and certainly most people would consider that gastric atrophy involves the loss of gastric glands and their replacement by metaplastic epithelium and fibrosis. Some might add that this process is irreversible, which was, in the main, the conclusion of Dixon[1], after an exhaustive review of the literature up to 1998. Others might confine the definition to the loss of specialized, oxyntic glands, although of course atrophy of mucus-secreting glands in the pylorus is also a feature of multifocal or pan-gastritis. While perhaps a tautology, still others add that the process is due to repeated or continuing mucosal injury due, *inter alia*, to *Helicobacter pylori* infection.

MECHANISMS OF GLAND LOSS

How are gastric glands destroyed? A great deal has been said about the inflammation caused by *H. pylori* destroying the stem cell zone in the gastric gland[1]. That the 'foveolitis' caused by *H. pylori* infection can indeed involve the neck and isthmus of the gastric gland, where the stem cells are housed, is a matter of common histopathological observation and certainly, if the cells in this area are indeed destroyed, then the gland will be irretrievably lost. There is considerable evidence that *H. pylori* induces apoptosis in gastric epithelial cells both *in vitro* and *in vivo* (see ref. 2 for review) and this is accompanied by a prominent compensatory proliferative response. However, whether such destruction of glands is caused by such direct bacterial effects, or as a result of host inflammatory or immune responses, is as yet unclear, since bacterial colonization itself is confined to the surface and foveolar epithelium. In *H. pylori*-associated gastritis, neutrophil polymorphs are frequently seen in the gland isthmus and neck, and release of proteases and reactive oxygen metabolites from such cells, damaging and killing the epithelial cells, is a distinct possibility: there is evidence that infection with the more virulent VacA-, CagA-positive strains, which are thought to be pro-inflammatory, are more likely to be associated with atrophy[3-5]. Indeed, a significant association is seen between CagA-posivity and the activity of gastritis and the presence of atrophy. However, infection with both CagA and VacA mutants both produced an early onset of apoptosis, with later induction of cell proliferation, and did not differ from wild-type *H. pylori* strains, albeit in Mongolian gerbils, suggesting that early events, at least, are not dependent on these genes[7]. However, there is a general perception that the progression of atrophic gastritis is determined more by host-related factors, a view reinforced by studies of animal models of *H. pylori* infection[1,8] where oxyntic gland atrophy is unrelated to bacterial colonization density, whereas the activity of the antral gastritis is so related. Such observations raise the possibility that immune mechanisms, such as the production of autoantibodies to foveolar and parietal cell canaliculi, are mediators of glandular loss, possibly produced by antigenic mimicry by the lipopolysaccharide component of some 80% of *H. pylori* strains of Lewis x and y host antigens[9,10]. There are certainly reports that the presence of anti-canalicular antibodies correlate with both the severity of corpus inflammation and the degree of atrophy[11]. Moreover, such immune mechanisms may not be confined to antibody-mediated damage, since lymphocytic infiltration of the epithelium associated with apoptosis has been reported, and there is increasing evidence of a role for cell-mediated cytoxicity in type A gastritis[12]. Furthermore, the HLA-DQ type of the host appears to modulate the progression of atrophy in *H. pylori* infection[13].

It is usual also to mention the role of bile reflux in accelerating the rate of development of atrophy in *H. pylori*-associated gastritis[14], the role of NSAIDs, a high-salt diet[15,16], cigarette smoking[17], and ammonia, in advancing the degree of atrophy. Conversely, antioxidants such as vitamin C may protect against atrophy. Ascorbic acid levels in gastric juice from *H. pylori*-infected individuals are lower than in controls, and the levels are inversely proportional to the degree of gastritis, gastric atrophy and metaplasia[18]. Moreover, CagA-positive infected patients had lower ascorbic acid concentrations than those infected with CagA-negative organisms.

Because the onset of cell proliferation is delayed after the early onset of apoptosis, and is associated with increased gastrin levels[7], the role of gastrin in the induction of atrophy has been examined. Insulin-gastrin transgenic mice were infected with *H. felis*[19], and after an initial increase in the number of parietal cells, gastric atrophy and intestinal metaplasia ensued, followed by invasive gastric carcinoma. Thus, chronic hypergastrinaemia may advance the progression of atrophic gastritis.

While not necessarily related to the mild hypergastrinaemia which accompanies therapeutic acid suppression, and possibly more dependent on the ability of *H. pylori* to colonize the oxyntic mucosa when the pH is raised, it has been proposed that acid-suppression therapy also advances the rate of gastric atrophy in *H. pylori* infection[20]. This has been strongly disputed[21] (see Chapters 28 and 29).

THE MUCOSAL RESPONSE

Obviously the gastric mucosa does not merely sit there and do nothing in the face of epithelial cell loss and gland destruction. The apoptotic cell loss, which accompanies *H. pylori* infection, is accompanied by a prominent proliferative response in an attempt to repopulate the depleted gastric glands. However, patients who later develop atrophic gastritis did not show increased cell proliferation and apoptosis, and the ratio of apoptosis (nick end labelling) to cell proliferation (Ki67) was not a determinant for the risk of developing atrophy 31 years later[22]. Moreover, gastric epithelial proliferation does not correlate with the degree of atrophy[23], although we have seen that current thinking involves the destruction of gastric glands by deletion of the stem cell compartment in the neck-isthmus in the generation of atrophy. However, there are mechanisms for replacing gastric glands, even in the adult. The healing of gastric ulcers involves the production of new glands which fill the mucosal defect during the healing process. *En passant*, it is worthwhile noting that it is a matter of conjecture where the new glands involved in the repair of gastric ulcers are derived, whether from glandular neogenesis from the epithelium migrating over the granulation tissue of the ulcer bed, or from gastric gland fission at the margins of the ulcer. Certainly, in development, and also in the adult animal, there is a well-defined mechanism for the increase in the number of gastric glands through glandular fission. In the neck of the gastric gland there is hyperplasia, which increases the number of cells in the gland circumference followed by the formation of a bud which grows downwards initially and, accompanied by local remodelling of the connective and vascular tissue in the lamina propria, the bud grows into a new tubule, which becomes detached from the parent gland[24].

So, we might ask why we get atrophy at all in the presence of a mechanism which is apparently capable of reproducing new glands, apparently at will. There are perhaps three mechanisms which might prevent such indefinite gland production. First, histological observation (Figure 1) shows that the lamina propria is increased in extent with proliferation of fibroblasts and myofibroblasts, and even an increased complement of smooth muscle cells, apparently from the muscularis mucosae. Rationalizing, it would be possible that the degree of fibrosis and distortion within the lamina propria might be such as to prevent glandular reproduction by fission. The deposition of extracellular matrix (ECM) during the healing of gastric mucosal defects is well documented[25]. Around each gastric gland is a closely applied meshwork of myofibroblasts which exist in intimate contact with the epithelial cells of the gastric gland and are thought to provide important crosstalk which partially provides proliferation and differentiation cues. Myofibroblasts are almost certainly involved in the process of gland fission, and disturbance to this intimate relationship could, of course, be pivotal in preventing gland fission. Against this proposal might be put the ability of epithelial cells to produce a range of matrix metalloproteinases and other enzymes which degrade the ECM, so such a hypothesis might also have to incorporate defective ECM degrading mechanisms. Moreover, it is well known that, even in the lamina propria of ulcerative Crohn's disease, where there is

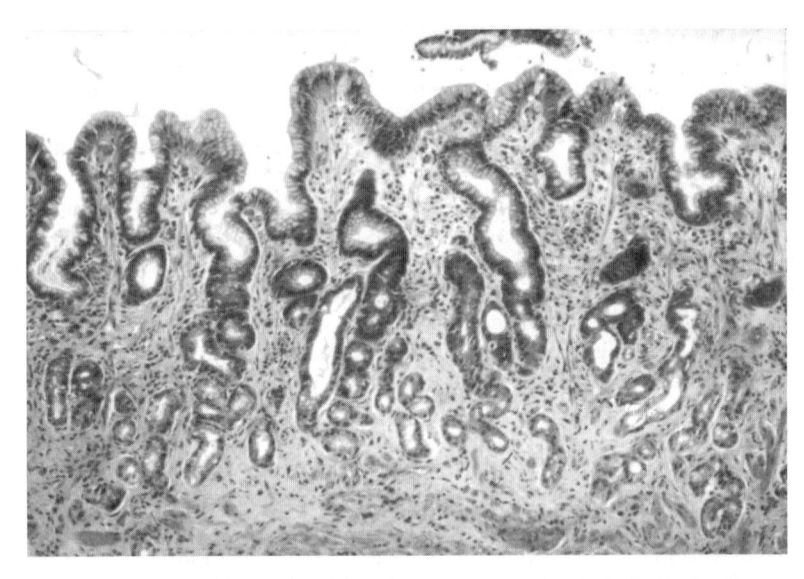

Figure 1. Chronic atrophic gastritis. Note the dense connective tissue in the lamina propria and the increased smooth muscle.

massive proliferation of myofibroblasts, neo-tubulogenesis still occurs, in the form of the ulcer-associated cell lineage (UACL), whose tubules penetrate the dense connective tissue[26]. Moreover, *H. pylori* infection is not associated with changes in α6 integrin of ECM proteins such as collagen IV, laminin and fibronectin, although E-cadherin, a molecule involved in cell–cell attachment and epithelial mobility, is down-regulated[27].

Secondly, a very interesting concept has recently emerged from studies of the clonal architecture of gastric glands. Initial observation in tetraparental allophenic mice indicated that gastric glands were clonal populations[28], but studies in human gastric glands, using the HUMARA (human androgen receptor gene) polymorphism on the X chromosome[29] suggested that, while pyloric glands were clonal, i.e. derived from a single cell at some stage in development, a proportion – up to 45% – of oxyntic glands showed a complex clonal architecture. While the cells of the foveola and fundus of the glands were monophenotypic, i.e. showed the same HUMARA allele, the neck and isthmus was polyphenotypic, presaging a polyclonal derivation.

More recent studies by Nomura *et al.*[30], using a mouse model in which the *lacZ* gene was engineered into one X chromosome, showed that at birth both pyloric and oxyntic gastric glands were polyclonal, but that in the first 6–12 weeks of life the glands undergo a sorting process which leaves the great majority, between 85% and 90%, as clonal populations. Nomura *et al.*[30] suggested that the sorting process might involve gland fission, with segregation of the two populations by the fission process in the same way that Park *et al.*[31] proposed for the sorting of partially mutated intestinal crypts after ethylnitrosourea-induced stem cell mutations.

So, in the mouse, some 10–15% of oxyntic gastric glands are polyclonal, and Nomura et al.[30] suggested that these were the glands which were capable of continued self-renewal by fission in adult life. We have seen that some 45% of human oxyntic glands are polyclonal and, if this proposal is true, it would suggest that loss of a critical fraction of gastric glands would deplete the regenerative reserve of the mucosa, since only a minority of glands can enter the gland cycle in adult life. While of course oxyntic glands are conceptually much more complex systems than the intestinal crypt, crypts are all apparently able to enter the crypt cycle[32], and these are clonal populations. So, if Nomura et al.'s[30] proposal, and the extrapolation as it applies to the progression of atrophy, is correct, then gastric glands differ diametrically in their behaviour vis-à-vis fission.

The third reason that gastric glands are not able to repopulate the mucosa might be because their place has been taken by metaplastic epithelium.

METAPLASIA AS A COMPONENT OF ATROPHY

While it is usual to concentrate on intestinal metaplasia (IM) as the only metaplastic process in atrophic gastritis, there are several other processes, unrelated to IM, loosely described under the umbrella of 'pseudopyloric metaplasia' (PPM). This occurs when the specialized cells of the oxyntic glands are replaced by simple mucus-secreting cells of foveolar-pit type. Such changes have been described in human autoimmune gastritis and in animal models of autoimmune gastritis and H. pylori infection[1]. Similarly, the process of 'antralization', in which the antral mucosa progresses proximately at the expense of the oxyntic mucosa, has been recognized as a component of atrophic gastritis, which advances with age, either on a broad front, or as part of a multifocal atrophic process[1]. Indeed, antralization at the incisura is a common event in H. pylori infection, and is associated with an increased risk of atrophic gastritis and intestinal metaplasia[33]. Further insight has been gained into this process by the study of ulcers occurring unequivocally in oxyntic mucosa, in most cases associated with H. pylori infection. Initially, there is a hyperplasia of mucous neck cells, which move both upwards and particularly downwards in the oxyntic tubule, replacing the specialized parietal and chief cells. The mucous neck cells are themselves replaced by cells of foveolar-pit phenotype. This can occur focally, occupying a single oxyntic tubule, groups of tubules, or processed on a fairly massive scale with many tubules involved (Figure 2). Dixon[1] has proposed that the UACL also contributes to the mass of glands of pyloric phenotype, but Wong et al.[34] have shown that this occurs only when intestinal metaplasia is also a component, where it is quite clear that PPM unequivocally occurs in the absence of IM.

Interestingly, Schmidt et al.[35] have proposed a relationship between a similar cell lineage – termed SPEM (spasmolytic peptide-expressing metaplasia) and the histogenesis of dysplasia/carcinoma in the antrum, as an alternative to the widely accepted IM/dysplasia/carcinoma sequence for the intestinal type of gastric carcinoma. The relationship of SPEM to PPM has

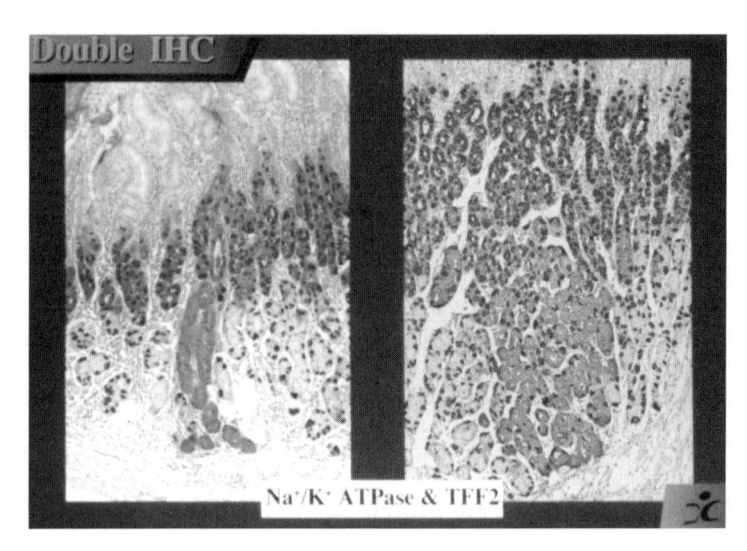

Figure 2. Sections of gastric fundus double-stained with antibodies against the H/K ATPase and hSP/TFF2. Note the appearance of pseudopyloric metaplasia in single glands, groups of glands and in large areas.

yet to be determined[34]. However, it is clear that *H. pylori* infection is very much associated with the induction of PPM and associated lesions.

The morphology and clinical correlates of IM have been elegantly reviewed[1], but very recently a remarkable insight into the mechanisms of induction of IM has come from the study of *Cdx2*, a gene in the Parahox cluster of genes with a homeo domain. *Cdx2* is a transcription factor, which is found in the adult mouse colon in maximum concentration in the caecum, with a diminishing concentration distally as the rectum, is reached[36]. Studies *in vitro* suggest that the *Cdx2* gene product is involved in the determination of epithelial cell polarity and the control of gene expression in villus epithelial cells. It has been reported that CDX-1, a related protein, is expressed in IM, suggesting a role in gastrointestinal cell lineage determination[36]. Direct evidence was lacking until the gene was deleted in mice by gene targeting[37,38]. $Cdx2-/-$ mice are lethal, dying *in utero*, but $Cdx2-/+$ mice show a fascinating phenotype. Polypoid lesions appear mainly in the proximal colon, which show, on histological examination, consecutively, small intestinal, followed by gastric antral, oxyntic and cardiac mucosa (Figure 3). The small intestinal phenotype is easily identified by the presence of Paneth cells, the antral mucosa by the presence of hSP/TFF$_2$ (human spasmolytic polypeptide/trefoil factor family) in the deeper glands and the oxyntic mucosa by the presence of numerous H^+K^+-ATPase-positive parietal cells.

The earliest lesions appear *in utero*, as a small, sometimes depressed, area of stratified squamous epithelium (recall that the proximal part of the mouse stomach is so lined) and the lesions develop, from this, cardiac, oxyntic, antral and small intestinal mucosae. There is no increase in the number of lesions with age, and the proliferative status of the colonic mucosa appears

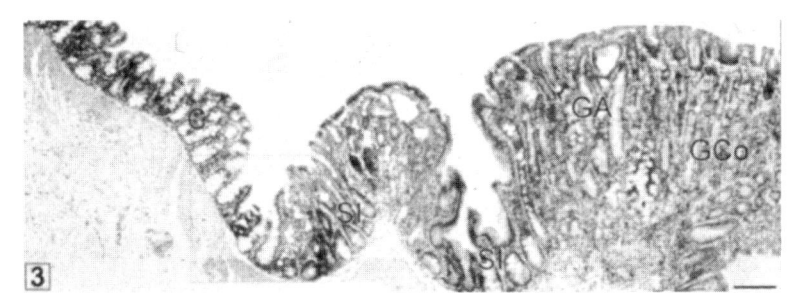

Figure 3. A polyp from a $Cdx2-/+$ mouse. Note the colonic mucosa giving rise to small intestine, gastric antrum and gastric corpus.

normal[39]. The remaining wild-type allele in the colonic mucosa shows no evidence of a mutation, and the $Cdx2$ gene product is not demonstrable in the gastric component of the polyps.

This experiment shows that haploid insufficiency, leading to a reduction in Cdx2 protein, leads to the colonic mucosa acceding to rostral influences, which encourage gastric differentiation. Once this signal is received in colonic stem cells, squamous stomach differentiation is switched on the gastric and small intestinal differentiation ensue through a process of intercalation. Thus LOH in a homeobox gene, without loss of the other allele by mutation, can give rise to different gastrointestinal lineage determination. It is thus easy to conceive how LOH in the gastric mucosa, possibly in association with a dominant negative effect, could then lead to differentiation along the intestinal lineage pathway. It is relevant to note that haploid insufficiency, without mutation in the other allele, does not lead to progression of the gastric phenotype with age: this might suggest that, for such metaplastic changes to occur in adult tissues, disabling of the other allele by mutation might be necessary. Thus, when we turn to the vexatious question of regressibility of IM, it would be interesting to see if homeo domain genes such as $Cdx2$, $Cdx1$ and $Pdx1$ are mutated in animal models of intestinal metaplasia.

CONCLUSION

We now widely accept that gastric atrophy is not merely loss of glands and their replacement by fibrous connective tissue, but also by metaplastic epithelium. While we can identify those organismal and host factors which are associated with atrophy, we cannot state down with any conviction the reasons why gastric glands are lost and are not replaced. However, insight on the molecular level into the origins of metaplasia are now finally emerging, and the next few years should prove very interesting in this respect.

References

1. Dixon MF. Atrophy, metaplasia and dysplasia – a risk for gastric cancer: are they reversible? In: Hunt R, Tytgat G, editors. *Helicobacter pylori*. Basic Mechanisms to Clinical Cure. Lancaster: Kluwer; 1998:336–53.

2. Moss SF. Epithelial cell turnover and apoptosis. In: Hunt R, Tytgat G, editors. *Helicobacter pylori*. Basic Mechanisms to Clinical Cure. Lancaster: Kluwer; 1998:110–22.
3. Fox JG, Correa P, Taylor WS et al. High prevalence and persistence of cytotoxin-positive *Helicobacter pylori* strains in a population with high prevalence of atrophic gastritis. Am J Gastroeneterol. 1992;87:1154–60.
4. Beales IL, Crabtree JE, Sennesa D, Coracci A, Calam J. Antibodies to CagA protein are associated with gastric atrophy in *Helicobacter pylori* infection. Eur J Gastroenterol Hepatol. 1998;8:645–9.
5. Ito S, Azunna T, Murakita H et al. Profile of *Helicobacter pylori* cytotoxin derived from two areas of Japan with different prevalence of atrophic gastritis. Gut. 1996;39:800–6.
6. Maaroos H-I, Vorobjora T, Sipponen T et al. An 18-year follow-up study of chronic gastritis and *Helicobacter pylori*: association of CagA positivity with development of atrophy and activity of gastritis. Scand J Gastroenterol. 1999;34:864–9.
7. Peck HM, Wirth H-P, Moss SF et al. *Helicobacter pylori* alters gastric epithelial cell cycle events and gastrin secretion in Mongolian gerbils. Gastroenterology. 2000;118:48–59.
8. Sahagami T, Dixon M, O'Rourke J et al. Atrophic gastric changes in both *Helicobacter felis* and *Helicobacter pylori*-infected mice are host-dependent and separate from antral gastritis. Gut. 1996;39:639–48.
9. Simoons-Smit IM, Appelmelk BJ, Verboom T et al. Typing of *Helicobacter pylori* with monoclonal antibodies against Lewis antigens in lipopolysaccharide. Role in autoimmunity. Gastroenterology. 1996;64:2031–40.
10. Negrini A, Savio R, Poiesi C et al. Antigenic mimicry between *Helicobacter pylori* and gastric mucosa in the pathogenesis of body atrophic growth. Gastroenterology. 1998; 116:655–65.
11. Faller G, Steininger H, Krauzkin J et al. Antigastrin autoantibodies in *Helicobacter pylori* infection: implication of histological and clinical parameters of gastritis. Gut. 1997; 41:619–23.
12. Eidt S, Oberhuber G, Schneider A, Stolte M. The histopathological spectrum of type A gastritis. Pathol Res Pract. 1996;192:101–6.
13. Azunna T, Konishi J, Tanka K et al. Contribution of HLA-DQA gene to host's response to *Helicobacter pylori*. Lancet. 1994;343:542–3.
14. Sobala GM, O'Connor HJ, Dewar GP, King RF, Axan AT, Dixon MF. Bile reflux in the intact stomach. J Clin Pathol. 1990;43:303–6.
15. Correa P, Cuello C, Fajardo LF, Haenzel W, Bolanos O, De Ramirez B. Diet and gastric ulcer: nutrition survey in a high risk area. J Natl Cancer Inst. 1983;70:693–8.
16. Fox JG, Dungler CA, Taylor NS, King A, Voh TJ, Wang TC. High salt diet induces gastric epithelial hyperplasia and parietal cell loss and enhances *Helicobacter pylori* colonisation in C57BL/6 mice. Cancer Res. 1999;59:4823–8.
17. Stemmerman GN, Nomura AMY, Chijou P-H, Hankin J. Impact of diet and smoking on risk of developing intestinal metaplasia of the stomach. Dig Dis Sci. 1990;35:433–8.
18. Jhang JW, Patchett SW, Perreu D, Katelaris PH, Domizio P, Farthing MJG. The relation between gastric vitamin C concentrations, mucosal histology and CagA seropositivity in the human stomach. Gut. 1998;43:322–6.
19. Wang TC, Dangler CA, Chen D et al. Synergistic interaction between hypergastrinaemia and *Helicobacter* infection in a mouse model of gastric cancer. Gastroenterology. 2000;118:36–47.
20. Logan RP, Walker MM, Misiewicz GJJ, Gummett PA, Karim QN, Baron JA. Changes in the intragastric distribution of *Helicobacter pylori* during treatment with omeprazole. Gut. 1995;36:12–16.
21. Lundnell L, Meittenen P, Myrold JE et al. Lack of effect of acid suppression therapy on gastric atrophy. Gastroenterology. 1999;117:319–26.
22. Moss SF, Valle J, Abdalla AM, Wang S, Siarala M, Sipponen P. Gastric cell turnover and the development of atrophy after 31 years of follow up: a case control study. Am J Gastroenterol. 1999;94:2109–14.
23. Lynch DA, Mapstone NP, Clarke AM et al. Correlation between epithelial cell proliferation and histological grading in gastric mucosa. J Clin Pathol. 1999;52:367–71.
24. Fujita S, Hattori T. Cell proliferation and differentiation in gastric mucosa: a study of the background for carcinogenesis. Pathophysiology of Carcinogenesis in Digestive Organs. Baltimore: University Park Press; 1977:22–31.

25. Shahin M, Gillessen A, Phole T et al. Gastric ulcer healing in the rat: kinetics and localisation of *de novo* procollagen synthesis. Gut. 1997;41:187–94.
26. Wright NA, Pike C, Elia G. Induction of a novel epidermal growth factor-secreting cell lineage by mucosal ulceration in gastrointestinal stem cells. Nature. 1990;340:82–5.
27. Gettisseu A, Vos B, Rauterberg J, Domschke W. Distribution of collagen types I, III and IV in peptic ulcer and normal gastric mucosa in man. Scand J Gastroenterol. 1993;28:688–9.
28. Thompson M, Fleming K, Evans DJ, Wright NA. Gastric endocrine cells share a clonal origin with other gastric epithelial cells. Development. 1990;110:477–81.
29. Nomura S, Kaminishi M, Sugiyama K, Oohara T, Esumi H. Clonal analysis of isolated single fundic and pyloric glands of stomach using X-linked polymorphisms. Biochem Biophys Res Commun. 1996;226:385–90.
30. Nomura S, Esumi H, Job C, Tan SS. Lineage and clonal development of gastric glands. Dev Biol. 1998;204:124–35.
31. Park H-S, Goodlad RA, Wright NA. Crypt fission in the small intestine and colon: a mechanism for the emergence of mutagen induced transformed crypts in mice. Am J Pathol. 1995;146:1416–27.
32. Bjerknes M. Expansion of mutant stem cell populations in the human colon. J Theor Biol. 1996;178:381–5.
33. Hua-Xiang H, Kalantar JS, Tolley NJ et al. Antral type mucosal mucosa in the gastric incisura, body and fundus (antralisation): a link between *Helicobacter pylori* infection and intestinal metaplasia? Am J Gastroenterol. 2000;95:114–21.
34. Wong R, Poulsom R, Garcia SB et al. The histogenesis of pseudopyloric metaplasia in the human gastric corpus. Human Pathol (Submitted).
35. Schmidt PH, Lee JR, Joshi V et al. Identification of a metaplastic cell lineage associated with human gastric adenocarcinoma. Lab Invest. 1999;79:639–46.
36. Silberg DA, Furtin EE, Taylor JK, Schenk T, Chiou T, Traber P. CDX1 protein expression in normal, metaplastic and neoplastic human alimentary tract epithelium. Gastroenterology. 1997;113:478–86.
37. Beck F, Chamensansophak K, Waring P, Playford RJ, Furness JB. Reprogramming of intestinal differentiation and intercalary regeneration in Cdx2 mutant mice. Proc Natl Acad Sci. 1999;96:7318–23.
38. Tamai Y, Nakajima R, Ishikama T, Selden MF, Taketo NM. Colonic haematoma development by anomalous reduplication in Cdx2 knockout mice. Cancer Res. 1999;59:2965–70.
39. Playford RJ, Goodlad RA, Beck F, Wright NA. Cell proliferation in Cdx2 knockout mouse colon. J Pathol. (In press).

27
Intestinal metaplasia: types, mechanisms of origin, and role in gastric cancer histogenesis

E. SOLCIA, O. LUINETTI, L. VILLANI, P. QUILICI,
C. KLERSY and R. FIOCCA

TYPES OF METAPLASIA

Intestinal metaplasia (IM) is by far the most frequent metaplastic change occurring in the gastric mucosa. True pyloric type metaplasia of oxyntic glands and pancreatic metaplasia of the cardia and oxyntic glands is relatively infrequent and focally restricted. So-called 'pseudopyloric metaplasia' of oxyntic glands, a prominent component of diffuse corpus–fundus (type A) atrophic gastritis, is better interpreted as mucous-neck cell hyperplasia with lack of acid-peptic differentiation, rather than as true metaplasia[1]. Three types of IM are usually considered: (1) type I or complete or small intestine type, composed of columnar crypt/absorptive enterocytes with sparse globet cells, with or without Paneth cells and intestinal type endocrine cells; (2) type II or incomplete sulphomucin-negative type, consisting of goblet cells scattered among gastric foveolar and neck cells; and (3) type III or incomplete sulphomucin-positive type, showing goblet cells scattered among sulphomucin-producing columnar cells. The latter cells show gastric or hybrid gastric/intestinal cell patterns under histochemical and ultrastructural investigation and overlie a relatively immature proliferative component, often sulphomucin-negative but CAR-5 (an intestinal oncofetal antigen) positive, whose expansion apparently leads to dysplasia[2]. Cytokeratin 7-positive glands or microcysts, mainly non-proliferative, are sometimes found at the bottom of type III or mixed complete/incomplete types of metaplasia, often combined with Brunner-type glands.

MECHANISMS OF ORIGIN OF INTESTINAL METAPLASIA

Available evidence is provided by numerous studies of the association of *Helicobacter pylori* infection and IM in human material and a few experimental investigations. An important role of *H. pylori* infection, especially with cagA-positive strains, and related active gastritis in the genesis of IM and associated gastric gland atrophy is strongly supported by serological and histological observations[3-6] and confirmed by experimental findings in *H. pylori*-infected Mongolian gerbils[7]. It seems likely that a mechanism of inappropriate differentiation is involved during repair of *H. pylori*-associated epithelial lesions, due to bacterial toxins or secondary to active inflammation. IM of the incomplete type has been observed experimentally in rats during repair of superficial erosions caused by NaOH treatment[8].

Little information is available concerning which factor(s) may lead to altered differentiation of gastric epithelial stem cells, possibly through activation of CDX1 and/or CDX2 transcription factors, known to be involved in the development of the intestinal phenotype[9]. However, one factor may well be increased: luminal pH. Indeed, several treatments leading to selective parietal cell loss, such as X-ray irradiation[10] or injection of 'xenogenic' gastric antigen[11], promoted the appearance of IM of complete or mixed complete and incomplete type. This effect, which seems to be enhanced by antisecretory drugs[12], may fit with the occurrence of focal IM in the antral mucosa of the human fetal and rat postnatal stomach, in association with poorly developed parietal cells and rather high luminal pH[13], and appears to be similar to the frequent occurrence of superficial-foveolar type gastric metaplasia in the duodenum seen under clinical or experimental conditions associated with high acidity[14,15]. Apparently this interpretation would seem in contrast with the development of IM in Barrett's oesophagus which occurs under acid reflux. However, it should be recalled that Barrett's IM is, as a rule, of incomplete type and shows, in addition to a few goblet cells, predominant populations of columnar cells with sulphated mucin resembling foveolar cells of type III gastric IM, normal oesophageal gland epithelium or fetal oesophageal epithelium[16]. In addition, gastric-type epithelium in the absence of goblet cells may also occur in reflux oesophagitis.

Enterogastric reflux of bile in operated and non-operated stomachs has also been proposed as an important cause of IM developing in the gastric stump or in the antrum of the intact stomach. Some experimental evidence, and a strong association of IM with increased bile acids in the gastric juice, support this suggestion[17], which might also have some implication in the genesis of IM of the oesophagus and cardia.

ROLE IN GASTRIC CANCER HISTOGENESIS

Whatever its mechanism of origin, IM is a rather persistent lesion, which survives *H.* pylori eradication[6] and, especially when extensive or type III and under the influence of endogenous or exogenous mutagens, may progress to dysplasia and cancer, at least of gland-forming, so-called 'intestinal', histological type[2]. However, the precise relationship of IM types with cancers of different histology and cell phenotype is not known. Therefore, we decided to reinvestigate peritumour IM and tumour tissue in a series of 71 early gastric cancers, histologically classified as glandular (tubular or papillary), diffuse or mixed (glandular and diffuse) according to previous criteria[18,19].

Table 1. Tumour cell phenotype versus histology in 71 early gastric cancers

	Phenotype			
	Intestinal	Mixed	Gastric	Total
Tubular (a)	15	6	6	27
Papillary (b)	1	3	5	9
Mixed (c)	7	2	7	16
Diffuse (d)	3	3	9	15
Total	26	14	27	67

Fisher's exact: a vs $b + c + d$, $p = 0.029$; a vs b, $p = 0.042$; a vs d, $p = 0.037$. In four of the 71 cases the phenotype remained undefined.

Table 2. Peritumour IM by tumour histology

IM total	Tubular (a)	Papillary (b)	Mixed (c)	Diffuse (d)	Total
Positive	27	9	11	8	55
Negative	3	0	5	8	16
Total	30	9	16	16	71

Fisher's exact: overall, $p = 0.004$; $a + b$ vs $c + d$, $p = 0.001$; $a + b$ vs d, $p = 0.001$; $a + b$ vs c, $p = 0.038$.

Table 3. Peritumour incomplete IM by tumour histology

IM incomplete	Tubular (a)	Papillary (b)	Mixed (c)	Diffuse (d)	Total
Positive	17	6	5	3	31
Negative	13	3	11	13	40
Total	30	9	16	16	71

Fisher's exact: overall, $p = 0.030$; $a + b$ vs $c + d$, $p = 0.008$; $a + b$ vs d, $p = 0.008$; b vs d, $p = 0.031$; a vs d, $p = 0.027$.

The predominant phenotype of tumour cells and peritumour IM was assessed with tests for M1 antigen, for gastric foveolar cells, periodic acid concanavalin A-positive mucin, for mucous-neck and pyloric gland cells, CAR-5 antigen (colorectal goblet and columnar cells, immature intestinal crypt cells and primitive fetal gut epithelium), M3 antigen (intestinal goblet cells) and CD10 antigen (CALLA; absorbing enterocytes) as previously reported[18–21].

RESULTS

The results are outlined in Tables 1–4. A significant correlation appears between tumour histological type and tumour phenotype, with a higher prevalence of the intestinal phenotype among tubular cancers and gastric phenotype among papillary and diffuse cancers (Table 1). Total (complete and incomplete) IM was significantly more represented in the mucosa sur-

Table 4. Peritumour IM extension by tumour histology

IM type	Tubular (a)	Papillary (b)	Mixed (c)	Diffuse (d)
Incomplete, mean (SD)	15.0 (19.03)	30.6 (30.87)	7.4 (16.11)	1.1 (2.02)
Total, mean (SD)	37.3 (25.28)	65.6 (26.51)	17.5 (22.36)	6.1 (7.49)

		Incomplete	Total
Kruska–Wallis test:	$p =$	0.0157	0.0001
Mann–Whitney U-test:	a vs c, $p =$	0.0782	0.0080
	a vs d, $p =$	0.0130	0.0000
	b vs c, $p =$	0.0315	0.0004
	b vs d, $p =$	0.0072	0.0000
	$a + b$ vs $c + d$, $p =$	0.0011	0.0000

rounding tubular and papillary tumours compared with that surrounding histologically mixed and, especially, diffuse tumours (Table 2). A similar pattern was shown by incomplete type IM alone (Table 3). Mean extension in the peritumour mucosa of incomplete or total IM was highest in papillary cancer cases and lowest in diffuse cases, with intermediate figures for tubular and mixed tumours (Table 4). No significant correlation was found between peritumour IM (total or incomplete) and tumour phenotype, either in terms of the presence/absence or extension. However, compared with both intestinal and mixed phenotypes, the gastric phenotype showed more extensive peritumour IM of incomplete type (mean 17.0, SD 26.8, versus 8.3, SD 13.71 and 8.2, SD 13.24, respectively).

From this investigation, it clearly appears that in early cancer a correlation exists between histological structure and tumour cell phenotype, with the highest prevalence of intestinal phenotype in tubular tumours and of gastric phenotype in diffuse as well as papillary tumours. These findings confirm previous histochemical studies showing mostly gastric-type mucins in a subset of well-differentiated intramucosal adenocarcinomas and carcinomas arising in hyperplastic polyps often showing papillary structure[22]. The phenotype divergence between papillary and tubular cancer is noteworthy in that the two types are commonly grouped together among glandular or 'intestinal' cancers, an approach which might prevent the detection of other relevant differences between these two tumour subsets. The above findings might also anticipate a higher contribution of intestinal metaplasia to tubular cancer, mostly intestinal in phenotype, than to tumours of predominantly gastric phenotype, such as diffuse or papillary cancers. Analysis of peritumour IM confirmed this prediction for tubular and diffuse cancers, whereas IM was unexpectedly found to be very prominent around papillary tumours, with the incomplete type accounting for nearly half the total IM. However, as gastric cell lineages, with special reference to superficial-foveolar and pyloric gland cell lines, predominate in incomplete IM[2], this finding may fit with the predominance of the gastric phenotype among tumour cells of papillary cancer, and may support a special role of incomplete IM in the histogenesis of such neoplasia. Although when type, prevalence and extension of peritumour IM were compared with tumour phenotype, no significant correlation was found, peritumour IM of incomplete type was twice as prominent around cancers of the gastric phenotype when compared with those of intestinal or mixed phenotype.

CONCLUSION

In conclusion, peritumour intestinal metaplasia seems to predict more the histological type of gastric cancer than its phenotype, which might be largely influenced by the high differentiation plasticity of neoplastic cells. The tendency of tumours arising in a background of extensive IM to retain glandular structure more than those arising mainly in non-metaplastic gastric mucosa, likely to be related to the molecular differences found in their carcinogenic process. This is particularly true for early structural or functional changes in genes coding for junctional proteins, for example, E. cadherin[23]. In IM-related carcinogenesis factors controlling cell proliferation seem to be affected earlier and more selectively than those involved in structural differentiation (cell to cell and cell to basal membrane junction, cell polarity, etc.) and secretory function[2].

Acknowledgements

The research of the authors was supported in part by grants from the Italian Ministry of Health (to IRCCS Policlinico S. Matteo), Italian Ministry of University and Research, and the Universities of Pavia and Genova.

References

1. Solcia E, Capella C, Fiocca R et al. Exocrine and endocrine epithelial changes in type A and B chronic gastritis. In: Malfertheiner P, Ditschuneit H, editors. *Helicobacter pylori*, Gastritis and Peptic Ulcer. Heidelberg: Springer-Verlag; 1990;245–58.
2. Solcia E, Fiocca R, Luinetti O et al. Intestinal and diffuse gastric cancers arise in a different background of *Helicobacter pylori* gastritis through different gene involvement. Am J Surg Pathol. 1996;20(Suppl. 1):8–22.
3. Fiocca R, Villani L, Luinetti O et al. *Helicobacter* colonization and histopathological profile of chronic gastritis in patients with or without dyspepsia, mucosal erosion and peptic ulcer. A morphological approach to the study of ulcerogenesis in man. Virchows Arch A (Pathol Anat). 1992;420:489–98.
4. Cho C, Murthy UK, Linscheer WG, Perez-Perez GI, Blaser MJ. Is intestinal metaplasia a consequence of *H. pylori* gastritis? Gastroenterology. 1994;106.A62 (abstract).
5. Kuipers EJ, Perez-Perez GI, Meuwissen SG, Blaser MJ. *Helicobacter pylori* and atrophic gastritis: importance of the cagA status. J Natl Cancer Inst. 1995;87:1731–2.
6. Van der Hulst R, Van der Ende A, Dekker F et al. Effect of *Helicobacter pylori* eradication on gastritis in relation to cagA: a prospective 1-year follow-up study. Gastroenterology. 1997;113:25–30.
7. Watanabe T, Tada M, Nagai H et al. *Helicobacter pylori* infection induces gastric cancer in Mongolian gerbils. Gastroenterology. 1998;115:642–8.
8. Oohara T, Sadatsuki H, Kaminishi M, Mitarai Y. Simple alkaline treatment induces intestinal metaplasia in the stomach of rats. Pathol Res Pract. 1982;175:365–72.
9. Silberg DG, Furth EE, Taylor JK et al. CDX1 protein expression in normal, metaplastic, and neoplastic human alimentary tract epithelium. Gastroenterology. 1997;113:478–86.
10. Watanabe H. Experimentally induced intestinal metaplasia in Wistar rats by X-ray irradiation. Gastroenterology. 1978;75:796–9.

11. Watanabe H; Hirose F, Takizawa S, Terada Y, Fujii I. Morphological and biochemical changes in the gastric mucosa of A/IIcJ mice injected with a xenogeneic stomach antigen. Acta Pathol Jpn. 1977;27:869–76.
12. Watanabe H, Kamikawa M, Nakagawa Y, Takahashi T, Ito A. The effects of ranitidine and cysteamine on intestinal metaplasia induced by X-irradiation in rats. Acta Pathol Jpn. 1988;38:1285–96.
13. Watanabe H, Naito M, Kawashima K, Ito A. pH-related differentiation in the epithelia of the gastric mucosa of postnatal rats. Acta Pathol Jpn. 1985;35:569–76.
14. James AH. Gastric epithelium in the duodenum. Gut. 1964;5:285–94.
15. Rhodes J. Experimental production of gastric epithelium in the duodenum. Gut. 1964;5:454–8.
16. Solcia E, Villani L, Trespi F et al. Cardia mucosa gastritis (carditis): pathogenesis, correlation with gastritis of other sites and clinicopathological relevance. In: Hunt RH, Tytgat GNJ, editors. *Helicobacter pylori*: Basic Mechanisms to Clinical Cure 1998. Kluwer; 1998;224–31.
17. Sobala GM, O'Connor HJ, Dewar EP et al. Bile reflux and intestinal metaplasia in gastric mucosa. J Clin Pathol. 1993;46:235–40.
18. Fiocca R, Villani L, Tenti P et al. The foveolar cell component of gastric cancer. Hum Pathol. 1990;21:260–70.
19. Luinetti O, Fiocca R, Villani L et al. Genetic pattern, histological structure, and cellular phenotype in early and advanced gastric cancers: evidence for structure-related genetic subsets and for loss of glandular structure during progression of some tumors. Hum Pathol. 1998;29:702–9.
20. Fiocca R, Cornaggia M, Villani L et al. Expression of pepsinogen II in gastric cancer. Its relationship to local invasion and lymph node metastases. Cancer. 1988;61:956–62.
21. Fiocca R, Villani L, Tenti P et al. Widespread expression of intestinal markers in gastric carcinoma: a light and electron microscopic study using BD-5 monoclonal antibody. J Clin Pathol. 1988;41:178–87.
22. Kushima R, Hattori T. Histogenesis and characteristics of gastric-type adenocarcinomas in the stomach. J Cancer Res Clin Oncol. 1993;120:103–11.
23. Becker KF, Atkinson MJ, Reich U et al. E-cadherin gene mutations provide clues to diffuse type gastric carcinomas. Cancer Res. 1994;54:3845–52.

28
Long-term proton pump inhibitor therapy accelerates the onset of atrophic gastritis in *Helicobacter pylori*-positive patients

E. J. KUIPERS and S. G. M. MEUWISSEN

INTRODUCTION

In 1967 Astra Hässle started a research project aiming at the development of an acid-suppressive drug for peptic ulcer disease[1]. After many hurdles and development problems this project eventually led, in 1979, to the synthesis of a benzimidazole with very powerful acid-inhibitory capacities. The first clinical results obtained with this drug, called omeprazole, were presented a few years later, showing healing of duodenal ulcers within 4 weeks in 25 of 26 patients treated with 40 mg omeprazole once daily[2]. Since then, proton pump inhibitors (PPIs) were proven to have a high efficacy for the treatment of acid-related disorders with few side-effects or intolerance. These properties have led to the very common use of PPIs. In countries such as the Netherlands 1–2% of the total population uses PPI maintenance therapy[3]. Together with the demonstration of powerful inhibition of acid secretion came the concerns about any related side-effects of this acid inhibition. These concerns were, in particular, fed by the observation of development of gastric carcinoids in rats after prolonged treatment with very high doses of omeprazole. For this reason, maintenance treatment in humans was initially allowed only in clinical trials with monitoring of serum gastrin levels and gastric histology by repeated endoscopy with biopsy sampling. These trials showed that gastric argyrophil cell hyperplasia developed in a proportion of patients in relation to hypergastrinaemia, but also confirmed that carcinoid formation did not occur. These trials did not focus on gastritis, but did report that a subgroup of patients developed active body gastritis after the start of omeprazole treatment, which was accompanied by development of gland loss during follow-up[4]. No explanation was given for these observations, and they were considered to relate to the normal progression of gastritis with ageing[5,6]. However, insight into these observations gradually came with the increasing knowledge of *Helicobacter pylori* and its effect on gastritis.

H. PYLORI GASTRITIS AND PPI TREATMENT

H. pylori gastritis usually predominates in the antrum with a strong decrease over the antral–corpus transitional zone[7]. Initial studies on the effect of profound acid suppression on *H. pylori*, therefore, focused only on the antrum, and it was enthusiastically reported that omeprazole monotherapy led to bacterial eradication. Unfortunately, patients became *H. pylori*-positive again soon after withdrawal of antisecretory therapy. It appeared that, although acid suppression led to a decrease of bacteria in the antrum, it had no effect on bacterial counts in the corpus, but in fact was associated with more severe corpus gastritis with influx of neutrophils and mononuclear cells[8–10]. This effect was consistently reported in many studies and explained historical observations of increased body gastritis after vagotomy for duodenal ulcer disease[11–14]. It was related to the optimal pH for *H. pylori*, a neutralophil with pronounced acid tolerance due to combined effects of *urease* A and B and a panel of other genes[15]. *In vitro*, in the presence of urea but limited availability of some bacterial nutrients such as iron and nickel, the optimal growth of *H. pylori* occurs in the pH range between 4.5 and 6. In the normal stomach this condition is present in the antrum and the luminal side of the mucus layer in the body of the stomach, thus explaining the predominant colonization in these locations under these circumstances. Profound acid suppression changes the intragastric pH but does not change the availability of urea and other nutrients. As such the optimal site of colonization shifts to the mucosal side of the corpus mucus layer. The lower bacterial density in the antrum leads to healing of gastritis; the closer contact with the body mucosa with bacterial toxins and ammonia, however, exacerbates corpus gastritis. This process reverses after return of acid secretion, although the time frame of this recovery is still unclear. In one report a rapid reversal was noted within a few weeks to months[8,16]; others, however, suggested that this recovery may take many months[17]. If so, this might be related to the fact that body gastritis impairs the return of acid production after PPI withdrawal, an effect which it has also been suggested may prevent rebound acid secretion as observed in *H. pylori*-positive but not in *H. pylori*-negative subjects[18].

Once this interaction between acid production and *H. pylori* gastritis became clear, the potential long-term implications of PPI therapy shifted from hypergastrinaemia and argyrophil cell hyperplasia to *H. pylori* gastritis. The next question then became whether the induction of a corpus-predominant pangastritis during PPI therapy in *H. pylori*-positive patients had any long-term implications.

GASTRITIS AND THE PROGRESSION TO ATROPHY

Ever since the first cohort studies on gastritis, it has been recognized that chronic inflammation of the gastric mucosa could lead to gland loss or atrophy. These conditions rarely developed in the absence of inflammation. Because of the ubiquitous high prevalence of gastritis, and the failure to recognize the role of *H. pylori*, the process of inflammation and gland loss was considered a normal effect of ageing. Based on an abundance of cross-sectional and follow-up data, Correa proposed 25 years ago a model of gastric carcinogenesis, according to which the predominant intestinal type of gastric cancer occurred via a multistep pathway of gland loss or atrophy, followed by intestinal metaplasia and dysplasia[19]. The data allowed calculations for the rate of development of atrophy as the first step in this process. Less than 1 per 100 subjects without mucosal inflammation would annually develop signs of atrophic gastritis, whereas 1–3 per 100 with gastritis would do so; thus corresponding to annual rates of progression to atrophy of 0–1% and 1–3%, respectively. These data originally came from the Baltic region in northern Europe[20], but remarkably similar findings later came from South America[21], western Europe[22] and recently Africa[23]. They also fitted with the age-dependent increase in both the prevalence of *H. pylori* infection and of atrophic gastritis in many countries all over the world. This age-dependent increase in the prevalance of atrophic gastritis in most countries is very gradual without steepening of the curve with ageing. This reflects a gradual progression to atrophy irrespective of age. No cohort data so far have shown a relation between age and the incidence of atrophic gastritis. The rate of progression to atrophy depends not only on the presence of gastritis, but also on the severity of the inflammatory response to *H. pylori*. This was already known from the older data, but was supported by observations of more severe gastritis and more rapid progression to gland loss in those colonized with *cagA*-positive *H. pylori* strains compared to those with *cagA*-negative strains[24–30]. Moreover, *cagA*-positive infection appeared to increase the risk for development of gastric cancer over *cagA*-negative infections. The correlation between *cagA* and atrophic gastritis was stronger for the corpus than for the antrum. Some authors observed improvement of antral histology during deterioration of body gastritis with gland loss, which is in agreement with data showing improvement of antral gastritis during loss of acid secretion whatever the cause[26]. The correlation between the severity of gastritis and the rate of progression to atrophy formed the basis for discussions on the long-term effect of PPI treatment in *H. pylori*-positive patients.

ACID SUPPRESSION ACCELERATES THE PROGRESSION TO ATROPHIC GASTRITIS

With the first follow-up studies on PPI treatment came reports of atrophic gastritis in a subgroup of patients. Solcia *et al.* observed the development of atrophic gastritis in 12% of 202 patients, mainly with gastro-esophageal reflux disease (GERD), treated with omeprazole for a mean of 1.5 years[4]. Half of them also developed micronodular argyrophil cell hyperplasia, while only 6% of those with non-atrophic gastritis, and 2% of those without gastritis, did so. A German group reported similar findings of atrophic gastritis during omeprazole treatment for duodenal and gastric ulcer disease, as well as for GERD[5,31]. They observed that 19% of their 74 patients developed atrophic gastritis of the body mucosa during periods of treatment up to 5 years. Klinkenberg-Knol et al. reported that 24% of 91 GERD patients developed atrophic gastritis during a mean of 4 years of maintenance treatment with omeprazole[32]. None of these studies made any reference to H. pylori infection, but an increased severity of body gastritis was invariably reported. Also, development of atrophic gastritis was confined to those with active body gastritis during treatment. Even though the rate of progression to atrophic gastritis in each of these studies was considerably faster than the previously reported 1-3% in general populations, no serious concerns were raised. First, the focus was on the behaviour of argyrophil cells, and the absence of any progression beyond micronodular hyperplasia was very reassuring. Second, no attention was given to H. pylori infection and nothing was then known about the acid-dependent nature of this organism. Third, a comparison was never made with data from general populations, but only with data from studies on the development of atrophic gastritis in vagotomized patients or those with gastric ulcer disease[5,6,33]. The patients with gastroduodenal disorders were considered more appropriate controls for omeprazole-treated patients, whereas no attention was given to the fact that vagotomy and gastric ulcer disease, like PPI treatment, are associated with low-acid states. Several older follow-up studies on vagotomized patients and those with gastric ulcer disease consistently reported an accelerated progression to atrophic gastritis, usually at a rate of 4-8% annually[11,12,34]. The PPI data did not differ from these reports, and this was considered the natural progression of gastritis in the presence of gastroduodenal disorders. This interpretation changed with the recognition that H. pylori infection is a key factor in the development of atrophic gastritis and that the severity of gastritis associated with this infection is not only strain-, but also acid-dependent. This recognition shed new light on the observation of an increase in body gastritis after the start of PPI therapy, and also made clear that the development of atrophic gastritis during treatment should be studied in relation to H. pylori infection and that comparisons should be made with subjects with normal acid secretion[35].

We performed a follow-up study of two GERD cohorts, one treated with omeprazole and one treated with fundoplication without any further acid-suppressive therapy[36]. In both cohorts the progression to atrophic gastritis in the absence of H. pylori infection was less than 2% per year. This important observation showed that PPI treatment alone does not induce gland loss, even when given for years. In fundoplication patients with H. pylori infection, the development of atrophic gastritis was also similarly slow. However, H. pylori-positive patients treated with omeprazole showed an increase in the severity of body gastritis after the start of omeprazole therapy and approximately one-third developed signs of atrophic gastritis within the first 5 years of treatment. This was significantly different from those with a fundoplication, and corresponded with an annual incidence of atrophic gastritis of 6.1%[36]. We concluded that this was in agreement with the previous data and the concepts of the acid-dependent behaviour of H. pylori gastritis and the relationship between the severity of gastritis and the rate of progression to atrophy. A minority of our patients also developed intestinal metaplasia in the oxyntic mucosa, invariably type I. Others soon confirmed our findings. Eissele et al. observed, albeit in a small trial, that lansoprazole treatment also increased the severity of chronic active corpus gastritis in *H. pylori*-infected individuals, which led to the development of atrophy in the oxyntic mucosa of 54% of *H. pylori*-colonized non-antrectomized patients within 5 years of treatment[37]. The authors stated that atrophy mainly developed in the first 2 years of therapy and then remained stable. However, this conclusion was based not on a standard survival analysis, but on a simple comparison of different patient groups at different time points, which therefore did not allow sequential comparisons of proportions. Further support came from a Norwegian study, which showed that lansoprazole treatment changed the kinetics of epithelial cell proliferation in the body mucosa of *H. pylori*-positive GERD patients[38], suggesting that this might play a specific role in the process of gland loss. In November 1996, during an FDA meeting on this issue, Astra data on file were presented, which showed that 20% of the patients monitored worldwide with sequential endoscopy and biopsy sampling had developed moderate to severe atrophy of their corpus mucosa after a maximum of 7 years treatment with omeprazole for GERD (G. Neil, personal communication). It was suggested that the absence of such findings in 80% of those patients refuted the previous findings. However, the results were not stratified for *H. pylori* status. As all these patients came from Western societies it can be assumed that no more than 50% of them were *H. pylori*-positive given the overall prevalence of *H. pylori* infection in these countries and the negative association between *H. pylori* colonization and GERD. As all studies consistently showed that atrophic gastritis during PPI treatment almost always occurs in *H. pylori*-positives, the 20% prevalence of moderate to severe atrophic gastritis after a maximum of 7 years omeprazole treatment for GERD would equal a 40% prevalence in *H. pylori*-positives, again confirming previous data. This is further supported by the results of the larger PPI maintenance treatment study with a follow-up to 11 years incorporating almost 1500 patient treatment years[39]. All patients were treated with omeprazole for severe H_2-blocker-resistant GERD. In this study from Australia, Canada, Sweden and the Netherlands, the annual incidence of atrophic gastritis was 0.7% in *H. pylori*-negative patients, but 4.7% in *H. pylori*-positives. Three patients also developed type I intestinal metaplasia although type II and III were again not observed. In agreement with cohort studies in healthy controls[24,26], atrophic gastritis in these PPI maintenance studies occurred in patients with moderate to severe inflammation of the oxyntic mucosa[36,39]. In the large multinational study, 94% of the patients with atrophic gastritis had previous signs of moderate to severe gastritis[39]. In our own study, development of atrophic gastritis during omeprazole treatment corresponded with the presence of *cagA*-positive *H. pylori* strains[40].

ACID SUPPRESSION DOES NOT ACCELERATE THE PROGRESSION TO ATROPHIC GASTRITIS

Unlike the studies mentioned above, several studies have reported no accelerated progression to atrophy in *H. pylori*-positive GERD patients treated with PPIs. One cross-sectional study observed a similar prevalence of atrophy among omeprazole-treated GERD patients as among dyspeptic controls[41]. However, the investigators had no baseline histology and, therefore, were not able to compare any rates of progression to atrophy. Also, the duration of omeprazole therapy prior to evaluation was relatively short and the selection of GERD cases versus dyspeptic controls introduced a bias with a potential higher prevalence of atrophy at baseline in the controls. Second, unpublished data presented at the FDA meeting on this issue described that only one of 99 *H. pylori*-infected GERD patients developed atrophy during treatment with lansoprazole for 15 months (J. W. Freston, personal communication). However, the limited size and follow-up of this study led to such a large confidence limit for the incidence of atrophic gastritis that the findings were not different from any of the previous PPI studies. Also, the protocol allowed a single pathologist to diagnose non-atrophic gastritis, but if she considered a diagnosis of atrophic gastritis, repeated evaluation by a second and sometimes third pathologist was required before this diagnosis could be made. This policy may have induced a selection against the diagnosis of atrophy. A third study also did not observe any progression to atrophic gastritis during PPI treatment. The investigators followed 62 duodenal ulcer patients during treatment with 15 mg lansoprazole daily, approximately half of whom were studied after 12 months of treatment and none had developed signs of gastric atrophy[16]. However, the investigators, unlike others, scored for the presence or absence of gastric atrophy, or a complete loss of glands. Such complete loss of glands would have been a very rapid phenomenon within 1 year of treatment. Also, as with the previous study, the sample size was too limited to narrow the confidence limit for the incidence of atrophic gastritis to levels below the incidence of atrophy observed in the earlier larger studies. For example, a study with a 1% incidence of atrophic gastritis would require at least 200 patient-years of follow-up before the upper limit of the incidence of atrophic gastritis would not be greater than 3%, i.e. the maximum reported incidence in a general population cohort not treated with vagotomy or acid suppression[21]. As such, this study, with approximately 30 patient-years of follow-up, had a six-fold too small sample size to allow conclusions about differences in the progression to atrophic gastritis in comparison with previous studies. The same group also followed 60 GERD patients during 1 year of treatment with either 20 mg omeprazole or 15 or 30 mg lansoprazole once daily[42]. Again, no development of gastric atrophy was observed, but 12% of the patients treated with 30 mg lansoprazole developed intestinal metaplasia of the corpus mucosa as a sign of atrophic gastritis.

The strongest evidence against an association between PPI treatment and accelerated progression to atrophic gastritis in *H. pylori*-positive patients was claimed in a multicentre Scandinavian study developed to compare the efficacy of omeprazole and surgical fundoplication for the control of GERD symptoms[43]. Analysis of sequential gastric biopsy specimens in these patients observed the development of moderate to severe atrophy in only two (4.5%) of 44 *H. pylori*-positive fundoplication patients without this condition at baseline, compared with seven (17.9%) of 39 omeprazole-treated patients[44].

Atrophic gastritis was usually preceded by moderate to severe corpus gastritis. These findings correspond to an annual progression to atrophy of 1.5% during presumed normal acid secretion, and 6.0% during acid suppression, which is in agreement with the other studies on this issue[10]. Nevertheless, as this difference was not significant, the authors claimed that their results showed that omeprazole treatment is not associated with an accelerated progression to atrophic gastritis in *H. pylori*-positive patients[44]. This claim was criticized by several European experts[45-48]. First, it was concluded, that this study simply lacked the necessary size to demonstrate significance for the difference in progression to atrophy between populations with normal and those with reduced acid secretion. In other words, before starting out with any analysis the investigators could already have predicted a non-significant result. Second, the fundoplication 'controls' in the Lundell study might simply not have the required normal acid output throughout the period of observation. All were treated with omeprazole until surgery, and 25% of them were also treated with a vagotomy or with omeprazole postoperatively. An increase in atrophy scores was observed in three (7.5%) of the 40 controls without versus four (31%) of the 13 controls with vagotomy or postoperative omeprazole ($p = 0.05$; Fisher exact). Similarly, a decrease in atrophy scores was observed in six (15%) of the controls without and none of the controls with vagotomy or postoperative omeprazole ($p = 0.3$; Fisher exact). Third, although the authors did attempt to randomize the patients, they failed, like others, to study patient groups with the same age. Finally, the data had been presented at various previous meetings[49] and the data in the paper differed from those presented previously, leading to a reduction of patients with atrophic gastritis. In the original abstract, six patients ended up with severe atrophic gastritis, four during omeprazole treatment[49]. In the full paper only one fundoplication patient did so, despite the same follow-up, number of patients and experienced pathologist involved[44]. This discrepancy could not be due to a change in classification since severe atrophy is a straightforward diagnosis ((sub)total loss of glands with specialized cells) within each classification and the investigators could not account for it. A further spontaneous reduction of atrophic gastritis was noted after 5 years follow-up, as presented recently[50]. This is the first cohort study to show spontaneous net regression of atrophic gastritis in the absence of *H. pylori* eradication. No explanation for this phenomenon was suggested.

ACID SUPPRESSION AND THE ONSET OF ATROPHIC GASTRITIS; POTENTIAL CONFOUNDERS

The issue of *H. pylori*, acid, and gastritis has been extensively debated in the past 4 years. A major concern has been that scoring of atrophic gastritis is compromised by the presence of inflammation, suggesting that the increase of corpus inflammation associated with PPI use in *H. pylori*-infected patients may give a false impression of gland loss[51]. As such, it has been suggested that 'atrophy' development during PPI use is a non-existent phenomenon. Although this issue may cause difficulty for the pathologist in individual cases, it seems overemphasized for study cohorts as a whole, in particular if the histology is read by experienced pathologists who know not to diagnose atrophy on the distribution of glands alone, but consider the presence of fibrosis or metaplasia a prerequisite for the diagnosis of gland loss. This is supported by several factors. First, the intra- and inter-observer reproducibility for the diagnosis of atrophic gastritis is generally good[52-54], even when disputable cases are selected[53]. Secondly, PPI therapy is associated with an immediate increase of body gastritis, which then remains stable[36,39]. If such gastritis would lead to a false diagnosis of atrophic gastritis, one might expect PPIs to be associated with an immediate and stable onset of atrophic gastritis, reversible after withdrawal of therapy. However, there is no follow-up study which describes such a pattern or onset of atrophic gastritis in the first few months of therapy. Likewise, we did not observe any change in atrophy scores by the Sydney system during short-term treatment with 40 mg of omeprazole[10]. Finally, we recently quantitatively measured the volumes of gland epithelium, infiltrate and stroma in histological slides[55]. The atrophy scores given by two experienced pathologists using the updated Sydney system closely correlated with the measured volumes of specialized epithelium. Increasing grades of atrophy correlated with a four-fold greater decrease in epithelial volume than the accompanying increase in infiltrate volume. Thus, increasing grades of atrophy correspond to a true loss of epithelial volume instead of a surrogate loss due to an increase of inflammatory infiltrate. This was accompanied by a gradual decrease of serum vitamin B_{12} levels in *H. pylori*-positive patients, who developed moderate to severe corpus atrophy during PPI use[56].

A second potential confounder is age. In two cohort studies the omeprazole-treated patients were older than those treated without acid suppression[36,44]. The highest incidence of atrophic gastritis in the omeprazole-treated patients might therefore be related to age rather than acid suppression. Atrophy can occur at any time during adult life. Once it has occurred, it will generally not regress unless *H. pylori* eradication therapy is given. Therefore, increasing age is associated with an increasing *prevalence* of atrophy. However, these studies focused on the prospective annual *incidence* of atrophy; the proportion of subjects in a cohort that annually develops atrophy when prospectively followed. There are so far no cohort follow-up data to suggest that this incidence of atrophic gastritis is age-dependent. The available cohort studies that analysed the data by age, the long-term Finnish study[57], the large Columbian study[21], our own volunteer study[22], and the multinational large omeprazole study[39] did not show that the incidence of atrophic gastritis was age-dependent. In our PPI study there was no difference in age between those that developed atrophy and those that did not[36].

ACID SUPPRESSION AND THE ONSET OF ATROPHIC GASTRITIS, MECHANISMS AND CONSEQUENCES

The development of atrophy is mostly preceded by moderate to severe inflammation, but the exact mechanisms leading to gland loss are unclear; it is most likely due to a direct damaging effect of chronic inflammation.

However, in a recent elegant animal study, Wang et al. suggested that gland loss may also result from hypergastrinaemia[58]. Transgenic mice with moderate hypergastrinaemia showed progression to atrophic gastritis and gastric cancer even in the absence of chronic gastritis. This process was accelerated if the mice were colonized with H. felis. The authors hypothesized that increased gastrin levels up-regulate growth factors such as transforming growth factor alpha, which would then play a role in the development of foveolar hyperplasia and loss of parietal cells and gastric glands.

Not only the exact mechanisms, but also the consequences of gland loss in H. pylori-positive GERD patients during PPI treatment remain unclear. Apart from the potential long-term effects on vitamin B_{12} levels, a loss of gastric glands with specialized cells may be beneficial for reflux disease, as reduction of acid facilitates GERD treatment. Concern and speculation has focused on the potential for an increased risk for gastric cancer. In this respect it is considered reassuring that only a few patients develop intestinal metaplasia during the first years of PPI treatment, and this has always been type I metaplasia of the incomplete type[51]. However, the true importance of this finding is still speculative. First, the follow-up after development of gland loss in all these studies is short and no more than a few years. The natural progression to atrophy and subsequent metaplasia is known to take much longer. Whether or not gland loss in H. pylori-positive GERD patients treated with PPIs will facilitate the later development of metaplasia is unknown. Furthermore, it is also unclear whether intestinal metaplasia is the actual precursor of gastric adenocarcinoma or a bystander. For example, the complete or type III intestinal metaplasia, in retrospective studies, is found in only a small minority of resection specimens for gastric cancer[59]. Although one cohort study originally reported an increased risk for cancer in the presence of type III metaplasia[60], the archival diagnosis of metaplasia subtypes was used. If, after revision, only the samples were used in which the earlier diagnosis could be confirmed, no significant differences were observed in cancer incidence between subjects with atrophy without metaplasia and subjects with atrophy with different subtypes of metaplasia[61]. This is in agreement with another study[62]. In this context some authors consider not the presence of atrophy or metaplasia *per se*, but the presence of a corpus-predominant pangastritis as a risk factor for later development of gastric cancer[7,63,64]. This hypothesis does not consider the nature or diagnostic pitfalls of atrophic gastritis or the importance of subtypes of intestinal metaplasia, but simply links gastric cancer risk with the severity and distribution of gastritis.

CAN *H. PYLORI* ERADICATION PREVENT THE DEVELOPMENT OF ATROPHIC GASTRITIS DURING PPI THERAPY?

The worsening of body gastritis and the associated onset of atrophy in H. pylori-positive patients treated with PPIs has led to the suggestion to eradicate H. pylori infection when prescribing long-term PPI maintenance therapy[42,65]. However, even though it is plausible to assume that such a strategy would heal gastritis and prevent atrophy, these assumptions need to be proven, and it is also necessary to show that such intervention would not be associated with adverse effects such as worsening of reflux symptoms or the need for higher doses of acid suppression therapy. These concerns were based on the observation of a negative association between *H. pylori* and both the development and severity of GERD, and the observation that *H. pylori* augments the antisecretory effects of PPI treatment.

In a small 1-year follow-up study of GERD patients, treated with omeprazole, Moayyedi *et al.* observed the development of atrophic gastritis only in *H. pylori*-positive patients, but not in *H. pylori*-negative or in *H. pylori*-positive patients treated with eradication therapy[66]. In a similar study we observed that *H. pylori* eradication could prevent the increase of corpus gastritis associated with omeprazole therapy[67]. In this study no dose adjustment of the PPI was necessary after eradication. Finally, a large multicentre international study is currently being performed to determine whether *H. pylori* eradication can prevent atrophic gastritis during PPI treatment.

In conclusion, acid suppression accelerates the onset of atrophic gastritis in *H. pylori*-infected patients. This phenomenon is biologically plausible and explained by the interaction between *H. pylori* and pH, the consistent report of pangastritis during profound acid suppression, and the demonstration that the distribution and severity of gastritis are related to atrophy. The conclusion is based on an extensive literature, which shows that the effect is not related to age, country of origin or pathologist involved in the studies. This necessitates further studies into the effect of *H. pylori* eradication in GERD patients treated with PPI maintenance therapy.

References

1. Sjöstrand SE, Olbe L, Fellenius E. The discovery and development of the proton pump inhibitor. In: Olbe L, editor. Proton Pump Inhibitors. Basel: Birkhäuser Verlag; 1999:3–20.
2. Bonnevie O, Nielsen AM, Matzen P *et al.* Gastric acid secretion and duodenal ulcer healing during treatment with omeprazole. Scand J Gastroenterol. 1984;19:882–4.
3. Hurenkamp GJB, Grundmeyer HGLM, Bindels PJE, Tytgat GNJ, van der Hulst RWM. A population-based inventarisation of longterm acid suppressant use in 24 general practices in the Netherlands. Digestion. 1998;59(Suppl. 3):101.
4. Solcia E, Fiocca R, Havu N, Dalväg A, Carlsson R. Gastric endocrine cells and gastritis in patients receiving long-term omeprazole treatment. Digestion. 1992;51(Suppl. 1):82–92.
5. Lamberts R, Creutzfeld W, Strüber HG, Brunner G, Solcia E. Long-term omeprazole therapy in peptic ulcer disease: gastrin, endocrine cell growth, and gastritis. Gastroenterology. 1993;104:1356–70.
6. Modlin IM, Goldenring JR, Lawton GP, Hunt R. Aspects of the theoretical basis and clinical relevance of low acid states. Am J Gastroenterol. 1994;89:308–18.
7. Veldhuyzen van Zanten SOJ, Dixon MF, Lee A. The gastric transitional zones: neglected links between gastroduodenal pathology and *Helicobacter* ecology. Gastroenterology. 1999;116:1217–29.
8. Solcia E, Villani L, Fiocca R *et al.* Effects of eradication of *Helicobacter pylori* on gastritis in duodenal ulcer patients. Scand J Gastroenterol. 1994;29(Suppl. 201):28–34.
9. Logan RPH, Walker MM, Misiewicz JJ, Gummett PA, Karim QN, Baron JH. Changes in the intragastric distribution of *Helicobacter pylori* during treatment with omeprazole. Gut. 1995;36:12–16.
10. Kuipers EJ, Uyterlinde AM, Peña AS *et al.* Increase of *Helicobacter pylori* associated corpus gastritis during acid suppressive therapy: implications for long-term safety. Am J Gastroenterol. 1995;90:1401–6.

11. Roland M, Berstad A, Liavåg I. A histological study of gastric mucosa before and after proximal gastric vagotomy in duodenal ulcer patients. Scand J Gastroenterol. 1975; 10:181–6.
12. Jorde R, Johnson JA, Bostad LH, Burhol PG. An endoscopic study of ulcer recurrence and mucosal changes following vagotomy and excision of gastric ulcer. Acta Chir Scand. 1987;153:297–302.
13. Äärimaa M, Söderström KO, Kalimo H, Inberg M. Morphology and function of the parietal cells after proximal selective vagotomy in duodenal ulcer patients. Scand J Gastroenterol. 1984;19:787–97.
14. Hart Hansen O, Larsen JK, Svendsen LB. Changes in gastric mucosal cell proliferation after antrectomy or vagotomy in man. Scand J Gastroenterol. 1978;13:947–52.
15. Rektorschek M, Weeks D, Sachs G, Melchers K. Influence of pH on metabolism and urease activity of *Helicobacter pylori*. Gastroenterology. 1998;115:628–41.
16. Meining A, Kiel G, Stolte M. Changes in *Helicobacter pylori*-induced gastritis in the antrum and corpus and after 12 months of treatment with ranitidine and lansoprazole in patients with duodenal ulcer disease. Aliment Pharmacol Ther. 1998;12:735–40.
17. Hackelsberger A, Miehlke S, Len N et al. *Helicobacter pylori* eradication vs short term acid suppression: long term consequences for gastric body mucosa. Gastroenterology. 1996; 110:A127 (abstract).
18. Gillen D, Wirz AA, Ardill JE, McColl KEL. Rebound hypersecretion post-omeprazole and its relation to on-treatment acid suppression and *Helicobacter pylori* status. Gastroenterology. 1999;116:239–47.
19. Correa P, Haenszel W, Cuello C, Tannenbaum S, Archer M. A model for gastric cancer epidemiology. Lancet. 1975;2:58–9.
20. Villako K, Kekki M, Tamm A et al. Epidemiology and dynamics of gastritis in a random sample of an Estonian urban population. Scand J Gastroenterol. 1982;17:601–7.
21. Correa P, Haenszel W, Cuello C et al. Gastric precancerous process in a high-risk population: cohort follow-up. Cancer Res. 1990;50:4737–40.
22. Kuipers EJ, Uyterlinde AM, Peña AS et al. Long term sequelae of *Helicobacter pylori* gastritis. Lancet. 1995;345:1525–8.
23. McFarlane GA, Wyatt J, Forman D, Lachlan GW. Trends over time in *H. pylori* gastritis in Kenya. Eur J Gastroenterol Hepatol. 1999;12 (In press).
24. Kuipers EJ, Pérez-Pérez GI, Meuwissen SGM, Blaser MJ. *Helicobacter pylori* and atrophic gastritis: importance of the *cagA* status. J Natl Cancer Inst. 1995;87:1777–80.
25. Ponzetto A, DeGiuli M, Sanseverino P, Soldati T, Bazzoli F. *Helicobacter pylori* and atrophic gastritis: importance of the *cagA* status. J Natl Cancer Inst. 1996;88:465–6.
26. Maaroos HI, Vorobjova T, Sipponen P et al. An 18-year follow-up study of chronic gastritis and *Helicobacter pylori*: association of CagA positivity with development of atrophy and activity of gastritis. Scand J Gastroenterol. 1999;34:864–9.
27. Beales ILP, Crabtree JE, Scunes D, Covacci A, Calam J. Antibodies to CagA protein are associated with gastric atrophy in *Helicobacter pylori* infection. Eur J Gastroenterol Hepatol. 1996;8:645–9.
28. Sozzi M, Valentini M, Figura N et al. Atrophic gastritis and intestinal metaplasia in *Helicobacter pylori* infection: the role of CagA status. Am J Gastroenterol. 1998;93:375–9.
29. Yamaoka Y, Kita M, Kodama T, Sawai N, Kashima K, Imanishi J. Induction of various cytokines and development of severe mucosal inflammation by *cagA* gene positive *Helicobacter pylori* strains. Gut. 1997;41.442–51.
30. Warburton VJ, Everett S, Mapstone NP, Axon AT, Hawkey P, Dixon MF. Clinical and histological association of *cagA* and *vacA* genotypes in *Helicobacter pylori* gastritis. J Clin Pathol. 1998;51–55–61.
31. Brunner GHG, Lamberts R, Creutzfeldt W. Efficacy and safety of omeprazole in long-term treatment of peptic ulcer and reflux oesophagitis resistant to ranitidine. Digestion. 1990; 47(Suppl. 1):64–8.
32. Klinkenberg-Knol EC, Festen HPM, Jansen JBMJ et al. Efficacy and safety of long-term treatment with omeprazole for refractory reflux esophagitis. Ann Intern Med. 1994; 121:161–7.
33. Freston JW. Omeprazole, hypergastrinemia, and gastric carcinoid tumors. Ann Intern Med. 1994;121:232–3.

34. Jönsson KÅ, Ström M, Bodemar G, Norrby K. Histologic changes in the gastroduodenal mucosa after long-term medical treatment with cimetidine or parietal cell vagotomy in patients with juxtapyloric ulcer disease. Scand J Gastroenterol. 1988;23:433–41.
35. Kuipers EJ, Lee A, Klinkenberg-Knol EC, Meuwissen SGM. Review article: The development of atrophic gastritis – *Helicobacter pylori* and the effects of acid suppressive therapy. Aliment Pharmacol Ther. 1995;9:331–40.
36. Kuipers EJ, Lundell L, Klinkenberg-Knol EC et al. Atrophic gastritis and *Helicobacter pylori* infection in patients with reflux esophagitis treated with omeprazole or fundoplication. N Engl J Med. 1996;334:1018–22.
37. Eissele R, Brunner G, Simon B, Solcia E, Arnold R. Gastric mucosa during treatment with lansoprazole: *Helicobacter pylori* is a risk factor for argyrophil-cell hyperplasia. Gastroenterology. 1997;112:707–17.
38. Berstad AE, Hatlebakk JG, Maartmann-Moe H, Berstad A, Brandtzaeg P. *Helicobacter pylori* gastritis and epithelial cell proliferation in patients with reflux oesophagitis after treatment with lansoprazole. Gut. 1997;41:740–7.
39. Klinkenberg-Knol EC, Nelis F, Dent J et al. Experience with omeprazole in the treatment of resistant gastroesophageal reflux disease: efficacy, safety and influence on gastric mucosa. Gastroenterology. 2000;118:661–9.
40. Kuipers EJ, Schenk BE, Pérez-Pérez GI, Roosendaal R, Meuwissen SGM, Blaser MJ. The relation of *H. pylori* CagA and HspA serum antibodies with age and development of atrophic gastritis during profound acid suppressive maintenance therapy. Gastroenterology. 1997;112:A185 (abstract).
41. Diebold M-D, Richardson S, Duchateau A et al. Factors influencing corpus argyrophil cell density and hyperplasia in reflux esophagitis patients treated with antisecretory drugs. Dig Dis Sci. 1998;43:1629–35.
42. Stolte M, Meining A, Schmitz JM, Alexandridis T, Seifert E. Changes in *Helicobacter pylori*-induced gastritis in the antrum and corpus during 12 months of treatment with omeprazole and lansoprazole in patients with gastro-oesophageal reflux disease. Aliment Pharmacol Ther. 1998;12:247–53.
43. Lundell L, Abrahamsson H, Ruth M, Rydberg L, Lönroth H, Olbe L. Long-term results of a prospective randomized comparison of total fundic wrap (Nissen–Rossetti) or semifundoplication (Toupet) for gastro-oesophageal reflux. Br J Surg. 1996;83:830–5.
44. Lundell L, Miettinen P, Myrvol HE et al. Lack of effect of acid suppression therapy on gastric atrophy. Gastroenterology. 1999;117:319–26.
45. Pounder RE, Williams MP. Omeprazole and accelerated onset of atrophic gastritis. Gastroenterology. 2000;118:238–9.
46. McColl KEL, Murray LS, Gillen D. Omeprazole and accelerated onset of atrophic gastritis. Gastroenterology. 2000;118:239.
47. Kuipers EJ, Klinkenberg-Knol EC, Meuwissen SGM. Omeprazole and accelerated onset of atrophic gastritis. Gastroenterology. 2000;118:239–40.
48. Stolte M, Meining A. Lack of effect of acid suppression therapy on gastric atrophy. Gastroenterology. 2000;118:242–3.
49. Lundell L, Havu N, Andersson A et al. Gastritis development and acid suppression therapy revisited. Results of a randomized clinical study with long-term follow-up. Gastroenterology. 1997;112:A771.
50. Lundell L, Havu N, Miettinen P et al. No effect of acid suppression therapy over five years on gastric glandular atrophy. Results of a randomised clinical study. Gut. 2000;118:A214.
51. Genta RM. Acid suppression and gastric atrophy: sifting fact from fiction. Gut. 1998; 43(Suppl. 1):S35–8.
52. Plummer M, Buiatti E, Lopez G et al. Histological diagnosis of precancerous lesions of the stomach: a reliability study. Int J Epidemiol. 1997;26:716–20.
53. Offerhaus GJA, Price AB, Haot J et al. Observer agreement on the grading of gastric atrophy. Histopathology. 1999;34:320–5.
54. Guarner J, Herrera-Goepfert R, Mohar A et al. Interobserver variability in application of the revised Sydney classification for gastritis. Hum Pathol. 1999;30:1431–4.
55. van Grieken NCT, Weiss MM, Meijer GA et al. Rapid quantitative assessment of gastric corpus atrophy in tissue sections. J Clin Pathol. 2000 (in press).
56. Schenk BE, Kuipers EJ, Klinkenberg-Knol EC et al. Atrophic gastritis during long-term omeprazole therapy affects serum vitamin B12 levels. Aliment Pharmacol Ther. 1999; 13:1343–6.

57. Valle J, Kekki M, Sipponen P, Ihamäki T, Siurala M. Long-term course and consequences of *Helicobacter pylori* gastritis. Scand J Gastroenterol. 1996;31:546–50.
58. Wang TC, Dangler CA, Chen D *et al*. Synergistic interaction between hypergastrinemia and *Helicobacter* infection in a mouse model of gastric cancer. Gastroenterology. 2000; 118:36–47.
59. Sipponen P, Seppälä K, Varis K *et al*. Intestinal metaplasia with colonic-type sulphomucins in the gastric mucosa; its association with gastric carcinoma. Acta Pathol Microbiol Scand. 1980;88:217–24.
60. Filipe MI, Muñoz N, Matko I *et al*. Intestinal metaplasia types and the risk of gastric cancer: a cohort study in Slovenia. Int J Cancer. 1994;57:324–9.
61. Dixon MF. Atrophy, metaplasia and dysplasia – a risk for gastric cancer: are they reversible? In: Hunt RH, Tytgat GNJ, editors. *Helicobacter pylori*. Basic Mechanisms to Clinical Cure. Dordrecht: Kluwer; 1998:336–53.
62. Ectors N, Dixon MF. The prognostic value of sulphomucin positive intestinal metaplasia in the development of gastric cancer. Histopathology. 1986;10:1271–7.
63. Meining A, Bayerdörffer E, Müller P *et al*. Gastric carcinoma risk index in patients infected with *Helicobacter pylori*. Virch Arch. 1998;432:311–14.
64. El-Omar EM, Oien K, El-Nujumi A *et al*. *Helicobacter pylori* infection and chronic acid hyposecretion. Gastroenterology. 1997;113:15–24.
65. Malfertheiner P. Current European concepts in the management of *Helicobacter pylori* infection: the Maastricht consensus report. Gut. 1997;41:8–13.
66. Axon ATR, Bardhan K, Moayeddi P, Dixon MF. Does eradication of *H. pylori* influence the recurrence of symptoms in patients with symptomatic gastro-oesophageal reflux disease? – A randomised double blind study. Gastroenterology. 1999;116:A117 (abstract).
67. Schenk BE, Kuipers EJ, Nelis GF *et al*. Effect of *Helicobacter pylori* eradication on chronic gastritis during omeprazole therapy. Gut. 2000;46:615–21.

29
Proton pump inhibitors do not accelerate the development of gastric atrophy in *Helicobacter pylori* gastritis

J. W. FRESTON

INTRODUCTION

Kuipers and colleagues[1] suggested in 1996 that long-term acid suppression by omeprazole accelerates the development of atrophic gastritis in patients infected with *Helicobacter pylori*. This, in turn, may facilitate the development of intestinal metaplasia, dysplasia, and gastric adenocarcinoma. This report received widespread media attention because of the public perception, particularly in the United States, that the increasing use of proton pump inhibitors (PPIs), already suspected to be carcinogenic, would cause even more cancer, given the ubiquity of *H. pylori* infection and gastro-oesophageal reflux disease (GERD) in the general population. The Food and Drug Administration (FDA) convened an urgent meeting to determine if PPIs should be removed from the market or have substantial changes in approved indications and directions for use.

Many observers, including this author[2], embraced the Kuipers hypothesis, and the European *H. pylori* consensus conference in Maastricht recommended that patients with GERD be tested and treated for *H. pylori* infection before undergoing chronic PPI treatment[3]. This 'bandwagon' effect did not seem inappropriate at the time, given the supporting information about the development of atrophic gastritis in low acid states. It was evident by then that the rate of progression to atrophy of gastric glands is associated with the severity and distribution of gastritis, which are, in turn, dependent on the degree of acid secretion[4]. Also evident was the fact that the intensity of the inflammatory response to *H. pylori* infection is altered during PPI therapy, becoming more intense in the corpus and less intense in the antrum[5,6].

In this setting the Kuipers hypothesis began to be accepted as definitive proof. Second thoughts on the part of some crept in by 1997, largely because some new information did not support the hypothesis[7,8]. The subsequent discussion has featured claims and counterclaims about the validity of key studies on both sides of the issue. The purpose of this report is to analyse the available data to determine whether the evidence does or does not prove that chronic PPI therapy accelerates the progression of *H. pylori* gastritis to atrophic gastritis and, thereby, increases the risk of developing intestinal metaplasia and gastric cancer. This issue seemed moot previously, given the ease with which *H. pylori* infection can be eradicated. However, the wisdom of eradicating the organism in all infected people, regardless of their clinical condition, has been challenged recently, largely because of the apparent protective effect of *H. pylori* infection against the development of GERD and its complications, including Barrett's oesophagus, dysplasia and adenocarcinoma of the oesophagus[9–12]. This development complicates the question of whether *H. pylori* should be eradicated in patients with GERD.

STUDIES WITH CONTROLS

The Kuipers study[1]

This study featured a comparison of the rate of progression to atrophic gastritis in two cohorts of patients. One cohort consisted of 105 Dutch patients with GERD treated with omeprazole, 20–40 mg daily, the other cohort consisted of 72 Swedish patients with GERD resistant to H_2-receptor antagonists who were treated with fundoplication. They did not receive acid-suppressive therapy after surgery. The mean age of the Dutch and Swedish patients was 62 and 53 years, respectively. The presence of *H. pylori* infection was established before omeprazole treatment by serology and histology on corpus biopsies obtained by endoscopy. *H. pylori* infection was established in the surgery patients by histology. The infection was not treated in any patient. All patients had repeated corpus biopsies during the follow-up period of 3–8 years. *H. pylori* gastritis was evaluated according to the Sydney System[13]. The criteria for the diagnosis of atrophic gastritis were not stated. (The term glandular atrophy has largely replaced atrophic gastritis and will be used throughout this chapter.)

The point prevalence of corpus glandular atrophy at the beginning and end of the observation period is depicted in Figure 1. No glandular atrophy was present at baseline in the infected patients treated with omeprazole, but 18 of the 59 had atrophy at the conclusion. In the surgery cohort none of the 31 infected patients developed atrophy. None of the patients in either cohort developed intestinal metaplasia. The authors concluded that omeprazole treatment increased the risk of *H. pylori*-infected patients developing glandular atrophy.

The Lundell study[14]

This was a randomized study of the comparative efficacy and safety of antireflux surgery and chronic omeprazole therapy in patients with GERD. All patients had been treated initially with omeprazole 20–40 mg daily for no more than 4 months. Those who experienced symptom relief were ran-

Percentage of patients with corpus atrophy

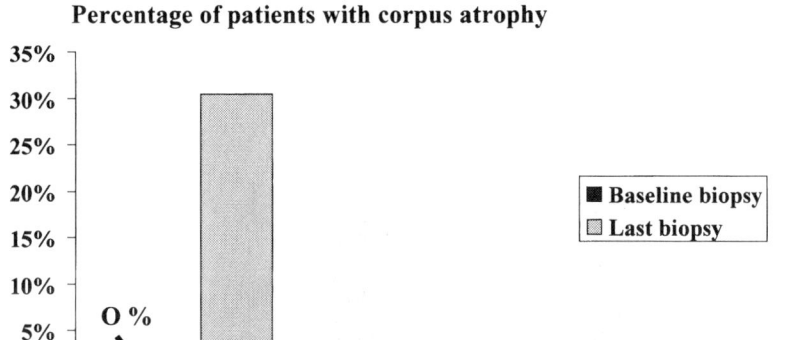

Figure 1. Prevalence of corpus glandular atrophy at baseline and after 5 years in patients with *H. pylori* infection treated continuously with omeprazole (left) or anti-reflux surgery (right). The difference in the prevalence at 5 years between the omeprazole and antireflux cohorts is statistically significant ($p = 0.001$). Data from ref. 1.

domized to omeprazole maintenance therapy or antireflux surgery. The mean age of patients in the omeprazole group and surgery group was 56 and 51 years, respectively. Gastric biopsies were obtained for histological evaluation at the beginning of the study and periodically during the 5-year follow-up period. All biopsies were evaluated by a single pathologist who, incidentally, was the same pathologist in the Kuipers study. According to the authors[15], the degree of glandular atrophy was first determined according to Whitehead[16], but subsequently according to the Sydney System[14]. A planned interim analysis at 3 years compared the intensity of inflammation and the prevalence of glandular atrophy and intestinal metaplasia in the two groups.

In this study 155 patients were randomized to the omeprazole group; 40 of these had *H. pylori* infection. A total of 144 patients were randomized to the surgery group; 53 of these had *H. pylori* infection. The point prevalence of glandular atrophy at baseline and after 3 years is shown in Figure 2. There was no difference in the progression to atrophy. In the omeprazole group, seven infected patients had atrophy at the beginning, compared to 10 at the end. In the surgery group, nine had atrophy at the beginning and 10 at the end. Most of the atrophy at baseline in the two groups was of mild severity, and there was no difference in the two groups with respect to progression to moderate or severe grades of atrophy. There also was no increase in the prevalence of intestinal metaplasia in either group. The authors concluded that long-term omeprazole therapy did not accelerate the progression of glandular atrophy.

Because most of the debate has focused on these two studies, their relative strengths and weaknesses will be compared. Various aspects of the results of the two studies are compared in Table 1. The major strength of the Kuipers study is its relatively large number of *H. pylori*-infected patients

Percentage of patients with corpus atrophy

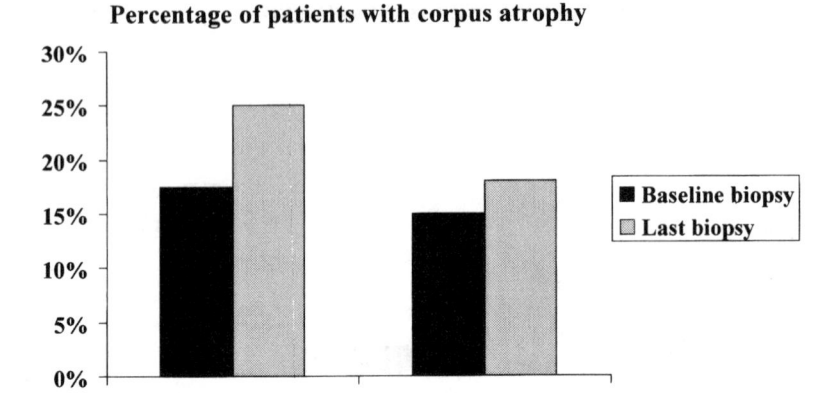

Figure 2. Prevalence of corpus glandular atrophy at baseline and after 3 years in patients with *H. pylori* infection treated continuously with omeprazole (left) or anti-reflux surgery (right). The difference in prevalence between the two groups after 3 years is not statistically significant ($p = 0.57$). Data from ref. 14.

Table 1. Comparison of the Kuipers[1] and Lundell[14] studies (modified from ref. 15, with permission)

	Kuipers	Lundell
Study duration	5 (range 3–8)	3
Antireflux surgery		
Patients (n)	72	144
Ratio of Hp$^+$/Hp$^-$	31/41	53/90
Mean age at baseline (years)	53 (range 25–73)	51 (range 18–77)
Hp$^+$ subjects		
Gastritis prevalance from start to end (n)	24 → 42	42 → 37
Atrophy prevalence from start to end (n)	1 → 1	8 → 10[a]
Omeprazone treatment		
Patients (n)	105	155
Ratio of Hp$^+$/Hp$^-$	59/46	40/115
Mean age at baseline (years)	62 (range 16–83)	56 (range 21–76)
Hp$^+$ subjects		
Gastritis prevalance from start to end (n)	35 → 48	34 → 32
Atrophy prevalance from start to end (n)	0 → 18	7 → 10

n = Number of patients.
[a] Excludes patients with acid-lowering surgery, e.g. vagotomy.
Hp$^+$ = *H. pylori*-positive; Hp$^-$ = *H. pylori*-negative.

studied for an average of 5 years. In addition, the corpus biopsies were evaluated by the same experienced pathologist. Its major shortcoming is its lack of an appropriate control group. The omeprazole cohort was studied in the Netherlands independently of the surgery cohort. Only later, apparently at the request of the *New England Journal of Medicine*, to which the uncontrolled omeprazole paper was submitted, was a surgery cohort identified in Sweden and incorporated as a comparator group. This introduced bias. The mean age of the omeprazole group was 9 years higher than in the surgery group. This is important because the development of atrophy increases with ageing, having a prevalence twice as high in *H. pylori*-infected subjects in the 57–68-year cohort than in the 46–56-year age cohort[17]. The fact that two different populations were compared may also be significant, given the genetic, socioeconomic, nutritional and dietary factors that influence the development of atrophy. Possibly the most troubling aspect of the Kuipers study was the total absence of atrophy at baseline in the omeprazole cohort, combined with the absence of any increase in atrophy over a period of 5 years in the surgery cohort. These findings differ from all other studies that show at least some atrophy in populations with *H. pylori* gastritis and at least some progression over time if the infection is untreated (see below). This combination of unusual findings may have been responsible for the difference reaching statistical significance.

The strengths of the Lundell study include its randomization, the systematic collection of biopsies according to a protocol, and their histopathological interpretation by an experienced pathologist (N. Havu, also the pathologist in the Kuipers study). It is not, however, without its flaws[81-20]. Some patients had a vagotomy and should be excluded because their low-acid state resembles that of patients treated with omeprazole. Their exclusion does not change the conclusions, but does contribute to what is probably the most serious deficiency: the relatively small number of patients with *H. pylori* infection in the two cohorts. It has been argued that this could have prevented the detection of a real difference between the groups[20]. The surgery patients in the Lundell study were treated with omeprazole[14] or with omeprazole or H_2-receptor antagonists[15] for up to 4 months before surgery. It has been argued that this set in motion an inflammatory process that eventually led to a high rate of atrophy in the surgery group, thereby preventing the detection of a difference between the groups[18]. However, the inflammatory changes induced by acid suppression are reversible[21].

Controlled studies analysed by the FDA[8]

The widespread publicity generated by the *New England Journal of Medicine*'s press release of the Kuipers study prompted the FDA to convene an advisory committee to evaluate the evidence linking PPI therapy to gastric glandular atrophy or other risk factors for gastric cancer[10]. Dr Kuipers presented this study and the results of earlier studies linking low-acid states to gastric atrophy. Preliminary data from the Lundell study were presented. The FDA also directed sponsors of PPIs to present all long-term data from their US and European trials; these are summarized in Tables 2–5.

The studies consisted of randomized, controlled trials of PPI maintenance therapy of erosive oesophagitis for 12–60 months and duodenal ulcer disease for up to 2 years. The comparator groups were placebo, ranitidine, and antireflux surgery. The patients included had corpus biopsies at baseline and final visit. The incidence of *H. pylori* infection was estimated to be 20–40% in the GERD patients and more than 90% in the duodenal ulcer patients. Corpus glandular atrophy was present at baseline in all groups

Table 2. Corpus glandular atrophy in controlled omeprazole maintenance trials of erosive oesophagitis followed for 12–60 months reviewed by FDA

Treatment	n	Baseline (%)	Last biopsy (%)	Fold increase
Omeprazole ≥ 20 mg q.d.	398	1.3	5.0	4.0
Omeprazole 10 mg q.d.	123	4.1	5.7	1.4
Omeprazole 20 mg 3/7 days	41	0.0	2.4	2.4
Ranitidine ≥ 150 mg q.d.	237	0.4	3.0	7.0
Anti-reflux surgery	121	3.3	6.6	2.0

Table 3. Corpus glandular atrophy in controlled omeprazole maintenance trials of duodenal ulcer for up to 24 months reviewed by FDA

Treatment	n	Baseline (%)	Last biopsy (%)	Fold increase
Omeprazole 20 mg q.d.	441	1.7	4.1	2.4
Omeprazole 10 mg q.d.	344	3.8	3.8	1.0
Ranitidine 150 mg q.d.	247	1.2	2.8	2.3
Placebo	78	2.6	3.8	1.5

Table 4. Corpus intestinal metaplasia in controlled omeprazole maintenance trials of erosive oesophagitis for 12–60 months reviewed by FDA

Treatment	n	Baseline (%)	Last biopsy (%)	Fold increase
Omeprazole > 20 mg q.d.	365	1.1	1.7	1.5
Omeprazole 10 mg q.d.	123	1.6	4.1	2.5
Ranitidine > 150 mg q.d.	198	1.0	2.0	2.0
Anti-reflux surgery	121	1.7	1.7	1.0

Table 5. Corpus intestinal metaplasia in controlled omeprazole maintenance trials of duodenal ulcer for up to 24 months reviewed by FDA

Treatment	n	Baseline (%)	Last biopsy (%)	Fold increase
Omeprazole 20 mg q.d.	306	1.0	2.0	2.0
Omeprazole 10 mg q.d.	245	1.6	1.6	1.0
Ranitidine 150 mg q.d.	247	0	2.0	2.0
Placebo	59	1.7	1.7	1.0

except the small group treated with omeprazole for 3 days each week. The prevalence of atrophy was increased in every group in the last biopsy; the increase was expressed as a 'fold increase'. Fold increases ranged from 3 to 7 in the oesophagitis patients; the highest increase was in the ranitidine group. No significant differences were found in the rate of progression to atrophy. The long-term lansoprazole randomized trials, which were smaller in number and generally of shorter duration than the omeprazole trials, also showed no increase in the prevalence of atrophy or intestinal metaplasia.

On the basis of the controlled trials the FDA concluded that PPIs did not accelerate the development of gastric atrophy, intestinal metaplasia or cancer[8]. The FDA also concluded that approved PPI indications should not be changed, nor should there be changes in labelling instructions for their

Table 6. Development of corpus glandular atrophy during PPI therapy in uncontrolled studies

Author/ref.	Country	PPI	Mean duration (years)	n	Baseline atrophy (%)	End atrophy (%)	Annual increase (%)
Eissele et al.[23]	Germany	Lansoprazole	5	38	10.5	37	5.3
Berstad et al.[24]	Germany	Omeprazole	1	43	0	9	9
Mulder et al.[25]	Netherlands	Lansoprazole	5	39	2	2	0
Freston et al.[22]	USA	Lansoprazole	1.25	99	0	1	1

use, e.g. testing for and treating *H. pylori* is not necessary in GERD patients on PPIs.

Uncontrolled studies

Uncontrolled studies cannot discern if an increase in the prevalence of gastric atrophy is more or less than what might have occurred in a comparable group of patients treated with something other than a PPI. The studies are summarized in Table 6. In 99 patients with *H. pylori* gastritis treated with lansoprazole for at least 1 year, there was one case of corpus glandular atrophy[22]. While this was a relatively short follow-up, it should be noted that the Kuipers study showed an increase of 13% in the first year. Statisticians at the FDA Advisory Committee meeting estimated the probability of the lansoprazole study missing an increase of this magnitude to be 1 in 100.

The Eissele study[23] examined the effects of lansoprazole in 38 *H. pylori*-infected patients with GERD treated for 5 years. The prevalence of corpus glandular atrophy increased from 10.5% to 37%. In the Berstad study[24] of GERD maintenance therapy with lansoprazole for 1 year in 43 patients, no patients had atrophy at baseline but nine had grade 1 atrophy on the last biopsy. Moderate or marked atrophy was not observed. The annual increase in the prevalence of atrophy was estimated to be 15%. In contrast, the recent Mulder study[25] from the Netherlands found no increase in the prevalence of glandular atrophy in 39 *H. pylori*-infected patients treated with lansoprazole for 5 years. Clearly, no conclusions can be drawn from these uncontrolled and conflicting studies.

THE ISSUE OF INTESTINAL METAPLASIA

Intestinal metaplasia of the III type (colonic) is closely linked to gastric carcinoma[26-28]. Persistent inflammation fosters the development of mucosal cells with the appearance of intestinal metaplasia, and dysplasia seems to arise from areas of intestinal metaplasia. Therefore, the detection of a high prevalence of intestinal metaplasia in patients treated with PPIs would be more significant than the finding of mere atrophy. None of the controlled or uncontrolled studies detected such an increased prevalence. The controlled studies that addressed this issue in the FDA analysis are shown in Tables 4 and 5.

THE ISSUE OF ANTRAL GLANDULAR ATROPHY

Most of the studies described previously included only corpus biopsies. This limits the accuracy of assessing changes that predispose to dysplasia and cancer, as discussed recently by Genta[29]. The primary sites for intestinal metaplasia as well as dysplasia and intestinal-type adenocarcinoma are the gastric antrum and angulus[30-32]. Moreover, intestinal metaplasia usually occurs in the antrum in patients infected with *H. pylori*[33]. During treatment with PPIs the intensity of inflammation increases in the corpus and decreases in the antrum[5,6,29,34]. A more accurate assessment of mucosal changes that predispose to cancer would take into account changes in both the antrum and corpus. It is possible that the *net* effect of any increase in atrophy and intestinal metaplasia in the corpus is cancelled by a decrease in these findings in the antrum. This consideration undermines the significance of reported increases in corpus atrophy during PPI therapy.

COMMENTARY ON THE STRENGTH OF THE EVIDENCE

All studies are not of equal value; uncontrolled studies are particularly limited in their ability to discern causes of time-dependent changes, such as the occurrence of gastric atrophy. Therefore, it is not surprising that the uncontrolled studies reached contradictory conclusions. Such studies, and the Kuipers study, which is, for practical purposes, uncontrolled, are useful in developing hypotheses for eventual testing in a controlled fashion. Similarly, uncontrolled pilot studies of the efficacy of a new drug guide the development of definitive randomized, controlled studies which establish if the drug is truly effective. Only the Lundell study and those analysed by the FDA were controlled. They must be given more credence, despite their shortcomings, which are dwarfed by the inherent flaws of the uncontrolled studies. The controlled studies do not support the hypothesis. Either the hypothesis is incorrect or the changes are so small, or develop so slowly, that their clinical meaning strains credulity. Given the current popularity of 'evidence-based medicine', it is surprising that many who jumped on the Kuipers 'bandwagon' have not re-evaluated their position in light of the evidence from controlled studies.

WHAT IS THE HARM IN ERADICATING *H. PYLORI*-POSITIVE PATIENTS WITH GERD?

Possibly none, but new evidence suggesting that *H. pylori* infection, particularly by CagA-positive strains, protects against GERD and its complications has prompted a reassessment of the wisdom of eradicating the organism in conditions that lack a valid scientific rationale. This development is prescient in light of the recommendation by some to eradicate the organism in GERD patients before undertaking chronic PPI therapy.

Epidemiological observations

Studies from Japan[35], Germany[36] and China[37] showed a significantly *lower* incidence of *H. pylori* infection in patients with reflux oesophagitis than in matched controls, and a US study found that patients infected with cagA-positive strains were less likely to have severe GERD, including its complications, Barrett's oesophagus and adenocarcinoma of the distal oesophagus[12]. A more recent study showed that the VacA 1 strain was most strongly associated with protection against GERD[38]. These observations have been made against the background of a decreasing prevalence of *H. pylori* infection in developed countries and, with it, dramatic reductions in peptic ulcers and gastric cancers, while the prevalence of GERD, Barrett's oesophagus and adenocarcinoma of the oesophagus is increasing[10,39]. Supporting the belief that these observations may be linked are studies showing that Asians and blacks are more likely than their white counterparts to be infected, particularly with CagA-positive strains, but are significantly less likely to develop adenocarcinoma of the oesophagus[40]. Moreover, a recent study suggests that infection with CagA-positive strains may protect against cancer of the cardia[39].

Effect of *H. pylori* eradication on GERD

Studies from Germany, Japan, and the US showed an increased prevalence of erosive oesophagitis after *H. pylori* eradication. The German study, by Labenz *et al.*[41], was in infected patients with duodenal ulcers. Nearly a quarter of patients developed endoscopically documented erosive oesophagitis within 3 years of successful *H. pylori* eradication, a significantly higher proportion than in a control group with persistent infection. In 70 infected Japanese patients with duodenal ulcer, gastric ulcer or atrophic gastritis, 14.3% had erosive oesophagitis 7 months after eradication[42]. Friedman *et al.*[43] reported that 37% of US duodenal ulcer patients developed GERD symptoms or oesophagitis after *H. pylori* eradication, compared to 13% in those failing eradication; the difference was highly statistically significant. A dissenting study is that of the GU-MACH and DU-MACH trial in which Malfertheiner *et al.*[44] analysed the impact of *H. pylori* eradication on heartburn. There was a reduction in the prevalence of heartburn after 6 months in both the *H. pylori*-positive and *H. pylori*-negative groups. In addition, McColl and colleagues[45] recently found no evidence that eradicating *H. pylori* in patients with peptic ulcers induced *de-novo* GERD symptoms.

Effect of *H. pylori* infection on GERD treatment

Hallerback *et al.*[46] found that *H. pylori*-positive patients with erosive oesophagitis on maintenance omeprazole therapy had significantly fewer relapses in 1 year than did *H. pylori*-negative patients. In contrast, more recent studies found no effect of eradication on the omeprazole dose required for successful maintenance therapy[47]. It is not known whether the many GERD patients on H_2-receptor antagonist maintenance therapy will require PPIs after *H. pylori* eradication. In terms of GERD healing, a large, prospective and controlled trial showed that pantoprazole was significantly more effective in healing erosive oesophagitis in *H. pylori*-positive patients than in *H. pylori*-negative patients, although the difference was less than 5%[48]. It would not be surprising to find GERD management with antisecretory drugs to be more effective in *H. pylori*-infected patients. Healing of oesophagitis is directly correlated to the number of hours the intragastric pH is held above 4, and the time during which the pH is above 4 nearly doubles in the presence of *H. pylori* infection[11]. Graham and Yamaoka[49] described *H. pylori* infection as a biological antisecretory agent.

H. pylori and GERD complications

Compelling evidence links *H. pylori* corpus gastritis, particularly that associated with the *cagA* gene, and protection against GERD and its complications. Mihara *et al.*[35] found that patients with moderate to severe *H. pylori* gastritis involving the corpus had less severe GERD than did age- and sex-matched controls. Vicari *et al.*[12] recently reported that the CagA-positive *H. pylori* infection was associated with less severe oesophagitis and fewer occurrences of Barrett's oesophagus and dysplasia or adenocarcinoma, all complications of GERD. The putative beneficial effect of *H. pylori* infection in GERD is probably due to reduced gastric acid secretion in some patients with corpus gastritis. They may have decreased acid secretion even in the absence of atrophy; this change is reversible after eradication[9,42,50,51].

Overall, the evidence supports the concept that at least some *H. pylori* strains confer protection against GERD, or its complications. This does not necessarily translate into a recommendation to avoid testing for the infection and eradication in GERD patients. That recommendation will require a more careful analysis of all the risks and benefits, including weighing the risk of developing gastric cancer if *H. pylori* is not eradicated versus the risk of developing oesophageal adenocarcinoma if it is. This analysis is tilted towards eradication because gastric cancer is more prevalent worldwide than oesophageal adenocarcinoma. However, the latter tumour is now the more prevalent among men in the US[52,53], suggesting yet again that blanket recommendations to eradicate *H. pylori* infection may be inappropriate compared to more targeted recommendations based on hard scientific evidence. Specifically, the recommendations to test all patients with GERD before treating them with maintenance PPI therapy is premature, if not inappropriate, in light of the evidence.

References

1. Kuipers EJ, Lundell L, Klinkenberg-Knoll EC *et al*. Atrophic gastritis and *Helicobacter pylori* infection in patients with reflux esophagitis treated with omeprazole or fundoplication. N Engl J Med. 1996;334:1018–22.
2. Freston JW. *Helicobacter pylori*, acid, gastritis, atrophy and progression to cancer: a critical view. In: Hunt R, Tytgat GNJ, editors. *Helicobacter pylori*: Basic mechanisms to clinical cure 1996. Dordrecht: Kluwer; 1996:245–54.
3. The European *Helicobacter pylori* Study Group (EHPSG). Current European concepts in the management of *Helicobacter pylori* infection. The Maastricht Consensus Report. Gut. 1997;41:8–13.
4. Kuipers EJ, Lee A, Klinkenberg-Knol EL, Meuwissen SGM. The development of atrophic gastritis – *Helicobacter pylori* and the effects of acid suppressive therapy. Aliment Pharmacol Ther. 1995;9:331–40.
5. Solcia E, Villani I, Fiocca R *et al*. Effects of eradication of *Helicobacter pylori* on gastritis in duodenal ulcer patients. Scand J Gastroenterol. 1994;29 (Suppl. 201):28–34.

6. Logan RPH, Walker MM, Misiewicz JJ et al. Changes in the intragastric distribution of *Helicobacter pylori* during treatment with omeprazole. Gut. 1995;36:12–16.
7. Lundell L, Navu H, Andersson P et al. Gastritis development and acid suppression therapy revisited: results of a randomized clinical study with long-term follow-up. Gastroenterology. 1997;112:A28.
8. Freston JW. Long-term acid control and proton pump inhibitors: interactions and safety issues in perspective. Am J Gastroenterol. 1997;92(Suppl.):51–7S.
9. Blaser MJ. Not all *Helicobacter pylori* strains are created equal: should all be eliminated? Lancet. 1997;349:1020–2.
10. Blaser MJ. Science, medicine, and the future – *Helicobacter pylori* and gastric diseases. Br Med J. 1998;316:1507–10.
11. Labenz J, Tillenburg B, Peitz U et al. Efficacy of omeprazole one year after cure of *Helicobacter pylori* infection in duodenal ulcer patients. Am J Gastroenterol. 1997;92:576–8.
12. Vicari JJ, Peek RM, Falk GW et al. The seroprevalence of *cagA*-positive *Helicobacter pylori* strains in the spectrum of gastroesophageal reflux disease. Gastroenterology. 1998;115:50–7.
13. Price AB. The Sydney System: Histological Division. J Gastroenterol Hepatol. 1991;6:209–22.
14. Lundell L, Miettinen P, Myrvold HE et al. Lack of effect of acid suppression therapy on gastric atrophy. Gastroenterology. 1999;117:319–26.
15. Lundell L. Omeprazole and accelerated onset of atrophic gastritis. Gastroenterology. 2000;118:240–2.
16. Whitehead R. Gastritis – histopathological background. Scand J Gastroenterol. 1982;79(Suppl):40–3.
17. Hackelsberger A, Günther T, Schultze V, Peitz U, Malfertheiner P. Role of aging in the expression of *Helicobacter pylori* gastritis in the antrum, corpus, and cardia. Scand J Gastroenterol. 1999;34:138–43.
18. Pounder RE, Wiliams MP. Omeprazole and accelerated onset of atrophic gastritis. Gastroenterology. 2000;18:238–9.
19. McColl KEL, Murray LS, Gillen D. Omeprazole and accelerated onset of atrophic gastritis. Gastroenterology. 2000;118:239.
20. Kuipers EJ, Klinkenberg-Knol EC, Meuwissen SGM. Omeprazole and accelerated onset of atrophic gastritis. Gastroenterology. 2000;118:239–40.
21. Stolte M, Meining A, Koop H et al. Eradication of *Helicobacter pylori* heals atrophic corpus gastritis caused by long-term treatment with omeprazole. Wirchows Arch. 1999;434:91–4.
22. Freston JW, Rose PA, Heller CA, Haber M, Jennings D. Safety profile of lansoprazole: the US clinical trial experience. Drug Safety. 1999;20:195–205.
23. Eissele R, Brunner G, Simon B, Solcia E, Arnold R. Gastric mucosa during treatment with lansoprazole: *Helicobacter pylori* is a risk factor for argyrophil cell hyperplasia. Gastroenterology. 1997;112:707–17.
24. Berstad AE, Hatlebakk JG, Maartmann-Moe H, Berstad A, Brandtzaeg P. *Helicobacter pylori* gastritis and epithelial cell proliferation in patients with reflux oesophagitis after treatment with lansoprazole. Gut. 1997;41:740–7.
25. Mudler CJJ, Dekker W, Geboes K. Lansoprazole maintenance treatment for GERD (5 years). Do we have to eradicate all Hp-positive patients? Gastroenterology. 2000 (In press).
26. Solcia E, Fiocca R, Luinetti O et al. Intestinal and diffuse gastric cancers arise in a different background of *Helicobacter pylori* gastritis through different gene involvement. Am J Surg Pathol. 1996;20(Suppl. 1):S8–22.
27. Correa P, Cuello C, Duqque E. Carcinoma and intestinal metaplasia in the stomach of Columbian migrates. J Natl Cancer Inst. 1970;44:297–306.
28. Fililpe MI. Borderline lesions of the gastric epithelium. New indications of cancer risk and clinical implication. In: Fenoglio, Priser M, Wulff, Rilke F, editors. Progressive Surgical Pathology, Vol. 12. New York: Field & Wood; 1992:269–90.
29. Genta RM. Acid suppression and gastric atrophy: sifting fact from fiction. Gut. 1998;43 (Suppl. 1):S35–8.
30. Eidt S, Stolte M. Prevalence of intestinal metaplasia in *Helicobacter pylori* gastritis. Scand J Gastroenterol. 1994;29:607–10.
31. Rugge M, Di Marri F, Casaro M et al. Pathology of the gastric antrum and body associated with *Helicobacter pylori* infection in nonulcerous patients: is the bacterium a promoter of intestinal metaplasia? Histopathology. 1993;22:9–15.

32. You WC, Blot WJ, Chang YS et al. Comparison of the anatomic distribution of stomach cancer. Jpn J Cancer Res. 1992;83:1150–3.
33. Xia Hua-Xiang H, Kalanter JS, Talley NJ et al. Antral-type mucosa in the gastric incisura, body and fundus (antralization): a link between Helicobacter pylori infection and intestinal metaplasia? Am J Gastroenterol. 2000;95:114–21.
34. Solcia E, Fiocca R, Havu N, Dalvag A, Carlsson R. Gastric endocrine cells and gastritis in patients receiving long-term omeprazole treatment. Digestion. 1992;51(Suppl. 1):82–92.
35. Mihara M, Haruma K, Kamada T et al. Low prevalence of Helicobacter pylori infection in patients with reflux esophagitis. Gut. 1996;39(Suppl. 2):A94.
36. Hackelsberger A, Schultze V, Gunther T, Labenz J, Kahl S, Dominguez-Munoz JE. H. pylori prevalence in reflux esophagitis – a case–control study. Gastroenterology. 1997;112:A137.
37. Wu JCY, Go MYY, Chan WB, Choi CL, Chan FKL, Sung JY. Prevalence and distribution of H. pylori in gastro–esophageal reflux disease: a study in Chinese. Gastroenterology. 1998;114:A334.
38. Fallone CA, Barkun AN, Gottke MU et al. Association of Helicobacter pylori genotype with gastroesophageal reflux disease and other upper gastrointestinal diseases. Am J Gastroenterol. 2000;95:659–69.
39. Chow WH, Blaser MJ, Blot WJ et al. An inverse relation between $cagA^+$ strains of Helicobacter pylori infection and risk of esophageal and gastric cardia adenocarcinoma. Cancer Res. 1998;58:588–90.
40. Grimley CE, Loft DE, Morris AG, Nwokolo CU. Virulent Helicobacter pylori in patients with gastric and esophageal adenocarcinoma. Gastroenterology. 1997;112:A571.
41. Labenz J, Blum AL, Bayerdorffer E, Meining A, Stolte M, Borsch G. Curing Helicobacter pylori infection in patients with duodenal ulcer may provoke reflux esophagitis. Gastroenterology. 1997;112:1442–7.
42. Koike T, Ohara S, Sekine H et al. Increase of gastric acid secretion after H. pylori eradication caused the development of reflux esophagitis. Gastroenterology. 1998;114:A183.
43. Friedman G, Fallone CA, Mayrand S et al. Is Helicobacter pylori eradication associated with the endoscopic development of esophagitis? Gastroenterology. 1998;114:A124.
44. Malfertheiner P, Veldhuyzen van Zanten S, Dent J et al. Does cure of Helicobacter pylori infection induce heartburn? Gastroenterology. 1998;114:A212.
45. McColl KEL, Dickson A, El-Nujumi A, El-Omar E, Kelman A. Symptomatic benefit 1–3 years after H. pylori eradication in ulcer patients: impact of gastroesophageal reflux disease. Am J Gastroenterol 2000;95:101–5.
46. Hallerback B, Unge P, Carling L et al. Omeprazole or ranitidine in long-term treatment of reflux esophagitis. The Scandinavia Clinics for United Research Group. Gastroenterology. 1994;107:1305–11.
47. Schenk BE, Kuipers EJ, Klinkenberg-Knol EC, Eskes SA, Meuwissen SGM. H. pylori and the efficacy of omeprazole for gastroesophageal reflux disease. Am J Gastroenterol. 1999;94:867–9.
48. Holtmann G, Cain C, Malfertheiner P. Gastric Helicobacter pylori infection accelerates healing of reflux esophagitis during treatment with the proton pump inhibitor pantoprazole. Gastroenterology. 1999;117:11–16.
49. Graham DY, Yamaoka Y. H. pylori and cagA: relationships with gastric cancer, duodenal ulcer, and reflux esophagitis and its complications. Helicobacter. 1998;3:145–51.
50. El-Omar EM, Oien K, El-Nujumi A et al. Helicobacter pylori infection and chronic gastric acid hyposecretion. Gastroenterology. 1997;113:15–24.
51. El-Omar EM, Penman ID, Ardill JE, Chittajallu RS, Howie C, McColl KE. Helicobacter pylori infection and abnormalities of acid secretion in patients with duodenal ulcer disease. Gastroenterology. 1995;109:681–91.
52. Blot WJ, Dervesa SS, Kneller RW, Fraumeni JF Jr. Rising incidence of adenocarcinoma of the esophagus and gastric cardia. J Am Med Assoc. 1991;265:1287–9.
53. American Cancer Society Surveillance Report, 1999.

30
Autoimmune gastritis via mimicking does occur

M. STOLTE, S. RAPPEL and H. MÜLLER

INTRODUCTION

Parietal cell antibody-induced atrophic autoimmune gastritis of the oxyntic mucosa with complete loss of the parietal cells, and focal intestinal metaplasia, achlorhydria and thus induced G cell hyperplasia of the antral mucosa, hypergastrinaemia and the resulting ECL cell hyperplasia of the corpus mucosa with possible development of carcinoid tumours, is a recognized entity of gastritis, which can lead to pernicious anaemia[1-4].

In 1992 we described for the first time that it is possible to diagnose the active pre-atrophic stage of autoimmune gastritis, with diffuse periglandular infiltration of the corpus mucosa by lymphocytes, lymphocytic destruction of corpus glands, parietal cell hypertrophy and focal atrophy[5].

At that time we already noted that parietal cell antibodies were detectable in the serum in only about 40% of patients with active autoimmune gastritis.

INCIDENCE OF NON-ATROPHIC AUTOIMMUNE GASTRITIS

The incidence of non-atrophic autoimmune gastritis in our material is about 36% of autoimmune gastritis overall. In common with atrophic autoimmune gastritis, the non-atrophic form is found predominantly in women, and *Helicobacter pylori* infection is detectable in almost 30% of cases, as compared with only 0.5% of patients with atrophic autoimmune gastritis (see Table 1).

In a further study done by our group, in which the state of the antral mucosa in atrophic autoimmune gastritis was investigated, it was found that non-active low-grade superficial gastritis, similar to that found after *H. pylori* eradication, was frequently present in the antrum[6].

Table 1. Incidence of atrophic and non-atrophic autoimmune gastritis in our biopsy material of the year 1997 ($n = 581$)

	Atrophic	Non-atrophic
Patients	64.1%	35.9%
H. pylori-positive	0.5%	29.7%
Age (m)	67.3 years	64.8 years
Male:female	1:2.4	1:1.8

HELICOBACTER PYLORI-INDUCED AUTOIMMUNE GASTRITIS

Subsequently, Negrini et al.[7], Faller et al.[8] and Claeys et al.[9] published reports showing that autoimmune gastritis also occurs in patients infected with *H. pylori*, and that the antigen of the gastric autoantibodies[10], as is the case of parietal cell antibody-induced gastritis, is the H^+K^+-ATPase of the parietal cells.

Patients with anticanalicular antibodies develop parietal cell atrophy, leading to an increase in serum gastrin and a decrease in the pepsinogen I/II ratio[11].

Steininger et al. have shown that the T-cell-mediated autoimmune mechanism triggered by the anticanalicular antibodies leads to apoptotic parietal cell loss[12].

This raises the question as to whether there are two, or even three, types of autoimmune gastritis. These would be the classical, parietal cell-antibody-induced autoimmune gastritis, *H. pylori*-induced autoimmune gastritis and, perhaps, a mixed form of the two.

Open questions that still remain to be answered are what host factors and what bacterial factors trigger autoimmunity, and whether *H. pylori* eradication leads to healing of the *H. pylori*-induced autoimmune gastritis[13].

H. PYLORI ERADICATION: HEALING OF AUTOIMMUNE GASTRITIS?

One possible piece of evidence for the existence of *H. pylori*-induced autoimmune gastritis would be the observation that eradication of the *H. pylori* infection results in healing of this gastritis. In patients with no histological evidence of *H. pylori* infection, a positive serological finding could be used to justify eradication treatment.

We have published a 'key' case that provides evidence for such a hypothesis. In a patient with active autoimmune gastritis with lymphocytic glandular destruction partial atrophy and nodular ECL cell hyperplasia, 9 months after *H. pylori* eradication, we found complete healing of the gastritis, with normalization of the partial atrophy of the corpus glands[14]. Table 2 shows a brief summary of the course of this case prior to and following *H. pylori* eradication, demonstrating an increase in atrophy together with a rise in serum gastrin level prior to eradication, and normalization of the histological findings and serum gastrin following eradication of the infection.

Table 2. Summary of the course of a patient with autoimmune gastritis prior to and following *H. pylori* eradication

	Prior to H. pylori-*eradication*			Following H. pylori-*eradication*	
	1988	1990	1994	1995	1996
H. pylori	+++	+	+	−	−
Degree of gastritis	++	+++	+++	+	+
Activity of gastritis	++	++	++	−	−
Corpus atrophy	−	−	++	+	−
Autoimmune infiltrates	−	++	+++	+	−
ECL-cell hyperplasia	−	−	+++	+	−
Parietal cell hyperplasia	+	+++	+++	+	−
Gastrin (pg/ml)	59	126	650	95	75

RESULTS OF A RETROSPECTIVE STUDY

On the basis of this experience, and experience with subsequent cases[15,16], we later carried out *H. pylori* eradication treatment in 80 patients with active autoimmune gastritis. In 36 of these patients we had also investigated the gastric mucosa, on average 39.3 months prior to eradication treatment, and in 35 of these patients biopsy material from the antrum and corpus on average 7.7 months after eradication treatment.

The results of this study are submitted for publication. Here we only show the most important results. Following *H. pylori* eradication, not only is there a significant decrease in the grade of gastritis in the corpus (see Figure 1), and, in the activity of the gastritis (see Figure 2), but the periglandular lymphocytic infiltrates have also disappeared (see Figure 3), thus leading to a significant reduction in focal lymphocytic glandular destruction (see Figure 4), and finally to an improvement in the grade of the atrophy – even to complete normalization of the corpus mucosa (see Figure 5).

CONCLUSION

In conclusion, the positive effect of *H. pylori* eradication treatment in our study shows that active, not yet atrophic, autoimmune gastritis, can be induced not only by parietal cell antibodies, but also by the *H. pylori* infection, and can be healed by eradication of *H. pylori*. Of course, there are numerous questions yet to be answered, and we are currently working to clarify these in a prospective, controlled diagnostic and therapeutic trial that includes additional serological, functional and immunohistochemical investigations.

References

1. Rappel S, Altendorf-Hofmann A, Stolte M. Prognosis of gastric carcinoid tumors. Digestion. 1994;56:455–62.
2. Rindi G, Luinetti O, Cornaggia M, Capella C, Solcia E. Three subtypes of gastric argyrophil carcinoid and the gastric neuroendocrine carcinoma: a clinicopathologic study. Gastroenterology. 1993;104:994–1006.

Corpus: Grade of gastritis

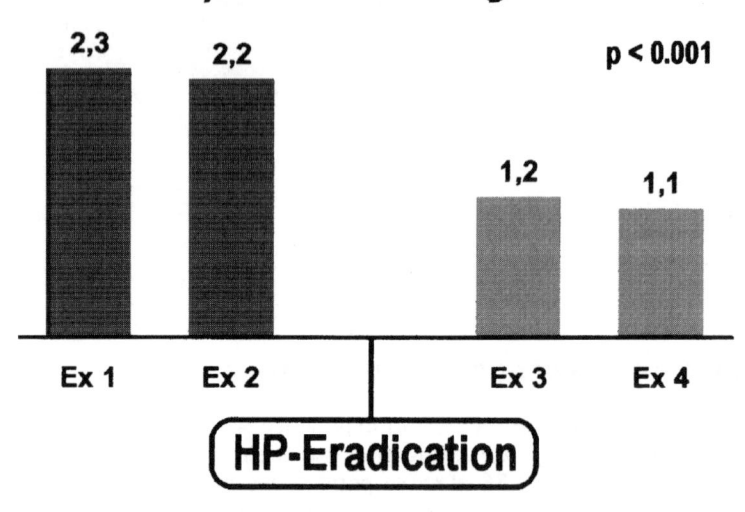

Ex 1: 2,3 Ex 2: 2,2 Ex 3: 1,2 Ex 4: 1,1 $p < 0.001$

HP-Eradication (between Ex 2 and Ex 3)

Figure 1. Grade of gastritis of the corpus mucosa before and after *H. pylori* eradication treatment (Ex 1 = examination on average 39.3 months prior to eradication, Ex 2 = examination prior to eradication, Ex 3 = examination 8 weeks after eradication, Ex 4 = examination on average 7.7 months after eradication treatment).

Corpus: Activity of gastritis

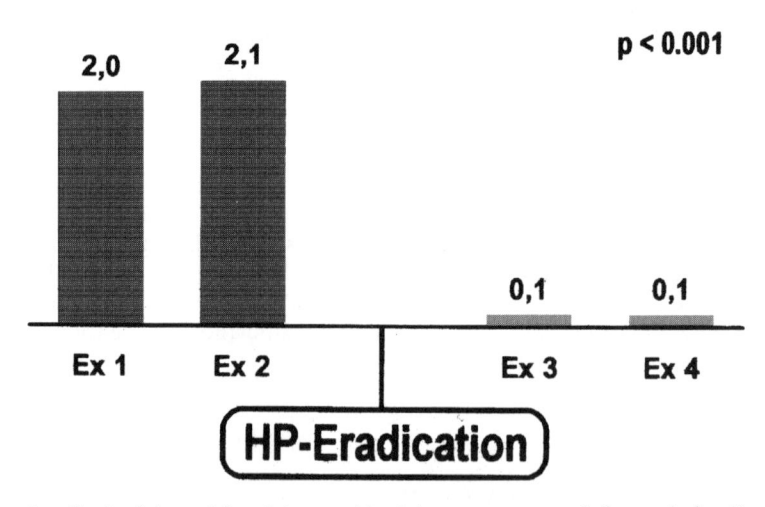

Ex 1: 2,0 Ex 2: 2,1 Ex 3: 0,1 Ex 4: 0,1 $p < 0.001$

HP-Eradication (between Ex 2 and Ex 3)

Figure 2. Grade of the activity of the gastritis of the corpus mucosa before and after *H. pylori* eradication treatment.

Corpus: Lymphocytic gland-infiltration

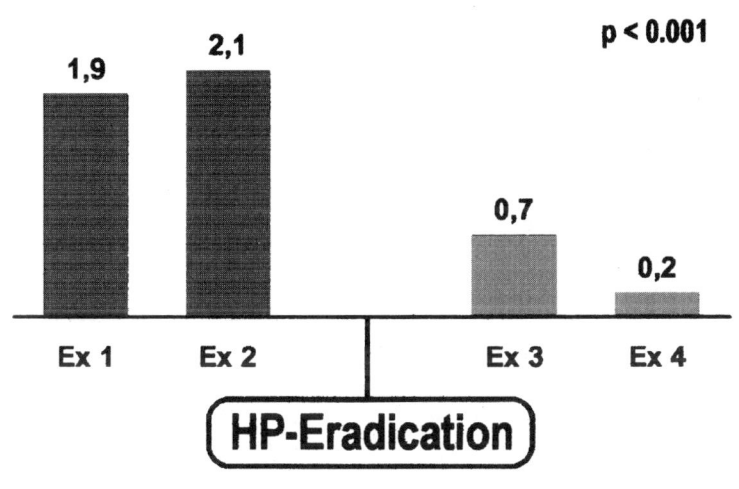

Ex 1: 1,9
Ex 2: 2,1
Ex 3: 0,7
Ex 4: 0,2

$p < 0.001$

HP-Eradication (between Ex 2 and Ex 3)

Figure 3. Grade of periglandular lymphocytic infiltration of the corpus mucosa before and after *H. pylori* eradication treatment.

Corpus: Focal gland-destruction

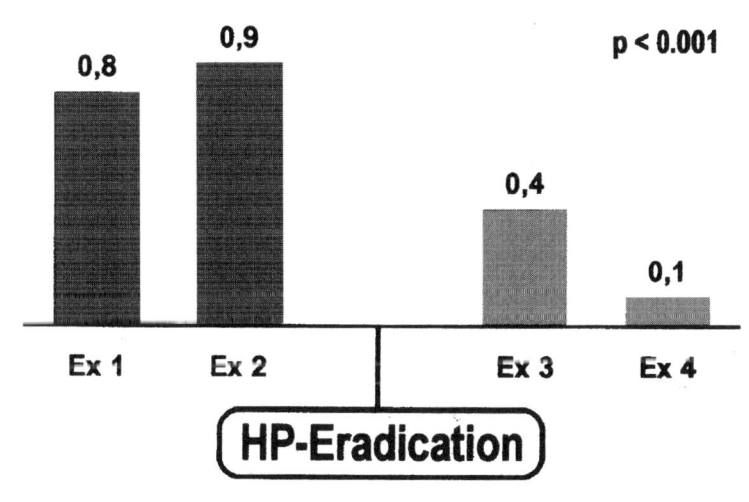

Ex 1: 0,8
Ex 2: 0,9
Ex 3: 0,4
Ex 4: 0,1

$p < 0.001$

HP-Eradication (between Ex 2 and Ex 3)

Figure 4. Grade of focal lymphocytic glandular destruction of the corpus mucosa before and after *H. pylori* eradication treatment.

Corpus: Grade of Atrophy

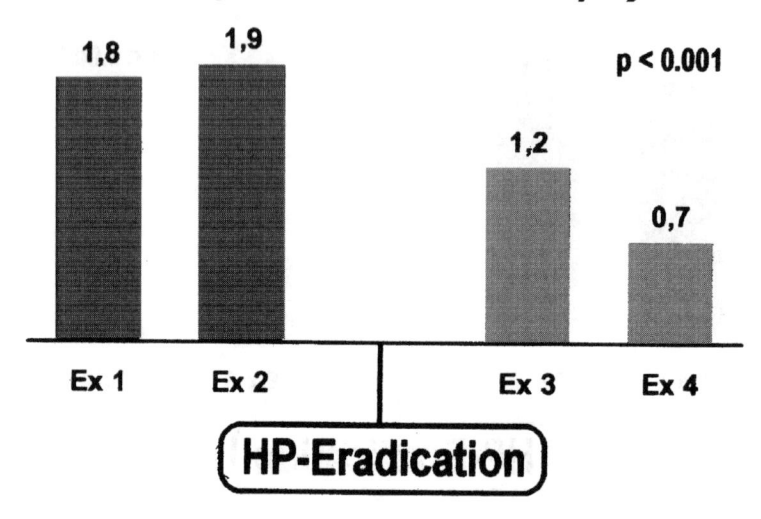

1,8   1,9   p < 0.001

                          1,2
                                        0,7

Ex 1   Ex 2   Ex 3   Ex 4

HP-Eradication

Figure 5. Grade of atrophy of the corpus mucosa before and after *H. pylori* eradication treatment.

3. Rindi G, Bordi C, Rappel S, La Rosa S, Stolte M, Solcia E. Gastric carcinoids and neuroendocrine carcinomas: pathogenesis, pathology, and behavior. World J Surg. 1996;20:168–72.
4. Capella C, Heitz PU, Höfler H, Solcia E, Klöppel G. Revised classification of neuroendocrine tumors of the lung, pancreas and gut. Digestion. 1994;55(Suppl. 3):11–23.
5. Stolte M, Baumann H, Bethke B, Lauer E, Ritter M. Active autoimmune gastritis without total atrophy of the glands. Z Gastroenterol. 1992;30:729–30.
6. Oberhuber G, Püspök A, Dejaco C et al. Minimal chronic inactive gastritis: indicator of preexisting *Helicobacter pylori* gastritis? Pathol Res Pract. 1996;192:1016–21.
7. Negrini R, Savio A, Poiesi C et al. Antigenic mimicry between *Helicobacter pylori* and gastric mucosa in the pathogenesis of body atrophic gastritis. Gastroenterology. 1996;111:655–65.
8. Faller G, Steininger H, Eck M, Hensen J, Han EG, Kirchner T. Antigastric autoantibodies in *Helicobacter pylori* gastritis: prevalence, *in-situ* binding sites and clues for clinical relevances. Virchows Arch. 1996;427:483–6.
9. Claeys D, Faller G, Appelmelk, BJ, Negrini R, Kirchner T. The H^+,K^+-ATPase is a major autoantigen in chronic *Helicobacter pylori* gastritis with body mucosa atrophy. Gastroenterology. 1998;115:340–7.
10. Burmann P, Mardh S, Nordberg L, Karlsson FA. Parietal cell antibodies in pernicious anemia inhibit H^+,K^+-adenosine triphosphate, the proton pump of the stomach. Gastroenterology. 1989;96:1434–8.
11. Faller G, Steininger H, Kränzlein J et al. Antigastric autoantibodies in *Helicobacter pylori* infection: implications of histological and clinical parameters of gastritis. Gut. 1997;41:619–23.
12. Steininger H, Faller G, Deweld E, Brabletz T, Jung A, Kirchner T. Apoptosis in chronic gastritis and its correlation with antigastric autoantibodies. Virchows Arch. 1998;433:13–18.
13. Appelmelk BJ, Faller G, Claeys D, Kirchner T, Vandenbroucke-Grauls CMJE. Bugs on trial: the case of *Helicobacter pylori* and autoimmunity. Immunol Today. 1998;19:296–9.
14. Stolte M, Meining A, Koop H, Seifert E. Eradication of *Helicobacter pylori* heals atrophic corpus gastritis caused by long-term treatment with omeprazole. Virchows Arch. 1999;434:91–4.

15. Stolte M, Meier E, Meining A. Cure of autoimmune gastritis by *Helicobacter pylori* eradication in a 21-year-old male. Z Gastroenterol. 1998;36:641–3.
16. Oberhuber G, Wündisch T, Rappel S, Stolte M. Significant improvement of atrophy after eradication therapy in atrophic body gastritis. Pathol Res Pract. 1998;194:609–13.

31
Autoimmune gastritis and antigenic mimicking

F. FRANCESCHI and R. M. GENTA

INTRODUCTION

Autoimmune gastritis is defined as a chronic atrophic gastritis of the corpus–fundus mucosa, which is associated with diffuse atrophy of the oxyntic mucosa and thus accompanying achlorhydria[1]. The presence of serum antibodies directed against parietal cell antigens and intrinsic factor is a specific feature of the disease. The advanced phases of this immunopathological spectrum are often associated with pernicious anaemia, a condition resulting from the impaired absorption of vitamin B_{12} caused by the unavailability of intrinsic factor[2].

Several studies reported the presence of antibodies directed against at least three autoantigens of the gastric mucosa of patients with autoimmune gastritis: intrinsic factor, cytoplasmic (microsomal–canalicular) and plasma membrane surface antigens of parietal cells[2]. However, the α and β subunits of H^+,K^+-ATPase located in the secretory canalicular system, which is the essential instrument in acid production by the stomach, represent the major parietal cell autoantigen[3,4]. These findings have been reproduced and confirmed in animal models. In particular, studies on murine autoimmune gastritis after neonatal thymectomy showed that the murine disease is cell-mediated because it can be transferred to syngeneic nude mice by spleen cells, but not by circulating antibodies[5]. The same studies also showed that autoimmune gastritis can be specifically induced by autoreactive T cells specific for H^+,K^+-ATPase[1].

Helicobacter pylori is the major cause of chronic gastritis and multifocal atrophic gastritis worldwide[6,7]. The bacterium induces histologically detectable damage to the gastric mucosa through a complex and as yet incompletely clarified combination of virulence factors (motility, production of cytotoxic enzymes, expression of *CagA* and *VacA* genes) and inflammatory responses induced in the host's mucosa[8–10]. The discovery of *H. pylori* and its recognition as the agent of chronic active gastritis have profoundly changed our understanding of the pathogenesis of gastroduodenal disease. The correlation of *H. pylori* infection with autoimmune gastritis has been suspected since the presence of antibodies apparently reacting with both bacterial and host gastric antigens had been demonstrated. Although an association may exist, however, the existence of a causal relationship remains controversial, since evidence exists both in favour of and against a pathogenetic association between these two entities.

EVIDENCE IN FAVOUR OF *H. PYLORI* AS A CAUSE OF AUTOIMMUNE GASTRITIS

Several authors have investigated the prevalence of *H. pylori* infection in patients with autoimmune gastritis and/or pernicious anaemia[11-13]. Interestingly, while studies based on the assessment of the infection by identification of specific IgG in the serum showed higher infection rates in patients than in controls[12,13], no significant differences were reported when attempts were made to evaluate the presence of the infection by histopathological methods[11]. This discrepancy could be easily explained by the fact that, as the destruction of the oxyntic glands proceeds, and intestinal metaplasia replaces the native gastric mucosa, the increased gastric pH would create an unfavourable environment for *H. pylori* and the infection would eventually disappear. Thus, while histology may document accurately the presence or absence of current infection, it does not provide information on the possibility of a past (and now presumably self-cured) infection. Therefore, one could tentatively accept the idea that a history of *H. pylori* infection is more common in subjects with autoimmune gastritis. Treatment trials seem to support the hypothesis of a *H. pylori*-related autoimmune gastritis. Stolte et al.[14], in a retrospective study on the effect of *H. pylori* eradication in 80 subjects with pre-atrophic corpus-predominant autoimmune gastritis (diagnosed histopathologicaly based on the predominance of peri-oxyntic lymphocytic infiltrates), reported a significant improvement in the grade of parietal cell hypertrophy and atrophy of the corpus mucosa.

A proportion of patients infected with *H. pylori* have been shown to develop antibodies against the conformational peptides of H^+,K^+-ATPase[15,16] (Figure 1). In 1996 Negrini et al.[15] reported a high prevalence of antibodies with high specificity for gastric mucosal antigens among patients with *H. pylori*-associated gastritis. Interestingly, pre-absorption of the serum from these patients with *H. pylori* removed most of these autoantibodies. Nineteen per cent of the subjects, moreover, showed autoantibodies reacting with the secretory canalicular structures of the parietal cell, which is one of the major targets in autoimmune gastritis. Two years later, Claeys et al.[16] reported a high prevalence of anti-H^+,K^+-ATPase antibodies both in *H. pylori*-positive patients (25%) and in infected patients with the previously demonstrated presence of anti-canalicular antibodies (47%); in this study the prevalence of such antibodies in non-infected control subjects was lower than 3%. Furthermore, it has been demonstrated that *H. pylori* lipopolysaccharides express Lewis x and y blood group antigens, which are also expressed by either H^+,K^+-ATPase or gastric epithelial cells[17]. The collective information gathered from these findings provides support for the concept

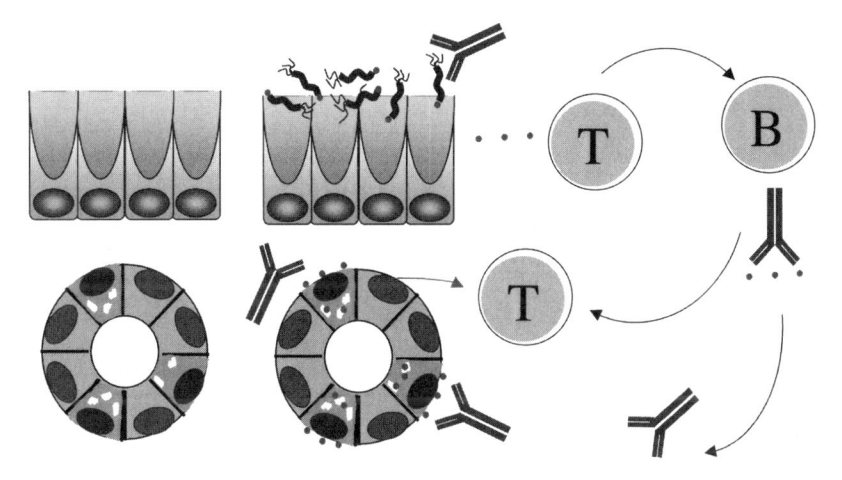

Figure 1. Pathways of the gastric autoimmune mechanisms evoked by *H. pylori* infection. Stimulation of T lymphocytes by the bacterium determines the activation of B lymphocytes and thus the production of specific antibodies anti-H^+,K^+ATP-ase. The same antibodies cross-react with the oxyntic mucosa, contributing to the gastric inflammation.

that a cross-mimicking mechanism between *H. pylori* and gastric mucosal antigens may be responsible for, or at least participate in, the pathogenesis of autoimmune gastritis.

EVIDENCE AGAINST *H. PYLORI* AS A CAUSE OF AUTOIMMUNE GASTRITIS

The presence in *H. pylori*-infected patients of a variety of antibodies reacting simultaneously with both gastric mucosal antigens and bacterial antigens provides the basis for a reasonable pathogenetic hypothesis to explain the damage that occurs in the oxyntic mucosa. However, the mere presence of such cross-reacting antibodies is no proof that a process of pathogenetic significance is under way. Autoantibodies could originate from tissue damage, in this case induced by *H. pylori*, which exposes antigens shielded from the immune system when tissues and cells are intact ('ignorant antigens'). In fact, antigenic mimicry has not been proven to be the pathogenetic mechanism in any of the many autoimmune diseases – for example, rheumatoid arthritis, autoimmune thyroiditis, Sjögren's syndrome – for which a precipitating infection has been proposed as the triggering event[18].

Furthermore, a critical evaluation of the pertinent literature reveals that experimental studies on the cross mimicking between *H. pylori* and gastric mucosal antigens also showed conflicting results. In particular, since the cross-reactivity between anti-*H. pylori* antibodies and secretory canalicular structures of the parietal cells (identified in H^+,K^+-ATPase) has been demonstrated[16], attempts have been made to absorb these autoantibodies with *H. pylori* antigens. A recent study showed that a *H. pylori* pre-absorption test can neutralize antibodies against secretory canalicular structures of the parietal cells in serum of infected subjects, except in patients affected by corpus-restricted atrophic gastritis (also referred to as antrum-sparing atrophic type I gastritis)[15]. This finding suggests that even if H^+,K^+-ATPase has been recognized to be a common target in either *H. pylori*-induced autoimmune gastritis or classical type A gastritis, the autoantibodies that characterized those two different entities bind different epitopes of the same molecule.

The role of antibodies against parietal cells as the pathogenic determinant of atrophic autoimmune gastritis has not yet been demonstrated. One issue that remains difficult to explain is related to the location and accessibility of the β subunit of H^+,K^+-ATPase. This subunit is located in the membranes of the intracellular canaliculi and the apical surface of parietal cells, but not in the basolateral cell membrane. Thus, it is unclear how circulating autoantibodies, with apparently limited access to the proton pump of intact parietal cells, could reach and promote damage to these cells *in vivo*. Furthermore, the cytotoxic activity of these antibodies in the gastric acid environment – a fundamental premise to the entire theory – has not been established.

CONCLUSIONS

The correlation between *H. pylori* infection and autoimmune gastritis is still controversial. Factors such as the high prevalence of the infection in patients with autoimmune gastritis and the evidence of autoimmune mechanisms against the gastric mucosa evoked by *H. pylori* suggest an association. On the other hand, *H. pylori*-induced anti-canalicular antibodies and classical anti-parietal cell antibodies described in autoimmune (type A) gastritis do not recognize the same epitope. Finally, several factors have to be examined critically before the 'antigenic mimicry theory' can be embraced. While billions of people are chronically infected with *H. pylori*, only a few develop a pure corpus-restricted atrophic gastritis that can be demonstrated to be autoimmune. In some populations a large percentage of the infected subjects develop atrophic gastritis which involves both the antrum and the corpus (atrophic pangastritis or multifocal atrophic gastritis). Although no-one knows what acts in concert with chronic *H. pylori* infection to cause this type of atrophic gastritis, the geographical distribution of the different types of gastritis suggests that environmental factors, such as diet, are of paramount importance. Before one can confidently make a case for *H. pylori* being the cause of autoimmune gastritis, much more biological, clinical, and epidemiological evidence is needed.

Nevertheless, as Stolte's study indicates[14], early treatment of *H. pylori* infection in subjects with non-atrophic, or pre-atrophic, corpus-restricted gastritis arrests the development of atrophy and reduces the risk for a variety of *H. pylori*-associated conditions. Therefore, even if this therapeutic approach still rests on attractive but untested theoretical foundations, its practical aspects make it entirely justifiable.

References

1. Cappella C, Fiocca R, Cornaggia M, Rindi G, Moratti R, Solcia E. Autoimmune gastritis. In: Graham DY, Genta RM, Dixon MF, editors. Gastritis. Philadelphia: Lippincott, Williams & Wilkins; 1999:79–96.

2. Wittingham S, Mackay IR. Pernicious anemia and gastric atrophy. In: Rose NR, Mackay IR, editors. The Autoimmune Diseases. London: Academic Press; 1985:243–5.
3. Karlsson FA, Burman P, Loof L, Mardh S. Major parietal cell antigen in autoimmune gastritis with pernicious anemia is the acid producing H,K adenosine triphosphatase of the stomach. J Clin Invest. 1988;81:475–9.
4. Toh BA, van Driel IR, Gleeson PA. Autoimmune gastritis: tolerance and autoimmunity to the gastric H/K-ATPase (proton pump). Autoimmunity. 1992;13:165–72.
5. Fukuma K, Sakaguchi S, Kuribayashi K et al. Immunologic and clinical studies on murine experimental autoimmune gastritis induced by neonatal thymectomy. Gastroenterology. 1998;94:274–83.
6. Marshall BJ, Warren JR. Unidentified curved bacilli in the stomach of patients with gastric and peptic ulceration. Lancet. 1984;1:1311–15.
7. Graham DY, Dixon MF. Acid secretion, *Helicobacter pylori* infection, and peptic ulcer disease. In: Graham DY, Genta RM, Dixon MF, editors. Gastritis. Philadelphia: Lippincott/Williams & Wilkins; 1999:177–87.
8. Figura N, Valassina M. *Helicobacter pylori* determinants of pathogenicity. J Chemother. 1999;11:591–600.
9. Shimoyama T, Crabtree JE. Bacterial factors and immune pathogenesis in Helicobacter pylori infection. Gut. 1998;43(Suppl. 1):S2–5.
10. Covacci A, Telford JL, Del Giudice G, Parsonnet J, Rappuoli R. *Helicobacter pylori* virulence and genetic geography. Science. 1999;284:1328–33.
11. Gonzalez JD, Sancho FJ, Sainz S, Such J, Fernandez M, Mones Xiol Y. *Helicobacter pylori* and pernicious anemia. Lancet. 1988;1:57.
12. Faisal MA, Russel RM, Samloff IM, Holt PR. *Helicobacter pylori* infection in atrophic gastritis in the elderly. Gastroenterology. 1990;99:1543–4.
13. Karnes WE, Samloff IM, Siurala M et al. Positive serum antibody and negative tissue staining for *Helicobacter pylori* in subjects with atrophic body gastritis. Gastroenterology. 1991;101:167–74.
14. Stolte M. Autoimmune gastritis via mimicking does occur. Chapter 30, this volume.
15. Negrini R, Savio A, Poiesi C et al. Antigenic mimicry between *Helicobacter pylori* and gastric mucosa in the pathogenesis of body atrophic gastritis. Gastroenterology. 1996;111:655–65.
16. Clayes D, Faller G, Appelmelk BJ, Negrini R. The gastric H^+,K^+-ATPase is a major autoantigen in chronic *Helicobacter pylori* gastritis with body mucosa atrophy. Gastroenterology. 1998;115:340–7.
17. Appelmelk BJ, Faller G, Clayes D, Kirchner T, Vandenbroucke-Grauls CMJE. Bugs on trial: the case of *Helicobacter pylori* and autoimmunity. Immunol Today. 1998;19:296–9.
18. Albert LJ, Inman RD. Molecular mimicry and autoimmunity. N Engl J Med. 1999;341:2068–74.

32
Carditis and intestinal metaplasia of the cardia is reflux related

M. B. FENNERTY

INTRODUCTION

Recently, there has been much controversy over the issue of carditis and intestinal metaplasia of the cardia. The real issue is where did all this controversy start and, more relevant, is it important? One of the driving forces in the interest in inflammation of the cardia has been related to the rising incidence of adenocarcinoma of the cardia and distal oesophagus over the past 30 years. Blot *et al.*, in their seminal paper in 1991, demonstrated that oesophageal and cardia adenocarcinomas showed the most rapidly rising incidence of any cancer over the past few decades[1]. Spechler *et al.* noted a high prevalence of intestinal metaplasia at the gastro-oesophageal junction[2]. These two reports were, in part, the genesis of the heightened awareness of the cardia and its potential of malignancy, as well as the premalignant pathology represented by intestinal metaplasia and its precursor lesion, carditis.

THE SAGA OF SPECHLER

In 1994 Spechler *et al.* reported on 142 patients, without endoscopicaly apparent Barrett's oesophagus, who had undergone biopsy at the junction during routine endoscopy[2]. Surprisingly, 18% of these patients had intestinal metaplasia observed in biopsies from this region. All of these patients were white, and the male to female ratio was 0.8. Interestingly, GERD symptoms did not discriminate between those patients with or without intestinal metaplasia. However, some investigators theorized that these patients had an ultra-short segment of Barrett's oesophagus, and this prevalent pathology could, in part, account for the rapidly rising incidence of cancer in this region.

Following these reports, a controversy developed regarding whether cardia mucosa was a normal finding, or arose as a consequence of gastro-oesophageal reflux disease. Oberg *et al.* reported in 1997 that cardia mucosa was not a normal finding but developed in response to gastro-oesophageal reflux[3]. More recently a substantial amount of evidence confirms that cardia mucosa is not an acquired epithelium but is a normal finding in 99% of adults, and most children[4,5].

Within cardia mucosa, inflammation, or carditis, can be observed as well as goblet cells representing intestinal metaplasia. More recently, controversy surrounding the cardia has focused on whether carditis and/or intestinal metaplasia of the cardia is related to reflux disease or *H. pylori* infections.

IS IT GERD OR IS IT *H. PYLORI*?

The simple answer is that it can be due to either *H. pylori* infection or reflux disease. However, this discussion will focus on the evidence that gastro-oesophageal reflux disease alone can result in inflammation and/or intestinal metaplasia of the cardia.

Hirota, in a study of 889 consecutive patients undergoing biopsy of the gastro-oesophageal junction, demonstrated that the prevalence of specialized intestinal metaplasia of the junction was approximately 13%[6]. Nearly half these patients had intestinal metaplasia at a normal-appearing gastro-oesophageal junction (a gastric cardia lesion), while the other half had intestinal metaplasia of the oesophagus, either short segment or long segment Barrett's oesophagus. Of further interest in this study was the demographics of these patients. As has been demonstrated with traditional Barrett's oesophagus, the majority of patients with intestinal metaplasia at the gastro-oesophageal junction were white and male. Although significantly more patients had coexistent *H. pylori* infection the prevalence was still only a little over 20% in these patients. Therefore, the majority of patients with intestinal metaplasia at the gastro-oesophageal junction or intestinal metaplasia of the cardia, were not infected with *H. pylori* and had demographic characteristics more similar to Barrett's oesophagus, which is related to gastro-oesophageal reflux disease (GERD).

There have been a number of studies supporting the concept that carditis and/or intestinal metaplasia of the cardia can occur secondary to GERD alone without *H. pylori* infection: Goldstein *et al.* reported 150 consecutive patients who had endoscopic biopsies from the cardia[7]. Forty-two of these patients were infected with *H. pylori*. In the *H. pylori*-negative patients cardia inflammation was correlated with the presence of squamous inflammation of the oesophagus, i.e. GERD, In those infected with *H. pylori*, cardia inflammation was correlated with antral inflammation and the presence of *H. pylori* in the cardia. This study clearly demonstrated that cardia inflammation could occur in the absence of *H. pylori* infection and was observed in the setting of gastro-oesophageal reflux disease. Similarly, Csendes *et al.* examined 500 patients for evidence of carditis in relation to GERD[8]. The prevalence of carditis in patients with reflux disease was 50% whereas the prevalence of carditis in patients without reflux disease was less than 10%. Intestinal metaplasia was seen in over 10% of patients with reflux disease, and in only 2% of patients in the control population. Thus, the presence of GERD was highly correlated with the finding of carditis and/or intestinal metaplasia of the cardia, and these histological findings were unusual in the control patients without gastro-oesophageal reflux disease.

Voutilainen examined 1053 subjects and found carditis in 75% of patients[9]. Thirty per cent of these patients were negative for *H. pylori* infection, indicating that carditis could exist in the absence of *H. pylori* infection. Confirming these findings Chen *et al.* were able to correlate the carditis grade with the presence or absence of *H. pylori* infection[10]. In patients with mild to moderate carditis, only 10% and 40%, respectively, of patients were infected with *H. pylori*. Even in those with severe carditis only a little over half the patients were infected with *H. pylori*. These data confirm that infection with *H. pylori* is not required for carditis, and GERD alone can result in this pattern of histology. Supporting this observation is the study by Bowery *et al.* in 150 patients with GERD[11]. Carditis was seen in 90% of the patients when cardia mucosa was found on biopsy. While carditis was more frequently found in those infected with *H. pylori*, it was also seen in 50% of patients who were *H. pylori*-negative.

Perhaps some of the differences in the prevalence of carditis in patients with GERD, seen in these above studies, can be explained by the study of Lembo *et al.*, which indicates that the location of the biopsies appears to be critical in determining whether carditis is detected[12]. When a biopsy bridging the squamocolumnar junction, which includes the most proximal region of the cardiac mucosa bordering the squamous mucosa, was obtained, the mean carditis score was substantially higher than when the biopsy was obtained from either just distal to this site or was one taken further distally, 1-2 cm below the Z-line. Thus, the more proximal the biopsy, the greater the likelihood of detecting carditis.

CONCLUSIONS

These data confirm that carditis and intestinal metaplasia of the cardia can be associated with gastro-oesophageal reflux disease alone. However, carditis is also associated with *H. pylori* infection and the presence of *H. pylori* may be an important determinant of the prevalence and degree of inflammation found in the cardia of a patient with reflux disease.

These data also underscore the need to closely scrutinize the methodology used in studying the cardia, in order to avoid even more confusion in this ongoing controversy.

References

1. Blot WJ, Devesa SS, Kneller RW, Fraumeni JF. Rising incidence of adenocarcinoma of the esophagus and gastric cardia. J Am Med Assoc. 1991;265:1287-9.
2. Spechler SJ, Zeroogian JM, Antonioli DA, Wang HH, Goyal RK. Prevalence of metaplasia at the gastro-oesophageal junction. Lancet. 1994;344:1533-6.
3. Oberg S, Peters JH, DeMeester TR *et al.* Inflammation and specialized intestinal metaplasia of cardiac mucosa is a manifestation of gastroesophageal reflux disease. Ann Surg. 1997; 226:522-30.
4. Kilgore SP, Ormsby AH, Gramlich TL *et al.* The gastric cardia is not a metaplastic mucosa secondary to gastroesophageal reflux disease (GERD). Gastroenterology. 1999;116:A213 (abstract).

5. Ormsby AH, Goldblum JR, Kilgore SP et al. The frequency and nature of cardiac mucosa and intestinal metaplasia (IM) of the esophagogastric junction (EGJ): a population based study of 223 consecutive autopsies. Gastroenterology. 1999;116:A273 (abstract).
6. Hirota WK, Loughney TM, Lazas DJ et al. Specialized intestinal metaplasia, dysplasia, and cancer of the esophagus and esophagogastric junction: prevalence and clinical data. Gastroenterology. 1999;116:277–85.
7. Goldstein NS, Karim R. Gastric cardia inflammation and intestinal metaplasia: association with reflux esophagitis and *Helicobacter pylori*. Mod Pathol. 1999;12:1017–24.
8. Csendes A, Smok G, Burdiles P et al. 'Carditis': an objective histologic marker for pathologic gastroesophageal reflux disease. Dis Esophagus. 1998;11:101–5.
9. Voutilainen M, Farkkila M, Mecklin JP et al. Chronic inflammation at the gastroesophageal junction (carditis) appears to be a specific finding related to *Helicobacter pylori* infection and gastroesophageal reflux disease. Am J Gastroenterol. 1999;94:3175–80.
10. Chen YY, Antonioli DA, Spechler SJ et al. Gastroesophageal reflux disease versus *Helicobacter pylori* as the cause of gastric carditis. Mod Pathol. 1998;11:950–6.
11. Bowery DJ, Clark GW, Williams GT. Patterns of gastritis in patients with gastro-esophageal reflux disease. Gut. 1999;45:798–803.
12. Lembo T, Ippoliti AF, Ramers C, Weinstein WM. Inflammation of the gastro-esophageal junction (carditis) in patients with symptomatic gastro-esophageal reflux disease: a prospective study. Gut. 1999;45:484–8.

33
Carditis and cardia intestinal metaplasia are *Helicobacter pylori*-related

W. M. WEINSTEIN

WHY DO WE CARE ABOUT THE GASTRIC CARDIA?

There are two reasons:

1. To determine whether the precursor lesions can be identified in relation to cancer of the gastric cardia.
2. As a marker for, or diagnostic test for, gastro-oesophageal reflux disease (GERD), in the setting where such a test is needed.

The two sides of the argument concerning the role of *Helicobacter pylori* are not mutually exclusive or necessarily confounding. *H. pylori* causes carditis and intestinal metaplasia and so does GERD. When the two occur together the injury may or may not be greater than either alone. *H. pylori* is a predictable cause of carditis whereas GERD is not. Moreover, the GERD connection cannot be rationalized until we know during how much of each day the gastric contents normally bathe the squamo-columnar junction. This is not physiological reflux; rather it is physiological contact with gastric contents. In one study of 10 volunteers it was found that cardia acid exposure was intermediate between that of the oesophagus and stomach[1].

We should first define what the cardia represents, and review some key study design issues in regard to morphological studies of this region.

WHAT IS THE GASTRIC CARDIA?

The term gastric cardia is used in two contexts: anatomical and histological.

Anatomical definition

Gastric cardia is often used as a synonym for gastro-oesophageal junction (GEJ) in relation to carcinomas in this region[2-4]. The GEJ or cardia is usually defined with certain boundaries within a few centimetres of the GEJ, both above and below. Anyone analysing or comparing research studies of GEJ tumours needs to determine whether the boundaries have been defined and whether the boundaries are in line with other studies.

Histological definition

Histologically the stomach consists of three zones, each named after the differing appearances of their gland types[5]:

1. antral glands of mucous type;
2. oxyntic glands (occupying the body and fundus) with glands containing parietal and chief cells;
3. the cardiac glands of mucous type.

The junctions between the gland zones consist of segments of variable length where the glands of the adjoining gland types are mixed[6].

The cardiac gland zone is a very narrow segment at and just below the GEJ that generally does not extend distal to the GEJ more than 2 cm. Its glands are of the mucous gland type, similar in appearance to those of the gastric antrum and the duodenal Brunner's glands. Much or all of the cardiac gland zone is actually a mix of the cardiac mucous glands and oxyntic gland elements, either parietal cells alone, or both parietal and chief cells. This appearance resembles that of the gastric antrum where oxyntic gland elements commonly extend all the way to the pylorus.

Pancreatic metaplasia or heterotopia

Nests of exocrine pancreatic glands may be present right at the region of the lower oesophageal sphincter, both in patients with and without Barrett's oesophagus. In two biopsy studies the prevalence was 9% and 24%[7,8] and in a resection study it was 14%[9]. It is not known whether these glands are acquired (metaplastic), or congenital (heterotopia), or whether they might contribute to mucosal disease at the GEJ.

IS THE CARDIAC GLAND MUCOSA ACQUIRED?

An autopsy study by Chandrasoma *et al.*, and a comparison study of cardiac gland extent with 24 h pH-metry in short and long segment Barrett's oesophagus have led to their proposal that the cardia is an acquired gland zone[10,11]. In their autopsy study approximately half had pure cardiac glands and the rest had mixed cardia/oxyntic glands. In 50% the cardiac glands did not extend around the circumference of the oesophagus and in 75% the length was less than 0.5 cm. There was a tendency for the cardiac gland zone to expand somewhat with age. Chandrasoma *et al.* propose that the cardiac gland zone in GERD could represent a useful histological definition for assessing the presence and severity of reflux. However, in patients with GERD, without Barret's oesophagus, even a putatively expanded cardiac gland zone is still very short, thus making biopsy mapping to define its extent difficult, if not impossible.

Table 1. Checklist for readers of studies assessing carditis with or without IM at a normally located Z-line

---
1. What is the definition of a normally located Z line? Should not permit columnar epithelium above the LES region to be considered 'normal'
2. Biopsy technique
   (a) Where were biopsies obtained? The term cardia by itself is not specific enough
   (b) How many biopsies were taken in each patient, how many ended up as interpretable?
3. What proportion of biopsies in the study contained only squamous epithelium, both squamous and columnar lined or columnar lined alone? In the columnar-lined mucosa what proportion were cardiac (with or without parietal cells) and which were pure oxyntic?
4. Demographics of the population: did they include the following and were the results analysed in part according to the applicable variables here?
   (a) Race?
   (b) Treatment – e.g. acid suppression, recent withdrawal of acid suppression, recent *H. pylori* eradication therapy?
   (c) If controls were used were they appropriate; retrospective or prospective?
   (d) Erosive oesophagitis or normal Z lines?
   (e) Associated disorders, i.e. dyspepsia, GERD, peptic ulcer?
5. How were carditis and IM defined? Were H&E–alcian blue stains done to avoid overdiagnosis of goblet cells?
6. Were histological results given as 'yes/no' for carditis or expressed at the type of abnormality and grade of severity?

In an autopsy study of the squamocolumnar junction in 49 pre-viable fetuses, stillbirths, infants and young children, small zones were identified that resembled cardiac glands[12]. Whether these are the same mucous gland types as seen in adulthood, or whether they regress and reappear in some other form, is unknown.

There is ample precedent to support the proposal from Chandrasoma and co-workers that some of the cardiac gland mucosa might be metaplastic, i.e. acquired. In severe atrophic gastritis of the oxyntic mucosa, mucous glands may replace oxyntic glands. The ingrained term for this is pseudopyloric (meaning pseudoantral) metaplasia, but the origin of these metaplastic glands is unknown. This phenomenon is also seen outside of the stomach in some small bowel mucosal diseases, especially Crohn's disease[13] and of course scattered throughout the length of Barrett's oesophagus, underlying the metaplastic surface columnar epithelium.

THE HISTOLOGIC ABNORMALITIES

Table 1 gives a checklist of items that one might look for in studies of carditis. Some of the items in the table seem patently obvious but are not uncommonly omitted. One not-uncommon practice is to list the system used for the histological analysis as either the Sydney or updated Houston systems, but then the results for histology are given only as a yes/no for carditis and intestinal metaplasia[14,15]. This practice, and a near-universal failure to provide photographs of what the different grades look like, is also a not-uncommon occurrence in studies of gastritis distal to the cardia.

Carditis

This term is meant to refer to inflammatory infiltrates as well as to epithelial cell damage.

The potential histological spectrum of carditis is similar to that of gastritis elsewhere in the stomach. The inflammatory infiltrate may be chronic or chronic active with or without epithelial cell changes. Sometimes epithelial cell change is the only or dominant feature, similar to reactive gastropathy elsewhere in the stomach.

Intestinal metaplasia

Intestinal metaplasia (IM) is considered part of the potential spectrum of carditis. For the purposes of this discussion IM refers to the finding of intestinal-type goblet cells, and is verified with a haematoxylin and eosin–alcian blue pH 2.5 stain. The purpose of this stain is to avoid overdiagnosis, because bloated gastric cardia cells may resemble goblet cells but will be negative-staining with alcian blue.

Other types of metaplastic cells may be present, as is seen in incomplete intestinal metaplasia of the stomach. A common pattern of incomplete metaplasia is where cells look gastric but stain like goblet cells. In addition to the stomach, this can also be seen in Barrett's oesophagus[16].

Variables that may affect the results of survey studies of carditis and cardia IM

Most of the studies to date have omitted some critical information. Retrospective pathology studies may offer interesting descriptive pathology but without any relevant clinical, therapeutic or endoscopic data[17].

Biopsy site

Since the cardia does not have discrete endoscopic boundaries it is important to know where biopsies were taken, and also where the best site would be to detect maximal mucosal injury. In a biopsy study of the cardia in GERD patients without erosive oesophagitis we found that biopsies intended to straddle the Z line only (taken on turnaround in the stomach) yielded both squamous and columnar epithelium in approximately half. The reason for this is probably that the biopsy forceps is parallel to the Z line and is difficult to rotate into a 90 degree angle relative to the Z line, where there is a better opportunity to obtain both squamous and columnar epithelium in the same biopsy specimen. This had a profound effect on the results. In Z line biopsies with both epithelia the prevalence of goblet cells was approximately 30%, whereas it was half that in Z line biopsies containing only columnar epithelium[18]. The cardia injury scores paralleled the goblet cell prevalence.

Recent studies have focused on biopsy 'just below' the squamocolumnar junction. One must be sure what that means. For example in one study of the cardia up to 3 cm of columnar mucosa above the lower oesophageal sphincter region was taken to be within the range of a normal Z line. Most would now consider anyone with IM in that zone to have short segment Barrett's oesophagus rather than IM in a normally located Z line[19].

The study population

The prevalence of *H. pylori* infection in GERD may vary widely. In the US, Caucasians with GERD may have prevalence rates between 15% and 25%, whereas in an overall analysis of all studies it was found to be in the range of 40%.

Is erosive oesophagitis present and are patients on acid-suppressive therapy?

If a GERD population is included in any survey of carditis it is important to know how many of the patients had erosive oesophagitis, and to see the study results analysed for that variable among the other parameters that are analysed. There are several reasons. If one purpose is to use the presence of carditis as a diagnostic aid in GERD, then the key patients are those *without* erosive oesophagitis since the presence of erosive oesophagitis makes the diagnosis. Secondly, not until erosive oesophagitis is healed does it become apparent how many patients actually have short segment Barrett's oesophagus. Thus, the prevalence of IM could be magnified if edges of inapparent short segment Barrett's oesophagus are biopsied in patients with erosive oesophagitis. In preliminary data from a US multicentre study of 603 patients with GERD, treated with either pantoprazole or placebo, we found that 17 cases of short segment Barrett's oesophagus were present at baseline and an additional 16 became apparent after healing of the esophagitis at 4 or 8 weeks[20]. None of the placebo-treated patients had any additional cases of Barrett's oesophagus detected after the baseline evaluation. These data do not mean that, in every study of oesophagitis after healing, the numbers of Barrett's oesophagus patients would double, but some number would be uncovered.

H. PYLORI CAUSES CARDITIS WITH IM

The odds ratio for the connection between *H. pylori* infection and cardia cancer is less than one, i.e. in one nested case–control study[3] as low as 0.4. Thus, although *H. pylori* is a predictable cause of carditis with or without IM it does not carry a cancer risk.

Unlike GERD or any other cause of cardia injury *H. pylori* is a predictable cause of carditis with or without IM[21-23]. Genta *et al.* studied the severity of inflammation in the cardia of 42 patients with *H. pylori* infection[21]. Forty of the 42 (95%) had *H. pylori* detected in the cardia. The inflammation in the cardia paralleled that of the antrum, with both being more severe than the gastric body. However, there were fewer lymphoid aggregates in the cardia[21]. Others have not found *H. pylori* as easily in the cardia region as in this study. That may relate to a variety of factors that are included in Table 1.

One interesting observation was made by Voutilainen *et al.* in a large prospective study from Finland[23]. Incomplete IM was present when carditis-associated IM was not associated with inflammation elsewhere in the stomach. In looking at prevalence in this study and others, one must always keep in mind the possibility that the endogenous *H. pylori* rates of infection and prevalences of cardia IM may be different on environmental or racial grounds.

Goldblum and associates studied 27 controls and 58 GERD patients[24]. It is not known how many of the GERD patients had erosive oesophagitis. The prevalence of *H. pylori* infection was high in the controls at 48% and was 40% in the GERD group. The prevalence of carditis was 100% in the controls and 96% in the GERD patients. Seven of the eight patients with IM were *H. pylori*-positive. Six of 27 controls and two of 58 GERD patients had IM. Although IM appears to be weighted in the controls, the total number is very small.

The prevalence of IM may vary according to the underlying *H. pylori*-associated conditions. This was illustrated in a study by Hackelsberger *et al.*[25] in which the prevalence of cardia IM in *H. pylori* infections varied from 10% in duodenal ulcer to 44% in gastric ulcer, with GERD being intermediate. The numbers in the disease groups were small but the study illustrates the need to detail which *H. pylori*-associated condition is being studied.

THE REAL DEBATE ABOUT CARDITIS AND IM

In regard to GERD, the main problem is that which plagues all oesophageal function tests. Namely it is difficult to distinguish between pathological GERD and physiological GERD. This is compounded further in regard to the cardia because there are very few data[1] to define the proportion of a normal person's day during which the squamocolumnar junction is exposed to gastric contents. Five centimetres up from the GEJ we accept that 4% of the day can have a pH less than 4. How much is that magnified right at the GEJ in health? Biopsy of the squamous mucosa in asymptomatic volunteers demonstrated that the regenerative hyperplasia changes described in GERD (basal cell hyperplasia, elongated dermal papillae) were commonly present in the distal 2.5 cm of the oesophagus[26]. This probably reflects the considerable physiological contact with gastric contents at and near the GEJ.

Goldblum *et al.* have used cytokeratin markers to distinguish between the IM of *H. pylori* infection and that not associated with *H. pylori*[27]. Their intriguing observation remains to be confirmed in other laboratories. However, one would still be left with the daunting task of stratifying risk from that point on. Also, theoretically, the IM of *H. pylori* infection and that of GERD and that of physiological contact could all coexist.

With regard to cancer of the cardia, carditis and GERD, the problem is similar to that of IM of the stomach; namely it is potentially sensitive but thoroughly non-specific. The prevalence of IM in African Americans and women appears to be the same in GERD and non-GERD as in white males without Barrett's oesophagus[28–30]. Yet they have much lower (women) to non-existent (African Americans) rates of cardia and Barrett's cancer. Thus, the key gender and race factors (white males) in cardia and Barrett's cancers must become operative after the development of intestinal metaplasia. There is no way to stratify this risk when IM of the cardia is encountered, and hence no reason to biopsy the normally located Z line outside of studies, no reason to enter those with IM into surveillance and certainly no reason to call IM at a normally located Z line ultrashort Barrett's oesophagus. Barrett's oesophagus has an oncological implication and, given the caveats above, use of the term ultrashort Barrett's oesophagus condemns a patient for life with worry about cancer risk, and attendant difficulties with life and disability insurance.

There is an understandable great drive to be able to use carditis as a marker of GERD and IM of the cardia as a marker of increased risk of cancer of the cardia. Optimism for this has outstripped reality with a rush to judgement in some quarters. We need to be able to define the interactions between the carditis and IM of life (wear and tear), GERD, and of *H. pylori* infection. Once the latter is excluded then we need predictors of risk for carcinoma just as we need them for IM of the stomach and Barrett's oesophagus[31,32]. It promises to be an exciting journey.

References

1. Katzka DA, Gideon RM, Castell DO. Normal patterns of acid exposure at the gastric cardia: a functional midpoint between the esophagus and stomach. Am J Gastroenterol. 1998;93:1236–42.
2. Hansen S, Melby KK, AAse S, Jellum E, Vollset SE. *Helicobacter pylori* infection and risk of cardia cancer and non-cardia gastric cancer – a nested case–control study. Scand J Gastroenterol. 1999;34:353–60.
3. Pera M. Epidemiology of esophageal cancer, especially adenocarcinoma of the esophagus and esophagogastric junction. Recent Results Cancer Res. 2000;155:1–14.
4. Cameron AJ, Lomboy CT, Pera M, Carpenter HA. Adenocarcinoma of the esophagogastric junction and Barrett's esophagus. Gastroenterology. 1995;109(5):1541–6.
5. Lewin KJ, Riddell RH, Weinstein WM. Stomach and proximal duodenum: inflammatory and miscellaneous disorders. In: Lewin KJ, Riddell RH, Weinstein WM, editors. Gastrointestinal Pathology and its Clinical Implications. New York, Tokyo: Igaku-Shoin; 1992:506–69.
6. Van Zanten SJ, Dixon MF, Lee A. The gastric transitional zones: neglected links between gastroduodenal pathology and *Helicobacter* ecology. Gastroenterology. 1999;116:1217–29.
7. Krishnamurthy S, Dayal Y. Pancreatic metaplasia in Barrett's esophagus. An immunohistochemical study. Am J Surg Pathol. 1995;19:1172–80.
8. Wang HH, Zeroogian JM, Spechler SJ, Goyal RK, Antonioli DA. Prevalence and significance of pancreatic acinar metaplasia at the gastroesoophageal junction. Am J Surg Pathol. 1996;20:1507–10.
9. Polkowski W, van Lanschot JJ, Ten Kate FJ *et al.* Intestinal and pancreatic metaplasia at the esophagogastric junction in patients without Barrett's esophagus (In Process Citation). Am J Gastroenterol. 2000;95:617–25.
10. Chandrasoma PT, Der R, Ma Y, Dalton P, Talra M. Histology of the gastroesoophageal junction: an autopsy study. Am J Surg Pathol. 2000;24:402–9.
11. Chandrasoma PT, Lokuhetty DM, DeMeester TR *et al.* Definition of histopathologic changes in gastroesoophageal reflux disease (In Process Citation). Am J Surg Pathol. 2000;24:344–51.
12. Ellison E, Hassall E, Dimmick JE. Mucin histochemistry of the developing gastroesophageal junction. Pediatr Pathol Lab Med. 1996;16:195–206.
13. Wright NA. Aspects of the biology of regeneration and repair in the human gastrointestinal tract. Phil Trans R Soc Lond B Biol Sci. 1998;353:925–33.
14. Dixon MF, Genta RM, Yardley JH *et al.* Classification and grading of gastritis – the updated Sydney System. Am J Surg Pathol. 1996;20:1161–81.
15. Price AB. The Sydney System: histological division. J Gastroenterol Hepatol. 1991;6:209–22.

16. Offner FA, Lewin KJ, Weinstein WM. Metaplastic columnar cells in Barrett's esophagus: a common and neglected cell type. Hum Pathol. 1996;27:885–9.
17. Goldstein NS, Karim R. Gastric cardia inflammation and intestinal metaplasia: associations with reflux esophagitis and *Helicobacter pylori*. Mod Pathol. 1999;12:1017–24.
18. Lembo T, Ippoliti AF, Ramers C, Weinstein WM. Inflammation of the gastroesoophageal junction (carditis) in patients with symptomatic gastroesophageal reflux disease: a prospective study. Gut. 1999;454:484–8.
19. Spechler SJ, Zeroogian JM, Antonioli DA, Wang HH, Goyal RK. Prevalence of metaplasia at the gastroesophageal junction. Lancet. 1994;344:1533–6.
20. Weinstein, WM. Erosive esophagitis impairs accurate detection of Barrett's esophagus: a prospective randomized double blind study. Gastroenterology. 1999;116:A352 (abstract).
21. Genta RM, Huberman RM, Graham DY. The gastric cardia in *Helicobacter pylori* infection. Hum Pathol. 1994;25:915–19.
22. Morales TG, Sampliner RE, Bhattacharyya A. Intestinal metaplasia of the gastric cardia. Am J Gastroenterol. 1997;92:414–18.
23. Voutilainen M, Farkkila M, Mecklin JP, Juhola M, Sipponen P. Chronic inflammation at the gastroesophageal junction (carditis) appears to be a specific finding related to *Helicobacter pylori* infection and gastroesophageal reflux disease. Central Finland Endoscopy Study Group. Am J Gastroenterol. 1999;94:3175–80.
24. Goldblum JR, Vicari JJ, Falk GW et al. Inflammation and intestinal metaplasia of the gastric cardia: the role of gastroesophageal reflux and *H. pylori* infection. Gastroenterology. 1998;114:633–9.
25. Hackelsberger A, Gunther T, Schultze V, Labenz J, Roessner A, Malfertheiner P. Prevalence and pattern of *Helicobacter pylori* gastritis in the gastric cardia. Am J Gastroenterol. 1997;92:2220–4.
26. Weinstein WM, Bogoch ER, Bowes KL. The normal human esophageal mucosa: a histological reappraisal. Gastroenterology. 1975;68:40–44.
27. Ormsby AH, Goldblum JR, Rice TW et al. Cytokeratin subsets can reliably distinguish Barrett's esophagus from intestinal metaplasia of the stomach. Hum Pathol. 1999;30:288–94.
28. Pereira AD, Suspiro A, Chaves P et al. Short segments of Barrett's epithelium and intestinal metaplasia in normal appearing oesophagogastric junctions: the same or two different entities? Gut. 1998;42:659–62.
29. Nandurkar S, Talley NJ, Martin CJ, Ng TH, Adams S. Short segment Barrett's oesophagus: prevalence, diagnosis and associations. Gut. 1997;40:710–15.
30. Hirota WK, Loughney TM, Lazas DJ, Maydonovitch CL, Rholl V, Wong RK. Specialized intestinal metaplasia, dysplasia, and cancer of the esophagus and esophagogastric junction: prevalence and clinical data. Gastroenterology. 1999;116:277–85.
31. Jankowski JA, Wright NA, Meltzer SJ et al. Molecular evolution of the metaplasia–dysplasia–adenocarcinoma sequence in the esophagus. Am J Pathol. 1999;154:965–73.
32. Fitzgerald RC, Triadafilopoulos G. Recent developments in the molecular characterization of Barrett's esophagus. Dig Dis. 1998;16:63–80.

34
Is gastric metaplasia in *Helicobacter pylori* really gastric?

N. A. WRIGHT

INTRODUCTION

There are really two questions in the title to this chapter: what is the relationship of 'gastric metaplasia' to the epithelium it so morphologically resembles, the gastric foveolar-pit mucus-secreting epithelium? And, of course, where does it come from?

THE PHENOTYPE

There is no doubt that, morphologically speaking, gastric metaplasia distinctly resembles the gastric foveolar-pit epithelium (Figure 1). The cells also stain positively with the diastase/periodic acid Schiff (D/PAS) method, reflecting the neutral mucin content of the cells, as opposed to the acid sialomucin of the goblet cells. Ultrastructurally, the metaplastic cells contain multiple apical mucous secretory droplets which are characteristic of gastric foveolar mucous cells[1]. In terms of mucin gene expression, gastric metaplasia shows MUC5AB, as do the foveolar-pit cells[2]. As we might expect, the gastric metaplasia also shows pS2/TFF1 expression (trefoil family factor 1) which is often co-expressed with MUC5AB in the gastric foveolar-pit cells[2,3] (Figure 1). Perhaps the only differences which have been reported between gastric metaplasia and foveolar-pit cells are in their lectin-binding profiles, reflecting differences not in mucin gene expression, but in the type of oligosaccharide side-chains[4].

So, as judged by morphology and gene expression profiling, at least thus far, gastric metaplasia appears identical to gastric foveolar epithelium.

THE ORIGINS OF GASTRIC METAPLASIA

There are basically four theories which attempt to account for the histogenesis of gastric metaplasia:

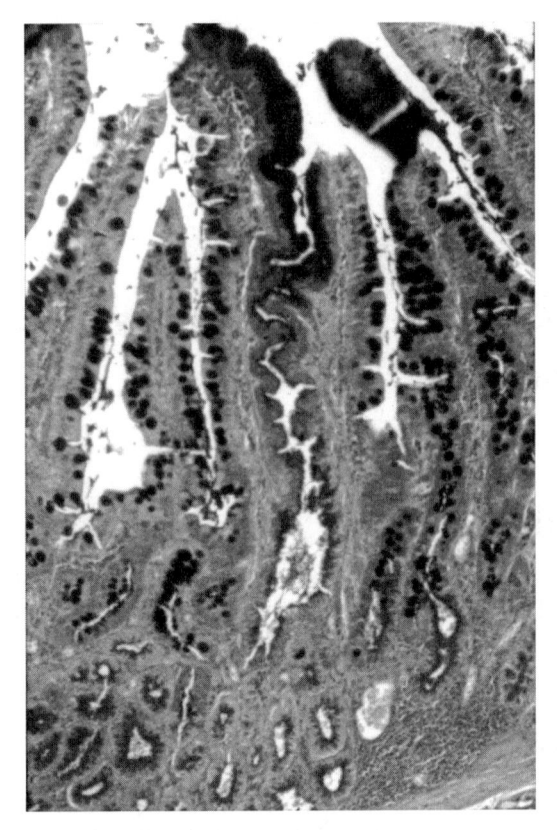

Figure 1. Illustration to show that gastric metaplasia in the duodenum has typical foveolar-pit morphology, is D/PAS positive, and expresses TFF1 MRNA.

1. direct transformation of goblet cells to foveolar-pit cells in the villi;
2. upward migration of Brunner's gland duct epithelium[5];
3. a true repetitive and presumably metaplastic cell lineage of Brunner's glands[6];
4. a true metaplastic change in the duodenal crypt stem cells.

What prerequisites does the theory have to satisfy? Obviously (1) the appearance of foveolar-pit cells on the villus; (2) the distribution of gastric metaplasia in the first and second part of the duodenum[1]; (3) the migration characteristics of gastric metaplasia, which appear to occupy right cohorts, appearing on the villus and migrating in thin ribbons to reach the villus tip, where the ribbons coalesce (Figure 2); and (4) the presence of so-called 'intermediate cells', purportedly transitional forms between goblet and foveolar-pit cells[7].

GASTRIC METAPLASIA IN *H. PYLORI*

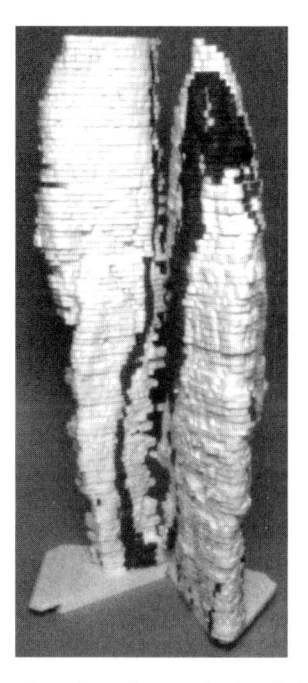

Figure 2. The pathway of migration of gastric metaplastic cells in duodenal villi. Serial sections were stained with D/PAS and the models reconstructed in polystyrene.

1. Direct goblet cell – foveolar pit cell transformation

This view has recently been championed by Shaoul et al.[2], and is based on a series of observations of MUC and TFF gene expression in developing established gastric metaplasia. They point to several observations supporting this hypothesis: (1) that in fact mucin secretory granules are heterogeneous in appearance in gastric metaplasia, with appearances which resemble those of intestinal and gastric cells; (2) that some (? early) metaplastic cells contain MUC2 core protein – i.e. MUC2 without oligosaccharide residues, which are usually confined to the Golgi of goblet cells; (3) the granules contain gastric (MUC5AC) and intestinal mucins (MUC2); (4) local goblet cells around areas of gastric metaplasia elaborate both intestinal and gastric mucins, (5) these goblet cells also express hSP/TFF1, a foveolar-pit cell marker. Moreover, the number of goblet cells with a mixed phenotype diminishes with distance away from the gastric metaplasia patches, and they are more numerous in early gastric metaplasia, before it becomes generalized.

This hypothesis certainly does account for the appearances of transitional forms, well described in the earlier literature. On the other hand, it does not account for the appearance of migrating cells in ribbons, nor for the distribution of gastric metaplasia in only the first and second part of the duodenum. It also puts great store on the proposal that MUC5AB and TFF1 are purely gastric markers, whereas it has previously been shown that goblet cells in the neighbourhood of the ulcer-associated cell lineage (UACL) express TFF1, possibly in response to the EGF thought to be secreted by the UACL[8].

The TFF1 gene has an EGF responsive enhancer sequence upstream of the start site. Moreover, MUC5AB is certainly not confined to the stomach and is seen in goblet cells in the colon and small intestine[9].

2. Upward migration of Brunner's duct epithelium

This was probably first proposed by James[10] to account for the localization of gastric metaplasia in the duodenum, where Brunner's glands are found, and also the frequent observation that gastric metaplasia is seen in direct continuity with cells apparently in the process of migrating from Brunner's gland ducts. Liu and Wright[5], by three-dimensional reconstruction of serial sections, traced the migration of gastric metaplasia cells upward from the crypt orifices onto duodenal villi (Figure 2). This draws parallels between the Brunner's gland duct and the duct of the UACL, from which cells with the morphological and molecular phenotype of foveolar-pit cells migrate onto the villi[11].

This proposal certainly accounts for the migration pattern and the duodenal localization, but it does not account for the formation of the so-called transitional goblet cells. Hanby et al.[3] showed that the TFF profile of gastric metaplasia resembled gastric foveolar cells, and also claimed that TFF1 was seen in Brunner's gland ducts, a view disputed by Shaoul et al.[2] and Rio (quoted by Shaoul et al.[2]). Shaoul et al.[2] also consider that this migration hypothesis is flawed, since MUC5AC is not apparently seen in Brunner's gland ducts, but of course in these lineages gene expression changes as cells migrate (e.g. the TFF and MUC gene expression programme of the UACL, which modulates with position in the lineage[8,12]).

3. A reparative metaplastic lineage of Brunner's glands

This is a new hypothesis proposed by Kushima et al.[6]. They employed a series of antibodies – M1 which stains foveolar cells and is thought to recognize a protein epitope of MUC5AB; M2, which stains deep pyloric glands, Brunner's glands and UACL, recognizing the truncated O glycan GalNaC (and corresponds to MUC6 distribution) while M3 recognizes intestinal goblet cells.

In the duodental crypts in inflamed and ulcerated mucosa, single and continuous groups of M1-positive cells were seen extruding from the M2-positive Brunner's glands. In some areas an organized growth, resembling a gastric gland with a defined proliferative zone and surface M1 and deep M2 staining, as seen in pyloric glands, was seen. This pattern was reproduced in longer, more tenuous ducts migrating through granulation tissue.

Kushima et al.[6] proposed that in duodenitis or duodenal ulceration a new generative zone, the 'neo G zone', is established in Brunner's glands. This produces M1-positive foveolar cells, which migrate towards the lumen with elongation of the generative zone, and an organoid gastric gland is produced. This hypothesis certainly provides the distribution of gastric metaplasia, and the migration pathways, but again not the transitional goblet cells on the villi. This proposal differs from (2) in that a true metaplasia of Brunner's gland (? of the duct) is proposed.

4. A true metaplasia

This proposal would state that the duodenal crypt stem cells alter their differentiation pathway to the gastric phenotype possibly by a change in Hox or Parahox genes, as discussed by Wright in Chapter 26. This would explain the migration characteristics, but not the duodenal localization or the transitional goblet cells.

CONCLUSION

It is clear that no hypothesis fits all the prerequisites we laid down at the outset. Perhaps the closest come proposals 3 and 2, which involve Brunner's glands and its ducts in the hypothesis. This leaves the problem of transitional goblet cells; however, these might be a finding in any area where EGF is secreted. It is clear that further studies, looking for more markers and also using current markers in serial sections, are required before we finally have an answer.

References

1. Walker MM, Dixon MF. Gastric metaplasia: its role in duodenal ulceration. Aliment Pharmacol Ther. 1998;10:119–28.
2. Shaoul R, Marcon P, Okada Y, Cutz E, Forstner G. The pathogenesis of duodenal gastric metaplasia: the role of local goblet cell transformation. Gut. 2000;30:397–403.
3. Hanby AM, Poulsom R, Elia G et al. The expression of the trefoil peptides pS2 and hSP in gastric metaplasia of the proximal duodenum. J Pathol. 1993;169:355–60.
4. Kuhl P, Baczako K, Nilucs M, Malfertheimer P. How does gastric metaplasia in the duodenum differ from gastric epithelium? Gut. 1995;37(Suppl. 1):A29.
5. Liu KC, Wright NA. The migration pathway of epithelial cells on human duodenal villi: the origin and fate of gastric metaplastic cells in duodenal mucosa. Epith Cell Biol. 1992;1:53–8.
6. Kushima R, Manabe R, Hattori T, Burckard F. Histogenesis of gastric foveolar metaplasia following duodenal ulcer: a definite reparative lineage of Brunner's glands. Histopathology. 1999;35:38–43.
7. Gregory MA, Spitaels JM. Variation in the morphology of villus epithelial cells within 8 mm of untreated duodenal ulcers. J Pathol. 1987;153:109–19.
8. Wright NA, Poulsom R, Stamp G et al. Trefoil peptide gene expression in gastrointestinal epithelial cells in inflammatory bowel disease. Gastroenterology. 1993;104:12–20.
9. Wright NA, Longman R, Poulsom R et al. Co-ordinated TFF and MUC gene expression in the gut. Gastroenterology. 2000 (In press).
10. James AH. Gastric epithelium in the duodenum. Gut. 1964;5:285–94.
11. Wright NA. Migration of the ductular elements of gut-associated glands gives clue to the histogenesis of lesions associated with responses to acid hypersecretory states. Yale J Biol Med. 1996;69:147–53.
12. Longman R, Poulsom R, Corfield A et al. TFF and MUC gene expression in the ulcer-associated cell lineage. Gut. 2000 (In press).

Section VII
Helicobacter pylori and Clinical Consequences

35
Extragastric manifestations of *Helicobacter pylori* – are they relevant?

C. W. HOWDEN and G. I. LEONTIADIS

INTRODUCTION

Helicobacter pylori has been linked conclusively to various disorders of the upper gastrointestinal tract. In addition, it has been proposed to be associated with a variety of conditions outside of the alimentary tract. The list of proposed 'extragastric' associations continues to grow despite the fact that *H. pylori* is a non-invasive organism whose infection is essentially confined to the surface of gastric-type mucosa.

Association does not necessarily imply causation. The prevalence of *H. pylori* infection is high in many communities around the world and so it may coexist by chance in some patients who are being investigated or treated for another prevalent condition. While this should stress the need for adequately controlled studies, it is clear that these are the exception rather than the rule[1]. Sackett and others have proposed a set of nine 'diagnostic criteria' to aid the assessment of whether an association is likely to be causal[2]. These are listed, in decreasing order of importance, in Table 1. Applying these criteria, we concluded that there was little hard evidence in support of *H. pylori* as a cause of most of the proposed non-gastrointestinal conditions

Table 1. Nine proposed diagnostic criteria to help determine whether a proposed association is causal (from Sackett et al.[2])

1	Is there evidence from true experiments in humans?
2	Is the association strong?
3	Is the association consistent from study to study?
4	Is the temporal relationship correct?
5	Is there a dose–response relationship?
6	Does the association make epidemiological sense?
7	Does the association make biological sense?
8	Is the association specific?
9	Is the association analogous to a previously proven causal association?

with which it had been preliminarily linked[1]. The aims of this chapter are to review and update the information linking *H. pylori* to those conditions already covered[1], and to some other conditions for which an association has been suggested.

CORONARY HEART DISEASE (CHD)

In view of its tremendous importance in clinical medicine, CHD would certainly be the most relevant association of *H. pylori* infection were it to be confirmed, and would easily dwarf peptic ulcer disease and gastric neoplasia combined! However, and as reviewed previously[1], an association that once seemed plausible has not been seen consistently, and has been less likely to be demonstrated in prospective, controlled studies. Both *H. pylori* infection and CHD are encountered more frequently in patients from lower socioeconomic strata, and many studies have not adequately controlled for this.

It has been speculated that the epidemiology of CHD has behaved like that of a chronic infectious disease. Recently, attention has increasingly been focused on the inflammatory component to atherosclerosis, whether in the coronary circulation or elsewhere[3–5]. Since *H. pylori* is non-invasive, it is of no surprise that it has not been found in association with atherosclerotic plaques[6]. However, its presence in the stomach could theoretically influence inflammatory and thrombotic processes elsewhere by modulating levels of circulating factors or by alterations in lipid profiles. Some pertinent theories are listed in Table 2.

Much attention has focused on any possible effect of chronic *H. pylori* infection on serum lipid levels. While the results of different studies have been inconsistent, we concluded that *H. pylori* infection might be associated with a reduction in levels of high-density lipoprotein (HDL)-cholesterol,

Table 2. Proposed explanation for the possible association between *H. pylori* infection and coronary heart disease

Mechanism	Comment	Highest level of evidence in support
Raised fibrinogen levels	Inconsistently observed; not seen in large studies or in meta-analyses	Cross-sectional study
Altered platelet function	Chance laboratory finding	No epidemiological evidence
Elevated serum lipids	Statistically significant differences of small magnitude; inconsistently observed	Cross-sectional study
Antibodies to heat shock proteins (hps)	Biological significance unclear; correlation between anti-hps and anti-*H. pylori* IgG	Cross-sectional study
Hyperhomocysteinaemia	Independent risk factor but no correlation with *H. pylori* infection	No epidemiological evidence

A full discussion of the above points appears in refs 1, 4 and 7.

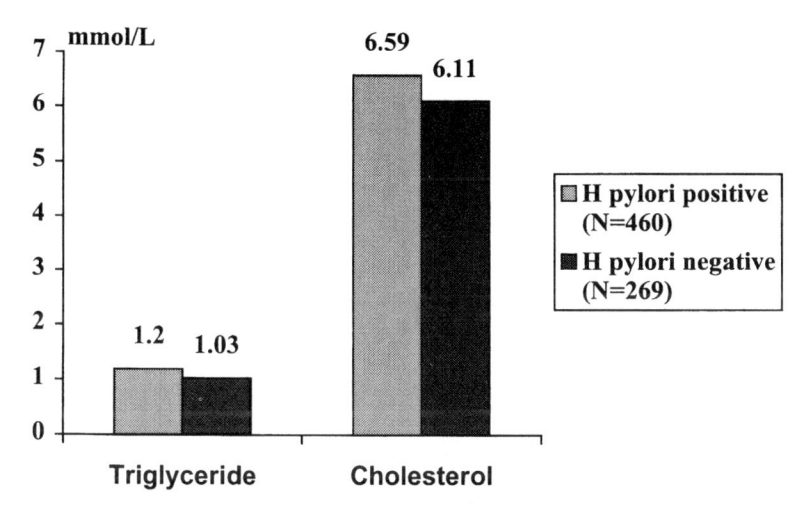

[Chart: Bar chart titled with y-axis "mmol/L" showing Triglyceride (1.2 vs 1.03) and Cholesterol (6.59 vs 6.11) for H pylori positive (N=460) and H pylori negative (N=269)]

Figure 1. Mean serum triglyceride and total serum cholesterol levels according to *H. pylori* status from Finnish nested case–control study[8]. There were statistically significant differences for both triglyceride and total cholesterol between *H. pylori*-positive and -negative subjects ($p < 0.001$ for both).

although the magnitude of the effect was small[1,4,7]. More recently, a large nested case–control study from Finland has reported significantly higher serum triglyceride and total cholesterol levels in men seropositive for *H. pylori* than in those who were seronegative[8]. These differences persisted despite adjustment for age, body mass index and social class. The principal results are depicted in Figure 1. Again, although highly statistically significant, the absolute magnitude of the differences was small. The investigators did not report levels of HDL- and LDL-cholesterol.

Danesh and colleagues in the UK performed a case–control study of 1122 survivors of suspected acute myocardial infarction aged between 30 and 49[9]. Forty-two per cent of the cases were seropositive for *H. pylori* infection compared with 24% of age- and sex-matched controls (OR = 2.28; 95% Cl = 1.80–2.90; $p < 0.0001$). When adjustment was made for smoking and socioeconomic status, the odds ratio fell to 1.87 (95% Cl = 1.42–2.47; $p > 0.001$). When further adjustment was made for blood lipid levels and obesity, the odds ratio fell to 1.75 (95% Cl = 1.29–2.36). Although, and as would be expected, the cases had higher total cholesterol levels than the controls, there were no statistically significant differences between *H. pylori*-positive and *H. pylori*-negative individuals with respect to total cholesterol, apolipoproteins A_1 or B, fibrinogen or C-reactive protein levels, consistent with this group's previous meta-analysis[7].

The same group also performed a sibling pairs study examining *H. pylori* status in 510 survivors of acute myocardial infarction and 510 age- and sex-matched siblings without a history of CHD[9]. Only 158 pairs out of 510 were discordant for *H. pylori* status. Of these, 91 cases and 67 controls were seropositive for *H. pylori* infection (OR = 1.33; 95% Cl = 0.86–2.05).

Danesh and colleagues have concluded that these two studies are consistent with a moderate association between H. pylori infection and CHD that is not fully explained by other known risk factors. However, based on their previous meta-analysis[7] and on the other accumulated literature[1], it is safe to conclude that these recent results are also incompatible with a major association between H. pylori infection and CHD. As is true for all the proposed non-gastrointestinal manifestations of H. pylori infection, there have been no direct experiments in humans[1], which is the single most important diagnostic criterion proposed by Sackett et al.[2] (Table 1). However, in order to address whether there is even a small association between H. pylori infection and CHD – that could, perhaps, be explained by alterations in serum lipid levels – prospective studies of the effects of eradication on subsequent coronary events would be required. Needless to say, this would involve the randomization of large numbers of patients and subsequent prolonged and detailed follow-up. There is a major ethical dilemma in randomizing infected individuals to placebo eradication regimes followed by the long-term follow-up of untreated infection. This aspect, and the decreasing incidence of H. pylori infection in the population as a whole, makes it doubtful whether such studies could be justified or satisfactorily undertaken.

Survivors of acute myocardial infarction are significantly less likely to have used tetracyclines or quinolones than age- and sex-matched controls without a history of CHD[10]. However, there is currently no justification for advising antibiotic therapy to 'prevent' myocardial infarction[11]. Furthermore, previous use of macrolides and penicillins was no different between CHD patients and controls, suggesting indirectly that coincidental eradication of H. pylori did not explain the observed differences. However, the chance eradication of Chlamydia pneumoniae infection – with which there is much stronger and more consistent evidence for an association with CHD – might help explain the finding.

AUTOIMMUNE THROMBOCYTOPENIC PURPURA

In our previous review of the non-gastrointestinal associations of H. pylori infection[1], we concluded that there was at least some evidence in support of an association with autoimmune thrombocytopenic purpura (ATP). Franceschi and colleagues from Italy had reported a higher than expected prevalence of H. pylori infection in an uncontrolled study of patients with ATP[12]. Among 15 patients in whom known causes of thrombocytopenia had been excluded, the prevalence of H. pylori infection was 67%. The 10 patients with H. pylori infection were treated for it, and seven had successful eradication. In these patients platelet counts increased from a mean of $90 200/mm^3$ to a mean of $148 800/mm^3$ ($p < 0.05$). In seven, anti-platelet antibodies became undetectable six weeks after treatment. In infected patients who were treated for H. pylori infection, but in whom eradication was unsuccessful, there was no change in platelet count or in the levels of anti-platelet antibodies. The same investigators subsequently reported their 12-month results after treating H. pylori infection in 11 infected patients with ATP[13,14] Of these 11, eight (73%) had successful cure of *H. pylori* infection. After 1 year the mean platelet count in these patients had increased from 86 ± 25 to $168 \pm 68 \times 10^9/L$ ($p < 0.05$). Furthermore, anti-platelet antibodies were detectable in 100% of patients before treatment but in only 13% after 1 year ($p < 0.003$). There was no apparent change in platelet count or in the titre of anti-platelet antibodies in the infected patients with failed eradication or in the non-infected patients over this time. There has still been no prospective, randomized, placebo-controlled trial of the eradication of *H. pylori* infection in ATP patients.

IRON-DEFICIENCY ANAEMIA

In our initial overview of the non-gastrointestinal manifestations of *H. pylori*[1], we concluded that there was some biological plausibility for an association with iron-deficiency amenia, and that a relatively strong association had been demonstrated from a cross-sectional paediatric study[15].

In Australia, Peach *et al.* studied the iron status and *H. pylori* status of 160 women and 152 men in a single town[16]. Of those studied, 33% of the women and 28% of the men were *H. pylori*-positive. Non-infected women had a statistically significantly higher mean serum ferritin level than infected women (88.8 vs. 59.3 µg/L; $p < 0.02$). Dietary iron take was similar between the infected and non-infected groups.

In a prospective, open study from Italy, Annibale and colleagues reported correction of iron-deficiency anaemia in some patients following treatment of *H. pylori* infection[17]. They treated 30 patients with iron-deficiency anaemia and no evidence of occult gastrointestinal bleeding, with omeprazole, amoxicillin and metronidazole for 2 weeks. Eradication of *H. pylori* infection was assessed by endoscopy and biopsy 6 months after the conclusion of treatment. Cure of infection was confirmed in 25 patients, of whom one was excluded from further analysis because of the development of menorrhagia. Mean ($\pm$SD) haemoglobin concentrations in the remaining 24 increased from 10.2 ± 0.2 g/dl at baseline to 13.0 ± 0.3 at 6 months ($p < 0.001$) and to 13.3 ± 0.03 at 1 year ($p < 0.001$ compared to baseline). Furthermore, serum ferritin values increased by over 300% despite discontinuation of oral iron supplements. Most patients had chronic pangastritis before entering the study.

These studies in adult patients lend some support to the possible association between *H. pylori* infection and iron-deficiency anaemia in the absence of documented gastrointestinal blood loss. It is possible that *H. pylori* competes with the host for dietary iron; a number of genes on the *H. pylori* genome encode for proteins with iron-scavenging functions[18]. Furthermore, chronic pangastritis and its associated relative hypochlorhydria and reduced intragastric levels of ascorbate might reduce absorption of dietary iron. Conceivably, both of these possibilities might pertain in at least some individuals; furthermore, either or both could be reversible with successful eradication of the infection.

RAYNAUD'S PHENOMENON

In our initial overview[1] we concluded that there was no obvious biological rationale for an association between this condition and *H. pylori* infection and that the results of one uncontrolled treatment study added little, if anything, to the evidence base. Since, then, the uncontrolled treatment study has been published in full[19], with more patients than were included in the original abstract cited in our initial review. Gasbarrini and colleagues studied 46 patients with primary Raynaud's phenomenon, of whom 36 had *H. pylori* infection diagnosed by [^{13}C]UBT[19]. Severity of Raynaud's phenomenon was similar in the infected and non-infected patients. The 36 infected patients received lansoprazole, clarithromycin and amoxicillin for seven days[30]; 83% had successful eradication of *H. pylori* proven by repeat [^{13}C]UBT and histology. The authors reported that five of the patients with successful eradication had no subsequent episodes of Raynaud's phenomenon in a 3-month period of follow-up; of the remaining 25, they reported improvement in symptoms of Raynaud's phenomenon in 18. In those patients who had failed eradication, the authors reported that symptoms of Raynaud's phenomenon did not change. However, the combination of uninfected patients and those patients who failed treatment for *H. pylori* infection does not constitute an adequate control group. The investigators did not randomize infected patients to active or placebo eradication treatment, which might have offered a higher probability of establishing any real treatment effect. This uncontrolled study does not prove any association between Raynaud's phenomenon and *H. pylori* infection.

SCLERODERMA

In our initial review[1] we concluded that there was no firm evidence and no obvious biological rationale for an association between *H. pylori* infection and scleroderma. Subsequently, Yazawa and colleagues from Japan have published their findings in 124 patients with scleroderma and 50 age- and sex-matched controls with non-systemic skin disorders[20]. The seroprevalence of *H. pylori* infection was 56% among the scleroderma patients and 32% in the controls ($p < 0.01$). Within the scleroderma group the prevalence of heartburn was significantly higher in the *H. pylori*-positive patients than in those who were *H. pylori*-negative (51% vs. 33%; $p < 0.05$). Similarly, the presence of oesophageal involvement in the scleroderma process was significantly higher in the *H. pylori*-positive than in the *H. pylori*-negative patients (75% vs. 51%; $p < 0.05$). These findings are of interest but are difficult to explain, since *H. pylori* cannot colonize squamous oesophageal epithelium and the symptom of heartburn is not generally correlated with *H. pylori* infection.

IDIOPATHIC URTICARIA

Having initially reviewed six studies that had looked for an association between urticaria and *H. pylori* infection[1], we concluded that there was no

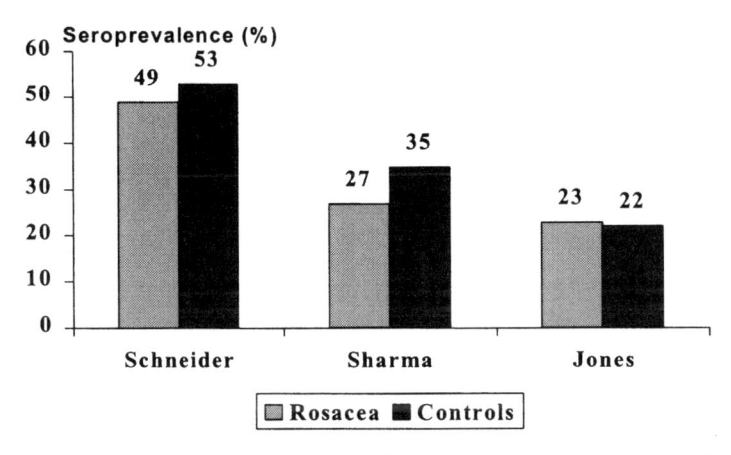

Figure 2. Results of three controlled studies of the seroprevalence of *H. pylori* infection in patients with rosacea (from refs. 24–26).

evidence for the association and no obvious biological rationale to explain it. The best evidence came from uncontrolled case series; treatment studies were of low quality and had added nothing to the evidence base. Since then, one study has been published in full[21]. This was an uncontrolled study of 42 patients with urticaria, of whom 23 (55%) had a positive [^{13}C]UBT. Infected patients received lansoprazole, clarithromycin and amoxicillin for 7 days; eradication of infection was checked by repeat [^{13}C]UBT 6 weeks later. It is unclear if the patients or the physicians following them were aware of post-treatment *H. pylori* status. Only 18 of the 23 infected patients completed the study; of these, 16 (88%) had successful eradication. In 3 months of follow-up there were no further episodes of urticaria in 13 of the 16 patients cured of the infection. The uninfected patients and the infected patients with failed eradication did not show any change in the severity of their urticaria. This inappropriately controlled study does not advance the case for an association between *H. pylori* infection and idiopathic chronic urticaria[22]. A single case report has documented improvement in the symptoms of hereditary angioedema after eradication of *H. pylori* infection[23].

ROSACEA

Three controlled studies, summarized in Figure 2, have not found any increased prevalence of *H. pylori* infection in patients with rosacea[24–26]. However, treatment for presumed *H. pylori* infection continues to be offered for this condition. In one US-based series of 230 patients undergoing serological testing for *H. pylori*, 22% were tested because of rosacea compared with only 10% for a past history of peptic ulcer and 9% for active peptic ulcer[27]. In recent US-based surveys, 12% of practising gastroenterologists and 4% of internal medicine residents would offer *H. pylori* testing to patients with rosacea[28,29]. However, not all would offer treatment based on a positive test result; they presumably felt that the patients' dermatologists would.

A study from Turkey included 23 patients with rosacea and 87 controls[30]. Servoprevalence of *H. pylori* infection was higher in the rosacea patients than controls (68% vs. 48%), although this was not statistically significant. The investigators reported significant improvements in erythema ($p < 0.01$), papule formation ($p < 0.01$) and pustule formation ($p < 0.05$) after treatment for *H. pylori* infection in rosacea patients. However, it is not clear if the investigators were blinded to treatment status, and there was apparently no post-treatment test to assess the effectiveness of eradication therapy.

There has now been one controlled study of the treatment of *H. pylori* infection in rosacea[31]. In a randomized, double-blind, placebo-controlled clinical trial, 44 patients with rosacea, positive *H. pylori* serology and a positive [^{13}C]UBT were randomized to treatment with omeprazole and clarithromycin or identical placebos for 2 weeks. Eradication rates were 75% and 9% in, respectively, the active treatment and placebo groups. Rosacea improved in all patients within the two treatment groups but there was no difference in the severity or activity of rosacea between the active treatment and control groups[31].

In summary, three controlled studies of the servoprevalence of *H. pylori* infection in rosacea have been negative[24–26] and one high-quality randomized, controlled trial has shown no added benefit over placebo of treating the infection in rosacea patients[31]. The prevalence of upper gastrointestinal symptoms in rosacea patients is similar to that in controls[25,31,32] – even in uncontrolled treatment studies that purport to show that patients with rosacea derive benefit from treatment for *H. pylori* infection[30]. Hopefully, the proposed association between rosacea and *H. pylori* infection – which seems to have been based on the erroneous interpretation of an older study of 'gastritis' in rosacea patients[32] – will now be put to rest.

MIGRAINE

In our initial review[1] we included one preliminary study examining a possible relationship between *H. pylori* infection and migraine that had been published only in abstract form. We concluded that there was no convincing evidence of an association. Since then, the study has been published in full[33]. Of 225 consecutive migraine patients, 90 (40%) had *H. pylori* infection diagnosed by the [^{13}C]UBT. Of these, 81 were treated with lansoprazole, clarithromycin and amoxicillin for 7 days, and 84% (68 of 81) had successful eradication demonstrated by a repeat [^{13}C]UBT performed 6 weeks after the end of therapy. Of the 81 treated patients, 19 reported complete disappearance of migraine during the subsequent 6 months of follow-up. The authors also reported reduction in migraine severity and frequency in 77% of the remainder. This study was uncontrolled. Although the 40% prevalence of *H. pylori* infection in the migraine patients appears high, it may not be significantly greater than in the age-matched control population in Italy, since the mean age of the migraine patients was 36. It is unclear from the description of the study if the patients and the investigators who assessed them were blinded to post-treatment *H. pylori* status. The treatment component to the study was similarly uncontrolled; again, uninfected patients and infected patients who failed eradication treatment were regarded as 'controls'.

In an open, uncontrolled paediatric study from Italy, *H. pylori* status was checked in 36 children with migraine using the [^{13}C] UBT[34]. The age range was 6–14 years with a mean age of 10. Only one child (2.7%) was infected, representing an appreciably lower rate of infection than in historical controls from the same geographic area of 8.1%.

These studies have demonstrated neither a link between *H. pylori* infection and migraine, nor an improvement in migraine symptoms following cure of *H. pylori* infection. Furthermore, there is no obvious biological rationale for any link between these two conditions. In a recent survey of internal medicine residents in the US, only 4% thought that migraine was an indication to test a patient for *H. pylori* infection[29]. In a similar survey among internal medicine trainees in Greece, the figure was 7%[35].

THYROIDITIS

In our initial review[1], we concluded that there was weak evidence of an association between *H. pylori* infection and autoiommune thyroid disease, but no obvious biological rationale to explain it. Subsequently, de Luis *et al.* in Spain studied the servoprevalence of *H. pylori* infection in 59 patients with various forms of autoimmune thyroid disease (21 had autoimmune atrophic thyroiditis, 20 had Graves' disease, and 18 had Hashimoto's thyroiditis)[36]. They also had two control groups – one consisted of 20 patients with non-toxic nodular goiter (a non-autoimmune thyroid disease) and the other consisted of 11 patients with Addison's disease (an autoimmune endocrine disease unrelated to the thyroid). Groups were well matched for age, sex and dyspepsia score. Of the patients with autoimmune atrophic thyroiditis, the *H. pylori* seropositivity was 86%, which was significantly higher than either of the control groups ($p < 0.01$). There was also a positive correlation between titres of anti-*H. pylori* IgG antibodies and thyroid antimicrosomal antibodies. This was a well-controlled study that demonstrated a significantly higher prevalence of *H. pylori* infection in one of the conditions studied. It suggests the possibility of some immunological cross-reactivity between anti-*H. pylori* antibodies and thyroid autoantibodies.

Centanni and colleagues in Italy studied the relationship between autoimmune thyroid disease and atrophic body gastritis[37]. Twenty-two (35%) of 62 patients with autoimmune thyroid disease had hypergastrinaemia, defined as a level that was over 2.5 times the upper limit of normal for the reference laboratory (80.2 pmol/L). Of these 22 (median serum gastrin 577, range 231–5250 pmol/L), all had histological evidence of atrophic body gastritis. Antiparietal cell antibodies were present in 68% of the patients with atrophic gastritis, and 82% were anaemic. *H. pylori* infection, assessed serologically and histologically, was found in 54% of those with atrophic body gastritis and in 46% of those without ($p = 0.42$). This study suggests that many patients with autoimmune thyroid disease may have atrophic gastritis. However, this is likely to be autoimmune-mediated in the majority, given the tendency for different organ-specific autoimmune endocrine diseases to coexist. There is no evidence for a major role of *H. pylori* in the gastritis, or of any role in the thyroid disease.

GUILLAIN-BARRÉ SYNDROME

Chiba and colleagues in Japan have studied the cerebrospinal fluid (CSF) of seven patients with Guillain–Barré syndrome and five control patients with multiple sclerosis (MS)[38]. Four of the seven Guillain–Barré patients had antibodies in their CSF that reacted to a variety of *H. pylori* antigens of molecular weight 60–70 kDa. None of the Guillian–Barré patients had CSF antibodies to *E. coli* or *Campylobacter jejuni* antigens. None of the MS patients had CSF antibodies that reacted against *H. pylori* antigens. Guillain–Barré syndrome may be precipitated by a number of infectious or immunological challenges including viral infection and immunization. While the results of Chiba and colleagues are of interest, it is difficult to imagine how antibodies to an infection that had presumably been present since childhood could contribute to an acute neurological condition of adulthood.

CONCLUSIONS

There has been considerable enthusiasm on the part of investigators to establish a link between *H. pylori* infection and a multitude of non-gastrointestinal disorders with which, at first sight, it would appear to be unrelated. In part this may be because *H. pylori* infection is still fairly prevalent, is easily diagnosed and can be effectively treated. However, much of the epidemiological research in this area has been uncontrolled or inadequately controlled. In many case series a seroprevalence rate for *H. pylori* infection is quoted without any knowledge of the prevalence in an age- and sex-matched control group. In general, treatment studies have – with some notable exceptions (e.g. ref. 31) – also been uncontrolled or inadequately controlled[19,21,30,33]. Infected patients with the condition under study should have been randomized to receive active or placebo treatment for *H. pylori* infection and the response to treatment made without knowledge of post-treatment *H. pylori* status. Instead, many studies treated all infected patients for the infection and used the combination of uninfected patients and the treated patients who failed eradication as the control group. In some studies no post-treatment check of *H. pylori* status was made.

Sufficient evidence from controlled studies now exists to disprove any association between *H. pylori* infection and several disorders – most notably rosacea[24–26,31]. However, treatment for *H. pylori* infection became rapidly accepted by practising dermatologists in the absence of any definitive evidence for the association, and despite a growing body of evidence against such an association. It is particularly unfortunate that, in one US study, more patients were referred to a specialist *H. pylori* clinic because of rosacea than because of peptic ulcer disease[27]. While it could be argued that it may be beneficial to treat *H. pylori* infection in any infected individual irrespective of the indication, there is also a potential disadvantage to jumping on to the 'extragastric bandwagon' that is now rapidly careering out of control. Primary-care physicians will rightly be sceptical of ever more elaborate claims for indications to test for – and treat – this infection. Patients consulting a physician because of, for example, a skin disorder, may be informed that their problem is the result of a bacterial infection of the stomach. They may then become alarmed at the prospect of another medical problem they were hitherto unaware of, or they may become irrationally optimistic about the prospect of both an explanation and a cure for their problem. Furthermore, the subsequent failure of the underlying condition to resolve following treatment for *H. pylori* infection is likely to promote disillusionment among practitioners and patients alike about the true significance and importance of *H. pylori* infection. This could have serious consequences for promoting effective testing for, and treatment of, the infection in patients with peptic ulcer disease. In addition, the increased use of antibiotics to treat *H. pylori* infection for unproven – or disproved – indications will undoubtedly increase the prevalence of resistant strains of this bacterium and – importantly – of others.

References

1. Leontiadis GI, Sharma VK, Howden CW. Non-gastrointestinal tract associations of *Helicobacter pylori* infection: what is the evidence? Arch Intern Med. 1999;159:925–40.
2. Sackett DL, Haynes RB, Tugwell P. Clinical Epidemiology: A Basic Science for Clinical Medicine. Boston, MA: Little Brown; 1985.
3. Saikku P, Leinonen M, Tankanen L et al. Chronic *Chlamydia pneumoniae* infection as a risk factor for coronary heart disease in the Helsinki heart study. Ann Intern Med. 1992;116:273–8.
4. Danesh J, Collins R, Peto P. Chronic infections and coronary heart disease: Is there a link? Lancet. 1997;350:430–6.
5. Meirer CR, Derby LE, Jick SS, Vasilakis C, Jick H. Antibiotics and risk of first-time acute myocardial infarction. J Am Med Assoc. 1999;281:427–31.
6. Malnick SDH, Goland S, Kaftoury A et al. Evaluation of carotid arterial plaques after endarterectomy for *Helicobacter pylori* infection. Am J Cardiol. 1999;83:1586–7.
7. Danesh J, Peto R. Risk factors for coronary heart disease and infection with *Helicobacter pylori*: meta-analysis of 18 studies. Br Med J. 1988;316:1130–2.
8. Laurila A, Bloigu A, Näyhä S, Hassi J, Leinonen M, Saikku P. Association of *Helicobacter pylori* infection with elevated serum lipids. Atherosclerosis. 1999;142:207–10.
9. Danesh J, Youngman L, Clark S, Parish S, Peto R, Collins R. *Helicobacter pylori* infection and early onset myocardial infarction: case–control and sibling pairs study. Br Med J. 1999;319.1157–62.
10. Meier CR, Derby LE, Jick SS, Vasilakis C, Jick H. Antibiotics and risk of subsequent first-time acute myocardial infarction. J Am Med Assoc. 1999;281:427–31.
11. Folsom AR. Antibiotics for prevention of myocardial infarction? Not yet! J Am Med Assoc. 1999;281:461–2.
12. Franceschi F, Gasbarinni A, Tartaglione R et al. Regression of autoimmune thrombocytopenic purpura after *Helicobacter pylori* eradication. Gastroenterology. 1998;114:A124 (abstract).
13. Franceschi F, Gasbarini A, Taratglione R et al. Healing of autoimmune thrombocytopenia after *H. pylori* eradication: 1 year of follow up. Gastroenterology. 1999;116:A164 (abstract).
14. Gasbarrini A, Franceschi F, Tartaglione R, Landolfi R, Pola P, Gasbarrini G. Regression of autoimmune thrombocytopenia after eradication of *Helicobacter pylori*. Lancet. 1998;352:878.
15. Bardhan PK, Hildebrand P, Sarker SA et al. *Helicobacter pylori* infection in children: is there an association with anemia? Gastroenterology. 1997;112: A65 (abstract).

16. Peach HG, Bath NE, Farish SJ. *Helicobacter pylori* infection: an added stressor on iron status of women in the community. Med J Aust. 1998;169:188–90.
17. Annibale B, Marignani M, Monarca B et al. Reversal of iron deficiency anemia after *Helicobacter pylori* eradication in patients with asymptomatic gastritis. Ann Intern Med. 1999;131:668–72.
18. Lee A. The *Helicobacter pylori* genome: new insights into pathogenesis and therapeutics. N Engl J Med. 1998;338:832–3.
19. Gasbarrini A, Massari I, Serricchio M et al. *Helicobacter pylori* eradication ameliorates primary Raynaud's phenomenon. Dig Dis Sci. 1998;43:1641–5.
20. Yazawa N, Fujimoto M, Kikuchi K et al. High seroprevalence of *Helicobacter pylori* infection in patients with systemic sclerosis: association with esophageal involvement. J Rheumatol. 1998;25:650–3.
21. Di Campli C, Gasbarrini A, Nucera E et al. Beneficial effects of *Helicobacter pylori* eradication on idiopathic chronic urticaria. Dig Dis Sci. 1998;43:1226–9.
22. Howden CW. No evidence for an association between *H. pylori* and idiopathic chronic urticaria. Dig Dis Sci. 1999;44:485–6 (Letter).
23. Rais M, Unzeitig J, Grant JA. Refractory exacerbation of hereditary angioedema with associated *Helicobacter pylori* infection. J Allergy Clin Immunol. 1999;103:713–14.
24. Schneider MA, Skinner RBJ, Rosenberg EW. Serological determination of *Helicobacter pylori* in rosacea patients and controls. Clin Res. 1992;40:831A (abstract).
25. Sharma VK, Lynn A, Kaminski M, Vasudeva R, Howden CW. A study of the prevalence of *Helicobacter pylori* and other markers of upper gastrointestinal disease in patients with rosacea. Am J Gastroenterol. 1998;93:220–2.
26. Jones MP, Knable AL Jr, White MJ, Durning SJ. *Helicobacter pylori* in rosacea: lack of an association. Arch Dermatol. 1998;134:511 (Letter).
27. Everhart AT, Jones MP. Use and misuse of *H. pylori* in primary care specialities: report from the field. Am J Gastroenterol. 1998;93:1633 (abstract).
28. Sharma VK, Vasudeva R, Howden CW. A survey of gastroenterologists' perceptions and practices related to *Helicobacter pylori* infection. Am J Gastroenterol. 1999;94:3170–4.
29. Sharma VK, Bailey DM, Raufman J-P et al. A survey of internal medicine residents' opinions and practices related to *H. pylori*. Am J Gastroenterol. 1999;93:1647 (abstract).
30. Uta S, Özbakir Ö, Turasan A, Uta C. *Helicobacter pylori* eradication treatment reduces the severity of rosacea. J Am Acad Dermatol. 1999;40:433–5.
31. Bamford JTM, Tilden RL, Blankush JL, Gangeness DE. Effect of treatment of *Helicobacter pylori* infection on rosacea. Arch Dermatol. 1999;135:659–63.
32. Marks R, Beard RJ, Clark ML. Gastrointestinal observations in rosacea. Lancet. 1967; 1:739–42.
33. Gasbarrini A, de Luca A, Fiore G et al. Beneficial effects of *Helicobacter pylori* eradication on migraine. Hepato-Gastroenterology. 1998;45:765–70.
34. Caselli M, Chiamenti CM, Soriani S, Fanaro S. Migraine in children and *Helicobacter pylori*. Am J Gastroenterol. 1999;94:1116–18 (Letter).
35. Leontiadis GI, Sharma VK, Howden CW, Kitis G. Comparison of the knowledge and practices of internal medicine trainees in Greece and the US concerning *H. pylori* infection. Gastroenterology. 2000;118 (In press) (abstract).
36. de Luis DA, Varela C, de la Calle H et al. *Helicobacter pylori* infection is markedly increased in patients with autoimmune atrophic thyroiditis. J Clin Gastroenterol. 1998;26:259–63.
37. Centanni M, Marignani M, Gargano L et al. Atrophic body gastritis with autoimmune thyroid disease: an underdiagnosed association. Arch Intern Med. 1999;159:1726–30.
38. Chiba S, Sugiyama T, Matsumoto H et al. Antibodies against *Helicobacter pylori* were detected in the cerebrospinal fluid obtained from patients with Guillain–Barré syndrome. Ann Neurol. 1998;44:686–8.

36
Peptic ulcer disease – the transitional zones are important

M. F. DIXON, A. LEE and S. J. O. VELDHUYZEN VAN ZANTEN

INTRODUCTION

In 1924 Konjetzny declared that 'an ulcer does not develop in a healthy mucosa'[1]. Over the next two decades it became increasingly apparent that peptic ulcers were complications of pre-existing chronic inflammation in the gastric and proximal duodenal mucosa. Indeed it emerged that different patterns of gastritis were associated with gastric and duodenal ulcers; the former was found in stomachs with diffuse chronic gastritis with multifocal atrophy whereas duodenal ulcers were associated with a non-atrophic antral-predominant gastritis in which the corpus showed little inflammation[2,3]. In the 1950s Oi and his colleagues in Tokyo examined large numbers of gastric resections for ulcer disease and made a meticulous study of the location of gastric and duodenal ulcers in relation to the border zones between adjacent mucosal types[4,5]. The relationship of peptic ulcers to these junctional zones has been a neglected topic which needs re-examination in the light of *Helicobacter pylori* ecology.

THE TRANSITIONAL ZONES

As the name implies, the transitional zones represent sites where one mucosal type merges with another. In the upper gastrointestinal tract they are found between the cardiac mucosa below the gastro-oesophageal junction and the corpus, between the antrum and corpus, and between antrum (pyloric) and duodenal mucosa (Figure 1). Where acid-secreting oxyntic glands of the corpus give way to simple mucous glands of the antrum or cardia there will be a parallel loss of parietal and chief cells as mucous/bicarbonate-secreting cells become the predominant type. However, the disappearance of parietal cells is not absolute. Scattered parietal cells may be found throughout the antrum. It is the absence of chief cells and the change from straight tubular to branched glands that characterizes the antrum. Likewise, the true cardia

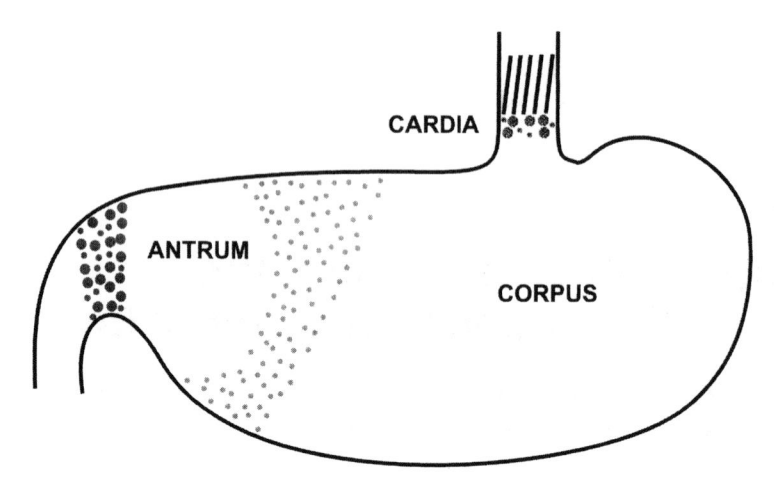

Figure 1. The normal transitional zones are found (i) where corpus mucosa merges with cardia – a narrow zone of columnar mucosa resembling gastric antrum and found immediately distal to the squamous epithelium (shaded) at the gastro-oesophageal junction, (ii) between corpus and antrum and (iii) between antral and duodenal mucosa.

is devoid of parietal cells but it is approached through a transitional zone which contains small numbers of parietal cells within the mucous glandular elements. In many instances the transitional zone is longer than the cardia proper. The cardia abuts directly onto the sharply demarcated distal margin of the squamous mucosa. This is therefore a squamo-columnar *junction* and not a transitional zone. As regards the antro-duodenal transitional zone, this is a narrow band of interdigitating gastric and small intestinal mucosa, which almost always corresponds to the crest of the pyloric muscle ring. In a small minority it is located a few millimetres distal to the crest[5].

LABILITY OF THE TRANSITIONAL ZONES

While there are anatomical definitions of the transitional zones, their locations are by no means fixed. Obviously the boundary between the antrum and corpus will be governed by the relative size of these compartments. Individuals who have a constitutionally enlarged parietal cell mass will have a relatively large corpus and the transitional zone will be shifted caudally. High acid output also provokes an adaptive response in the first part of the duodenum, in which the mucosa undergoes metaplasia to a gastric phenotype, i.e. a mucosa better suited to resist the adverse environment of high local acid levels. While this occurs as discrete patches, it may also develop as distal extension of antral-type epithelium into the duodenum. This may be more appropriately called 'substitution' rather than metaplasia, but whatever its histogenesis it has the effect of shifting the antro-duodenal transitional zone caudally (Figure 2). Likewise, acid regurgitation into the lower oesophagus may lead to columnar metaplasia of cardia-type replacing squamous epithelim. This would have the effect of enlarging both the cardia

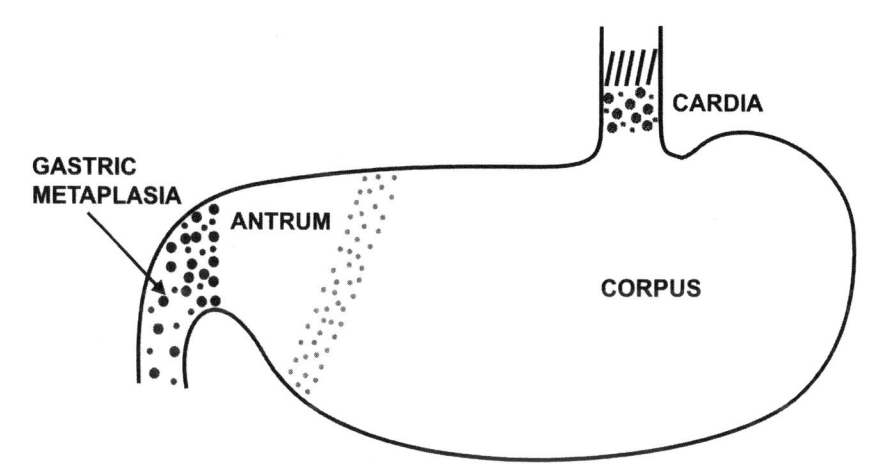

Figure 2. In high acid output states there is distal movement of the corpus–antrum transitional zone which is more 'abrupt' (narrower) than normal. The action of acid on the duodenal mucosa provokes gastric metaplasia. This can occur as discrete patches but can also arise by distal extension of antral-type mucosa into the first part of the duodenum. In *H. pylori*-infected individuals the presence of gastric epithelium now permits colonization (and inflammation) at this site.

and the transitional zone into the tubular oesophagus. On the other hand, subjects with low acid output will have a relatively larger antrum and proximal shift of the antral–corpus transitional zone. However, proximal displacement of this zone is usually an acquired change consequent upon inflammation, atrophy and metaplasia encroaching on the corpus.

It has been appreciated for many years that the boundary between non-atrophic corpus mucosa and atrophic antral mucosa is endoscopically visible. The boundary has been called the 'atrophic border', and Japanese investigators have demonstrated that it moves proximally with advancing age[6,7]. The dynamics of this migrating border are interesting. Inflammation in the transitional zone results in glandular atrophy. Loss of corpus glands at the interface with the transitional zone is followed by mucous cell and pyloric gland metaplasia. Thus, the original corpus type mucosa close to the boundary takes on an antral aspect. The gradual development of this 'pseudo-antrum', which is in continuity with the inflamed and atrophic true antrum, has the effect of progressively enlarging the 'antrum' at the expense of corpus (Figure 3). Over the years the expanding antrum comes to occupy the entire lesser curvature of the stomach and spreads out to involve ever greater areas of the anterior and posterior walls. Encroachment into the corpus could also result from chronic inflammation at the corpus–cardia transitional zone. The chronic inflammation at these sites is now known to be due to *H. pylori* infection. Differences in the degree of inflammation across the transitional zones could be a reflection of changes in *H. pylori* colonization density or the virulence of the organisms. Certainly, there is increased colonization immediately proximal to the atrophic border, and there is greater polymorph activity when compared to the mucosa immediately distal

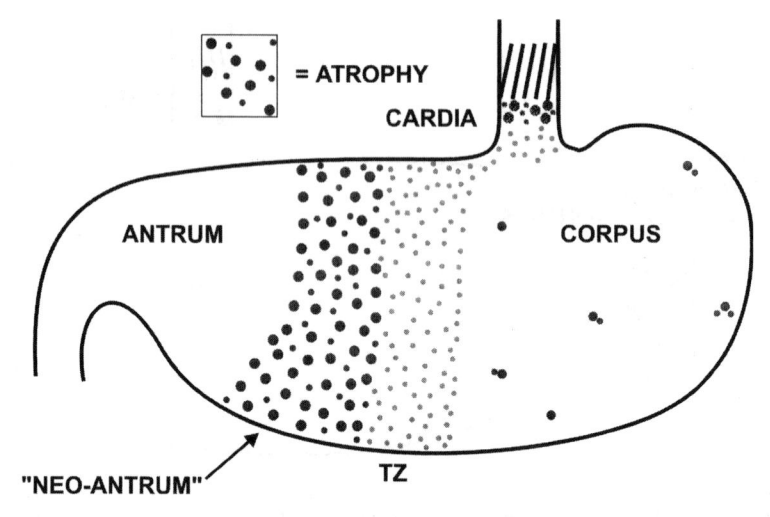

Figure 3. Over time the original corpus–antrum transitional zone in the *H. pylori*-infected stomach becomes the main site for atrophy and intestinal metaplasia. Associated mucous metaplasia in glands and pyloric metaplasia give rise to 'antralization' of the affected corpus and the transitional zone becomes displaced cephalad. Further antralization means that the 'atrophic border' advances progressively into the corpus which also contains separate discrete foci of atrophy – multifocal atrophic gastritis. This advancing zone is the favoured site for gastric peptic ulceration.

to the border[8]. Conversely, and in keeping with our concepts of causation, the mucosa distal to the border shows significantly more atrophy and intestinal metaplasia. It is likely that *H. pylori* colonization and virulence will be affected by the local acid levels prevailing across the transitional zones.

H. PYLORI AND ACID TOLERANCE

There is convincing evidence that *H. pylori* has evolved to survive in the acid environment of the human stomach[9–11]. Meyer-Rosberg *et al.*[10] have shown that in the pH range 3.5–8 the organism is able to maintain the so-called 'proton motive force' across its membrane, which ensures a continuous supply of energy through ATP synthesis. The major factor in the acid resistance of *H. pylori* is its urease enzyme. The urease gene cluster contains a gene, *ureI*, which encodes a membrane protein that functions as an acid-activated urea transporter[12]. Urea and hydrogen ions diffuse into the periplasm of the bacterium, probably through porins in this outer membrane. Acidification within the periplasm results in a conformational change in UreI, permitting the entry of urea into the cytoplasm, where it is rapidly hydrolysed to CO_2 and NH_3. The ammonia rapidly diffuses back into the periplasmic space where it becomes protonated, raising the pH to about 6.2 – a level consistent with survival and growth[13]. In contrast, the non-gastric *Helicobacter muridarum* or other weak urease producers, such as *Proteus vulgaris*, cannot survive at pH 2 even if urea is added[9]. *In-vitro*

H. pylori can grow in buffered media between pH 5 and 8, and is able to survive between pH 4 and 8, even if urea is absent[9–12]. There is also an upper limit of pH above which *H. pylori* cannot survive. If little or no acid is present the organism will self-destruct by continuing production of ammonia, which takes the pH above 8[14–17].

Definitive data on local acid levels in the gastric mucus layer and in the different regions of the mucosa itself are lacking[18–20]. Nevertheless, it is likely that *H. pylori* organisms within the mucus layer are exposed to different local acid levels in antrum and corpus. In the antrum local acid is derived entirely from the gastric lumen. By contrast, in the corpus the local acid levels are the sum of the protons diffusing via the acid channels from the glands and back-diffusion of H^+ ions from the lumen. Across the transitional zones there is likely to be a gradient in local acid levels, as the number of parietal cells in the transitional zone increases from absence or low density on the antral side to high density in body mucosa.

There are other observations which support the view that acid levels may dictate the behaviour of *H. pylori* at the transitional zones. If patients with recurrent duodenal ulcers undergo surgical reduction of acid production by either antrectomy, vagotomy or highly selective vagotomy, progression of atrophic gastritis in the body during follow-up is seen, supporting the concept that high acid output may be the limiting factor in the development of corpus gastritis in such patients[21–24]. Human and animal studies have demonstrated that acid suppression with the proton pump inhibitor omeprazole markedly changes the behaviour of *H. pylori*[25–29]. They show a reduction of *H. pylori* colonization levels in the antrum and an increase in the corpus. Concomitantly, the activity of gastritis improves in the antrum, whereas it deteriorates in the body. Further proof that acid output determines the geographic distribution of *H. pylori* comes from the few descriptions of acute *H. pylori* infection[30–32]. Acute *H. pylori* infection can temporarily induce a period of hypochlorhydria, which probably facilitates widespread colonization. During the acute stage a pangastritis is seen, which coincides with the period of hypochlorhydria, while in the later stages of infection the antrum becomes the main area of inflammation.

H. PYLORI AT THE ACID-GRADIENT TRANSITIONAL ZONES

There are two possible explanations for the apparent ability of *H. pylori* to induce a more intense inflammatory repose at the acid-gradient transitional zones which border the oxyntic (corpus) mucosa. The bacteria are either metabolizing and proliferating maximally because the local environment is at their pH optimum, or they are generating more inflammatory products due to induction of stress proteins. Bacteria tend to find their growth optimum when confronted with an environmental gradient. Thus, it is likely that at some point across the gradient of local acid found through the transitional zones, *H. pylori* finds optimal conditions and can maximize adhesion, growth and release of inflammatory products and induce a maximal cytokine production via signal transduction at the epithelial cell surface (Figure 4). These areas of peak inflammatory response are the preferential

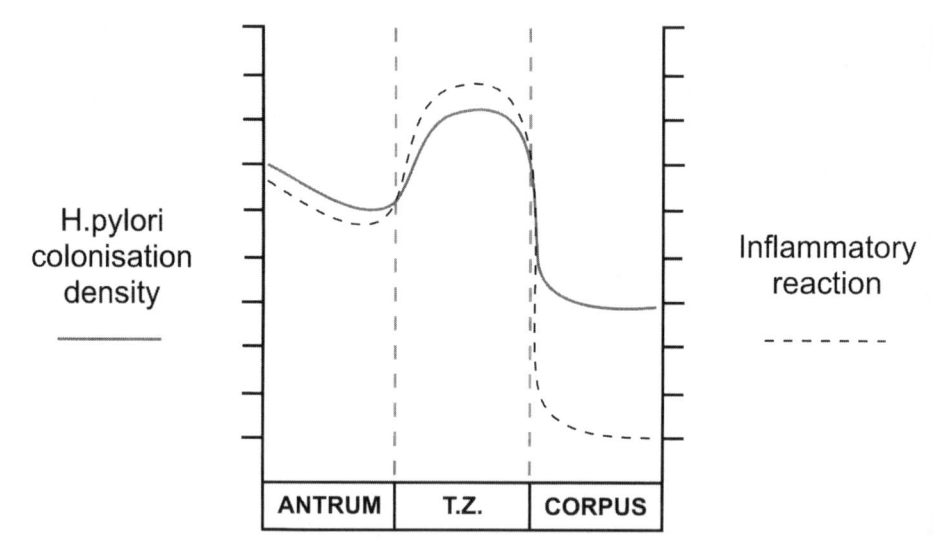

Figure 4. Hypothetical representation of the degree of *H. pylori* colonization and inflammatory cell response in moving across the acid gradient of the antrum–corpus transitional zone. There is likely to be a narrow pH range within this gradient that provides the optimum conditions for bacterial growth, and this could maximize the inflammatory response. On the other hand, in the proximal part of the transitional zone the bacteria will be subjected to increasing acid stress and could respond by liberating pro-inflammatory acid (heat) shock proteins. In either event the transitional zone represents an area of heightened inflammatory reaction.

sites for the development of atrophy and intestinal metaplasia and for ulceration. Alternatively, it is known that bacteria have a series of well-developed physiological mechanisms for dealing with environmental stress, among which is the acid-tolerance response[33]. Various genes are switched on which code for proteins that allow the bacterium to survive[34]. Examples of these molecules are acid (heat) shock proteins[35,36]. In the transitional zone there will be a 'watershed' area where the local acid environment is such that the acid-tolerance response of the bacterium becomes further stressed. It is conceivable that, at this site, novel proteins could be produced, which are more inflammatory than those produced elsewhere. Over the corpus proper the local acid levels are so high that colonization density falls, adhesion is inhibited and bacterial virulence factors are compromised, resulting in little, if any, inflammatory reaction.

Although we favour the first possibility; the reasons for the increased inflammatory potential of *H. pylori* at the transitional zones remain unknown and will only be discovered by close investigation of the bacterium *in vivo*.

Whatever the explanation, the increased inflammatory activity and the deleterious effects of antrophy and intestinal metaplasia on mucosal defence renders the transitional mucosa susceptible to ulceration.

PROXIMAL GASTRIC ULCERS

A distinction is made between distal ulcers occurring within the antrum, i.e. pre-pyloric ulcers, and more proximal ulcers in the stomach. The former share epidemiological characteristics with duodenal ulcer and the patients usually have raised acid levels. In such cases the site of ulceration may be determined by patches of atrophy in the antrum, making the mucosa more susceptible to acid attack. The transitional zones play a pivotal role in the pathogenesis of proximal gastric ulcers. Oi et al. in 1969[37], and Stadelmann et al. in 1971[38], brought attention to the importance of the antral–corpus transitional zone in the pathogenesis of gastric ulcers. Stadelmann demonstrated that progression of gastritis with increasing atrophy in the body at the proximal border of the transitional zone is crucial for the development of gastric ulcers.

In the study by Stadelmann et al. the pattern of gastritis and atrophy, especially in the area of the transitional zone, was evaluated in 176 stomachs resected for gastric ulcer[38]. The ulcer area itself, and the mucosa just proximal and distal to the ulcer, were carefully mapped. It was evident that with few exceptions the ulcers were located in the transitional zones in sections where atrophic corpus gastritis was present. Ulcers were never found in areas of uninflamed mucosa. The large Japanese study by Oi et al.[37] of 855 stomachs resected for gastric and/or duodenal ulcers confirms the importance of the transitional zone in gastric ulcers. They found that 475 of 499 gastric ulcers (95%) were located immediately adjacent (with 2 cm) to the antral–corpus transitional zone. The average distance was 0.38 cm. Interestingly, the authors measured the surface area of the stomachs and estimated that the transitional zone occupied 5%. The fact that the great majority of ulcers occur in such a small area of the stomach highlights the importance of the transitional zone in this process. As in other studies, Oi et al. also noted that there were marked differences in the distance of the gastric ulcers from the pylorus, but these differences coincided with the distance of the transitional zone from the pylorus. Another important finding in this study was that in 21 of the 26 ulcers not located close to the transitional zones (out of the total of 855 cases), there were coexisting duodenal and/or gastric ulcers in which the other ulcer was close to a transitional zone.

The relationship of *H. pylori* infection to the transitional zones now affords a plausible explanation for the finding of gastric ulcers at these sites. Colonization, particularly by the more virulent *CagA*-positive strains, leads to increased exfoliation of surface epithelial cells[39]. Accelerated cell exfoliation results in compensatory cell proliferation so that immature cells populate the foveolae and surface. Mucin and bicarbonate production is impaired and the integrity of the mucus barrier may be compromised. In addition, activation of complement via the alternate pathway and the release of chemical mediators by mast cells and activated polymorphs may lead to microvascular disturbances and focal ischaemic damage to the surface epithelium[40]. Apart from these inflammatory factors, ulcerogenesis may be promoted by the greater degree of atrophy and intestinal metaplasia found immediately distal to the transitional zone. Differences in mucus composition and bicarbonate production in metaplastic mucosa may lower the protection afforded by the mucous barrier. Indeed, metaplastic and atrophic mucosa also differs from normal mucosa in the local production of epithelial growth factors and regulatory (trefoil) peptides[41], and there may also be differences in the pattern of receptors for luminal growth factors (e.g. epidermal growth factor[42]. Diminished growth factor or regulatory peptide stimulation will adversely affect mucosal regeneration and exaggerate the effects of injury. However, there may also be bacterial factors at work. *H. pylori* infection down-regulates E-cadherin expression in gastric epithelial cells[43]. E-cadherin is involved in cell-to-cell adhesion and in epithelial cell proliferation, so that depressed production could adversely affect the resistance of the mucosa to acid attack. All these consequences of *H. pylori* infection conspire to make the acid-gradient transitional zones peculiarly susceptible to acid-peptic attack, and therefore the principal sites of peptic ulceration.

DUODENAL ULCERS

Acid is a necessary requirement for the development of a duodenal ulcer[44,45]. Baron documented that there is a threshold in peak acid output below which patients do not develop duodenal ulcers (in men 15 mEq per hour, in women 18 mEq per hour)[45]. There is a large body of evidence that patients with duodenal ulcers are on the high end of the spectrum of acid secretion[45–48]. As patients with duodenal ulcers do not have much corpus gastritis, maximal stimulation of acid secretion with pentagastrin provides an indirect measurement of the number of parietal cells[47,48]. Studies have consistently shown that patients with duodenal ulcers tend to have a high parietal cell mass[47–50]. A further consequence of a high acid output or un-neutralized acid reaching the duodenum is the development of gastric metaplasia at this site. Gastric metaplasia may be an essential factor in the pathogenesis of peptic duodenal ulcer, and the importance of the minimum acid threshold could be a level below which gastric metaplasia does not occur[51].

Most duodenal ulcers occur with 1–2 cm of the pylorus[52]. Oi and Sakurai looked carefully at the location of 136 surgically resected duodenal ulcers in relation to the antro-duodenal transitional zone[5], which was usually just inside the pyloric ring. Of the ulcers, 32% were located right at the transitional zone, 64% within 1 cm and 3% within 2 cm. In only 1% was the distance >2 cm. The mean distance between the ulcer and the transitional zone was 0.42 cm. A subsequent study by Oi et al.[37] confirmed that virtually all duodenal ulcers (335 of 353, 99%) were located immediately adjacent to the antro-duodenal transitional zone on the distal (i.e. duodenal) side. Schrager et al., in a study of 75 duodenal ulcers[52], made similar observations. Interestingly, they also noted that some ulcers extended from the antro-duodenal transitional zone into the distal antrum. This is one possible explanation for the formation of prepyloric ulcers.

As the duodenal ulcer itself destroys the mucosa it may be impossible to say that the ulcer occurred in an area of gastric metaplasia, but most of the evidence points towards this conclusion. Studies in which biopsies are taken from the edges of duodenal ulcers usually show gastric metaplasia[53,54]. We believe that patches of gastric metaplasia are often located immediately adjacent to, and confluent with, the antro-duodenal transitional zone, and can be viewed as a 'natural' extension of the normal transitional zone. This would explain why most acid-peptic duodenal ulcers occur within a few centimetres of the pyloric entrance, even though the actual size of the transitional zone may be narrow.

CONCLUSION

The transitional zones have long been recognized as having a close topographical relationship to peptic ulcers. Only with the discovery of *H. pylori*, and a greater understanding of its adaptation to an acidic environment, have plausible explanations for this relationship emerged. In an acid gradient *H. pylori* will either find its pH optimum, where it will maximize colonization and expression of virulence factors, or it will be subjected to acid stress and liberate novel pro-inflammatory proteins. In either case a more pronounced inflammatory response ensues. Greater degrees of inflammation will be followed by more atrophy and intestinal metaplasia, and mucosal defence will be further compromised. Peptic ulceration is most likely to occur in these sites.

Other factors may contribute to the susceptibility of the transitional zones to ulceration. For instance, in the antrum–corpus zone differences in blood supply could play a part. A meticulous study of gastric vasculature found that in the region of the lesser curve the mucosal vessels do not arise from the submucosal plexus, as is the case in the rest of the stomach, but instead stem directly from the arterial branches which run external to the gastric musculature[55]. This may render the lesser curve more prone to ischaemia and predispose to mucosal injury. There may also be a fundamental instability at mucosal junctions or border zones. It is well known that border zones between different types of epithelia are prone to chronic inflammation, ulceration and neoplasia. Examples of these are the squamo-columnar junction of the uterine cervix (the site of cervicitis, 'erosions' and dysplasia and carcinoma development), the transitional epithelium of the ano-rectal junction (inflammation and basaloid/squamous carcinomas) and the squamo-columnar junction at the upper margin of specialized metaplasia in Barrett's oesophagus (chronic inflammation/Barrett's ulcer/dysplasia). Nevertheless, these additional factors must be considered speculative.

We believe that the inevitable conclusion to be drawn from this amalgam of old histological studies and new knowledge of *H. pylori* ecology is that the transitional zones are sites of maximal *H. pylori*-related pathology, namely chronic inflammation, peptic ulcer and premalignant conditions (atrophy and intestinal metaplasia)[56]. We certainly concur with the dictum originally proposed over 40 years ago that 'peptic ulcer is *the ulcer of junction* between two different mucosal tissues'[5].

Acknowledgement

Our thanks are due to Michael Todd for the diagrams.

References

1. Konjetzny GE. Zur chirurgischen Beureilung der chronischen Gastritis. Arch Klin Chirurg. 1924;129:139–71.

2. Hebbel R. Chronic gastrits: its relation to gastric and duodenal ulcer and to gastric cancer. Am J Pathol. 1943;19:43–71.
3. Magnus HA. The pathology of simple gastritis. J Pathol Bacteriol. 1946;58:431–9.
4. Oi M, Oshida K, Sugimura S. The location of gastric ulcer. Gastroenterology. 1959;36:45–59.
5. Oi M, Sakurai Y. The location of duodenal ulcer. Gastroenterology. 1959;36;60–4.
6. Kimura K, Takemoto T. Endoscopic recognition of the atrophic border and its significance in chronic gastritis. Endoscopy. 1969;8:87–97.
7. Kimura K. Chronological transition of the fundic–pyloric border determined by stepwise biopsy of the lesser and greater curvatures of the stomach. Gastroenterology. 1972;63:584–92.
8. Yoshimura T, Shimoyama T, Fukuda S, Tanaka A, Axon ATR, Munakata A. Most gastric cancer occurs on the distal side of the endoscopic atrophic border. Scand J Gastroenterol. 1999;34:1077–81.
9. Ferrero RL, Lee A. The importance of urease in acid protection for the gastric-colonising bacteria *H. pylori* and *H. felis* sp. nov. Microbiol Ecol Health Dis. 1991;4:121–34.
10. Meyer-Rosberg K, Scott DR, Melchers K, Sachs G. The effect of environmental pH on the proton motive force of *H. pylori*. Gastroenterology. 1996;111:886–900.
11. McGowan CC, Cover TL, Blasr MJ. *Helicobacter pylori* and gastric acid: biological and therapeutic implications. Gastroenterology. 1996;110:926–38.
12. A H^+-gated urea channel: the link between *Helicobacter pylori* urease and gastric colonization. Science. 2000;287:482–5.
13. Scott DR, Marcus EA, Weeks DL, Lee A, Melchers K, Sachs G. Expression of the *Helicobacter pylori ureI* gene is required for acidic pH activation of cytoplasmic urease. Infect Immun. 2000;68:470–7.
14. Clyne M, Labigne A, Drumm B. *H. pylori* requires an acidic environment to survive in the presence of urea. Infect Immun. 1995;63:1669–73.
15. Greig MA, Neithercut WD, Hossack M, McColl KEL. Harnessing of urease activity of *H. pylori* to induce self-destruction of the bacterium. J Clin Pathol. 1991;44:157–9.
16. Neithercut WD, Williams C, Hossack M, McColl KEL. Ammonium metabolism and protection from urease mediated destruction in *H. pylori* infection. J Clin Pathol. 1993;46:75–8.
17. Wiliams C, Neithercut WD, Hossack M, Hair J, McColl KEL. Urease-mediated destruction of bacteria is specific for *Helicobacter* urease and results in total cellular disruption. FEMS Immunol Med Microbiol. 1994;9:273–80.
18. Schade C, Flemstrom G, Holm L. Hydrogen ion concentration in the mucus layer on top of acid-stimulated and -inhibited rat gastric mucosa. Gastroenterology. 1994;107:180–8.
19. Engel E, Peskoff A, Kaufman GL, Grossman MI. Analysis of hydrogen ion concentration in the gastric gel mucus layer. Am J Physiol. 1984;247:G321–38.
20. Bahari HMM, Ross IN, Turnberg LA. Demonstration of a pH gradient across the mucus layer on the surface of human gastric mucosa *in vitro*. Gut. 1982;23:513–16.
21. Roland M, Berstad A, Liavag J. Histological study of gastric mucosa before and after proximal gastric vagotomy in duodenal ulcer patients. Scand J Gastroenterol. 1975;10:181–6.
22. Watt PCH, Sloan JM, Kennedy TL. Changes in gastric mucosa after vagotomy and gastrojejunostomy for duodenal ulcer. Br Med J. 1983;287:1407–10.
23. Jonsson KA, Storm M, Bodemar G, Norby K. Histologic changes in the gastroduodenal mucosa after long term medical treatment with cimetidine or parietal cell vagotomy in patients with juxtapyloric ulcer disease. Scand J Gastroenterol. 1988;23:433–41.
24. Peetsalu A, Maaroos HI, Sipponen P, Peetsalu M. Long-term effect of vagotomy on gastric mucosa and *H. pylori* in duodenal ulcer patients. Scand J Gastroenterol. 1991;26 (Suppl. 186):77–83.
25. Logan RP, Walker MM, Misiewicz JJ *et al*. Changes in the intragastric distribution of *H. pylori* during treatment with omeprazole. Gut. 1995;36:12–16.
26. Kuipers EJ, Lee A, Klinkenberg-Knol, Meuwissen SGM. Review article: The development of atrophic gastritis – *Helicobacter pylori* and the effects of acid suppressive therapy. Aliment Pharmacol Ther. 1995;9:331–40.
27. Solcia E, Fiocca R, Villani L, Carlsson J, Rudback A, Zeijlon L. Effects of permanent eradication or transient clearance of *Helicobacter pylori* on histology of gastric mucossa

using omeprazole with or without antibiotics. Scand J Gastroenterol. 1996;31(Suppl. 215):105–10.
28. Kuipers EJ, Lundell L, Klinenberg-Knol EC et al. Atrophic gastritis and *Helicobacter pylori* infection in patients with reflux esophagitis treated with omeprazole or fundoplication. N Engl J Med. 1996;334:1018–22.
29. Danon SJ, O'Rouke JL, Moss ND, Lee A. The importance of local acid production in the distribution of *Helicobacter felis* in the mouse stomach. Gastroenterology. 1995;108:1386–95.
30. Graham DY, Alpert LC, Lacey Smith J, Yoshimura HH. Iatrogenic *Campylobacter pylori* infection is a cause of epidemic hypochlorhydria. Am J Gastroenterol. 1988;83:974–80.
31. Frommer DJ, Carrick J, Lee A, Hazell SL. Acute presentation of *Campylobacter pylori* gastritis. Am J Gastroenterol. 1988;83:1168–71.
32. Sobala GM, Crabtree JE, Dixon MF et al. Acute *Helicobacter pylori* infection: clinical features, local and systemic immune response, gastric mucosal histology, and gastric juice ascorbic acid concentrations. Gut. 1991;32:1415–18.
33. Rektorschek M, Weeks D, Sachs G, Melchers K. Influence of pH on metabolism and urease activity of *Helicobacter pylori*. Gastroenterology. 1998;115:628–41.
34. Olso ER. Influence of pH on bacterial gene expression. Mol Microbiol. 1993;8:5–14.
35. Kjelleberg S, editor. Starvation in Bacteria. New York: Plenum Press; 1993.
36. Goodwin S. *Helicobacters* shed new light on chaperonins. Lancet. 1995;346:653–5.
37. Oi M, Ito J, Kumagai F et al. A possible dual control mechanism in the origin of peptic ulcer: a study on ulcer location as affected by mucosa and musculature. Gastroenterology. 1969; 57:280–93.
38. Stadelmann K, Elster K, Stolte M et al. The peptic gastric ulcer – histotopographic and functional investigations. Scand J Gastroenterol. 1971;6:613–23.
39. Warburton VJ, Everett S, Mapstone NP, Axon ATR, Hawkey P, Dixon MF. Clinical and histological associations of cagA and vacA genotypes in *Helicobacter pylori* gastritis. J Clin Pathol. 1998;51:55–61.
40. Dixon MF. Pathophysiology of *Helicobacter pylori* infection. Scand J Gastroenterol. 1994; 26(Suppl. 201):7–10.
41. Hanby AM, Poulsom R, Singh S et al. Spasmolytic polypeptide is a major antral peptide: distribution of the trefoil peptides human spasmolytic polypeptide and pS2 in the stomach. Gastroenterology. 1993,105:1110–16.
42. Konturek PC, Ernst H, Konturek SJ et al. Mucosal expression and luminal release of epidermal and transforming growth factors in patients with duodenal ulcer before and after eradication of *Helicobacter pylori*. Gut. 1997;40:463–9.
43. Terres AM, Pajares JM, O'Toole D, Ahern S, Kelleher D. *H. pylori* infection is associated with down-regulation of E-cadherin, a molecule involved in epithelial cell adhesion and proliferation control. J Clin Pathol. 1998;51:410–12.
44. Graham DY. *Campylobacter pylori* and peptic ulcer disease. Gastroenterology. 1989; 96:615–25.
45. Baron JH. Studies of basal and peak acid output with an augmented histamine test. Gut. 1963;4:136–44.
46. Baron JH. An assessment of the augmented histamine test in the diagnosis of peptic ulcer: correlations between gastric secretion, age and sex of patients, and site and nature of the ulcer. Gut. 1963;4:243–53.
47. Card WI, Marks IN. The relationship between the acid output of the stomach following 'maximal' histamine stimulation and the parietal cell mass. Clin Sci. 1960;19:147–63.
48. Graham DY, Genta RM, Malaty H. Which is the most important factor in duodenal ulcer pathogenesis: the strain of *H. pylori* or the host? In: Hunt RH, Tytgat GNJ, editors. *Helicobacter pylori*: basic mechanisms to clinical cure. Lancaster: Kluwer;1996:85–91.
49. Wormsley KG. Progress report. The pathophysiology of duodenal ulcer. Gut. 1974;15:59–81.
50. Wormsley KG, Grossman MI. Maximal histalog test in control subjects and patients with peptic ulcer. Gut. 1965;6:427–35.
51. Wyatt JL, Rathbone BJ, Dixon MF, Heatley RV. *Campylobacter pyloridis* and acid induced gastric metaplasia in the pathogenesis of duodenitis. J Clin Pathol. 1987;40:841–8.
52. Schrager J, Spink R, Mitra S. The antrum in patients with duodenal and gastric ulcers. Gut. 1967;8:497–508.

53. Carrick J, Lee A, Hazell S et al. Campylobacter pylori, duodenal ulcer, and gastric metaplasia: possible role of functional heterotopic tissue in ulcerogenesis. Gut. 1989;30:790–7.
54. Steer HW. Surface morphology of the gastroduodenal mucosa in duodenal ulceration. Gut. 1984:25:1203–10.
55. Barlow TE, Bently FH, Walder DN. Arteries, veins and arteriovenous anastomoses in the human stomach. Surg Gynaecol Obstet. 1951;93:657–71.
56. van Zanten SJOV, Dixon MF, Lee A. The gastric transitional zones: neglected links between gastroduodenal pathology and *Helicobacter* ecology. Gastroenterology. 1999;116:1217–29.

37
What causes *Helicobacter pylori*-negative non-NSAID-related ulcers?

C. W. HOWDEN

INTRODUCTION

Although *Helicobacter pylori* infection is the single most common underlying cause of peptic ulceration, attention in the United States has recently focused on the apparently growing number of *H. pylori*-negative ulcers seen in clinical practice. Clearly, the epidemiology of *H. pylori* infection is changing; smaller family size and improvements in hygiene and sanitation mean less primary *H. pylori* infection in childhood. Incidence and prevalence rates of *H. pylori* infection are falling, at least in the developed world. The widespread eradication of *H. pylori* infection from adult patients with peptic ulcer disease and other conditions further reduces the opportunity for intra-familial transmission of the infection. Presumably, there has always been a subset of peptic ulcer disease that was unrelated to *H. pylori* infection. As the pool of *H. pylori* infection and *H. pylori*-related peptic ulcers has diminished, the proportion – although not, perhaps, the absolute number – of *H. pylori*-negative ulcers has risen.

PREVALENCE OF *H. PYLORI*-NEGATIVE ULCERS

The prevalence is highly variable geographically. In 10 studies from the USA, the proportion of ulcers that were *H. pylori*-negative was as high as 61%[1-10] (Table 1). In seven studies of patients with uncomplicated duodenal ulcer[1-3,6,8-10], 27% of 3122 were *H. pylori*-negative; in three studies of patients with uncomplicated gastric ulcer[1,8,9], 26% of 315 were *H. pylori*-negative.

In contrast, the reported prevalence of *H. pylori*-negative ulcers from elsewhere – and from Europe in particular – appears to be much lower[11-18] (Table 2). One exception to this is when complicated ulcers are studied in isolation. In a UK-based study of patients with perforated duodenal ulcer,

Table 1. Recent US-based studies of the prevalence of *H. pylori*-negative ulcers

Reference	n	Ulcer type	H. pylori-*negative (%)*
1	100	DU	1
	145	GU	8
2	183	DU	30
3	59	DU	52
4	80	PUD	61
5	166	PUD	40
6	201	DU	20
7	339	Bleeding DU	27
		Bleeding GU	36
8	144	DU	39
	127	GU	39
9	41	DU	39
	43	GU	47
10	2394	DU	27

Adapted, with permission, from Peura DA. The problem of *H. pylori*-negative idiopathic ulcer disease (in press).
DU = duodenal ulcer; GU = gastric ulcer; PUD = peptic ulcer disease.

Table 2. Recent non-US-based studies of the prevalence of *H. pylori*-negative ulcers

Reference	n	Ulcer type	H. pylori-*negative (%)*	Country
11	435	DU	3	UK
12	80	Perforated DU	53	UK
13	707	DU, pyloric	2	Finland
14	125	PUD	30	Finland
15	125	DU	45	Australia
16	774	DU	5	Spain
17	14	DU	43	Australia
	33	GU	58	
	7	DU + GU	43	
18	215	GU	3	Japan
	120	DU	2	

Adapted, with permission, from Peura DA. The problem of *H. pylori*-negative idiopathic ulcer disease (in press).

53% were *H. pylori*-negative[12] (Table 2). One other exception is Australia, where there is a high reported prevalance of *H. pylori*-negative duodenal ulcer[15] (Table 2). In that study, 40% of the patients with duodenal ulcer had been taking aspirin or another NSAID, and there was a trend towards higher NSAID use in *H. pylori*-negative patients ($p = 0.09$). Another study from Australia to have found a high prevalence of *H. pylori*-negative ulcers did not specifically report rates of aspirin or NSAID use[17].

The explanation for the higher prevalence of *H. pylori*-negative ulcers in the USA compared to Europe and Japan, but not apparently to Australia, is unclear. However, infection rates in the USA are probably lower than in some European countries, and may have been falling more rapidly.

Furthermore, aspirin or NSAID use – conscious, unconscious or surreptitious – may be a more substantial problem in the USA[19] and in Australia[15].

H. PYLORI-NEGATIVE ULCER DISEASE – ROLE OF ASPIRIN AND NSAIDs

Aspirin or NSAID use must always be considered in those patients with ulcer disease that is negative for *H. pylori* and in those patients whose ulcers appear slow or difficult to heal, or that relapse soon after treatment[19]. This may sometimes be overlooked in routine clinical practice. In the USA three non-aspirin NSAIDs (ibuprofen, naproxen and ketoprofen) are available for over-the-counter purchase, albeit in low doses. However, patients may take more than the recommended or approved doses of these drugs, and may combine them with aspirin or with various proprietary combinations that contain aspirin. They could, therefore, take a cumulatively large – and potentially ulcerogenic – dose of aspirin and NSAIDs.

Not all of the studies outlined in Tables 1 and 2 rigorously excluded surreptitious or unreported aspirin or NSAID use. Jyotheeswaran *et al.* from Rochester, NY, interviewed patients about use of these drugs; when admitted aspirin or NSAID use was excluded, 39% of ulcers were still unassociated with *H. pylori* infection[8]. Ciociola and colleagues reviewed six multi-centre US-based clinical trials in duodenal ulcer. Aspirin and NSAID use were specific exclusion criteria for these trials, in which the rate of *H. pylori*-negative ulcers ranged from 21% to 33%[10]. In McColl's initial series from Scotland[11], 12 of 435 patients with duodenal ulcer were *H. pylori*-negative; four of these were using NSAIDs. In the most recently reported European series, Gisbert *et al.* from Spain found that 95.3% of 774 consecutive duodenal ulcer patients were *H. pylori*-positive. If patients with admitted aspirin or NSAID use were excluded, the proportion of duodenal ulcer patients who were *H. pylori*-positive increased to 99.1%[16].

Assuming that use of aspirin and NSAIDs has been formally excluded, other possible aetiologies of *H. pylori*-negative ulcers need to be considered.

POSSIBLE CAUSES OF H. PYLORI-NEGATIVE, NSAID-NEGATIVE ULCER DISEASE

Zollinger–Ellison syndrome (ZES)

This probably accounts for only 1% of duodenal ulcers at most[20], and for even fewer gastric ulcers. A history of complicated ulcers, or ulcers at multiple or unusual sites, should raise suspicion of ZES, especially if tests for *H. pylori* are negative. The combination of duodenal ulceration and severe erosive oesophagitis, or duodenal ulcer and diarrhoea, are other possible presentations of ZES. A strong family history of peptic ulcer disease – perhaps suggesting multiple endocrine neoplasia (MEN) type I – is also suggestive. Hypercalcaemia may indicate underlying hyperparathyroidism, in MEN-I.

False-negative test(s) for H. pylori infection

A false-negative result of a test for *H. pylori* infection might be another explanation for apparent '*H. pylori*-negative' ulcers. The sensitivity of endoscopic methods and of urea breath and blood tests is reduced in patients on proton pump inhibitors (PPIs) and in those who are taking – or have recently been taking – antibiotics or bismuth-containing compounds. Laine and colleagues reported that 33% of 93 patients with known *H. pylori* infection had a false-negative ^{13}C-UBT while taking lansoprazole[21]. Sensitivity of the ^{13}C-UBT increased to 91%, 97% and 100% after, respectively, 3, 7 seven and 14 days off lansoprazole. Bravo and colleagues found that lansoprazole produced false-negative rates of 30–40% for the ^{13}C-UBT and of 15–25% for the HpSA™ stool antigen test[22]. Bismuth subsalicylate treatment was associated with false-negative rates of 45–55% for the ^{13}C-UBT and 10–15% for the HpSA™ stool antigen test[22]. Ranitidine had no significant effect on the sensitivity of either test.

Helicobacter heilmannii infection

H. heilmannii is a Gram-negative bacterium isolated from the human stomach and probably transmitted zoonotically. Previously called *Gastrospirillum hominis*, it is morphologically distinct from *H. pylori*. Infection is associated with a mild antral-predominant gastritis and has been preliminarily linked to peptic ulcer. In a retrospective study of gastric biopsies from 946 patients with duodenal ulcer, Jhala and colleagues found *H. heilmannii* in only four, all of whom had negative cultures for *H. pylori*[23]. Among the biopsies from 281 patients with NSAID-related gastric ulcers, only two had evidence of *H. heilmannii*[23]. The gastritis of *H. heilmannii* infection appears to be patchier and milder than that of *H. pylori*, and more likely to be confined to the gastric antrum[23,24]. In Stolte *et al.*'s series of 202 patients with *H. heilmannii* gastritis, only eight had ulceration, which was usually associated with NSAID use[24].

Crohn's disease

Oberhuber and colleagues in Austria examined gastric and duodenal biopsies from 792 patients with known intestinal Crohn's disease but without specific upper gastrointestinal manifestations[25]. They found histological features consistent with Crohn's disease in the gastric corpus in 37%, the antrum in 42%, the duodenal bulb in 13% and the descending duodenum in 12%. Overt Crohn's disease of the duodenum usually occurs in association with active disease elsewhere. In the series of Yamamoto and colleagues from England, 96% of 54 patients with gastroduodenal Crohn's had expression of the disease elsewhere in the gastrointestinal tract[26]. Ulceration was found in only four of the 54 patients; the commonest presentation was with stricture, which was present in 41 patients.

Hypercalcaemia

Steinberg and colleagues studied 268 elderly patients consecutively admitted to an acute-care geriatric medicine facility[27]. The mean age of the patients was 77 (range 61–98). Thirty-five patients (13%) had hypercalcaemia at the time of admission. Oesophagogastroduodenoscopy (OGD) was performed on all patients in whom there was clinical suspicion of peptic ulcer disease.

Forty-two patients had OGD, of whom 27 had peptic ulcer. Of the 27 with ulcer disease, six had normal serum calcium and *H. pylori*-positive duodenal ulcer, 10 had hypercalcaemia and *H. pylori*-positive duodenal ulcer, five had hypercalcaemia and *H. pylori*-positive gastric ulcer, and six had hypercalcaemia and *H. pylori*-negative gastric ulcer. This preliminary study highlights the unexpectedly high prevalence of hypercalcaemia in elderly patients. Most of the patients with ulcer disease were hypercalcaemic; however, most were also positive for *H. pylori* infection. Hypercalcaemia is therefore unlikely to contribute much to the high rate of *H. pylori*-negative ulcers seen in the USA.

CONCLUSIONS

There appears to be a major difference between the USA (and, possibly, Australia) and other regions of the world, including Europe and Japan, with respect to the prevalence of *H. pylori*-negative ulcers. The explanation for this is not entirely clear. Use of aspirin and other NSAIDs probably accounts for many of the *H. pylori*-negative ulcers encountered in clinical practice, and has not been definitively excluded in some published series. US-based clinical trials sponsored by pharmaceutical companies, and conducted to standards required by the Food and Drug Administration, have carefully tried to exclude patients taking aspirin or other NSAIDs. However, such trials still uncovered a substantial proportion of ulcers that were not apparently related to *H. pylori* infection[10]. Although many other conditions can produce ulceration in the upper gastrointestinal tract, most of these should be suggested by individual patients' clinical presentations. Crohn's disease, for example, usually only affects the duodenum in conjunction with lower intestinal disease and, even then, most often manifests with stricture rather than ulceration[26].

When faced with a patient with ulcer disease that is apparently *H. pylori*-negative, the clinician should first review the manner in which the patient had been tested for *H. pylori* infection, so as to exclude the possibility of a false-negative result. Then, consumption of aspirin, aspirin-containing products and other NSAIDs should be carefully explored. Ideally, a test of platelet cyclo-oxygenase function should be made if there is any doubt about surreptitious or unconscious aspirin use[28]. If aspirin or other NSAID use is confidently excluded, a fasting serum gastrin level should be checked when the patient is not taking any gastric antisecretory medicines. Consideration might then be given to other possible causes of ulceration, as reviewed here and listed in Table 3. Many of these will only be suggested by elements of the patient's clinical presentation. Lastly, there will remain a proportion of patients with ulcer disease that is *H. pylori*-negative, unrelated to aspirin or NSAID use and genuinely 'idiopathic'. The optimal management for such patients is unclear at this point. They will not benefit from treatment directed at *H. pylori* infection, and are likely to require indefinite treatment with gastric antisecretory drugs. While surgery might be a reasonable option in some, this has not been studied in an exclusively *H. pylori*-negative group of patients.

Table 3. Uncommon causes of peptic ulcer disease unrelated to *H. pylori* infection

Crohn's disease
Helicobacter heilmannii infection
Hypercalcaemia
Portal hypertension
Carcinoma
Tuberculosis
Lymphoma
Ischaemia
Cytomegalovirus infection
Herpes simplex infection
Systemic mastocytosis
Rare genetic syndromes – not always adequately characterized or defined (e.g. 'ulcer–tremor–nystagmus' syndrome, 'stiff-man' syndrome)

REFERENCES

1. al-Assi MT, Genta RM, Karttunen TJ, Graham DY. Ulcer site and complications: relation to *Helicobacter pylori* infection and NSAID use. Endoscopy. 1996;28:229–33.
2. Lanza F, Ciociola AA, Sykes D, Heath A, McSorley DJ, Webb DD. Ranitidine bismuth citrate plus clarithromycin is effective in eradicating *H. pylori*, healing duodenal ulcers, and preventing ulcer relapse. Gastroenterology. 1996;110:A172 (abstract).
3. Sprung DJ, Gano B. The natural history of duodenal ulcer disease and how it relates to *H. pylori* – a community study. Am J Gastroenterol. 1997;92:1655 (abstract)
4. Gislason GT, Emu B, Okolo P, Pasricha PJ, Kalloo AN. Where have all the *Helicobacter* gone? Etiologic factors in patients with duodenal ulcers (DU) presenting to a university hospital. Gastrointest Endosc. 1997;45:AB90.
5. Greenberg PD, Albert CM, Ridker PM et al. *Helicobacter pylori* as a risk factor for peptic ulcers in patients taking low-dose aspirin. Gastroenterology. 1997;112:A133.
6. Peterson WL, Ciociola AA, Sykes DL, McSorley DJ, Webb DD. Ranitidine bismuth citrate plus clarithromycin is effective for healing duodenal ulcers, eradicating *H. pylori* and reducing ulcer recurrence. Aliment Pharmacol Ther. 1996;10:251–61.
7. Jensen DM, Cheng S, Jensen ME et al. Risk factors and recurrence of ulcer hemorrhage. Gastroenterology. 1997;112:A160.
8. Jyotheeswaran S, Shah AN, Jin HO, Potter GD, Ona FV, Chey WU. Prevalence of *Helicobacter pylori* in peptic ulcer patients in greater Rochester, NY: is empirical triple therapy justified? Am J Gastroenterol. 1998;93:574–8.
9. Schubert M, DeWitt JM, Taylor CA. Prospective evaluation of the prevalence of *H. pylori* in duodenal and gastric ulcer: is its role overstated? Gastroenterology. 1999;116:A305.
10. Ciociola AA, McSorley DJ, Turner K, Sykes D, Palmer JB. *Helicobacter pylori* infection rates in duodenal ulcer patients in the United States may be lower than previously estimated. Am J Gastroenterol. 1999;94:1834–40.
11. McColl KEL, El-Nujumi AM, Chittajallu RS et al. A study of the pathogenesis of *Helicobacter pylori* negative chronic duodenal ulceration. Gut. 1993;34:762–8.
12. Reinback DH, Cruickshank G, McColl KEL. Acute perforated duodenal ulcer is not associated with *Helicobacter pylori* infection. Gut. 1993;34:1344–7.
13. Hyvarinen H, Salmenkyla S, Sipponen P. *Helicobacter pylori*-negative duodenal and pylori ulcer: role of NSAIDs. Digestion. 1996;57:305–9.
14. Kemppainen H, Raiha I, Sourander L. Clinical presentation of peptic ulcer in the elderly. Gerontology. 1997;43:283–8.
15. Henry A, Batey RG. Low prevalence of *Helicobacter pylori* in an Australian duodenal ulcer population: NSAIDitis or the effect of ten years of *H. pylori* treatment? Aust NZ J Med. 1998;28:345.
16. Gisbert JP, Blanco M, Mateos JM. *H. pylori*-negative duodenal ulcer prevalence and causes in 774 patients. Dig Dis Sci. 1999;44:2295–302.
17. Xia HH-X, Phung N, Kalandar J, Talley NJ. Characteristics of *Helicobacter pylori* positive and negative peptic ulcer disease. Gastroenterology. 1999;116:A359 (abstract).

18. Tsuji H, Kohli Y, Fukumitsu S. *Helicobacter pylori*-negative gastric and duodenal ulcers. J Gastroenterol. 1999;34:455–60.
19. Hirschowitz BI, Lanas A. Intractable peptic ulceration due to aspirin (ASA) abuse in patients who have not had gastric surgery. Gastroenterology. 1997;112:A149 (abstract).
20. Isenberg JI, Walsh JH, Grossman MI. Zollinger–Ellison syndrome. Gastroenterology. 1973;65:140–65.
21. Laine L, Estrada R, Trujillo M, Knigge K, Fennerty MB. Effect of proton-pump inhibitor therapy on diagnostic testing for *Helicobacter pylori*. Ann Intern Med. 1998;129:547–50.
22. Bravo LE, Realpe L, Campo C, Mera R, Correa P. Effects of acid suppression and bismuth medications on the performance of diagnostic tests for *Helicobacter pylori* infection. Am J Gastroenterol. 1999;94:2380–3.
23. Jhala D, Jhala N, Lechago J, Haber M. *Helicobacter heilmannii* gastritis: association with acid peptic diseases and comparison with *Helicobacter pylori* gastritis. Mod Pathol. 1999;12:534–8.
24. Stolte M, Kroher G, Meining A, Morgner A, Bayerdorrfer E, Bethke B. A comparison of *Helicobacter pylori* and *Helicobacter heilmannii* gastritis. A matched control study involving 404 patients. Scand J Gastroenterol. 1997;32:28–33.
25. Oberhuber G, Hirsch M, Stolte M. High incidence of upper gastrointestinal tract involvement in Crohn's disease. Virchow's Arch Pathol. 1998;432:49–52.
26. Yamamoto T, Allan RN, Keighley MR. An audit of gastroduodenal Crohn's disease: clinicopathologic features and management. Scand J Gastroenterol. 1999;34:1019–24.
27. Steinberg EN, Cho-Steinberg HM, Howden CW. Hypercalcemia is predictive of peptic ulcer disease in chronically ill, institutionalized, geriatric patients. Am J Gastroenterol. 1996;91:1926 (abstract).
28. Lanas A, Remacha B, Sáinz R, Hirschowitz BI. Study of outcome after targeted intervention for peptic ulcer resistant to acid suppression therapy. Am J Gastroenterol. 2000;95:513–19.

38
From the pump to the helix

I. M. MODLIN, J. FARHADI and M. KIDD

INTRODUCTION

The history of the evolution of bacteriology and microbiology is a long and complex subject. The nature of disease has long baffled mankind and in this respect the elucidation of the role of organisms has proved to be amongst the most challenging of areas. Initially there existed no medical concept of anything other than divine retribution or fate as a cause of disease. Subsequently the consideration of unpropitious omens, misalignment of the planets and stars, bad air, certain herbs and even contact with certain types of animals was deemed causative. The understanding that contact with diseased individuals could lead to disease was suggestive of an agent of transmission, but lack of evidence further propagated superstition and fear rather than rational analysis of the problem. The development of lenses allowed for the realization that there existed animalcules, but their relationship to disease remained unrecognized and unproven for some considerable time. The demonstration by Agostino Bassi (1773–1856) of transmissibility of disease in animal species was followed by the identification of specific classes of organisms and the evidence that they were related to a specific disease process. Nevertheless, much argument related to the source of bacteria and their mode of propagation. Indeed widespread belief in spontaneous generation and heterogenesis resulted in acrimonious controversy for many years. The precise roles of the numerous many individuals in the establishment of microbiology are too numerous to describe in this text but credit must be given to certain critical contributors. Girolamo Fracastoro (1478–1553) described disease and noted transmissibility, Antonj van Leeuwenhoek (1632–1723) first noted the existence of microscopic animalcules, Agostino Bassi described transmission by organisms and Christian Ehrenberg (1795–1876) classified them with use of stains provided by Wilhelm von Gleichen (1717–1783). John Snow (1813–58), in his classic epidemiology study of the Broad Street pump cholera event, demonstrated the concept of contamination and disease spread. F. G. Jacob Henle (1809–85) introduced rigour into the study of bacteria and produced the postulates of disease that were later assumed by Robert Koch (1843–1910).

Theodor Schwann (1810–82) reported that organisms (yeast) divided and produced chemicals, while Sir Edward Jenner (1749–1823) and thereafter Louis Pasteur (1822–95) and Robert Koch, added substantial contributions to the identification of organism-related disease and also introduced the concepts of therapy. Sir Ronald Ross (1857–1932), Walter Reed (1851–1902) and William Gorgas (1854–1920) proved the existence of animal vectors and demonstrated that sanitary measures were effective in the control of transmissible disease. Jules Bordet (1870–1939), Paul Ehrlich (1854–1915) and Elie Metchnikoff (1845–1916) defined complement, amboreceptors and phagocytosis respectively, leading to the delineation of immunity and laying the scientific foundation for a novel area of development. Gerard Domagk (1895–1964), Sir Alexander Fleming (1881–1955) and Sir Howard Florey (1898–1968) pioneered the concept of chemotherapy that has been so successfully extrapolated by synthetic chemists. The last decade of the 20th century has witnessed the delineation of the genome of organisms and the likelihood that therapeutic targeting will move from beyond the cell membrane and cytoplasmic processes to the nucleus itself.

This chapter seeks to describe the evolution of the understanding of bacteria as related to the elucidation of peptic ulcer disease, and to amplify and place into perspective the recent advances in the delineation of the role of *Helicobacter pylori* in this disease process.

EARLY CONCEPTS OF DISEASE

From the earliest of times, humans have battled with the concept of disease and its noxious effect on health. Initially, afflictions were thought to represent divine retribution for misdeeds or, alternatively, the invasion of the body by spirits or demons. The advent of religious doctrine resulted in the consideration of disease as a consequence of sin. Overwhelming episodes of illness such as the pestilence or plague, involving entire communities, were believed to be visitations from the gods. By 400 BC thoughtful physicians such as Hippocrates (460–375 BC) had already developed more rational thoughts regarding disease, and in his book *Airs, Waters and Places* he dealt with the influence of climate, winds, water supplies, the habitats of the people, and the nature of the soil on the illnesses prevalent in an area[1]. While such considerations were useful, they failed to explain the nature of transmission of illness from individuals in close proximity or by exposure to clothing and objects used by ill people. As a result of such observations it was postulated that animated particles invisible to the naked eye might be the cause of the disease. Varro (117–26 BC) proposed that disease was caused by tiny animals, which could not be seen by the naked eye and would carry through the air to the mouth and nose and thence to the body[2]. The recognition that the disease process may be transmissible was more apparent to the ancient Hebrews, who devised rules in regard to lepers (Book of Leviticus). Specific instructions regarding the isolation of the patient, washing and burning of infected clothing, and the disinfection of houses was advocated. The concept of isolation and quarantine, although harshly imposed under such circumstances, adequately demonstrated that disease spread could be managed.

A similar problem on a vaster scale was evident in consideration of the plague. This scourge is thought to have originated in the East between 900 and 1500 AD and documented to have attacked Europe more than 65 times[3]. The Black Death of the 14th Century began in the Far East, where millions died in India and China, before it spread to Europe in 1347. First noted in Venice it spread thereafter to France and finally England. In 1403, on an island adjoining the city of Venice, a detention hospital was open for all travellers from the Levant. A 40-day isolation period was required based on the biblical injunction. Similar institutions were opened in Genoa in 1467 and in 1476 in Marseilles. Although the Black Death decimated the European population, its intermittent nature was very different from that of syphilis and subsequently tuberculosis. The prolonged effects of these diseases would ravage the European population for almost four centuries and last well into the 20th century.

SYPHILIS

Syphilis was first recognized towards the end of the 15th century. Initially characterized by an acute onset of skin eruptions and ulcers, with widespread tissue destruction, the subsequent, chronic course of this disease reflected alterations in immunity, and possibly the evolution of the organism compared to its original infective form. Controversy existed as to the precise origin of syphilis and some scholars believe that the sailors of Columbus, infected by the natives of Haiti, transferred it to the Spanish occupants of Naples. Evidence exists, however, that it was present in Europe before the discovery of America. Other proposals maintain that Spanish sailors returning from the voyages to West Africa contaminated the population of Europe. Irrespective of the source, its effects on the early European population were so devastating that in 1495, at the siege of Naples, the army of Charles VIII of France was decimated by the disease. The subsequent return of the troops to France resulted in further dissemination of the disease which was then referred to by the French as the Neapolitan disease. The Spaniards, in contrast, regarded it as the French disease. In 1546 the Italian physician, Fracastoro, resolved the nomenclature by naming the disease syphilis[4]. Fracastoro was interested in the subject of disease spread, and given his knowledge of leprosy and the plague, was fascinated by a novel disease spread by sexual intercourse. Inspired by the punishment inflicted on the mythological shepherd Syphilus, Fracastoro wrote a poem about the disease in Latin hexameter[4]. He used as the central character Syphilus, the second son of Niobe, portrayed by Ovid as having been afflicted by a loathsome and contagious disease for offending Apollo, the sun god. Fracastoro proposed that the disease was transmitted by a perceptible particle which he called *Seminaria Contagionum* or the seeds of disease. His appreciation of this concept of the source of disease and its transmission earned him the later soubriquet of 'Father of Modern Epidemiology'.

HYGIENE AND CHOLERA

The general rules of hygiene were reasonably well known. In Deuteronomy (chapter XXIII, verse 13) Moses provided instructions for his soldiers to

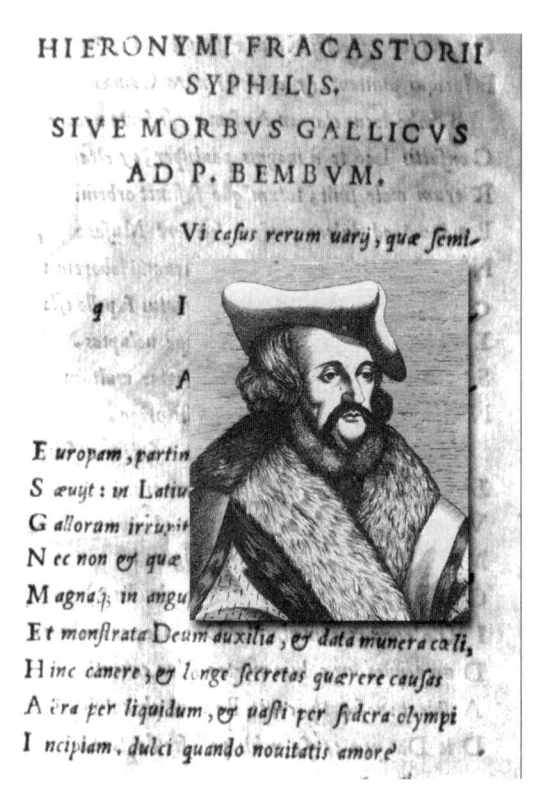

Figure 1. Girolamo Fracastoro (1478–1553), an Italian scholar and physician, was born in Verona and thereafter became professor of philosophy in Padua. While practising as a physician in Verona he propounded the theory that infection was due to passage of minute bodies, capable of self-multiplication. His development of the theory of contagion embraced one of the earliest concepts of the 'germ theory' of disease. An excellent geographer, astronomer and mathematician he was also a skilled musician and poet. As such his Latin poem on the novel venereal disease *Syphilis sive Morbus Glaciers*, of 1530, achieved widespread notoriety and Fracastoro has ever since been credited with the introduction of the term 'syphilis'.

carry a spade in order to bury their excreta and not defile the camp, 'and thou shalt have a paddle upon thy weapon; and it shall be, when thou wilt ease thyself abroad, thou shalt dig therewith and shall turn back and cover that which cometh from thee'[5]. The failure of inhabitants of medieval cities, even into the 18th and 19th centuries, to follow the Mosaic doctrine was responsible for widespread epidemics of cholera, typhoid and dysentery. Many homes lacked sanitation facilities and house home-dwellers often filled chamber pots with excreta which after days would be emptied out of a window into the street below with the cry of *'gardez l'eau'*. It was recognized by Edwin Chadwick (1800–90) that sanitary reform was necessary to control disease and that sewage disposal in particular was an important issue. His 1842 report on the sanitary conditions of the labouring population of Great Britain was further expanded upon by William Budd (1811–80) who, during

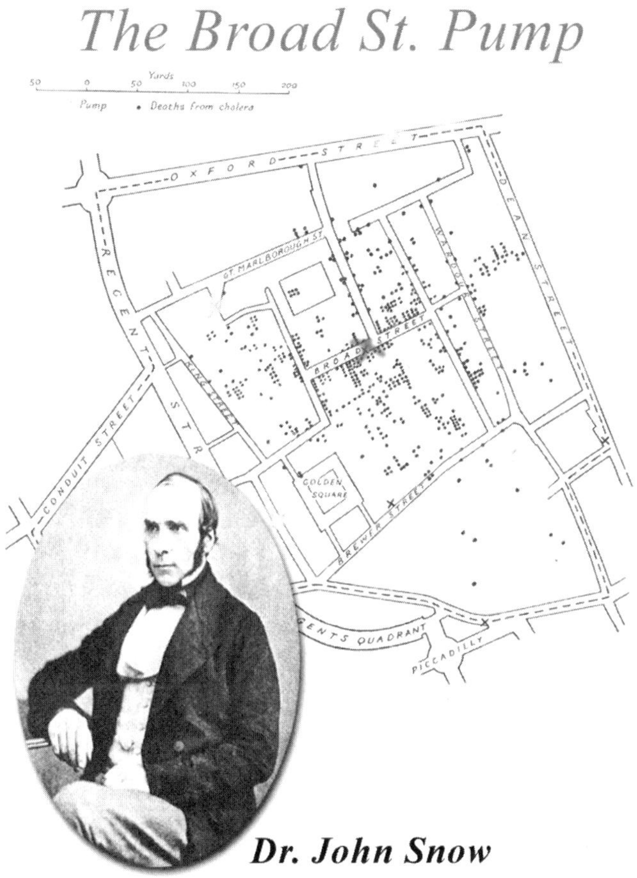

The Broad St. Pump

Dr. John Snow

Figure 2. John Snow (1813–58), an English anaesthetist and epidemiologist, was born in York. He was a young general practitioner in 1831 when cholera first appeared in Britain and became convinced that the disease spread through contaminated water. After 1836 he practised in London and during the cholera outbreaks of 1848 and 1854 undertook some brilliant epidemiological investigations, tracing one local outbreak to a sewage-contaminated well in Broad (now Broadwick) Street, Soho. To obviate the further spread of the disease he had the pump handle removed. His subsequent work implicated the Thames river, into which many of London's sewers drained, and from which much of the domestic water of the city was obtained. In addition to his epidemiological contributions, he undertook fundamental experimental work on chloroform, and also devised apparatus to administer anaesthetics. Such was his repute that he administered chloroform to Queen Victoria in 1853 during the birth of Prince Leopold.

the Great Stench of London in the summer of 1858, pointed out that organic putrefaction by itself was not enough to cause disease. The sewage of 19th-century London (almost three-quarters of a million people) collected in one vast cesspit in the middle of the city and during the summer the hot sun produced a stench so foul that even Parliament and the Lower Courts were closed. Dreading the onset of massive disease epidemics the populace were apprehensive, but, in fact a remarkable decrease in the proportion of fevers, dysentery and such like were noted during this time. It was thus obvious that some additional agency was necessary apart from organic putrefaction itself. Indeed these observations had already been made by John Snow in 1854 during the last great cholera epidemic in Great Britain[6]. Snow believed that contaminated water was responsible for the large number of outbreaks, and studied the water supply of each affected area. Although his initial proposals were ignored the study of the Broad Street epidemic confirmed his postulates. In this instance, 500 people living within 250 yards of the region where the first case was diagnosed died of the disease within 10 days. As a result the remaining inhabitants decamped, leaving the area almost deserted. Snow demonstrated that all the victims had used the pump connected to one particular well, and that a person suffering from cholera had been in the habit of using a certain cesspool which drained into this well. Having removed the handle of the pump, he noted no further cases of cholera. Although unable to demonstrate the microorganism responsible, he established by inference that the disease was spread by water which had been contaminated by excreta containing some noxious agent.

THE SPONTANEOUS GENERATION CONTROVERSY

Although the concept of contagion and the recognition of microorganisms were apparent, it was only in the last quarter of the 18th century that serious progress occurred. Efforts to arrange microorganisms into some sort of taxonomic scheme occupied the attention of many investigators, including Otto Friedrich Müller (1730–84) and the scheme was subsequently expanded by others, of whom Christian Gottfried Ehrenberg (1795–1876) was the most effective[7]. Although Leeuwenhoek was probably the first to see both gastrointestinal and oral bacteria, it was O. Müller (1730–84) of Copenhagen who provided the first definitive observations and descriptions of microorganisms; he also coined the terms 'bacillus' and 'spirillum'[8]. A problem in the elucidation of microbiology was the obscurity surrounding the origin of the animalcules in question. Although individuals as perspicacious as Carl Rokitansky (1804–78) had presumed that inert fluids possessed the capacity for generating viable body elements, this assumption was widespread, and held that living things could arise from organic but non-viable material. Indeed this concept of spontaneous generation was old (even C. Lucretius (98–55 BC) had been critical of it) and proposed that various noxious creatures arose *de novo* out of refuse. Bizarre notions of mice being generated from rags and maggots in garbage from the larva of flies were reported. Nevertheless, as has been noted by sage minds, 'obscurity flourishes in the realm of the invisible'. The observation by the Italian parliamentarian and cleric, Abbate Spallanzani (1729–99), that there was no vegetative power in inanimate matter (1765)[9] was contradicted by the Catholic priest, John Tuberville Needham (1713–81), and George LeClair Comte de Buffon (1707–88). The controversy continued to be widely argued during the first part of the 19th century when it became apparent that organic infusions could not develop animalcules if free access to the air was denied. Thereafter, it was demonstrated that air that had previously been subjected to heating, or passed through an acid, did not generate microorganisms, and it was proposed that the air so treated had been 'hopelessly vitiated'. Although Heinrich Schroder (1810–85) and Theodore von Dusch (1824–90) in 1854 attempted to refute this proposal, their research was not widely accepted. In 1859 Félix-Archmèdi Pouchett (1800–72) published a major text, *Hétérogénie*, that adumbrated upon the theory of spontaneous generation and gained much support. Fortunately, Louis Pasteur (1822–95) examined this issue with scientific rigour and proved conclusively that the agents of putrefaction did not develop *de novo* in organic solutions, but were either present *ab initio* or acquired by exposure to the air, as expressed in his 'Mémoire sur les corpuscules organisés qui existent dans l'atmosphère. Examen de la doctrine de générations spontanées'[10]. Although the controversy continued for a considerable time, it finally dissipated as attention was devoted to more specialized phases of bacteriology.

Agostino Bassi (1773–1856) of Lodi was responsible for a major contribution by demonstrating that microorganisms caused disease and fulfilled the postulates of an 'animate contagium'. In the study of silkworm disease he demonstrated that the causative agent was fungus and that the disease was transmissible. In so doing he fulfilled one of the initial three requisites which Jakob Henley had established in his essay on 'My Asthma and Contagia' as requisite for proving the causative relationship of a 'contagium' to any given disease[11]. This essay, published in 1840, was a critical advance in the field of bacteriology in establishing three criteria by which the causative association of a contagium to a disease could be tested. Bassi of Lodi proposed that the requirements should include: (1) to demonstrate the presence of the suspected organism in every instance of the given disease but in no other disease; (2) the isolation of the organism from other microorganisms and from all other extraneous matter; and (3) demonstration that the isolated organism was capable of inducing the disease from which it was originally taken. As Cecilia Mettler (1909–43) so aptly stated, these were in 1840 simply desiderata, not accomplishments[12]. It would remain for Louis Pasteur and Robert Koch to fulfil Henle's proposals and establish the theory of the germ causation of disease.

SCHWANN AND PASTEUR

By the beginning of the 19th century it was agreed that yeast was an aftereffect of fermentation, although chemists fought a long battle against the proponents of *vitalism*, who considered the round globules to be some type of chemical. In 1837 Theodore Schwann demonstrated that yeast was a living organism and called it '*Zuckerpilz*', from which the subsequent term *Saccharomyces* was developed[13]. Schwann also demonstrated that, in addition to yeast, fermentation of a sugar solution required the presence of a nitrogenous substance. He proposed that the yeast plant drew its nutrition from the sugar, azoic substance, producing alcohol and other compounds. In so doing he clearly demonstrated that yeast existed as an organism, and accepted that there were technical issues relating to the precise delineation of the process of fermentation. Unfortunately his work was not only ignored

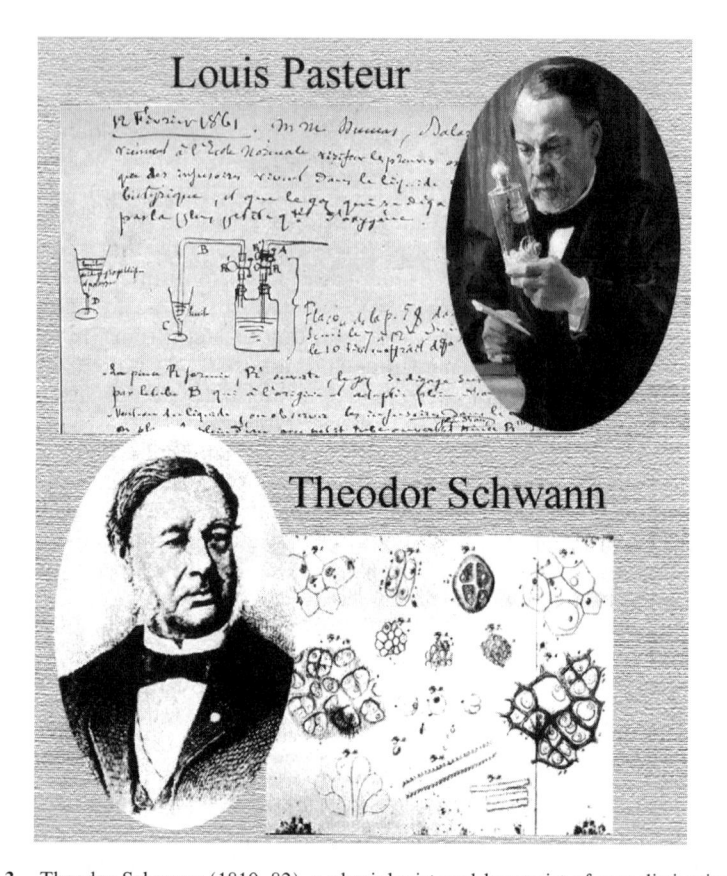

Figure 3. Theodor Schwann (1810–82), a physiologist and humanist of rare distinction, was born in Neuss, Germany. As a pupil of Müller in Berlin he undertook a series of fundamental experiments whose impact is still felt. These included the discovery of the enzyme pepsin, the delineation of muscle contraction, the role of microorganisms in putrefaction. He also brilliantly propounded the single-cell theory of disease for which he was subsequently awarded the Sydenham prize. As the victim of a scientific dispute with J. Liebig, the dominant chemist of the time (Schwann was ultimately proved correct) he departed Germany and in 1838 he became professor in Louvain and subsequently in 1848 at Liege. Louis Pasteur (1822–95), French chemist and bacteriologist, was born in Dôle. His work greatly extended the initial contributions of Schwann and vindicated the latter's proposals in regard to the cellular rather than chemical nature of fermentation and putrefaction. Pasteur's contributions to the making of wine, vinegar and beer, as well as his resolution of the problems of the silkworm disease and fowl cholera, led to his widespread acclaim. The development of vaccination for anthrax and rabies earned him international fame, and in 1888 the Institute Pasteur, of whom he was the first director, was founded to support the development of inoculation and the study of bacteriology.

by F. Wöhler (1800–82) and J. von Liebig (1803–73), but J. Berzelius (1779–1848) himself was critical of it, since both he and A. Lavoisier (1743–94) regarded yeast as a decomposition product of malt and therefore to be a chemical event.

Louis Pasteur, the son of a sergeant in Napoleon's army, was born into a modest family in Dôle in 1822. After qualifying from school he worked with the two great chemists, Jean Dumas (1800–84) and Antoine Balard (1802–76), and proved to be a fine pupil. Pasteur made fundamental contributions to the science of crystallography and his identification of enantiomers would in its own right have achieved him considerable fame if that were all he had ever undertaken. After finishing his studies in Paris he initially moved to Dijon in 1847, and thereafter became Acting Professor of Chemistry at the University of Strasbourg. Under the guidance of Pierre Bertin-Mourot, the Professor of Physics at Strasbourg, Pasteur was introduced not only to the world of science but to the appreciation of food and wine. In 1849 he married Marie Laurent, the daughter of the Director of the University. In seeking her hand Pasteur wrote a letter to the father indicating that, although he had no money, he could offer good health, courage, and a fine position at the university. He also informed him that he was possessed of a doctor's degree, had presented original work at the Academy of Science, and enclosed a report of an investigation that he had recently published. In 1854 the Minister of Education intervened in the life of Pasteur, appointing him as Professor of Chemistry at Lille. Since one of the main industries of this city was the fermentation of the beet sugar to produce alcohol, Pasteur rapidly developed an understanding of the relationship of microbes in this system. His wife, however, complained bitterly that 'Louis spends all his days in the distillery and is up to his neck in beet juice'[7].

The process of fermentation in the 19th century was regarded as a chemical event, whereby spirituous or acid substances were obtained from organic liquid, although the nature of the chemistry was ill-defined. Thus, the production of alcohol from beet juice was called alcoholic fermentation; wine into vinegar was called acidic acid fermentation,; and the souring of milk, during which lactic acid was produced, was called lactic acid fermentation. Indeed, it was thought the fermentation of liquids was probably brought about by changes similar to those which occurred in meats and eggs during decomposition and putrefaction. Unfortunately, the chemical thought leaders of the time, such as Thenard, Dumar, Gay-Lussac, and Lavoisier, considered that all changes in organic substances could be explained in terms of chemical reactions and expressed as chemical formulae. Thus, Lavoisier proposed that the production of alcohol from carbohydrates reflected a split into two parts of the latter, and transfer of oxygen from one part to the other. This failed to explain why carbohydrate underwent this change and ignored the fact that yeast was required to be present. By 1840 Theodore Schwann had demonstrated that yeast was not simply an organic substance but consisted of living cells, which could be observed to multiply by budding. The seminal work undertaken by Schwann was heavily criticized by leading chemists including Berzelius and Liebig, who were dedicated in their opposition to his theory. Although Pasteur might easily have conformed to this orthodox doctrine he confirmed in a number of experiments that the production of alcohol from sugar was brought about by the action of yeast cells, and that the amount of alcohol produced was directly proportional to the number of cells present[10].

Prior to the Renaissance it had been accepted that plants and animals could, under certain circumstances, derive from inanimate matter. The circumstance was described by numerous early writers including Aristotle (384–322 BC) and as late as the 16th century Jean Baptiste van Helmont (1577–1644), a celebrated chemist, reported that mice could be created by placing dirty linen together with a piece of cheese in a container. A further extrapolation of this proposal was defined by the concept of a biogenesis during the 17th century, whereby it was proposed that plants and certain small creatures such as flies and spiders and other insects could be produced. Francesco Reddi (1626–97) proposed this viewpoint, and conducted studies demonstrating that the theory of spontaneous generation did not apply at least for animals large enough to be observed with the naked eye. Nevertheless, it was widely accepted that living organisms of microscopic size found in large numbers in decaying organic matter could be produced by chemical reaction and thus be a form of spontaneous generation. The alternative viewpoint, that microbes were already present in the air and deposit on the substance, was bitterly argued until the work of Louis Pasteur. Initially he demonstrated the presence of bacteria in air by drawing air through a tube plugged by a cotton-wool filter. The filter was noted to contain numerous microorganisms, and when this dust was sprinkled on an organic substance previously heated to kill off any bacteria, and placed in a vacuum, there was a rapid growth of microorganisms. This demonstrated that microorganisms had been present in the dust from the air. In a subsequent experiment he utilized a number of flasks filled with liquid containing yeast and sugar, and drew out the neck of each to a fine point by heating it on a flame and then boiled the liquid to drive out the air, destroying any living substance in it. The flasks were then sealed off completely by heating the drawn-out ends with a blowpipe. Since they were now free of living material, they could remain sterile for as long as they were kept sealed. These flasks were then placed in widely different geographical locations and the neck of each broken with a long pair of pliers to allow the introduction of air. Meticulous attention was paid to detail, to ensure that the neck of the flasks and the pliers were first heated to kill the bacteria and that the air was not contaminated with dust from the clothes of the scientists. Once the neck of the flask was broken the surrounding air filled the vacuum and each flask was then resealed in a flame. By opening the flasks at different sites, and in areas of greater and greater altitude, Pasteur was able to demonstrate a relative abundance of microorganisms in different sites. Similarly he was able to produce irrefutable evidence that microbes would appear in an organic substance only when exposed to the air, unless they were already present in the air itself[10].

The identification by Pasteur that air contained bacteria was of particular interest to Joseph Lord Lister (1827–1912) who concluded that septic processes evident to surgeons were due to airborne bacteria in the operating rooms. His use of the carbolic spray to purify the air generated considerable controversy[14]. Issues that confounded the resolution of the problem at that time included the questions of whether bacteria were normally present in tissues or whether sepsis was due to the bacteria, as opposed to devitalized tissue that was subsequently contaminated by the bacteria.

Although it seemed reasonable to consider that microorganisms could engender such disease, the identification of such agents in disease tissue on the whole was interpreted as a secondary event. Otto Obermeier (1843–73) meanwhile had in 1868 noted the presence of large numbers of spiral-shaped organisms in the blood of patients suffering from a disease called relapsing fever. Although this seemed evidence of the cause of the disease, many physicians and scientists were of the opinion that tissue devitalized by the disease had been secondarily infected by such agents. It thus became vital not only to identify the presence of a microorganism, but also to determine that it was constantly associated with the disease and, if introduced into another animal, was capable of reproducing such a disease.

The subsequent focus of Louis Pasteur on chemistry, and thereafter the advancement of Schwann's work on fermentation, was important in focusing a coherent worldview in emerging bacteriology. In particular, the issue of contagion and its relationship to disease was still obscure. Although many scientists accepted that microorganisms might cause the disease the mechanism was uncertain, and some believed that organisms produced a specific poison in much the same way as yeast produced alcohol. It was, therefore, intuitive that the poison itself was responsible for the symptomatology of the disease. Others adhered to the belief that animalcules produced 'noxious vapors', while some believed that disease represented parasitism.

EARLY BACTERIOLOGY

A particular drawback in the identification of germs was the lack of appropriate methodology to identify them. Heinrich Robert Goeppert (1800–84) and Ferdinand Julius Cohn (1828–98) made major contributions in this area in 1849. Almost a decade later Joseph von Gerlach (1820–96) described the use of carmine for histological staining (in 1858) and a few years later, in 1863, H. Waldeyer (1836–1921) and Bohmer proposed that haematoxylin be similarly used. H. Hoffman was the first to attempt to stain bacteria in 1869, using carmine of fuchsine. These dyes had been prepared from aniline and coal tar since as early as 1856, and agents such as mauveine and fuchsine were available for study. In 1871 C. Weigert (1845–1904) noted that carmine could be used to stain cocci, and his subsequent observations in 1875 of the use of methyl violet to stain cocci in animal tissues marked the first successful studies to demonstrate these bacterial forms in animal tissues. In 1877 Salominosen was able to stain bacteria in a watery solution of fuchsin, and by 1884 Heinz Christian Joachim Gram (1853–1938) produced his seminal report upon the differential method of staining.

Ferdinand Cohn (1828–98) from Breslau, the botanist now regarded as one of the founders of bacteriology, classified microorganisms into several groups: bacterial (short, cylindrical cells), bacilli (longer cells), and spirilla (wavy or spiral forms) and coccoid (spherical), and noted the fixity of bacterial species[15]. Thus, even under varying conditions, he was never able to obtain cocci from bacilli or vice-versa. In 1870 Cohn established his own journal, *Beitrage zur Biologie der Pflanzen*, and in this communication hosted most of the original, classical bacteriology papers, authored by both himself and his young protégé, Robert Koch. The classic postulates of the latter would subsequently form the logical basis for the investigation and identification of the disease-causing potential of bacteria. In 1872 Cohn published his mature exposition on bacteriology entitled *Untersuchungen uber Bakteria*, wherein he further expanded the classification of bacteria into genera and species. He suggested an expanded classification into four groups: sphaerobacteria (cocci), microbacteria, desmobacteria (bacillus and vibrio) and spirobacteria (spirillum and spirochaete). This work was well received and became so popular that it was reprinted in 1875 and again in 1876.

In 1878 C. E. Sedillot (1804–83), a French surgeon who was responsible for undertaking the first gastrostomy, and may have unwittingly happened upon *H. pylori*, introduced the term 'microbe'. He proposed this term, derived from the Greek for 'small life', with the caveat that such 'small lives' must have the special ability to cause fermentation, putrefaction or a disease process. This was a proposal much favoured by T. Schwann (1810–82), who had himself not only discovered pepsin in 1834, but also written extensively on the role of fermentation, as well as the single-cell theory of disease.

THE RELATIONSHIP OF MICROORGANISMS TO SEPSIS

In 1878 Robert Koch (1843–1910) published his *Untersuchungen über dier Aetiologie der Wundinfektions-Kkrankheiten* and demonstrated that microorganisms and sepsis were interrelated[16]. This work was accomplished using staining methods (aniline compounds including methyl violet, fuchsine, and aniline brown) and the use of an oil emergence lens. Until his dramatic entry into the field of anthrax investigation, Koch had been an obscure country doctor. In April of 1876 he had written a letter to Ferdinan Cohn at Breslau and claimed that he had resolved the problem of anthrax and would be delighted to present it to the faculty. Although Pierre Rayer (1793–1867) in 1850 had reported the presence of small finely formed bodies in the blood of sheep with anthrax, the first observation of such agents had been by Casimir Davaine (1812–82). There had been consideration that these Deavaine bodies were the cause of anthrax for some years, but it was Koch, in a series of meticulous and rigorous experiments, who determined the principal morphological variations of the anthrax bacillus, its pathogenic potentialities, and its transmissibility from animal to animal. Pasteur subsequently became interested in the anthrax problem, and the attention of these two individuals on different issues of bacteriology led to major advances. Pasteur, as a representative of the French school of bacteriology, focused particularly on the elucidation of the manner in which bacteria caused disease, and to the underlying principles of recovery from and resistance to infection. German bacteriology as represented by Koch was more concerned with the biological characteristics of the bacteria and with the prevention of disease by the application of sanitary measures. In this respect the methods of cultivation devised by Koch in 1881 allowed for the identification of numerous species of bacteria, and in the words of William Bulloch (1868–1941) 'almost entire reconstruction of ideas on the causation of disease'[17]. While Koch established the biological basis of bacteriology, Pasteur

Table 1. A brief chronology of the individuals and the observations relevant to the identification and treatment of gastric bacteria. It is salutary that almost a century elapsed before confirmation of the original findings was achieved

Year	Individual	Observations
1875	G. Bottcher/M. Letulle	demonstrated bacteria in ulcer margins
1881	C. Klebs	bacterial colonization and 'interglandular small cell infiltration'
1888	M. Letulle	experimental induction of acute gastric lesions in guinea pigs (S. aureus)
1889	W. Jaworski	spiral organisms (Vibrio rugula) in gastric washings
1893	G. Bizzozero	identified spirochetes in gastric mucosa of dogs
1896	H. Salomon	spirochetes noted in gastric mucosa and experimentally transferred to mice
1906	W. Krienitz	spirochetes in gastric contents of patient with gastric carcinoma
1908	F.B. Turck	induced gastric ulcers in dogs by Bacillus (Escherichea) coli
1916	E.C. Rosenow	described streptococcus induced gastric ulcers
1917	L.R. Dragstedt	identified bacteria in experimental ulcers, no significant role identified
1921	J.S. Edkins	experimental physiology of S. regaudi (H. felis)
1924	J.M. Luck	discovered gastric mucosal urease
1925	B. Hoffman	described B. Hoffmani – putative ulcerous agent
1930	B. Berg	partial vagotomy inhibits secondary infections in ulcers
1938	J.L. Doenges	spirochetes/inflammation in Macacus monkey and man
1940	A.S. Freedberg/L. Barron	identified spirochetes in man – no etiologic role
1940	F.D. Gorham	postulated gastric acidophilic bacteria as an etiologic agent in ulcer disease
1954	E.D. Palmer	no spirochetes detected using HE in 1,180 suction biopsies
1975	H.W. Steer	polymorphonuclear migration in ulcers – isolated Pseudomonas aeruginosa
1983	J.R. Warren	identified Campylobacter (Helicobacter) pylori in human gastritis
1983	B. Marshall	isolated and cultured H. pylori
1985–1987	B. Marshall/A. Morris	ingested and proved the infectivity of H. pylori (Koch's 3rd postulate)

focused more on determining the virulence of the aetiological agents, and attempted to attenuate this capacity while maintaining the ability to establish immunity. In 1881 his Pasteur's success with immunization against anthrax established the prophylactic value of bacterial vaccines, and in 1884 he was able to report success in protecting against infection from rabies. His development of vaccines by a process of attenuation of the organisms was an important advance, but in 1884 and 1886 Daniel Elmer Salmon (1850–1914) and Theobold Smith (1859–1934) demonstrated, using hog cholera, that a dead vaccine was also capable of producing protective immunity.

EARLY GASTRIC BACTERIOLOGY

Careful analysis of gastric contents revealed that under fasting conditions the normal stomach contained mucus, a few bacilli and some yeast cells, whilst in stagnant gastric contents, obtained from patients with gastric disease, bacilli, micrococci, yeast and fungus could readily be seen. Such early observations supported speculations regarding a putative causative role of these 'foreign bodies' in gastric pathology. It was, however, unclear to these primordial, gastric bacteriologists whether a specific organism was the cause of a gastric disease entity or whether it was simply an abnormal accumulation of organisms in the stomach itself, which culminated in gastric disturbances.

One of these first gastric bacteriologists was the German, G. Bottcher, who, along with his French collaborator M. Letulle (1853–1929), demonstrated bacterial colonies in the ulcer floor and in its mucosal margins[18]. Bottcher's convictions in regard to the disease-causing potential of ingested organisms, were so ardent that by 1875 he had attributed the causation of ulcers to the bacterial forms demonstrated. This, however, was not a popular point of view and in spite of an 1881 report by the pathologist, C. Klebs, of a bacillus-like organism evident both free in the lumen of gastric glands and between the cells of the glands and the tunica propria with corresponding 'interglandular small round cell infiltration', the 'bacterial hypothesis' fell into disrepute[18]. Nevertheless, Bottcher was probably the first to report the presence of spiral organisms in the gastrointestinal tract of animals, although spiral organisms were already well known and had been described as early as 1838 by Ehrenberg. The pathogenic properties of these particular organismal forms had similarly been recognized by Obermeier of Berlin, who in 1872 demonstrated their presence in the blood of patients with relapsing fever. It is of considerable interest that an examination of the report of Klebs indicates that he had noted the presence of an inflammatory infiltration, although he made no specific comments in regards to its significance.

In 1889 Walery Jaworski, Professor of Medicine at the Jagiellonian University of Cracow, Poland, was the first to describe in detail spiral organisms in the sediment of washings obtained from humans. Amongst other things he noted a bacterium with a characteristic spiral appearance, which he named *Vibrio rugula*. He suggested that it might play a possible pathogenic role in gastric disease. Jaworski supposed that these 'snail' or 'spiral' cells were only to be found in rare cases. However, I. Boas (1858–1938), already a luminary for his gastrointestinal contributions and for the discovery of the 'Oppler–Boas' lactobacillus, found these cells quite constantly in all 'fasting' gastric contents containing hydrochloric acid. Further detailed analysis by Boas' assistant, P. Cohnheim, indicated that such 'cells' could be induced by the reaction of bronchial or pharyngeal mucus and hydrochloric acid. This led to the suggestion that Jaworski had consistently observed acid-altered myelin, and that similar secondary structures, threads and small masses could also be induced by these simple chemical reactions. Cohnheim and Boas, therefore, inferred from their experiments that Jaworski's 'cells' were most probably the product of gastric mucus and acid chyme[19].

The observations of Bottcher and Letulle had suggested a causative bacterial agent in ulcer disease, and by 1888 Letulle was actively searching for this postulated entity. A few years earlier, in 1881, the Scottish surgeon and bacteriologist Alexander Ogston (1844–1929) had identified *Staphylococcus pyrogenes aureus* both in acute and chronic abscesses. Noting the similarity of this bacterium to their postulated entity, Letulle, in the time-honoured tradition of his day, undertook a classical experiment. He used two modes of administration to guinea pigs: intramuscular injection of Ogston's pure, cultured *Staphylococcus* or oral intake of the agent. Not surprisingly, this resulted in the formation of acute gastric lesions perfectly consistent, at least to Letulle, with the predictable mode of generation of gastric ulcers. Matters were, however, somewhat complicated by the fact that he obtained similar results with dysentery organisms and with pyogenic streptococci. Letulle

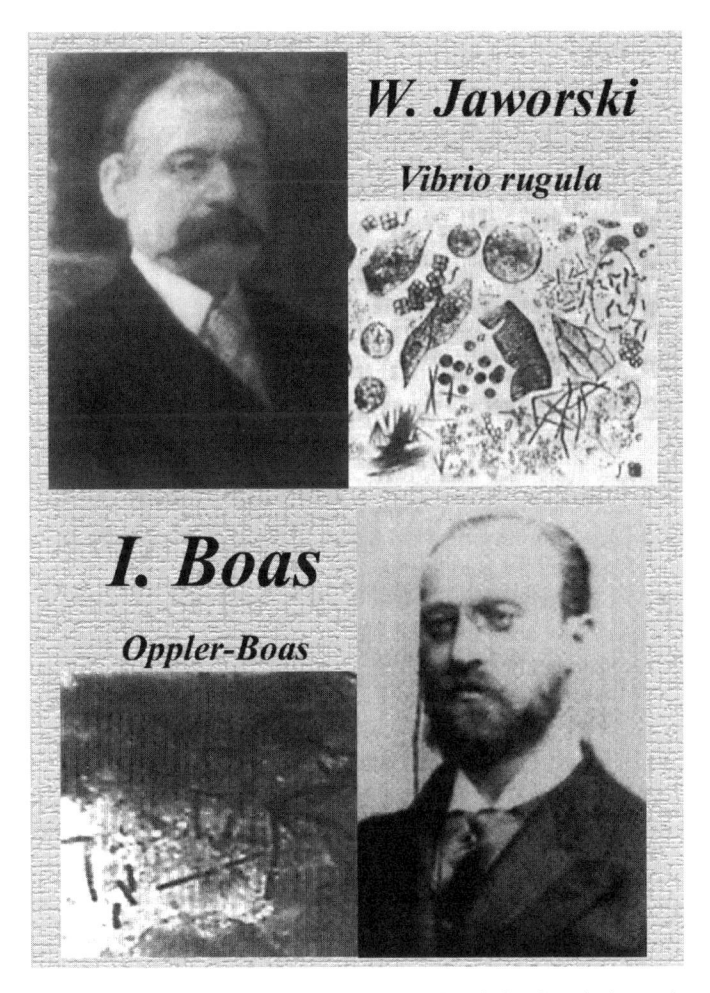

Figure 4. W. Jaworski of Poland postulated a pathogenic role for the spiral organisms (*Vibrio rugula*) that he had identified in gastric contents. Boas and his colleagues, however, maintained they could generate similar morphological forms chemically, and suggested that Jaworski's organisms were artefactual and the result of an inter reaction of gastric mucus and acid. The dispute also reflected the fact that Boas himself had opined that an agent that he and Oppler had described (the Oppler–Boas bacterium) was an infective agent of the stomach and implicated in the aetiology of gastric carcinoma.

was never able to experimentally discriminate between these different agents, and was therefore not able to conclusively prove a role for bacteria in ulcer disease. Nevertheless, the experimental work of Letulle inspired a number of other scientists to follow his lead, and similar results were obtained with *Lactobacillus*, diphtheria toxin, and *Pneumococcus*.

In a time frame contiguous to these sophisticated experiments, the Italian anatomist G. Bizzozero (1846–1901), was busily engaged in the extensive study of the comparative anatomy of vertebrate gastrointestinal glands with

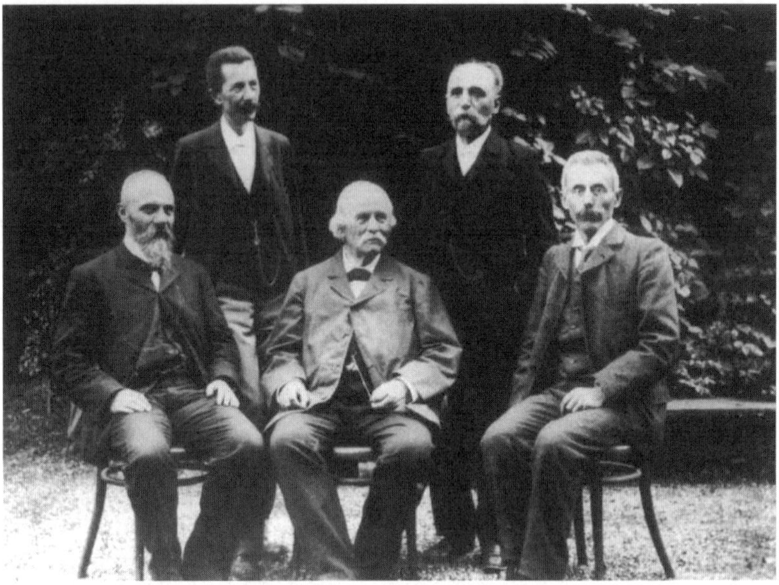

Figure 5. A group portrait taken at the holiday home of G. Bizzozero in Varese, Italy, during the visit of A. Kölliker of Würzberg 1900. From left to right (*back row*): G. Bizzozero and Camillo Golgi; (*front row*): A. Perroncito, A. Kölliker, and R. Fusari. Kölliker played a role in securing international recognition and a Nobel Prize for K. Röntgen of Würzberg, and would subsequently propose that R. y Cajal of Madrid and Golgi be similarly recognized for their contributions to the understanding of the neural system. Bizzozero and Golgi were both members of the same family and had in their early days worked closely on the stomach before Golgi embraced the area of neuroanatomy. It was during this period that Golgi defined the changes in the canalicular apparatus of the resting and stimulated gastric gland, and Bizzozero noted, but failed to pursue, the organisms evident in the histological preparations of the gastric mucosa. As a result he is best remembered for his identification of the platelets of the blood, and recognized amongst the cognoscenti only for his description of 'gastric spirochaetes'.

his adept and capable pupil, the future Nobel Prize winner, Camillo Golgi (1844–1926). In the specimens of the gastric mucosa of six dogs, Bizzozero noted the presence of a spirochaete organism in the gastric glands and in both the cytoplasm and vacuoles of parietal cells. He commented that this organism affected both pyloric and fundic mucosa, and its distribution extended from the base of the gland to the surface mucosa. Although he neglected to ascribe any clinical relevance to these observations, he nevertheless remarked upon their close association with the parietal cells.

Three years later, in 1896, in a paper entitled 'Spirillum of the mammalian stomach and its behaviour with respect to the parietal cells' H. Salomon reported spirochaetes in the gastric mucosa of dogs, cats and rats, although he was unable to identify them in other animals, including humans[21]. In this early paper Salomon undertook a series of somewhat bizarre experiments in which he tried to transmit the bacterium to a range of other animal species by using gastric scrapings from dogs. He failed to transmit it to owls, rabbits, pigeons and frogs, but the feeding of gastric mucus to white mice resulted in a spectacular colonization within a week, as evidenced by the series of drawings of infected gastric mucosa reproduced in the original paper. The lumen of the gastric pits of the mice was packed with the spiral-shaped bacteria, and invasion of the parietal cells was also noted. Almost two decades later, in 1920, K. Kasai and R. Kobayashi successfully repeated these experiments, and using spirochaetes isolated from cats, demonstrated pathogenic results in rabbits. Histological examination indicated both haemorrhagic erosion and ulceration of the mucosa in the presence of masses of the spirochaetes.

TWENTIETH-CENTURY EUROPE

By the beginning of the 20th century, physicians involved in the treatment of gastrointestinal disease were generally familiar with some infective processes of the digestive tract: the ulcerative processes of typhoid fever, a variety of dysenteric conditions and tuberculosis. Kiyoshi Shiga had discovered a bacterium, erroneously specified as *Shigella dystenteriae* in 1898, and an unspecified type of upper gastrointestinal (gastric) bacterial infection, not accompanied by signs of active inflammation, and designated as 'bacterial necrosis', had also been annotated and was described in detail in Hemmeter's text of 1902. This pathology was characterized by the invasion of bacteria, usually into the lower depths of the mucous membrane, followed by bacterial growth and subsequent tissue necrosis.

J. Cohnheim (1839–84), Professor of Pathology at Kiel, who as early as 1880 had prophesied that the young Koch would surpass all others in the field of medical bacteriology, had suggested that the formation of ulcers depended on chemical factors. Shortly thereafter, F. Reigel attributed hyperchlorhydria as the cause of chronic ulcers. The scientific foundations for the recognition of the role of gastric juice (acid) in the genesis of ulcer disease were laid first by A. Kussmaul (1822–1902), who had in 1869 developed a method of intubation of the stomach, and secondly by the creation of the experimental gastric pouch preparation by I. Pavlov (1849–1936)[22].

In 1906 Krienitz identified spirochaetes in the gastric contents of a patient with a carcinoma of the lesser curvature of the stomach and commented that, on microscopic examination, three types of spirochaetes, including *Spirochaete pallidum*, could be identified. He did not address the question of aetiology. Spirochaetal dysentery, as well as the presence of spirochaetes in the stool of healthy individuals, were known, and P. Muhlens (1874–1943) and, independently, Luger and Neuberger, had all reported these organisms to be evident in the stomach contents of patients with ulcerating carcinomas of the stomach. The latter authors also noted the rarity of these organisms in the gastric mucosa and gastric juice of healthy individuals. Experimental biology, however, dominated gastric research, and in the same year, Turcke had undertaken an experiment in which he fed broth cultures of *Bacillus coli* to dogs for a number of months. This resulted in the development of chronic gastric ulceration[23]. In an attempt to establish cause and effect, he thereafter cultured *B. coli* from the faeces of ulcer patients, which were then

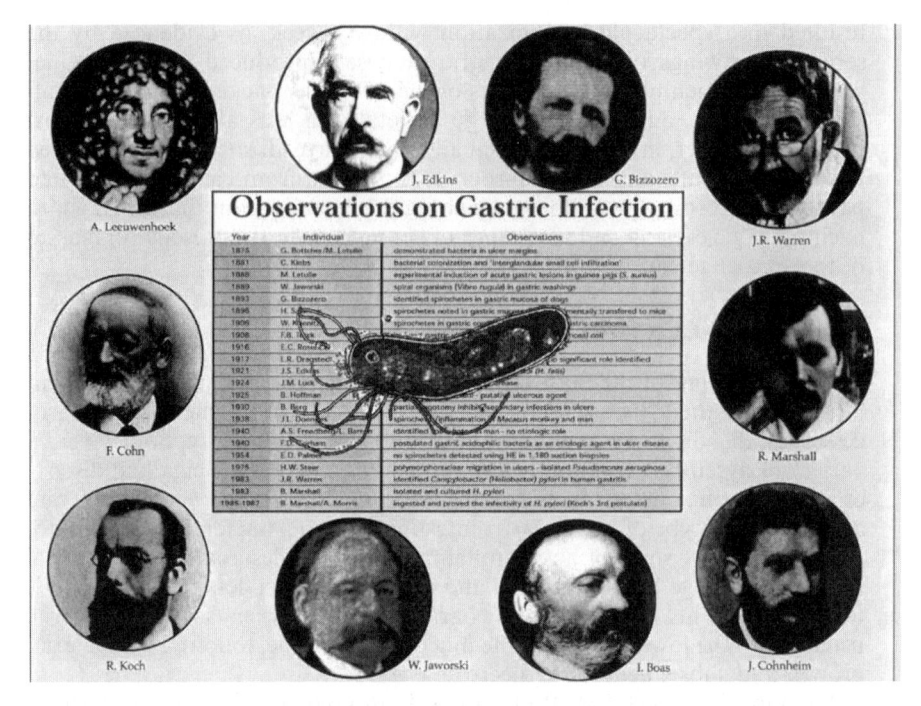

Figure 6. A diverse array of individuals each played a role in the evolution of microscopy, and thereafter microbiology and histology, that led to the identification and establishment of the role of *H. pylori* as a pathogen.

injected intravenously into dogs, without effect. However, when the animals ingested the microorganism, every single dog reacted with a spectrum of non-specific gastric and duodenal changes, which Turcke loosely called 'ulcers'. When Gibelli attempted to repeat this work, he could not confirm these results obtained by Turck.

TWENTIETH-CENTURY USA

In Cincinnati, Ohio, the American bacteriologist, E. C. Rosenow, over a decade from 1913 to 1923, strongly maintained that ulceration of the stomach could be reproduced in laboratory animals by *Streptococcus*[24]. He isolated this bacterium from foci of infection in humans with ulcer disease and injected the culture into a wide range of animals, including rabbits, dogs, monkeys, guinea pigs, cats and mice. A higher incidence of experimental lesions was identified using this particular inoculum than from cultures isolated from foci in other patients. Of additional interest was that streptococci isolated from jejunal ulcers in Mann–Williamson operated dogs also caused acute gastritis and duodenal ulcers, which were limited to the upper gastrointestinal tract in experimental animals. Based on these observations, Rosenow postulated that 'gastric ulcer producing Streptococci' had a selective affinity for the gastric mucosa and produced a local destruction of the glandular tissue. He further proposed that, consequent upon such damage, ulcers would thereafter form, given the autolytic capacity of gastric acid. Rosenow thought that the reservoirs for these bacteria were carious teeth, and advanced the idea that a haematogenous bacterial invasion would result in the formation of an ulcer. Hardt continued these experiments in dogs, and later McGown did so in guinea pigs, with analogous results.

One of the early scientific interests of L. R. Dragstedt (1893–1975) was the causation of gastroduodenal ulceration, although he would subsequently (1943) achieve renown as the surgeon who established the 'physiological' rationale for vagotomy as a treatment for duodenal ulcer disease. As early as 1917, as a young physiologist, he had attempted to define the different mechanisms by which gastric juice could affect healing of acute gastric and duodenal ulcers. Aware of Rosenow's work, and the question of the importance of the virulence of different bacterial strains in determining the chronicity of ulcers, he attempted to isolate and culture any bacteria he could find in the silver nitrate-induced ulcers of five experimental Pavlov pouch dogs. Bacteriological examination revealed *Streptococcus*, *Staphylococcus* and *Bacillus* species, which were similar to those types of bacteria isolated from clinical ulcers in humans.

Dragstedt concluded that these bacteria colonized the damaged mucosa following ulcer formation, and proposed that they had migrated up from the alimentary tract. He did not believe that they played a substantial role in the aetiology of the disease, and did not pursue these studies further, choosing rather to focus on the role of vagal innervation in acid-induced ulceration. Fifteen years later, at the Mount Sinai Hospital, B. Berg, utilized partial vagotomy to reduce 'secondary' infections in ulcer margins. Soon thereafter, however, he turned his attention to ulcers of the colon, and along with his collaborator Crohn, became more famous for his role in the discovery of the aetiology of this disease[25].

EDKINS AND *S. REGAUDI*

J. S. Edkins (1863–1940), of London, had made a significant contribution to the elucidation of gastric physiology by the discovery of gastrin[26]. The scientific doyens of his time declared it to be humbug, although time vindicated him. Motivated by his early disappointment, Edkins proceeded to investigate how the host itself might affect the prevalence and location of the spirochaete organisms in different parts of the stomach. The organisms were named *Spirochaete regaudi*, after Regaudi who considered that the organisms of the gastric mucus layer of cats were morphologically analogous to the syphilis spirochaete. Using the Giemsa stain to identify the organisms in stomach sections, Edkins identified them in both the fundus and the antrum, and noted specific invasion of the epithelial cells of the fundic glands. It was also evident that the organism appeared to have a preference for the surface epithelium, or for thick mucus of the feline experimental model. Of particular note was the demonstration of organisms not only in the subepithelial lymphoid tissue, but even located within the phagocytic cells. He also described a 'beaded form' of the organism in fasting cats, an observation consistent with the discovery of sporulation bodies. Gastric secretory activity did not appear to be compromised when the organisms were present and abundant; indeed, there appeared to be a parallelism between the degree of acid and the abundance of the organisms.

In 1925 A. Hoffman investigated whether the causative agent of ulcer disease was a member of the bacillus family by the injection of 5 cc of gastric contents from a peptic ulcer patient into guinea pigs. He successfully produced gastric ulcers from which he recovered Gram-negative, fine slender rods, which when inoculated into another guinea pig once again produced the same lesions. He modestly named his organism '*Bacillus hoffmani*', but it was evident after further study that the lesion-producing capabilities of this bacterium were non-specific. In 1930 E. Saunders demonstrated that the *Streptococcus* organism isolated from peptic ulcers in humans was of the alpha variety, and identified specific antibodies against this agent in serum from patients. However, he was not able to produce ulcers in animals by injecting the inoculum, and proposed that laboratory animals do not spontaneously form gastric ulcers, since they exhibited an innate resistance to this organism.

DOENGES AND GORHAM

Based to a certain extent on the recognition of the widespread scourge of luetic disease, at around the beginning of the Second World War, spirochaetes returned to gastric prominence. J. L. Doenges observed the organisms to invade the gastric glands of every single one of the *Macacus* rhesus monkeys he studied, and to be present in 43% of human gastric autopsy specimens[27]. In contrast to the monkey, the organisms appeared to be difficult to identify in human gastric mucosa and only 11 of the 103 specimens showed appreciable numbers. Doenges' specimens, however, were autolytic, which precluded the attachment of any major significance to his observations. Of especial note, however, was his observation that the organism was restricted to the gastric mucosa and not evident in the intestinal mucosa.

These reports prompted A. Freedberg and L. Barron in 1941 to investigate the presence of spirochaetes in the gastric tissue of patients who had undergone partial resection surgery. Both authors were familiar with the methods of identifying the organism, and used the silver staining method of DaFano, which they had previously successfully used (but not published) to identify spirochaetes in dogs. In spite of such expertise they were not able to identify the organisms, although they could demonstrate that spirochaetes were more frequently present in ulcerating stomachs as compared to non-ulcerated stomachs (53% vs. 14%). Based on their own difficulties with adequate identification, and the apparent histological differences noted in Doenges' observations in the *Macacus* mucosa, they concluded that no absolute aetiopathological role for these organisms could be defined[28]. It is with almost tragic irony that one reads that, in the report of the discussion of this paper, Frank D. Gorham, of St Louis, Missouri, noted: 'I believe that a further search should be made for an organism thriving in hydrochloric acid medium (and variations of hydrochloric acid are normal in all stomachs) as a possible factor of chronicity, if not an etiologic factor, in peptic ulcer.'

Of interest is that Gorham also wrote that he had, over the previous 10 years, successfully treated patients who had refractory ulcer disease with intramuscular injections of bismuth! Although Gorham may have seemed to be ahead of his time, as early as 1868 Kussmaul had advocated the use of bismuth subnitrate for the treatment of gastric ulcer. In fact, the oral use of bismuth for gastrointestinal symptoms was well accepted and, as early as the 18th century, reports of the therapy had begun to appear in the English literature. R. Sazerac and C. Levaditit (1874–1953) had already successfully exploited the antibacterial properties of bismuth, which may or may not have been known to Gorham, in 1921, who used it to cure experimental syphilis in rabbits. Gastric syphilis had also been described, the ulcers associated with this disease were well known, and the infective agent, *Spirochaete pallida*, had been successfully isolated and cultured from syphilitic abscesses.

The negative results of Freedberg and Barron, and the ambivalent results of Doenges, subsequently prompted E. D. Palmer, in the early 1950s, to investigate spirochaetes in human gastric samples. He obtained gastric mucosal biopsies from 1180 subjects using a vacuum tube technique, but using standard histological techniques failed to demonstrate either spirochaetes or any structures resembling them[29]. Although Palmer did not attempt to identify the organisms with the more reliable silver stain, he concluded (confidently) that the results of all previous authors could be best explained as a postmortem colonization of the gastric mucosa with oral cavity organisms. He also postulated that spirochaetes were normal commensals of the mouth. Palmer's work may thus be credited with setting back gastric bacterial research by a further 30 years.

AMMONIA AND GASTRIC UREASE

Ammonia had been noted in gastric juice as early as 1852, but it was not until 1924 that Luck discovered gastric mucosal urease[30]. His subsequent work, and the work of others, especially the Dublin biochemist E. J. Conway, who specialized in investigations of the redox mechanism of acid secretion, confirmed the presence of gastric urease in a number of mammals. Histochemical studies demonstrated that enzyme activity appeared to be concentrated in the surface layers of the mucosa, in close conjunction with oxyntic cells. In addition, tissues surrounding gastric ulcers were found to be particularly rich in urease, whilst cancerous or achlorhydric stomachs were devoid of urease activity. These observations, as well as the long-standing observation of ammonia in gastric juice, prompted the proposal that urease activity was somehow coupled to hydrochloric acid secretion. This hypothesis was, however, swiftly refuted by the demonstration that the mucosa could secrete acid in the complete absence of urea. Nevertheless, a clinical role for urea in gastric physiology was postulated by O. Fitzgerald (Conway's medical colleague), who postulated that gastric urease functioned as a mucosal protective agent by providing ions to neutralize acid. This led to a number of studies (usually on medical students) in which the ingestion of urea-containing solutions was utilized to alter histamine-stimulated gastric acid secretion. Notwithstanding the unpleasant side-effects of this administration (diarrhoea, headache, polyuria, painful urethritis), Fitzgerald further applied his hypothesis by treating ulcer patients with this regimen in 1949. Although he charitably summarized his results as 'in general, satisfactory', no further therapeutic studies were undertaken with this particular agent.

Within 5 years, investigators of gastric urease-containing tissue suspensions were also able to demonstrate the presence (contamination) of urea-splitting organisms. This led to the suggestion that gastric urease might actually be of bacterial origin. Preliminary feeding of antibiotics (penicillin and Terramycin) to animals resulted in reduced expiration of $^{14}CO_2$ from intraperitoneally injected [^{14}C] urea, as well as the abolition of urease activity in mucosal homogenates. Similar studies with analogous results were also performed in controls and subjects with uraemia. These observations, whilst establishing that gastric urease was of bacterial origin, failed to initiate an investigation of the relationship between urease-containing bacteria and ulcer disease. Indeed the prevailing notion by the end of 1955 was that neither the bacterial gastric urease nor the bacteria played any essential role in gastric pathology. Interestingly, at the time however, the clinical information derived suggested to some that antibacterial therapy could be utilized in patients with liver disease and elevated gastric ammonia levels. Antibiotic therapy was noted to reduce gastric urea and ameliorate the associated encephalopathy.

In 1975 H. Steer, while studying polymorphonuclear leucocyte migration in the gastric mucosa in a series of biopsy materials obtained from patients with gastric ulceration, identified bacteria in close contact with the epithelium, and suggested that white cells migrated in response to these bacteria[31]. In this seminal contribution he not only clearly demonstrated bacterial phagocytosis, but provided electron microscopic images consistent with ingestion of *Helicobacter*-like organisms. Steer also attempted to isolate and culture the organism but, being unfamiliar with micro-aerophilic techniques, succeeded only in growing and identifying *Pseudomonas aeruginosa*.

THE DISCOVERY OF *HELICOBACTER PYLORI*

By 1980, reports concerning an 'epidemic gastritis associated with hypochorhydria' had been published[18]. These observations coupled with Steer's findings of an apparent association between 'active gastritis' and a Gram-negative bacterium, suggested that the simultaneous occurrence of bacteria in the stomach and peptic ulceration might represent more than a correlatable epiphenomenon. Robin Warren, a pathologist at the Royal Perth Hospital, had for many years observed bacteria in the stomach of people with gastritis. Although he was convinced that they somehow played a role in gastric disease, in the light of the prevailing dogma of acid-induced ulceration and the scepticism of his colleagues, he had been reluctant to discuss this controversial observation in the wider gastroenterological community[32].

In 1982 a young gastroenterology fellow, Barry Marshall, was looking for a project to complete his fellowship. The iconoclastic hypothesis of Warren attracted Marshall, who persuaded Warren to allow him to investigate this further in the appropriate clinical setting. Later in the year Marshall submitted an abstract detailing their initial investigations to the Australian Gastroenterology Association. It was flatly rejected, along with a handful of other abstracts[32]. Unfazed, Marshall sought an alternative audience for the work and submitted the same abstract to the International Workshop of *Campylobacter* Infections, where it was accepted. Although the audience was sceptical of Marshall and Warren's results, some members became interested enough to attempt to repeat some of their observations. Soon after the meeting, both Warren and Marshall published their initial results as two modest letters in the *Lancet*. In the introduction to his seminal article on an S-shaped *Campylobacter*-like organism, Warren noted both the constancy of bacterial infection, as well as the consistency of the associated histological changes, which he had identified in 135 gastric biopsy specimens studied over a 3-year period[33]. He commented that these microorganisms were difficult to see with haematoxylin and eosin, but stained well in the presence of silver. Furthermore, he observed the bacteria to be most numerous in an 'active chronic gastritis', where they were closely associated with granulocyte infiltration. It is a mystery, he wrote, that bacteria in numbers sufficient to be seen by light microscopy were almost unknown to clinicians and pathologists alike! He presciently concluded: 'These organisms should be recognized and their significance investigated'.

Koch's second postulate states that 'the germ should be obtained from the diseased animal and grown outside the body'. In the same issue of the *Lancet*, Marshall described the conditions necessary to fulfil this requirement[34]. Utilizing the knowledge that these bacteria resemble the species of campylobacters rather than spirochaetes, he used *Campylobacter* isolation techniques (microaerophilic conditions) to successfully grow isolates on moist chocolate agar. It is interesting to note that no organism growth was detected after 2 days culture in the first 34 endoscopic biopsies Marshall tried to grow. The 35th plate, however, was left to culture over the long (6 days) Easter weekend, and resulted in luxuriant bacterial growth[32].

In order to substantiate that the microorganism was actually a disease-causing agent it was necessary to demonstrate that it could colonize normal mucosa and induce gastritis (Koch's third and fourth postulates). To prove pathogenicity, Marshall, looking back in time for guidance, decided to be his own guinea pig. Marshall, who had a histologically normal gastric mucosa and was a light smoker and social drinker, received, by mouth, a test isolate from a 66-year-old non-ulcer dyspeptic man[35]. Over the next 14 days a mild illness developed, characteristic of an acute episode of gastritis, and was accompanied by headaches, vomiting, abdominal discomfort, irritability and 'putrid' breath. The infectivity of the agent was then successfully confirmed when, after 10 days, histologically proven gastritis was endoscopically documented. The disease process later resolved on its own accord by the fifteenth day. A. Morris later followed Marshall's lead, and in a similar experiment ingested the same inoculum of *H. pylori*. Although this did not

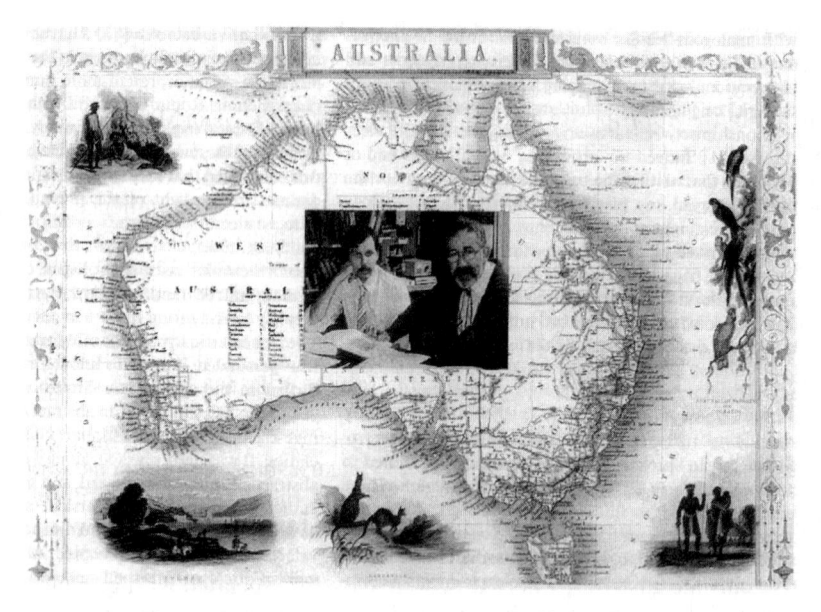

Figure 7. The pathologist J. R. Warren (*right*) and his research fellow, B. J. Marshall (*left*). Their seminal antipodean discovery helped resolve a problem with which numerous investigators had grappled unsuccessfully for more than a century. Warren's observation of the agent involved in gastritis, combined with Marshall's demonstration that it fulfilled the criteria of infectivity originally proposed by Henle, initiated the establishment of a novel discipline of gastric patho-biology.

establish itself, a repeat challenge of the mucosa with a different, local (New Zealand) inoculum was more successful[18]. In fact it was so successful that a 2-month treatment of an antibacterial agent and bismuth was required to 'eradicate' the organism. Morris and Nicholson established a direct effect of infection on acid secretion, but unfortunately for Morris, who had residual gastritis, a relapse was inevitable. Five years after the initial experiment, Morris, was finally cured. There has been no recorded third experiment. Marshall went on to describe the urease of the organism and recognized its role in enabling survival of the organism in acidic media. Subsequent work showed that eradication of the organism reduced recurrence of duodenal ulcer to or better than those seen with maintenance therapy with histamine H_2-receptor antagonists and acceptance of this organism as causative, in association with acid, is now universal.

The importance of these findings is enormous and must rank among the great iconoclasms in medicine[18]. Some 15 years after the start of the modern *Helicobacter* era, many of the important issues remain unresolved. There is still a lack of knowledge about many aspects of the organism itself. Thus, its mode of transmission (contamination of water sources has been suggested), how it causes disease, and why only a select few develop ulcers, and what the correct clinical management of this infection should be, both in practice and as a public health issue, are among the unanswered questions.

CODA

Bacteriology has progressed far beyond Snow's original observations of the Broad Street pump to the membrane-bound pumps of bacteria that facilitate survival and growth in hostile environments. Indeed *H. pylori* itself represents a measure of the advances that have been made in both the elucidation of the pathological basis of microbiological disease and the development of therapeutic strategies. Its effect on the gastric mucosa has been defined and the sophisticated nature of its biochemical armamentarium has been elucidated. Thus the H^+K^+ATPase pump of the parietal cell, the urease pump of the bacteria, may now not only be considered in terms of their function but as therapeutic targets. The helical nature of the organism mirrors the structure of DNA, and the concept of developing a genetic strategy for eradication may be only a short distance from achieving reality. The intertwining of the pump and the helix in the pathobiology and therapeutic strategy of the gastric mucosa lends itself to the consideration of the common origin of humans and their pathogens. Proliferation and contagion, neoplasia and metastasis may not be so very different after all! Exogenous agents of disease contrasted with endogenous agents all sharing common pumps, helical regulatory codes and mandated, each in their own unique fashion to seek a milieu in which they may successfully proliferate and procreate. Indeed the earliest history of human life may be viewed within this context. Who knows; perhaps the apple was contaminated or, as considered by Fracastoro, Eve nothing more than a transient contagion. The serpent was certainly a helical structure and there is little doubt that the first pump was the heart of Adam. Lest there be any doubt of the validity of the encoded message even the initial letters of *H. pylori* confirm the primal nature of the Helix and the Pump!

References

1. Hippocrates. The Genuine World of Hippocrates. London: Sydenham Society; 1899.
2. Garrison F. An Introduction to the History of Medicine. Philadelphia: W. B. Saunders; 1929.
3. Kiple K. Plague, Pox and Pestilence. Disease in history. New York: Barnes & Noble; 1997.
4. Fracastoro G. Syphilis sive morbus glaciers. Veronae: S. Niccolini da Sabbio; 1530.
5. Deuteronomy. Chap XXIII, verse 13.
6. Snow J. On the mode of communication of Cholera. 2nd edn. London, 1855.
7. Garrison F. Louis Pasteur. History of Medicine, 4th edn. Philadelphia, PA: W. B. Saunders, 1929:575–8.
8. Müller O. Animacula infusoria fluviatilia et marina, quae detexit, systematice descript et ad vivum delineari. Huaniae: N. Molleri; 1786.
9. Spallanzani L. Saggio di osservazioni microscopiche relative al sistema della generazione. Modena; 1767.
10. Pasteur L. Mémoire sur les corpuscles organisés qui existent dans l'atmosphère. Examen de la doctrine des generation spontanées. Ann Chim Phys. 1862;64:5–110.
11. Bassi A. Sui contagi in generale e specialmente su quelli che affligono l'umana specie. Lodi; 1844.
12. Mettler C. History of medicine. A correlative text arranged according to subjects. Philadelphia: Blakiston; 1947.
13. Schwann T. Mikroskopische Untersuchungen uber die Uebereinstimmung in der Struktur und dem Wachsthum der Thiere und Pflanzen. Berlin; 1839.

14. Lister J. On the effects of the antiseptic system of treatment upon the salubrity of a surgical hospital. Lancet. 1870;1:4–6.
15. Cohn F. Untersuchungen uber Bacterien. Beitr Biol Pflanzen. 1872;1:127–224.
16. Koch R. Untersuchungen uber die Aetiologie der Wundinfectionskrankheiten. Liepzig: FCW Vogel; 1878.
17. Bulloch W. The History of Bacteriology. London: Oxford University Press; 1938.
18. Kidd M, Modlin I. A century of *Helicobacter pylori*. Paradigms lost – paradigms regained. Digestion. 1998;59:1–15.
19. Boas I. Diseases of the stomach. Philadelphia: FA Davis; 1907.
20. Bizzozero G. Ueber die schlauchformigen Drusen des Magendarmkanals und die Beziehungen ihres Epithels zu dem Oberflachenepithel der Schleimhaut. Arch Mikr Anat. 1893;42:82.
21. Salomon H. Ueber das Spirillum des Saugtiermagens und sein Verhalten zu den Belegzellen. Zentralbl Bakteriol. 1896;19:433–42.
22. Pavlov I. The Work of the Digestive Glands. London: Griffin; 1902.
23. Turck FB. Experimental studies on round ulcers of the stomach and duodenum. J Med Res. 1908;17:365.
24. Rosenow E. The causation of gastric and duodenal ulcer by streptococci. J Infect Dis. 1916;19:333.
25. Crohn B. Regional ileitis. A pathologic and clinical entity. J Am Med Assoc. 1932;99:1323–9.
26. Modlin I, Kidd M, Marks I, Tang L. The pivotal role of John S Edkins in the discovery of Gastrin. W J Surg. 1997;21:226–34.
27. Doenges J. Spirochaetes in Gastric glands of *Macacus rhesus* and humans without definite history of related disease. Proc Soc Exp Biol Med. 1938;38:536–8.
28. Freedberg A, Barron L. The presence of spirochetes in human gastric mucosa. Am J Dig Dis 1940;7:443–5.
29. Palmer E. Investigation of the gastric mucosa spirochetes of the human. Gastroenterology. 1954;27:218–20.
30. Luck J. Gastric urease. Biochem J. 1924;18:1227–31.
31. Steer H. Ultrastructure of cell migration through the gastric epithelium and its relationship to bacteria. J Clin Pathol. 1975;28:639–46.
32. Marshall B. History of the discovery of *C. pylori*. In: Blaser M, editor. *Campylobacter pylori* in gastritis and peptic ulcer disease. New York: Igaku-Shoin; 1989:7–23.
33. Warren J. Unidentified curved bacilli on gastric epithelium in active chronic gastritis. Lancet. 1983;1273.
34. Marshall B. Unidentified curved bacilli on gastric epithelium in active chronic gastritis. Lancet 1983;1273–5.
35. Marshall B, Armstrong J, McGechie D, Glancy R. Attempt to fulfill Koch's postulates for pyloric *Campylobacter*. Med J Austr. 1985;142:436–9.

39
Mechanisms involved in the development of hypochlorhydria and pangastritis in *Helicobacter pylori* infection

K. E. L. McCOLL and E. EL-OMAR

INTRODUCTION

Helicobacter pylori infection exerts diverse effects on gastric physiology. It may increase gastric acid secretion, reduce it or result in no overall change in acid output[1]. The disturbance in acid secretion is related to the pattern of gastritis induced by the infection (Figure 1). In subjects with an antral-predominant non-atrophic *H. pylori* gastritis, acid secretion is normal or increased. This is the pattern of gastritis seen in patients who develop duodenal ulceration. In other subjects it produces an atrophic pangastritis or body-predominant gastritis. This results in markedly reduced acid secretion or achlorhydria and is seen in patients who develop non-cardia gastric cancer.

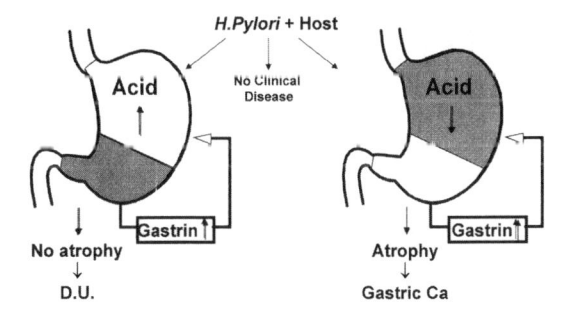

Figure 1. Association between pattern of *H. pylori* gastritis and disturbance in gastric physiology. An antral-predominant non-atrophic gastritis is associated with increased acid secretion (left). In contrast, an atrophic pangastritis or body-predominant gastritis is associated with reduced acid secretion or achlorhydria (right).

ASSOCIATION BETWEEN THE MORPHOLOGICAL AND FUNCTIONAL CHANGES INDUCED BY *H. PYLORI*

The association between the pattern of gastritis and disturbance in gastric physiology can be explained by the different functions of the antrum and body region of the stomach. The antral region contains the G cells which release the hormone gastrin. The more proximal body region of the stomach contains the acid-secreting parietal cells. When a meal is ingested, the protein component stimulates the G cells to release gastrin. This hormone circulates and stimulates the parietal cells in the body region to secrete acid. Gastrin does not directly stimulate the parietal cells but stimulates the adjacent ECL cells to release histamine, which then stimulates the parietal cells. As the acid accumulates and overcomes the buffering effect of the food, the fall in pH inhibits further release of gastrin and thus prevents secretion of excessive amounts of acid.

H. pylori-induced hyperchlorhydria

H. pylori infection of the antral region of the stomach disrupts the negative feedback control of gastrin release, resulting in inappropriately high and sustained levels of gastrin following a meal[2-4]. In subjects with an antral-predominant non-atrophic gastritis, this increased gastrin release stimulates the healthy body region of the stomach to secrete excessive amounts of acid[5-8]. The increased acid output produced by this pattern of gastritis results in an increased duodenal acid load and thus duodenal ulceration[9]. Eradicating *H. pylori* infection in subjects with this pattern of gastritis results in a fall in serum gastrin and a concomitant fall in acid secretion[5,6].

H. pylori-induced hypochlorhydria

In subjects with an atrophic pangastritis, or body-predominant gastritis, there is also increased antral gastrin release, but this is not accompanied by increased acid secretion. In such subjects, acid secretion is reduced or may be completely absent[10-12]. The low acid secretion despite increased gastrin levels indicates that the ability of the oxyntic mucosa to secrete acid in response to gastrin stimulation is markedly impaired. If you eradicate the infection in patients with this pattern of gastritis, then they show a recovery in acid secretion[10-12]. The degree of recovery in acid secretion is variable, with some patients resuming normal levels of acid output, whereas others show only a very small increase[10]. The recovery in acid output following eradication of the infection coincides with disappearance of the organism and with resolution of the inflammation of the body mucosa (Figure 2). There is little evidence of resolution of the atrophy of the body mucosa[10]. This observation suggests that the impairment of the body mucosa to secrete acid is related to either the presence of the organism in the body mucosa or the accompanying inflammation, or both.

Mechanism of *H. pylori*-induced hypochlorhydria

H. pylori-induced hypochlorhydria might be due to the bacterium releasing some substance which can directly inhibit acid secretion. Several candidate

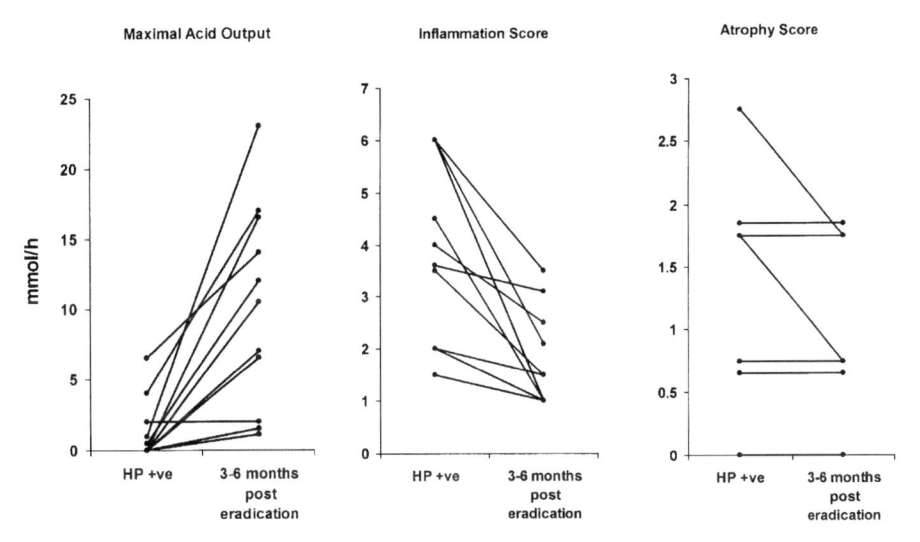

Figure 2. Changes in gastric acid secretion and mucosal histology following eradication of H. pylori in patients with hypochlorhydria (from ref. 20).

substances have been proposed, which inhibit parietal cell function *in vitro*[13-16], but the evidence that these are responsible for the *in-vivo* effect remains weak. *H. pylori* infection also produces ammonia, and it has been suggested that this may uncouple the proton pump[17,18]. The amount of ammonia produced by *H. pylori* infection in hypochlorhydria subjects is relatively small[19], although its ability to penetrate the mucosa will be increased in hypochlorhydric subjects due to a greater proportion being in the un-ionized form at neutral pH. Another problem with attributing the impairment of oxyntic mucosal function to the presence of *H. pylori* organisms is that the density of colonization of the body mucosa with *H. pylori* organisms is similar or lower in subjects with hypochlorhydria than in subjects with normal or high acid secretion[20,21] (Figure 3). It is possible, however, that the ability of some inhibitory factor produced by the organism to reach the epithelium may be greater in hypochlorhydric subjects due to the low acid secretion failing to flush such products away from the epithelium. However in the present state of knowledge it is difficult to attribute the impaired functioning of the oxyntic mucosa to a direct effect of some factor produced by the organism.

An alternative explanation for the impaired acid-secretory function seen in some patients with *H. pylori* infection is that it is a consequence of the inflammation of the oxyntic mucosa induced by the infection. Certainly the severity of inflammation of the body mucosa is more marked in subjects with *H. pylori*-associated hypochlorhydria than in subjects with *H. pylori* infection and normal or increased acid secretion[20,21] (Figure 3). This raises the possibility that a product of the inflammatory response might be resulting in the inhibition of acid secretion. One of the cytokines whose production within the gastric mucosa is stimulated by *H. pylori* infection is interleukin-

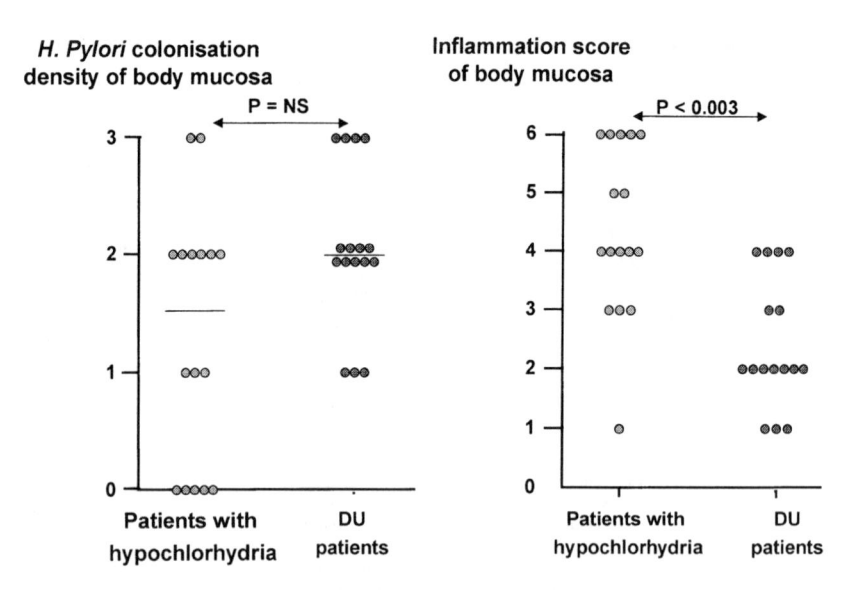

Figure 3. Compared to subjects with normal or increased acid secretion, subjects with hypochlorhydria have similar or lower density of H. pylori colonization of body mucosa but markedly greater severity of inflammation (from ref. 20).

1β[22-24]. The increased production of this cytokine may be important because it is a very powerful inhibitor of acid secretion. Indeed, on a molar basis it is 100 times more powerful than the most powerful pharmacological inhibitors of acid secretion, namely proton pump inhibitors[25-28]. The exact mechanism by which interleukin-1β inhibits acid secretion is unclear. One study found that it inhibits acid secretion in response to gastrin stimulation but not in response to histamine or acetylcholine stimulation, suggesting that it exerts its effect mainly at the level of the enterochromaffin-like cell (ECL cell)[25]. More recent studies have shown that interleukin-1β inhibits the biological functions of both ECL and parietal cells, and that both cell types express interleukin-1 type 1 receptors[29,30]. The cytokine has been shown to inhibit gastrin-stimulated histamine synthesis and secretion via activation of these interleukin-1 receptors[29,31,32]. One study suggests that the acid-inhibitory effect of interleukin-1β may be mediated via its stimulation of inducible nitric oxide synthase and nitric oxide production[28]. In addition, interleukin-1β-induces apoptosis in ECL cells, thus leading to sustained functional impairment[29,31]. Most recently, Mahr et al. showed that interleukin-1β-induced apoptosis in ECL cells is mediated by activation of nuclear factor-κB (NF-κB), inducible nitric oxide synthase (iNOS) and the proapoptotic Bax protein[33]. In view of the fact that it has been shown to be produced in excess by the H. pylori-infected gastric mucosa, and the fact that it is a very powerful inhibitor of acid secretion, this makes it a powerful candidate for mediating the inhibition of acid secretion associated with H. pylori infection.

WHY DOES *H. PYLORI* INFECTION PRODUCE DIFFERENT PATTERNS OF DISEASE?

One key question which has to be addressed is why *H. pylori* infection produces different patterns of gastritis, and consequently different disturbances of gastric physiology. Why do some people with *H. pylori* infection develop an antral-predominant non-atrophic gastritis with increased or normal acid secretion, whereas other people with the same infection develop an atrophic pangastritis with hypochlorhydria or achlorhydria? The two possible explanations which have received most attention are first that it may be related to different strains of *H. pylori* infection and secondly that it may be related to genetically determined differences in the host response to the infection.

Effect of bacterial CagA status on the pattern of gastritis and gastric acid secretion

We have recently studied the pattern of gastritis and disturbance in gastric acid secretion in 121 *H. pylori*-infected dyspeptic patients with no endoscopic evidence of ulcer disease. All subjects had discontinued any antisecretory medication at least 3 weeks prior to the examination. *H. pylori* CagA status was determined serologically.

We found that maximal acid output to gastrin stimulation fell linearly with increasing age and the level of acid output was lower in females than males. However, we found no evidence of any difference in acid secretion between the CagA-positive and -negative subjects. Acid output to gastrin-releasing peptide showed the same pattern.

The histological study showed that the severity of inflammation of both the antrum and body mucosa was greater in the CagA-positive subjects than in the CagA-negative subjects. However, the distribution of inflammation between the body and antral mucosa was similar in the CagA-positive and CagA-negative subjects. These studies therefore indicate that the CagA status of the *H. pylori* infection does not determine whether the subject develops hypochlorhydria or hyperchlorhydria, and also does not determine whether such patients develop an antral-predominant or body-predominant type of gastritis. This is consistent with CagA strains of the infection being associated with increased incidence of both duodenal ulcer and gastric cancer.

Effect of host genetic factors on pattern of gastritis and acid secretion

Could the fact that some subjects develop pangastritis and hypochlorhydria in response to *H. pylori* infection, and others develop an antral-predominant gastritis with normal or increased acid secretion, be due to genetically determined differences in the host response to the infection? If this were the case, then you would expect a familial tendency of one response or the other. Gastric cancer is known to occur in subjects who develop atrophic pangastritis and hypochlorhydria in response to *H. pylori* infection. If this is a genetically determined response, then close blood relatives of such subjects

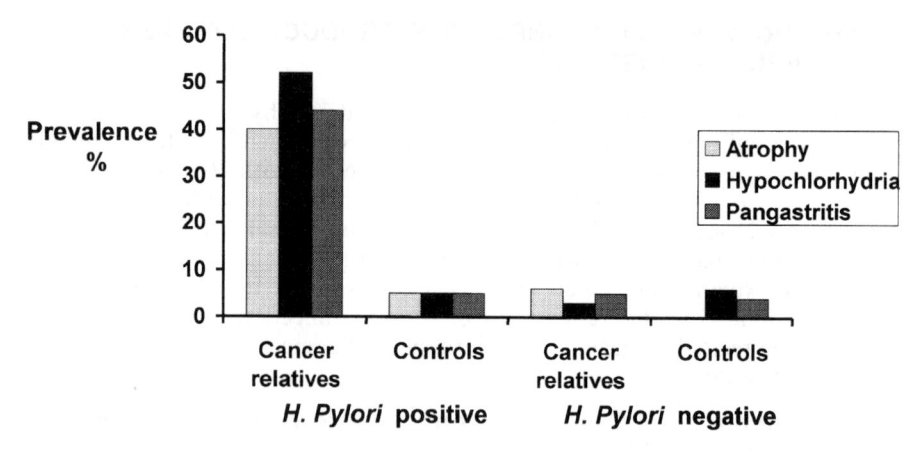

Figure 4. Prevalence of hypochlorhydria, atrophy and pangastritis in *H. pylori*-infected subjects with and without family history of gastric cancer (from ref. 21).

should be more likely to show this type of response than do the general population. We have recently investigated this by examining gastric function and morphology in *H. pylori*-infected first-degree relatives of patients with gastric cancer, and comparing them with *H. pylori*-infected control subjects without a history of gastric cancer[21].

The prevalence of *H. pylori* infection was similar in the gastric cancer relatives and controls. However, the gastric cancer relatives had a much higher prevalence of hypochlorhydria, atrophy and pangastritis than the controls (Figure 4). The increased prevalence of these abnormalities was due to their very high prevalence in the *H. pylori*-positive gastric cancer relatives. The gastric cancer relatives with *H. pylori* infection therefore had a much higher prevalence of hypochlorhydria (40%), pangastritis (21%) and atrophy (52%) than the *H. pylori*-infected controls (5%, 3%, and 5%, respectively). The magnitude of the increased prevalence of this hypochlorhydric response could not be attributed to any differences in the prevalence of CagA strains of infection. The two *H. pylori*-infected groups of subjects were also matched for socioeconomic class, making it difficult to attribute the responses to environmental or dietary factors. This therefore suggested that there may well be a host-genetic factor predisposing to the hypochlorhydric type of response to *H. pylori* infection.

A prime candidate for a genetically determined response, which could affect gastric secretory function, would be the interleukin-1 gene. This is due to the facts that: (1) interleukin-1β production within the gastric mucosa is induced in response to *H. pylori* infection[22–24] and (2) this cytokine is known to be a very powerful inhibitor of acid secretion[25–28]. Furthermore, there are well-recognized polymorphisms within the interleukin-1 gene cluster[34–39]. In order to investigate this, we have examined the interleukin-1 polymorphisms in our *H. pylori*-infected gastric cancer relatives with and without hypochlorhydria[40].

Table 1. IL-1 genotype frequencies in gastric cancer relatives with normal vs. low acid output

Locus	Genotype	Low acid (n = 45)	Normal (n = 58)	OR (95% CI)
IL-1B-31	C/C	5	30	1.0
	C/T	28	21	8.1 (2.0–33)
	T/T	12	7	13.6 (2.6–71)
IL-1RN	1/1	17	35	1.0
	1/2	14	14	2.4 (0.9–6.2)
	1/3, 4, 5	0	2	0
	2/2	14	7	5.6 (1.8–17)

From ref. 40.

Table 2. IL-1 genotype frequencies in gastric cancer cases and controls

Locus	Genotype	Cases (n = 366)	Controls (n = 429)	OR (95% CI)
IL-1B-31	C/C	128	219	1.0
	C/T	172	164	1.8 (1.3–2.4)
	T/T	66	46	2.5 (1.6–3.8)
IL-1RN	1/1	148	230	1.0
	1/2	117	152	1.2 (0.9–1.6)
	1/3, 4, 5	8	7	1.8 (0.7–4.8)
	2/2	93	39	3.7 (2.4–5.7)
	2/5	0	1	0

Population attributable fraction of gastric cancer related to these pro-inflammatory genotypes: IL-1B-31 = 31%; IL-1RN = 18%; Combined = 38% (El-Omar et al., Nature 2000).

The above studies have shown strong association between pro-inflammatory polymorphisms of the interleukin-1 gene and *H. pylori*-induced hypochlorhydria. The gastric cancer relatives with hypochlorhydria had a significantly higher frequency of the proinflammatory *IL-1RN*2* allele and the T-T haplotype of *IL-1β-31* and *IL-1β-511*, as compared to those without hypochlorhydria (Table 1). In a logistic regression model including both factors, the estimated age-adjusted ORs for *IL-1β-31T+* and *IL-1RN*2/*2* were 7.5 (95% CI 1.8–31) and 2.1% (95% CI 0.7–6.3, respectively).

Further evidence of the importance of the host-genetic polymorphisms was investigated by determining whether there was an association between them and development of gastric cancer in the general population[40]. In view of the fact that development of hypochlorhydria and pangastritis is important in the progression towards gastric cancer, one would expect any genetic factor predisposing to this form of response to be associated with the development of the cancer. In a large population of 700 patients we examined polymorphisms in 366 patients with gastric cancer and 429 controls[40]. This confirmed a similar association between the genotypes and gastric cancer (Table 2). In a logistic regression model including both genotypes the estimated ORs for *IL-1β-31T+* and *IL-1RN*2/*2* were 1.6 (95% CI 1.2–2.2) and 2.9 (95% CI 1.9–4.4), respectively.

These results therefore indicate that host pro-inflammatory *IL-1* genotypes are important in determining the functional response to *H. pylori* infection, the pattern of gastritis and the ultimate clinical outcome of gastric cancer. Our study suggests that the combined population-attributable fraction of gastric cancer due to those *IL-1* alleles is 38%.

RELATIONSHIP BETWEEN THE PATTERN OF GASTRITIS AND FUNCTIONAL DISTURBANCE IN ACID SECRETION

Pro-inflammatory polymorphisms involving the interleukin-1 gene may therefore explain why some subjects infected with *H. pylori* develop hypochlorhydria. However, one still has to explain why the subjects with the hypochlorhydria also have a different pattern of gastritis with the inflammation involving the body region of the stomach and usually being accompanied with atrophy. This can be explained by the fact that the pattern of gastritis is affected by the level of gastric acid secretion. In particular, marked suppression of acid secretion in *H. pylori*-positive subjects leads to the development of pangastritis and accelerates the development of atrophy[41-45]. If subjects with antral-predominant non-atrophic *H. pylori* gastritis are treated with proton pump inhibitor therapy which markedly suppresses their gastric acid secretion the distribution of gastritis changes from being antral-predominant to being body-predominant. With longer-term treatment a proportion of such subjects progress to develop atrophy of the body mucosa.

One can therefore see that there is a two-way interaction between *H. pylori* gastritis and gastric acid secretion. The pattern of gastritis affects the gastric acid secretion with an antral-predomiant non-atrophic gastritis resulting in increased acid secretion and an atrophic pangastritis producing reduced acid secretion. In addition, acid secretion affects the distribution of the gastritis: high acid secretion promoting antral-predominant, body-sparing gastritis and low acid secretion favouring the development of pangastritis and atrophy.

SEQUENCE OF EVENTS LEADING TO GASTRIC CANCER IN *H. PYLORI* INFECTION

It now appears that the genetically determined host response to *H. pylori* may be a key factor in determining the outcome of the infection. In subjects with one of the pro-inflammatory polymorphisms of the interleukin-1 gene, *H. pylori* infection will result in particularly high interleukin-1β activity within the gastric mucosa, resulting in marked suppression of gastric acid secretion. This suppression of acid secretion will allow development of a body-predominant, or pangastritis. Development of the body gastritis will further inhibit acid secretion and therby maintain the pattern of distribution of gastritis. This pattern of gastritis, along with persisting hypochlorhydria, will encourage the development of atrophic gastritis, a well-recognized precursor of carcinoma. The proportion of such subjects developing carcinoma

```
        H. Pylori Infection
                ↓
        Mucosal inflammation
                ↓
        IL-1B pro-inflammatory
            Host genotype
           /            \
        Yes              No
         ↓                ↓
→ Acid hyposecretion    Normal or high acid ←
         ↓                ↓                  |
⌐ Body predominant    Antral predominant ────┘
   gastritis              gastritis
         ↓                ↓
  Atrophic gastritis   D.U. or No Disease
         ↓
       Cancer
```

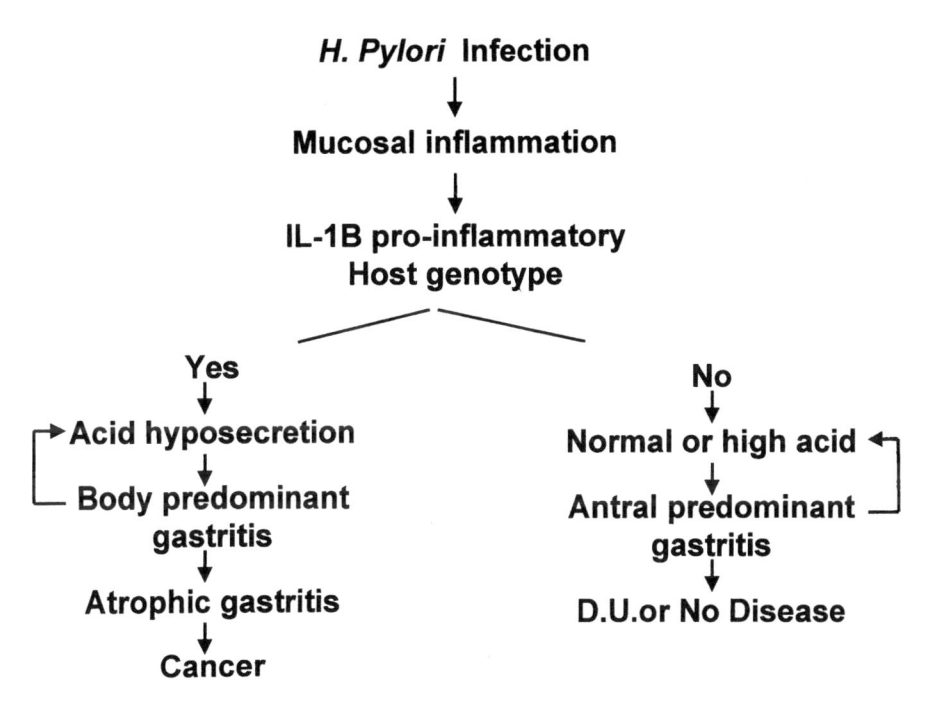

Figure 5. Interactions between host-genetic factor, *H. pylori* gastritis and gastric physiology determining outcome of *H. pylori* infection.

is likely to depend upon additional factors such as antioxidant intake (Figure 5).

In subjects without the pro-inflammatory polymorphisms of interleukin-1 gene the infection will not result in such a marked inhibition of acid secretion. In the absence of hypochlorhydria the inflammation will not extend into the acid-secreting mucosa, and these patients subsequently develop an antral-predominant body sparing gastritis. This pattern of gastritis will maintain acid secretion and thus maintain the body-sparing pattern of gastritis. In subjects with a genetically high parietal cell mass, the increased gastrin release will result in a markedly increased acid secretion, leading to duodenal ulceration (Figure 5).

CONCLUSIONS

We now recognize that complex interactions are involved in determining the long-term outcome of *H. pylori* infection. The virulence of the organism influences the likelihood of developing significant disease, but does not influence whether one develops duodenal ulcer disease or gastric cancer. The specific disease one develops appears to be largely dependent upon the genetically determined host response. In particular, pro-inflammatory polymorphisms of the interleukin-1β gene favour the development of hypochlorhydria and atrophy, and consequently gastric cancer. The two-way interaction between gastric acid secretion and the pattern of *H. pylori* gastritis is also important in maintaining either a hypochlorhydric or hyperchlorhydric response to the infection. Finally, dietary and environmental factors such as antioxidant and nitrate intake, and smoking, are likely to be important in influencing the incidence of atrophy and cancer in subjects who develop the hypochlorydric response to the infection.

References

1. McColl KEL, El-Omar E, Gillen D. Interactions between *H. pylori* infection, gastric acid secretion and anti-secretory therapy. Br Med Bull. 1998;54:121–38.
2. McColl KE., Fullarton GM, Chittajallu R et al. Plasma gastrin, daytime intragastric pH, and nocturnal acid output before and at 1 and 7 months after eradication of *Helicobacter pylori* in duodenal ulcer subjects. Scand J Gastroenterol. 1991;26:339–46.
3. Levi S, Beardshall K, Haddad G, Playford R, Ghosh P, Calam J. *Campylobacter pylori* and duodenal ulcers: the gastrin link. Lancet. 1989;1:1167–8.
4. Tarnasky PR, Kovacs TOG, Sytnik B, Walsh JH. Asymptomatic *H. pylori* infection impairs pH inhibition of gastrin and acid secretion during second hour of peptone meal stimulation. Dig Dis Sci. 1993;38:1681–7.
5. El-Omar E, Penman I, Dorrian CA, Ardill JES, McColl KEL. Eradicating *Helicobacter pylori* infection lowers gastrin mediated acid secretion by two thirds in patients with duodenal ulcer. Gut. 1993;34:1060–5.
6. El-Omar E, Penman ID, Ardill JES, Chittajallu RS, Howie C, McColl KEL. *Helicobacter pylori* infection and abnormalities of acid secretion in patients with duodenal ulcer disease. Gastroenterology. 1995;109:681–91.
7. Haris AW, Gummett PA, Misiewicz JJ, Baron JH. Eradication of *Helicobacter pylori* in patients with duodenal ulcer lowers basal and peak acid outputs to gastrin releasing peptide and pentagastrin. Gut. 1996;38:663–7.
8. Moss SF, Calam J. Acid secretion and sensitivity to gastrin in patients with duodenal ulcer: effect of eradication of *Helicobacter pylori*. Gut. 1993;34:888–92.
9. Hamlet A, Olbe L. The influence of *Helicobacter pylori* on postprandial duodenal acid load and duodenal bulb pH in humans. Gastroenterology. 1996;111:391–400.
10. El-Omar EM, Oien K, El-Nujumi A et al. *Helicobacter pylori* infection and chronic gastric acid hyposecretion. Gastroenterology. 1997;113:15–24.
11. Haruma K, Mihara M, Okamoto E et al. Eradication of *Helicobacter pylori* increases gastric acidity in patients with atrophic gastritis of the corpus – evaluation of 24-h pH monitoring. Aliment Pharmacol Ther. 1999;13:155–62.
12. Gutierrez O, Melo M, Segura AM, Angel A, Genta RM, Graham DY. Cure of *Helicobacter pylori* infection improves gastric acid secretion in patients with corpus gastritis. Scand J Gastroenterol Hepatol. 1997;32:664.
13. Cave DR, King WW, Hoffman JS. Production of two chemically distinct acid-inhibitory factors by *Helicobacter pylori*. Eur J Gastroenterol Hepatol. 1993;5(Suppl. 1):S23–7.
14. Beil W, Birkholz C, Wagner S, Sewing K-F. Interaction of *Helicobacter pylori* and its fatty acids with parietal cells and gastric H^+/K^+-ATPase. Gut. 1994;35:1176–80.
15. Cave DR, Vargas M. Effect of a *Campylobacter pylori* protein on acid secretion by parietal cells. Lancet. 1989;2:187.
16. Courillon-Mallet A, Launay J-M, Roucayrol A-M et al. *Helicobacter pylori* infection: physiopathologic implication of Na-methyl histamine. Gastroenterology. 1995;108:959–66.
17. Sachs G. *Helicobacter pylori* and proton pump inhibitors. Gastroenterology. 1997; 112:1033–5.
18. Lorentzon P, Jackson R, Wallmark B et al. Inhibition of proton potassium ATPase by omeprazole in isolated gastric vesicles requires proton transport. Biochim Biophys Acta. 1987;897:41–51.
19. Gillen D, Wirz AA, Neithercut WD, Ardill JES, McColl KEL. *Helicobacter pylori* infection potentiates the inhibition of gastric acid secretion by omeprazole. Gut. 1999;44:468–75.
20. El-Omar EM, Oien K, El-Nujumi A et al. *Helicobacter pylori* infection and chronic gastric acid hyposecretion. Gastroenterology. 1997;113:15–24.

21. El-Omar EM, Oien K, Murray LS et al. Increased prevalence of precancerous changes in relatives of gastric cancer patients: critical role of H. pylori. Gastroenterology. 2000; 118:22–30.
22. Noach LA, Bosma NB, Jansen J, Hoek FJ, van Deventer SJH, Tytgate GNJ. Mucosal tumor necrosis factor-α, interleukin-1β, and interleukin-8 production in Scand J Gastroenterol. 1994;29:425–9.
23. Yamaoka Y, Kita M, Kodama T, Sawai N, Kashima K, Imanishi J. Induction of various cytokines and development of severe mucosal inflammation by cagA gene positive Helicobacter pylori strains. Gut. 1997;41:442–51.
24. Crabtree JE, Farmery SM. Helicobacter pylori and gastric mucosal cytokines: evidence that CagA-positive strains are more virulent. Lab Invest. 1995;73:742–5.
25. Wallace JL, Cucala M, Mugridge K, Parente L. Secretagogue-specific effects of interleukin-1 on gastric acid secretion. Am J Physiol. 1991;261:G559–64.
26. Wallace JL, Cucala M, Mugridge K, Parente L. Cytokine inhibition of gastric acid secretion – a little goes a long way. Am J Physiol. 1991;261:G559–64.
27. Uehara A, Okumara T, Sekiya C, Okamura K, Takasugi Y, Namiki M. Interleukin-1 inhibits the secretion of gastric acid in rats: possible involvement of prostaglandin. Biochem Biophys Res Commun. 1989;162:1578–84.
28. Esplugues JV, Barrachina MD, Calatayud S, Pique JM, Whittle BJR. Nitric oxide mediates the inhibition by interleukin-1 beta of pentagastrin-stimulated rat gastric acid secretion. Br J Pharmacol. 1993;108:9–10.
29. Prinz C, Neumayer N, Mahr S, Classen M, Schepp W. Functional impairment of rat enterochromaffin-like cells by interleukin 1 beta. Gastroenterology. 1997;112:364–75.
30. Schepp W, Dehne K, Herrmuth H, Pfeffer K, Prinz C. Identification and functional importance of IL-1 receptors on rat parietal cells. Am J Physiol. 1998;275:G1094–105.
31. Mahr S, Neumayer N, Kolb HJ, Schepp W, Classen M, Prinz C. Growth factor effects on apoptosis of rat gastric enterochromaffin-like cells. Endocrinology. 1998;139:4380–90.
32. Prinz C, Zanner R, Gerhard M et al. The mechanism of histamine secretion from gastric enterochromaffin-like cells Am J Physiol. 1999;277:C845–55.
33. Mahr S, Neumayer N, Gerhard M, Classen M, Prinz C. IL-1 beta-induced apoptosis in rat gastric enterochromaffin-like cells is mediated by iNOS, NF-kappaB, and Bax protein. Gastroenterology. 2000;118:515–24.
34. Bidwell, JL et al. Cytokine gene polymorphism in human disease. http://www.pam.bris.ac.uk/services/GAI/cytokine4.htm.
35. Pociot F, Molvig J, Wogensen L, Worsaae H, Nerup J. A TaqI polymorphism in the human interleukin-1 beta (IL-1 beta) gene correlates with IL-1 beta secretion in vitro. Eur J Clin Invest. 1992;22:396–402.
36. Santtila S, Savinainen K, Hurme M. Presence of the IL-1RA allele 2 (IL1RN*2) is associated with enhanced IL-1 beta production in vitro. Scand J Immunol. 1998;47:195–8.
37. Andus T et al. Imbalance of the interleukin 1 system in colonic mucosa – association with intestinal inflammation and interleukin 1 receptor antagonist genotype 2. Gut. 1997;41:651–7.
38. Danis VA, Mililngton M, Hyland VJ, Grennan D. Cytokine production by normal human monocytes: inter-subject variation and relationship to an IL-1 receptor antagonist (IL-1Ra) gene polymorphism. Clin Exp Immunol 1995;99:303 10.
39. Tountas NA et al. Functional and ethnic association of allele 2 of the interleukin 1 receptor antagonist gene in ulcerative colitis. Gastroenterology. 1999;117:806–13.
40. El Omar EM, Carrington M, Chow W II et al. Interleukin-1 polymorphisms associated with increased risk of gastric cancer. Nature Med. (In press).
41. Stolte M, Meining A, Schmitz JM, Alexandridis T, Seifert E. Changes in Helicobacter pylori-induced gastritis in the antrum and corpus during 12 months of treatment with omeprazole and lansoprazole in patients with gastro-oesophageal reflux disease. Aliment Pharmacol Ther. 1998;12:247–53.
42. Kuipers EJ, Lundell L, Linkenberg EC et al. Atrophic gastritis and Helicobacter pylori infection in patients with reflux esophagitis treated with omeprazole or fundoplication. N Engl J Med 1996;334:1018–22.
43. Hackelsberger A, Miehlke S, Lehn N, Stotle M, Malfertheiner P, Bayerdorffer E. Helicobacter pylori eradication vs. short term acid suppression: longterm consequences for gastric body mucosa. Gastroenterology. 1996;110:A127.

44. Kuipers EJ, Uyterlinde AM, Pena AS *et al.* Increase of *Helicobacter pylori*-associated corpus gastritis during acid suppressive therapy: implications for longterm safety. Am J Gastroenterol. 1995;90:1401–6.
45. Hui Wm, Lam SK, Ho J *et al.* Effect of omeprazole on duodenal ulcer associated antral gastritis and *Helicobacter pylori*. Dig Dis Sci. 1991;36:577–82.

34
Effect of *Helicobacter pylori* infection on gastric acid control using proton pump inhibitors

P. O. KATZ

INTRODUCTION

Therapy for the patient with gastro-oesophageal reflux (GERD) is based on appropriate acid suppression; acid is responsible for the damage, so inhibition of acid is required for effective management. Healing of reflux oesophagitis and symptom relief are directly related to the percentage of time that the gastric pH is maintained above a pH of 4.0 over 24 h[1]. In effect, the amount of oesophageal acid exposure is inversely related to the degree of intragastric pH control.

Histamine H_2-receptor antagonists (H_2RA) provided the first effective medical therapy for GERD, but are limited by the need for frequent dosing, development of tolerance (tachyphylaxis)[2] and an important pharmacodynamic interaction with food intake[3]. H_2RAs suppress gastric acidity most effectively in a fasting patient, or at night, but during the day meals induce acid secretion in spite of medication. Standard doses of H_2RAs improve symptoms and heal oesophagitis after 8 weeks of therapy in 40–60% of patients[4]. In severe and refractory reflux disease, healing rates are lower, and increased doses do not improve results. These agents have been supplanted by proton pump inhibitors (PPIs) as the agents of choice to treat patients with difficult-to-manage GERD.

Once-daily dosing of a PPI, omeprazole 20 mg, lansoprazole 30 mg, pantoprazole 40 mg or rabeprazole 20 mg, will heal reflux oesophagitis in 80–90% of patients within 8 weeks with comparable symptom relief[5–8]. These same doses are effective for the long-term management of GERD, with maintenance therapy with PPIs keeping 80–90% healed and asymptomatic over 12 months[9]. Limited data are available on the efficacy of higher doses of PPIs. Omeprazole 40 mg or lansoprazole 60 mg daily marginally increases healing rates in unselected groups of GERD patients, but when used in patients with resistant disease, these or higher doses will most often heal reflux oesophagitis and control symptoms[10]. Recent studies have found that, when higher doses of PPI are needed, dosing with a twice-daily regimen – before breakfast and dinner – provides superior intragastric pH control compared with doubling the dose once a day[11,12]. However, even when treated with a PPI b.i.d., patients may still have extended periods when the intragastric pH is <4.0. This is most commonly seen during the night between the hours of midnight and 6 a.m. Approximately 70% of patients on a PPI twice daily have periods with the intragastric pH < 4 lasting for 60 min or longer during the night. This has been termed nocturnal gastric acid breakthrough[13]. This breakthrough period begins approximately 7 hours after the evening dose of PPI and as early as 10 p.m. if a once-daily PPI is given at 8 a.m. In patients with recumbent reflux, low LES pressure, and ineffective oesophageal motility, particularly those with Barrett's oesophagus, this is likely to result in prolonged oesophageal acid exposure[14]. and, potentially, treatment failure.

The reason for this overnight 'PPI failure' is multifactorial. Possibilities include:

1. The oral bioavailability of PPIs varies considerably between subjects, and may be decreased further when the drug is taken with food or antacids[15,16].
2. Only actively secreting H^+,K^+-ATPase molecules are inhibited by PPIs. The drug should, therefore, ideally be taken 15–30 min before a meal. In a crossover study pH control was compared when volunteers took a PPI in relation to a breakfast meal, with that when the drug was taken with no food until lunchtime, and demonstrated a significantly better effect when taken prior to breakfast[17].
3. PPIs are metabolized by the hepatic cytochrome P-450 2C enzymes, and while pharmacokinetic interactions are uncommon, considerable genetic variation in enzyme capacity has been seen. Reduced metabolic rate in slow or intermediate metabolizers of omeprazole will partly determine the effect of PPIs on gastric acidity[18]. Rapid metabolizers of omeprazole show lower effect of PPIs on gastric acidity than slow or intermediate metabolizers.
4. Hypersecretors may show a lower effect of PPIs; however, this is uncommon in GERD patients[19].
5. There are a small group of patients who are PPI-resistant despite normal blood levels of the drug, strongly suggesting an abnormality of the proton pump, which has, however, not been identified. These patients fail to show pH control both in daytime and at night[20].
6. The impact of *H. pylori* infection. Though there is some debate as to its clinical importance there are differences in control of intragastric pH during treatment with PPIs dependent on *H. pylori* status. The remainder of this chapter will review the available data on the differential effect of *H. pylori* infection on intragastric pH control while taking PPI.

H. PYLORI GASTRITIS: EFFECT ON ACID SECRETION

The impact of *H. pylori* infection on acid secretion is related to the pattern of gastritis and the degree of gastric atrophy caused by the infection. When gastritis is antral-predominant, such that no atrophy is present, acid secretion is often increased, a situation that might lead to exacerbation of GERD and perhaps a greater PPI requirement to control intragastric pH, although neither has been directly studied. When gastritis is body-predominant, a situation leading to gastric atrophy, *H. pylori* infection is a cofactor in reduced (or absent) gastric acid secretion, which might be protective against GERD (here there is evidence), and may reduce PPI requirement for intragastric pH control due to a higher basal pH, though again the latter has not been systematically studied. Finally when gastritis is mixed antral and body, *H. pylori* may have no effect on acid secretion, GERD or PPI effect, although this also has not been directly studied[21]. As no study has looked directly at the pattern of gastritis and its effect on intragastric control, this confounds much of the data evaluating the effect of *H. pylori* and intragastric pH control on PPIs.

The decrease in maximal acid output while on PPIs is significantly greater in *H. pylori*-positive patients compared to those that are negative, even when maximum acid output at baseline (when not on PPIs) is the same for both groups. There is a suggestion that PPI therapy in patients who are *H. pylori*-positive may actually change the pattern of gastritis from antral- to body-predominant, thus suggesting two effects of PPIs in infected patients: the ability to pharmacologically increase median pH when on therapy and possibly alter the pattern of gastritis to further reduce baseline acid output.

Studies have demonstrated that control of intragastric pH is significantly better in *H. pylori*-positive patients compared to *H. pylori*-negative patients when they are treated with PPIs, and that eradication of the infection reduces the ability of PPIs to control intragastric pH. Verdu *et al.* found that this effect was seen when normal subjects who are *H. pylori*-positive are compared to *H. pylori*-negative subjects treated with omeprazole. Significantly higher 24-h intragastric pH values were achieved in the infected individuals[22]. Two other studies comparing 24-h intragastric pH before and after eradication in patients treated with omeprazole showed an increase in median time pH > 4 before eradication. This effect was seen in normal individuals[23] as well as those with duodenal ulcer disease[24]. Pantoprazole has been found to increase 24-h intragastric pH to a greater degree in normal subjects who are *H. pylori*-positive compared to *H. pylori*-negative[25]. In a recent study by Van Harwaarden *et al.* the time of intragastric pH < 4 in normal subjects treated with lansoprazole was significantly decreased after successful *H. pylori* eradication. In this study normal subjects who were *H. pylori*-positive were treated with lansoprazole 30 mg a day or ranitidine 150 mg b.i.d. for 7 days and studied with 24-h intragastric pH monitoring. Subsequently they were randomized to receive antibiotic treatment to eradicate *H. pylori* (or placebo) and those successfully cured of the infection were restudied after 7 days of lansoprazole 30 mg or ranitidine. The time intragastric pH < 4 was significantly increased after eradication of *H. pylori* infection in subjects treated with lansoprazole[26]. Overall median pH dropped from 5.5 to 3.5 after treatment. The most pronounced effect on lansoprazole was overnight when the median pH dropped from 6.2 to 3.6 after eradication. Overall the pH control was superior on lansoprazole compared to ranitidine

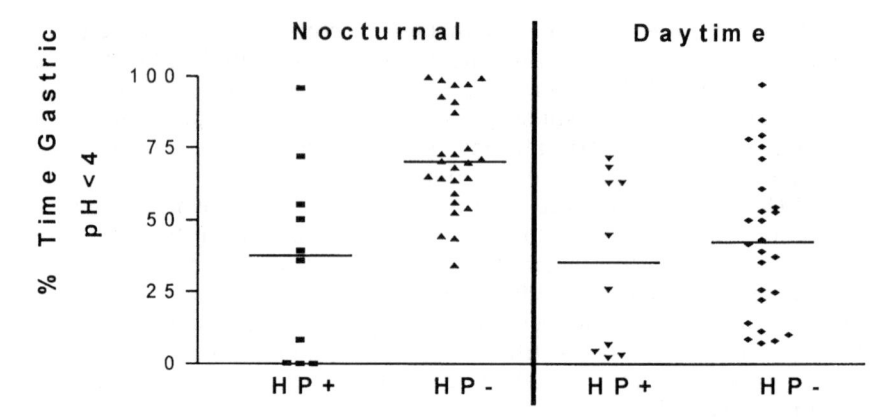

Figure 1. Difference in percentage time gastric pH < 4 on pantoprazole 40 mg in *H. pylori*-positive compared to *H. pylori*-negative subjects.

regardless of *H. pylori* status; however, intragastric pH on ranitidine was unaffected by *H. pylori* status[26].

Two recently performed intragastric pH studies suggest these differences in pH control occur predominantly overnight. In a study reported in abstract form data were extracted from a randomized double-blind crossover study assessing the efficacy of three different doses of pantoprazole in 36 normal subjects treated for 7 days, with a 24-h intragastric pH study performed on day 7. A 1-week washout period was included between studies. Subjects were studied in a clinical research unit and given three standardized meals on each study day. Time pH < 4 daytime and night (10 p.m.–6 a.m.) was analysed for each study. The median time pH < 4 overnight (10 p.m.–8 a.m.) was significantly less in the 26 *H. pylori*-positive subjects (median 35%) compared to the 10 *H. pylori*-negative subjects (70%, $p < 0.02$) (Figure 1) when given the highest dose of pantoprazole (40 mg)[27].

The second study was a randomized crossover study comparing omeprazole 20 mg twice daily with lansoprazole 30 mg twice daily in 21 normal subjects treated with each drug for 7 days, followed by 24-h intragastric pH monitoring. Subjects had a 1-week washout period between drugs, and all had the same meals on each study day. Sixteen were *H. pylori*-negative and five *H. pylori*-positive by serology. Median time pH < 4 overnight was significantly less in *H. pylori*-positive compared to negative subjects ($p < 0.05$) independent of which PPI was studied. The frequency of nocturnal acid breakthrough was decreased in the *H. pylori*-postive individuals compared to the *H. pylori*-negatives in both studies[28].

These intragastric pH studies support the findings of clinical studies which demonstrate that patients with erosive oesophagitis on maintenance omeprazole therapy had significantly fewer relapses in the first year when *H. pylori*-infected compared to uninfected patients[29]. *H. pylori*-infected patients with erosive oesophagitis healed more quickly and experienced earlier relief of symptoms compared to *H. pylori*-negative patients treated with pantoprazole[30]. This effect was most significant in the first 4 weeks, with the symptom advantage disappearing after 8 weeks, suggesting that over time this difference may not be crucial to patient outcome. Similar superior symptom relief was documented in *H. pylori*-infected compared to *H. pylori*-uninfected patients with non-erosive oesophagitis treated with omeprazole.

The data support the conclusion that *H. pylori* infection increases the ability of PPI to raise intragastric pH. This is a class effect having been documented with omeprazole, lansoprazole and pantoprazole, and this effect occurs in normal subjects, patients with gastro-oesophageal reflux and duodenal ulcer. Recent studies suggest that this effect is predominantly nocturnal, suggesting that *H. pylori* infection plays a key role in the recently described phenomenon of nocturnal gastric acid breakthrough seen in 70–80% of patients treated with PPIs, even when given twice daily[13]. It seems clear that the short-term effects of PPI therapy are enhanced in patients who are infected with *H. pylori* compared to those that are not. Whether *H. pylori* infection plays any role in long-term treatment of gastro-oesophageal reflux remains to be carefully studied; so while Graham's characterization of *H. pylori* as a biological antisecretory agent is probably correct, the clinical[31] importance of this is not clear.

References

1. Bell NJV, Burget D, Howden CW, Wilkinson J, Hunt RH. Appropriate acid suppression for the management of gastro-oesophageal reflux disease. Digestion. 1992;51 (Suppl. 1):59–67.
2. Hatlebakk JG, Berstad A. Gastro-oesophageal reflux during three months of therapy with ranitidine in reflux esophagitis. Scand J Gastroenterol. 1996;31:954–8.
3. Frislid K, Berstad A. Prolonged influence of a meal on the effect of ranitidine. Scand J Gastroenterol. 1984;19:429–32.
4. Huang J-O, Hunt RH. Meta-analysis of comparative trials for healing erosive esophagitis with proton pump inhibitors and H_2 receptor antagonists. Gastroenterology. 1998; 114:A154–5.
5. Castell DO, Richter JE, Robinson M et al. and the Lansoprazole Group. Efficacy and safety of lansoprazole in the treatment of erosive reflux esophagitis. Am J Gastroenterol. 1996;91:1749–57.
6. Hatlebakk JG, Berstad A, Carling L et al. Lansoprazole versus omeprazole in short-term treatment of reflux oesophagits. Scand J Gastroenterol. 1993;28:224–8.
7. Cloud ML, Enas N, Humphries TJ et al. and the Rabeprazole Study Group. Rabeprazole in the treatment of acid peptic diseases. Dig Dis Sci. 1998;43:993–1000.
8. Mossner J, Hoschler AH, Herz R et al. A double-blind study of pantoprazole and omeprazole in the treatment of reflux oesophagitis: a multicenter trial. Aliment Pharnacol Ther. 1995;9:321–6.
9. Hatlebakk JG, Berstad A. Lansoprazole 15 and 30 mg daily in maintaining healing and symptom relief in patients with reflux oesophagitis. Aliment Pharmacol Ther. 1997; 11:365–72.
10. Bate CM, Crowe, JP, Dickinson RJ et al. Reflux oesophagitis resolves more rapidly with omeprazole 20 mg once daily than with ranitidine 150 mg twice daily: omeprazole 40 mg once daily provides further benefit in unresponsive patients. Br J Clin Res. 1991;2:113–48.
11. Kuo B, Castell DO. Optimal dosing of omeprazole 40 mg daily: effects on gastric and esophageal pH and serum gastrin in healthy controls. Am J Gastroenterol. 1996;91:1532–8.
12. Hatlebakk JG, Katz PO, Kuo B, Casell DO. Nocturnal gastric acidity and acid breakthrough on different regimens of omeprazole 40 mg daily. Aliment Pharmacol Ther. 1998; 12:1235–40.
13. Katz PO, Anderson C, Khoury R, Castell DO. Gastro-oesophageal reflux associated with nocturnal gastric acid breakthrough on proton pump inhibitors. Aliment Pharmacol Ther. 1998;12:1231–4.

14. Fouad YM, Katz PO, Castell DO. Patients with refractory nocturnal gastroesophageal reflux (GER) have more prevalent esophageal motility abnormalities. Am J Gastroenterol. 1998;93:1615.
15. Delhotal-Landes B, Cournot A, Vermerie N et al. The effect of antacid and food on the bioavailability of lansoprazole in man. Eur J Drug Metab Pharmocokinet. 1990; 15(Suppl.):6.
16. Holloway RH, Downton J, Mitchell B et al. Effect of cisapride on postprandial gastro-esophageal reflux. Gut. 1989;30:1187–93.
17. Hatlebakk JG, Katz PO, Castell DO. Proton pump inhibitors: better before breakfast than without breakfast. Am J Gastroenterol. 1998;93:1636 (abstract).
18. Sagar M, Seensalu R, Tybring G et al. CYP2C19 genotype and phenotype determined with omeprazole in patients with acid-related disorders with and without *Helicobacter pylori* infection. Scand J Gastroenterol. 1998;33:1034–8.
19. Hirschowitz BI. A critical analysis, with appropriate controls, of gastric acid and pepsin secretion in clinical esophagitis. Gastroenterology. 1991;101:1149–58.
20. Leite LP, Johnston BT, Just RJ et al. Persistent acid secretion during omeprazole therapy: a study of gastric acid profiles in patients demonstrating failure of omeprazole therapy. Am J Gastroenterol. 1996;91:1527–31.
21. Metz DC, Kroser JA. *Helicobacter pylori* and gastroesophageal reflux disease. Gastroenterol Clin N Am. 1999;28:971–89.
22. Verdu EF, Armstrong D, Fraser R et al. Effect of *Helicobacter pylori* status on intragastric pH during treatment with omeprazole. Gut. 1995;36:539–43.
23. Verdu EF, Armstrong D, Idstrom J-P et al. Effect of curing *Helicobacter pylori* infection on intragastric pH during treatment with omeprazole. Gut. 1995;37:743–8.
24. Labenz J, Tillenburg B, Peitz U et al. *Helicobacter pylori* augments the pH-increasing effect of omeprazole in patients with duodenal ulcer. Gastroenterology. 1996;110:725–32.
25. Koop H, Kuly S, Flug M et al. Intragastric pH and serum gastrin during administration of different doses of pantoprazole in healthy subjects. Eur J Gastroenterol Hepatol. 1996;8:915–18.
26. VanHerwaarden MA, Samsom M, Van Nispen CHM, Mulder PGH, Smout AJPM. The effect of *Helicobacter pylori* eradication on intragastric pH during dosing with lansoprazole or ranitidine. Aliment Pharmacol Ther. 1999;13:731–40.
27. Katz PO, Silman J, Katzka D et al. *H. pylori* infection increases nocturnal acid control on proton pump inhibitors. Am J Gastroenterol. 1998;93:1641 (abstract).
28. Katz PO, HatlebakkJ, Castell DO. Omeprazole or lansoprazole twice daily intragastric pH profile on omeprazole or lansorpazole twice daily. Aliment Pharmacol Ther. 2000 (In press).
29. Holtman G, Cain C, Malfertheiner P. Gastric *Helicobacter pylori* infection accelerates healing of reflux esophagitis during treatment with the proton pump inhibitor pantoprazole. Gastroenterology. 1999;117:11–16.
30. Hallerback B, Unge P, Carling L et al. Omeprazole or ranitidine in long-term treatment of reflux esophagitis. The Scandinavia Clinic for United Research group. Gastroenterology. 1994;107:1305–11.
31. Graham DY, Yamaoka Y. *H. pylori* and *cagA*: relationships with gastric cancer, duodenal ulcer, and reflux esophagitis and its complications. Helicobacter. 1998;3:145–51.

41
Rebound acid hypersecretion after acid-suppressive therapy

D. GILLEN and K. E. L. McCOLL

H₂ ANTAGONISTS

Early studies suggested that there were no physiological sequelae to H$_2$-receptor antagonist-induced acid suppression after treatment was discontinued[1,2]. However, these early studies focused primarily on pentagastrin-stimulated maximal acid secretion. Since that time a number of studies have shown that there is significant rebound hypersecretion of gastric acid after H$_2$-receptor antagonist treatment, both basally[3-6] and in response to meal[7] and gastrin-releasing peptide (GRP) stimulation[6].

It was previously suggested that this rebound acid phenomenon after H$_2$-receptor antagonists was of physiological interest, but was unlikely to be of clinical importance. However, anecdotal clinical experience of a rapid resurgence of symptoms after stopping treatment with these agents suggested that it might be of clinical relevance. Furthermore, in a previous open physiological study we had noted the new onset of dyspeptic symptoms in a group of previously asymptomatic *Helicobacter pylori*-positive healthy subjects[6]. We have therefore since undertaken a double-blind, placebo-controlled study using a validated symptom questionnaire[8]. This showed that there is a significantly greater new onset of dyspeptic symptoms in the actively treated, previously asymptomatic group of subjects, when compared with the placebo group, at a time coincident with the physiological rebound phenomenon. This is therefore consistent with a symptomatic role for this phenomenon, seen after the use of these widely prescribed agents[9].

PROTON PUMP INHIBITORS

Proton pump inhibitors (PPIs) have very rapidly become one of the world's most frequently prescribed medications[9]. This is attributable to the profound suppression of gastric acid secretion which they induce[10,11] and which has made them of great use in the full spectrum of acid/peptic diseases[12-14].

Early in omeprazole's development, animal studies had shown that profound 24 hour acid inhibition led to oxyntic mucosal hypertrophy and associated rebound pentagastrin-stimulated maximal acid hypersecretion at 8 days after stopping treatment[15,16]. Human studies after the drug became available suggested that a similar hypersecretion phenomenon was not found in humans[17,18]. However, timing of acid secretion studies is vitally important. Taking this into account, Waldum's group have since shown that there is both basal and pentagastrin-stimulated maximal acid hypersecretion in a group of eight reflux oesophagitis patients studied at 14 days after stopping a 90-day course of omeprazole 40 mg/day[19]. However, their study included subjects of mixed *H. pylori* status, which precluded any comment on any potential influence for this parameter on the rebound phenomenon.

We have since studied this phenomenon further in a group of 12 *H. pylori*-negative and nine *H. pylori*-positive healthy, asymptomatic subjects using gastrin-17 (G-17) dose–response studies[20]. In these *H. pylori*-negative subjects, studied at 15 days after treatment with a 2-month course of omeprazole 40 mg/day, both significant rebound basal and G-17-stimulated maximal acid hypersecretion were found.

The dose–response studies allowed us to calculate sensitivity to gastrin stimulation. This parameter is the dose of gastrin which achieves 50% of the maximal acid secretion possible in a particular individual[21]. This was unaltered between pre- and post-omeprazole in these *H. pylori*-negative subjects, i.e. their rebound hypersecretion was not due to an increased sensitivity to the acid-stimulatory effects of gastrin after treatment. Similarly, the rebound hypersecretion was not due to increased gastrin secretion, since the on-treatment hypergastrinaemia had returned to normal by 2 weeks post-treatment. However, data had also been collected during omeprazole treatment for both fasting intragastric pH and fasting plasma gastrin. Gastrin stimulates acid secretion by releasing histamine[22] from the oxyntic enterochromaffin-like (ECL) cell[23,24], which acts on the H_2-receptor of the parietal cell[25]. This hormone also exerts trophic effects on both of these cell types. Prolonged acid inhibition is known to induce ECL cell and parietal cell hyperplasia in both animals[26] and humans[27,28]. This effect is thought to be mediated via increased gastrin concentrations because both antrectomy[29] and specific gastrin receptor antagonism[30] prevent its development in animal models. We were therefore able to correlate the degree of increase in post-treatment maximal acid output (MAO) with the measured on-treatment intragastric pH and on-treatment fasting plasma gastrin[20]. These proved to be significantly positively associated. This is consistent with the rebound phenomenon in the *H. pylori*-negative subjects being due to the hypergastrinaemia found during PPI treatment leading to hypertrophy/hyperplasia of the ECL and/or parietal cells. This increase in functional mass can then lead to rebound acid hypersecretion on withdrawal of the acid inhibition of PPI therapy.

However, the duration of this phenomenon remained unknown. We have therefore studied a further group of 12 *H. pylori*-negative subjects both before and at 7, 14, 28, 42 and 56 days after a 56-day course of 40 mg/day of omeprazole[31]. This study has shown that there is significant elevation of both submaximal and maximal pentagastrin-stimulated acid secretion at all time points to at least 56 days. Thus, there is a prolonged persisting rebound phenomenon after PPIs. This is consistent with the phenomenon being due to trophic effects on cells of the oxyntic mucosa.

The pattern found in the *H. pylori*-positive subjects at 15 days after omeprazole was different[20]. They had no significant increase (and in fact a trend towards a significant decrease) in basal acid output (BAO). This was associated with a significantly decreased sensitivity to gastrin stimulation. Similarly, there was no significant increase in MAO in the *H. pylori*-positives at 15 days after omeprazole. This was due to a heterogeneous response in this group, with some subjects showing a marked increase and others showing persisting suppression of acid secretion.

The reason for this lack of increase in the *H. pylori*-positive subjects is unknown. It is especially surprising, since they are known to have a greater degree of hypergastrinaemia during PPI therapy than uninfected subjects[32], due to a much more marked acid supression than *H. pylori*-negative subjects during treatment[33,34]. The cause of this itself is unclear. However, it is known that a greater intensity of oxyntic mucosal inflammation develops in *H. pylori*-positive subjects during PPI therapy[35]. Oxyntic mucosal inflammation has previously been associated with impaired acid secretion[36]. This effect may be mediated through the paracrine effect of inflammatory cytokines, such as interleukin-1[37]. The presence of persisting enhanced oxyntic gastritis in even a subgroup of these *H. pylori*-positve subjects at 15 days after omeprazole, thereby masking the rebound phenomenon, could explain why the *H. pylori*-positive subjects as a group do not show rebound acid hypersecretion after PPIs.

However, the lack of significant rebound at 2 weeks does not exclude the possibility of rebound hypersecretion occurring in the *H. pylori*-positive subjects at a later time-point, once the enhancement of the oxyntic gastritis may have resolved. Similarly, we cannot exclude that rebound phenomena might be unmasked by removal of the antigen driving the oxyntic gastritis, i.e. by eradication/suppression of *H. pylori* in the immediate post-treatment phase. Certainly, we have measured acid secretion in a 57 kg asymptomatic, *H. pylori*-positive woman who took amoxycillin incidentally at the end of a 2-month course of omeprazole. Her BAO rose from 6.7 mmol h^{-1} before treatment to 26.5 mmol h^{-1} at 14 days after treatment (which is in the Zollinger–Ellison range) and her MAO from 32.3 mmol h^{-1} to 54.9 mmol h^{-1}. Interestingly, she also developed new onset of dyspeptic symptoms, which lasted from 7 until 77 days after treatment. Both the possibility of rebound at later time-points in *H. pylori*-positive subjects and also the influence of *H. pylori* eradication/suppression on rebound will merit further investigation.

It is of interest to contrast the rebound phenomenon after H_2-receptor antagonsists with that found after PPIs. The rebound after H_2-receptor antagonists is more marked in *H. pylori*-positive subjects[6], whereas that after PPIs has only been shown to occur in *H. pylori*-negative subjects[20]. The basal rebound after H_2-receptor antagonists is seen early, occurring by 3 days after treatment[6], whereas that after PPIs is not seen at 6 days, but is seen by 14 days[19,20]. This is likely to reflect the non-competitive nature of the inhibition of the latter drugs. Finally, there is no significant increase in MAO seen after H_2-receptor antagonists[1,2], whereas there is a marked increase in MAO after PPIs[19,20]. This reflects an increase in functional oxyntic acid secretory capacity, which is probably mediated through the trophic effects of the more marked hypergastrinaemia due to the much more profound acid inhibition caused by PPIs.

The clinical relevance of the rebound hypersecretion after PPIs remains unknown. However, since there is symptomatic relevance of the much shorter-lived post H_2-receptor antagonist rebound phenomenon[8], it is not unreasonable to suggest that the post-PPI phenomenon may also be of some clinical importance. If so, this prolonged phenomenon may make it very difficult to withdraw treatment. This is therefore of potential long-term significance, both for the patient and also in terms of pharmacoeconomics.

CONCLUSION

In summary, there is significant rebound basal, submaximal and maximal acid hypersecretion at 2 weeks after treatment with omeprazole in *H. pylori*-negative subjects. Furthermore, their rebound hypersecretion is prolonged, lasting to at least 56 days after a 56-day treatment course. This rebound hypersecretion in *H. pylori*-negative subjects is likely to be due to the trophic effects on the oxyntic mucosa of the hypergastrinaemia, which occurs on PPI treatment. However, *H. pylori*-positive subjects do not demonstrate these rebound phenomena at 2 weeks after treatment with omeprazole. This may reflect persistence into the post-treatment phase of the enhanced oxyntic gastritis, which they are known to develop during PPI therapy. However, significant rebound at later time-points or under the influence of *H. pylori* eradication/suppression cannot be excluded, and will merit further investigation.

References

1. Forrest JAH, Fettes MR, McLoughlin GP, Heading RC. Effect of long-term cimetidine on gastric acid secretion, serum gastrin and gastric emptying. Gut. 1979;20:404–7.
2. Mohammed R, Holden RJ, Hearns JB, McKibben BM, Buchanan KD, Crean GP. Effects of eight weeks' continuous treatment with oral ranitidine and cimetidine on gastric acid secretion, pepsin secretion and fasting serum gastrin. Gut. 1983;24:61–6.
3. Fullarton GM, McLauchlan G, MacDonald A, Crean GP, McColl KEL. Rebound nocturnal hypersecretion after four weeks treatment with an H_2 receptor antagonist. Gut. 1989;30:449–54.
4. Fullarton GM, MacDonald AMI, McColl KEL. Rebound hypersecretion after H_2-antagonist withdrawal – a comparative study with nizatidine, ranitidine and famotidine. Aliment Pharmacol Ther. 1991;5:391–8.
5. Nwokolo CU, Smith JTL, Sawyerr AM, Pounder RE. Rebound intragastric hyperacidity after abrupt withdrawal of histamine H_2 receptor blockade. Gut. 1991;32:1455–60.
6. El Omar EM, Banerjee S, Wirz A, Penman I, Ardill JES, McColl KEL. Marked rebound acid hypersecretion after treatment with ranitidine. Am J Gastroenterol. 1996;91:355–9.
7. Frislid K, Aadland E, Berstad A. Augmented postprandial gastric acid secretion due to exposure to ranitidine in healthy subjects. Scand J Gastroenterol. 1986;21:119–22.
8. Smith AD, Gillen D, Cochran KM, El Omar EM, McColl KEL. Dyspepsia on withdrawal of ranitidine in previously asymptomatic volunteers. Am J Gastroenterol. 1999;94:1209–13.

9. Garner A, Fadlallah H, Parsons ME. 1976 and all that! – 20 years of antisecretory therapy. Gut. 1996;39:784–6.
10. Howden CW, Forrest JAH, Reid JL. Effect of single and repeated doses of omeprazole on gastric acid and pepsin secretion in man. Gut. 1984;25:707–10.
11. Walt RP, Gomes M de FA, Wood EC, Logan LH, Pounder RE. Effect of daily oral omeprazole on 24 hour intragastric acidity. Br Med J. 1983;287:21–14.
12. Co-operative Study. Omeprazole in duodenal ulceration: acid inhibition, symptom relief, endoscopic healing and recurrence. Br Med J. 1984;289:525–8.
13. Howden CW, Hunt RH. The relationship between suppression of acidity and gastric ulcer healing rates. Aliment Pharmacol Ther. 1990;4:25–33.
14. Koop H, Arnold MD. Long-term maintenance treatment of reflux esophagitis with omeprazole. Prospective study in patients with H_2 blocker resistant esophagitis. Dig Dis Sci. 1991;36:552–7.
15. Carlsson E, Larsson H, Mattson H, Ryberg B, Sundell G. Pharmacology and toxicology of omeprazole – with special reference to the effects on gastric mucosa. Scand J Gastroenterol. 1986;21 (Suppl. 118):31–8.
16. Larsson H, Carlsson E, Ryberg B, Fryklund J, Wallmark B. Rat parietal cell function after prolonged inhibition of gastric acid secretion. Am J Physiol. 1988;254:G33–9.
17. Prewett EJ, Hudson M, Nwokolo CU, Sawyerr AM, Pounder RE. Nocturnal intragastric acidity during and after a period of dosing with either ranitidine or omeprazole. Gastroenterology. 1991;100:873–7.
18. Bell N, Rohss K, Cederberg C, Hunt R. Does tachyphylaxis and/or rebound acid secretion occur during/after treatment with omeprazole or ranitidine? Gastroenterology. 1993; 104:A41.
19. Waldum HL, Arnestad JS, Brenna E, Eide I, Syversen U, Sandvik AK. Marked increase in gastric secretory capacity after omeprazole treatment. Gut. 1996;29:649–53.
20. Gillen D, Wirz AA, Ardill JES, McColl KEL. Rebound hypersecretion after omeprazole and its relation to on-treatment acid suppression and *Helicobacter pylori* status. Gastroenterology. 1999;116:239–47.
21. Gillen D, El-Omar EM, Wirz AA, Ardill JES, McColl KEL. The acid response to gastrin distinguishes duodenal ulcer patients from *H. pylori*-infected healthy subjects. Gastroenterology. 1998;114:50–7.
22. Sandvik AK, Waldum HL, Kleveland PM, Schulze-Sognen B. Gastrin produces an immediate and dose-dependent histamine release preceding acid secretion in the totally isolated, vascularly perfused rat stomach. Scand J Gastroenterol. 1987;22:803–8.
23. Brenna E, Waldum HL. Studies of isolated parietal and enterochromaffin-like cells. Scand J Gastroenterol. 1991;26:1296–306.
24. Prinz C, Kajimura M, Scott DR, Mercier F, Helander HF, Sachs G. Histamine secretion from rat enterochromaffin-like cells. Gastroenterology. 1993;105:459–61.
25. Black JW, Duncan WAM, Durant CJ, Ganellin CR, Parsons MC. Definition and antagonism of histamine H_2 receptors. Nature. 1972;236:385–90.
26. Creutzfeldt W, Stockmann F, Conlon JM, Folsch UR, Bonatz G, Wulfrath M. Effect of short and long-term feeding of omeprazole on rat gastric endocrine cells. Digestion. 1986;35 (Suppl. 1):84–97.
27. Klinkenberg Knol EC, Festen IIPM, Jansen JBMJ et al. Long-term treatment with omeprazole for refractory reflux esophagitis: efficacy and safety. An Intern Med. 1994;121:161–7.
28. Drimon D, Wright C, Tougas G, Riddell R. Omeprazole produces parietal cell hypertrophy and hyperplasia in humans. Gastroenterology. 1995;108:A85.
29. Larsson H, Carlsson E, Mattsson H et al. Plasma gastrin and gastric enterochromaffin-like cell activation and proliferation. Studies with omeprazole and ranitidine in intact and antrectomised rats. Gastroenterology. 1986;90:391–9.
30. Eissele R, Patberg H, Koop H et al. Effect of gastrin receptor blockade on endocrine cells in rats during achlorhydria. Gastroenterology. 1992;103:1596–601.
31. Gillen D, Wirz AA, McColl KEL. Rebound acid hypersecretion after omeprazole is a prolonged phenomenon. Gut. 2000;46:A51.
32. El-Nujumi A, Williams C, Ardill JE, Oien K, McColl KEL. Eradicating *H. pylori* reduces hypergastrinaemia during long-term omeprazole therapy. Gut. 1998;42:159–65.
33. Verdu EF, Armstrong D, Idstrom J-P, Cederberg C, Blum Al. Effect of *H. pylori* status on intragastric pH during treatment with omeprazole. Gut. 1995;36:539–43.

34. Gillen D, Wirz AA, Neithercut WD, Ardill JES, McColl KEL. *Helicobacter pylori* infection potentiates the inhibition of gastric acid secretion by omeprazole. Gut. 1999;44:468–75.
35. Kuipers EJ, Uyterlinde AM, Pena AS *et al*. Increase of *Helicobacter pylori*-associated corpus gastritis during acid suppressive therapy: implications for long-term safety. Am J Gastroenterol. 1995;90:1401–6.
36. El-Omar EM, Oien K, El-Nujumi A *et al. H. pylori* infection and chronic gastric hyposecretion. Gastroenterology. 1997;113:15–24.
37. Robert A, Olafsson AS, Lancaster C, Zhang W. Interleukin-1 is cytoprotective, antisecretory, stimulates PGE_2 synthesis by the stomach and retards gastric emptying. Life Sci. 1991;48:123–34.

42
Gastric consequences of proton pump inhibitor therapy and *Helicobacter pylori* eradication

G. SACHS, C. ATHMANN, D. WEEKS and D. SCOTT

INTRODUCTION

A medical marvel that mostly goes unheralded is the relegation of peptic ulcer disease to a minor ailment that can be cured and rapidly treated. Three steps were taken, in the last quarter of the twentieth century, that provided the fuel for this revolution. In the 1970s came the first medical means of controlling acid secretion that was well tolerated by patients, the H_2-receptor antagonist drug class[1]. The first of the class, cimetidine, had two drawbacks that were recognized early on by the development of its major competitor, ranitidine. These were a propensity for drug interaction due to inhibition of a cyP450 isozyme and a relatively low potency at the H_2-receptor. With ranitidine, probably the full benefit of reversible H_2 receptor antagonism was realized and its range of clinical usefulness defined, at first using twice-daily dosing, and now with only night-time dosing. The introduction of proton pump inhibitors (PPIs) as a more effective means of acid suppression provided the second step which resulted in effective acid control for treatment of gastro-oesophageal reflux disease (GERD)[2]. The recognition that a gastric denizen, *Helicobacter pylori*, was responsible, along with acid for peptic ulcer disease, was the third step, providing a means for curing most ulcer diseases where eradication uses PPIs accompanied by two antibiotics[3,4]. Now the focus of treatment has changed, from control of acid to prevent peptic ulcer disease to control of acid to prevent even symptoms of acid reflux.

Still there are concerns, with some acute effect of drugs used for the control of acid secretion, with chronic effects of the self-same drugs and with consequences of eradication of *H. pylori* infection. If acid control deteriorates either as an inherent effect of the drug, or because a change has occurred in the physiology of acid secretion, this can increase acid reflux and increase the risk of oesophageal cancer. Can the drug-related risks be reduced if the mechanism of acid rebound is understood? Is this increased exposure of the lower oesophagus to acid a risk sufficient to outweigh the risk of peptic ulcer disease and gastric cancer resulting from infection by *H. pylori*?

HISTAMINE-2 RECEPTOR ANTAGONISTS (H_2RA): EFFECTS AND SECRETORY PATHWAYS

These receptor antagonists (or inverse agonists, more precisely) were effective in healing duodenal ulcers, but required continuous therapy for prevention of relapse. Only after the beginning of this therapeutic approach did it become known that these ulcers were caused by an infection, not just by acid. This explained the need for maintenance therapy for ulcer prevention. These drugs were also effective in gastric ulcer treatment, whether caused by infection, excessive acid, stress or drugs such as NSAIDs; but again, usually maintenance therapy was required to prevent recurrence or to adequately treat.

As these drugs became a mainstay of gastrointestinal therapy, a surprise was in store for the clinical community. As peptic ulcer disease was declining, so the incidence of GERD was increasing and, along with it, oesophageal cancer. Although acid reflux is responsible for the erosions, symptoms and sequelae, the defect is in the lower oesophageal sphincter. In this disease the H_2-receptor class of drug, at standard dose (e.g. ranitidine 300 mg nocte) was considerably less effective as a therapeutic agent. This necessitated a four-times daily dose schedule.

We still do not understand the defects in the lower oesophageal sphincter that lead to reflux, nor the pain mechanisms leading in some to symptoms, in others to none. With widespread use of these drugs three other observations were made. First, that tolerance developed rapidly to these compounds; secondly that, after stopping treatment, a period of hyperacidity ensued, acid 'rebound'; and thirdly, they were less effective at daytime pH control as compared to night-time pH control.

Not only are the first two sets of phenomena, although well accepted, not explained, but there is little evidence that they have measurable clinical consequences. What evidence would one look for? Acid rebound, if clinically significant, should raise the incidence of ulcer disease after stopping treatment, or at the very least increase symptoms of hyperacidity such as frequency of pain or heartburn. Tolerance should lead to a crowd at the doctors' office complaining of recrudescence of the sickness that brought them there in the first place. The latter certainly has not taken place, perhaps because, as GERD was increasing, a different class of drug was entering the market-place that did not show tolerance and was more effective. This class provided significant pH elevation during the day and hence largely replaced H_2RA for daytime GERD sufferers.

Even today, many years after the recognition of the weak action of H_2RA, there is not a fully satisfactory explanation. Even with the publication of the first paper on these receptor antagonists, it became obvious that the action of gastrin on acid secretion was mediated by histamine release[1]. It was obvious that stimulation by carbachol, as a stand-in for acetylcholine, was much less sensitive to H_2-receptor blockade. This led to the proposal

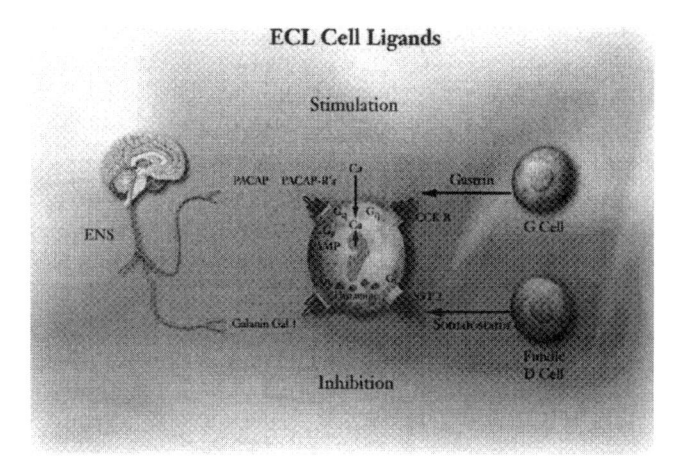

Figure 1. Complexity of peripheral pathways regulating gastric acid secretion. On the top are two pathways stimulating ECL cell release of histamine; on the bottom are two pathways inhibiting release of histamine from the ECL cell. Not shown is the direct cholinergic stimulation of the parietal cell.

that central stimulation of acid secretion was less sensitive to H_2-receptor antagonism than peripheral stimulation of acid secretion, and that daytime secretion was driven more by central stimulation than night-time secretion. However, this assumes that carbachol injection mimics central stimulation. That it really does not do so is shown by the finding that as much as 60% of acid secretion generated by central injection of TRH is blocked by H_2-receptor antagonists, a much greater effect than that exerted on carbachol-stimulated secretion[5].

To advance an explanation for the contrast between central and peripheral stimulation of acid secretion, a brief digression into the regulation of acid secretion is germane. Figure 1 illustrates the complexity of the situation as we understand it today, and this must be a simplified comprehension.

The central cell regulating acid secretion is the ECL cell or enterochromaffin-like cell. There are four well-defined receptor subtypes on this cell, activation of which leads to either stimulation or inhibition of histamine release. On the top are the two best-known activating receptors, i.e. those that lead to histamine release. These are (a) gastrin, the well-known peripheral endocrine stimulant of gastric acid secretion, that depends on release of histamine for its stimulatory action on acid secretion and (b) pituitary adenylate cyclase-activating peptide (PACAP) produced by post-ganglionic neurons in the gastric enteric nervous system[6].

CENTRAL VERSUS PERIPHERAL STIMULATION

The latter stimulant is somewhat of a surprise. Whereas it had been shown that PACAP injection inhibited gastric acid secretion[7], nevertheless PACAP was an effective stimulant of histamine release from ECL cells and of both cAMP and calcium signalling in these cells *in vitro*. In contrast, carbachol did not affect ECL cells, ruling out its participation in the H_2RA sensitive component of gastric acid secretion. However carbachol does stimulate the parietal cell directly.

Another *in-vitro* experiment provided even more compelling evidence that PACAP was a serious candidate as the neural mediator for stimulation of acid secretion. A rabbit gastric gland, after loading with Fluo-4 for measurement of intracellular calcium, when superfused with PACAP, shows a calcium signalling response in ECL cells and adjacent parietal cells. The ECL cell signal is not affected by the presence of a H_2RA, but the parietal cell signal is abolished[6].

The explanation for the *in-vivo* inhibitory effect of PACAP may be found in Figure 1. The fundic D or somatostatin cell is a potent inhibitor of ECL cell function as well as that of parietal cells. On its surface there are VIP or VPAC receptors, in contrast to the PACAP receptors (PAC1 receptors) on the ECL cell. The latter have a 1000-fold higher affinity for PACAP than VIP; the former have equal and low affinity for PACAP and VIP relative to PAC1. Hence a relatively high concentration of PACAP in the vicinity of D cells will tend to block acid secretion by somatostatin release. When PACAP was given along with a neutralizing concentration of anti-somatostatin antibody, stimulation of acid secretion was observed, rather than inhibition[6]. These new data have enabled an explanation of the sensitivity of central stimulation of acid secretion to H_2RA as well as the insensitivity of carbachol stimulation to the same compounds. Central stimulation uses post-ganglionic PACAP nerves for ECL cell stimulation and acetylcholine-containing nerves for direct parietal cell stimulation to give the mixed sensitivity of daytime acid secretion to H_2RA.

TOLERANCE AND REBOUND TO H_2RA

Tolerance

The loss of efficacy of acid inhibition by H_2RA is of the order of 50% within 7 days[8]. There are several defined mechanisms of drug tolerance, such as receptor up-regulation where insufficient antagonist is present to achieve maximal effect, changes in drug metabolism, activation of alternative pathways and many other possibilities.

In the case of tolerance to these receptor antagonists, this is not overcome by ever-higher doses of H_2RA. It is therefore not due to receptor up-regulation. It is also not due to increase in metabolism of the drug. It is not bypassed by high doses of gastrin; hence it is not due to alterations in patterns of histamine release.

H_2RA inhibit cAMP formation from adenylate cyclase even in the absence of histamine or other agonist. They are, by definition, inverse agonists where occupancy of their site on the cyclase also inhibits basal activity. It appears that there is not a H_2RA-insensitive cAMP production. With down-regulation of the histamine pathway, up-regulation of the acetylcholine pathway could occur, but attempts to obtain direct evidence that there is a change in cholinergic stimulation of the parietal cell are absent.

Rebound

The effect of H_2RA is to restore the acid pump to its resting configuration, i.e. no longer present on the secretory membrane of the cell. In that configuration it is not subject to the same rate of endocytosis as the normal stimulated pump. It has been shown that the half-life of the pump is about doubled with H_2RA infusion in rats[9]. If this happens with treatment in humans, then the stomach will show a higher secretory rate no matter what the simulus. So inhibitory adaptation by increase of pump level could account for H_2RA-induced acid rebound that would develop quite rapidly following H_2RA treatment. This is a hypothesis that can readily be tested using Western analysis of gastric biopsies.

PPIs AND THEIR EFFECTS

Even as the usefulness of H_2RA was penetrating doctors' consciousness, a new class of acid control drugs was being developed, the proton pump inhibitors, PPIs[10]. These, in contrast to the receptor-based drugs, inhibited the gastric acid pump, the final step of acid secretion, in a covalent manner. These were therefore more effective in controlling acid secretion. However, once more, treatment of peptic ulcer disease required maintenance therapy. As this was also being realized, *H. pylori* infection was becoming recognized as a major contributor to peptic ulcer disease[3,4]. Treatment of this gastric infection required not only acid suppression, but also antibiotics to eliminate the bacteria.

At first the concern around these drugs focused on ECL cell hyperplasia and possible gastric carcinoid formation. The past decade or so of experience have allayed these fears with maintenance therapy using omeprazole, lansoprazole or pantoprazole. The mechanism initially postulated for the hyperplasia and carcinoids seen in the rat appears to be the high levels of gastrin induced by the inhibition of acid secretion. However, there now appears to be a consensus that parietal cell hyperplasia develops fairly rapidly during PPI therapy, even within 1 month of beginning therapy[11]. The increased parietal cell mass can lead to acid hypersecretion after cessation of PPI therapy.

GASTRIN EFFECTS ON PARIETAL CELLS

The action of gastrin on parietal cells is to increase both cAMP and intracellular calcium levels due to the histamine liberated from the ECL cells in the vicinity of the parietal cell, since histamine antagonism at low levels of gastrin fully inhibits the parietal cell response. The different effects of gastrin are illustrated in the images of Figure 3, showing the ECL and local effects of 1 nM gastrin on gastric glands, and then the effects of ranitidine on that signal.

However, there are also effects of 10 nM gastrin on calcium signalling in the gastric gland that are insensitive to either ranitidine or somatostatin, suggesting a more complex role for gastrin in the gastric epithelium.

Ca^{2+}- signaling with with 100 nM PACAP

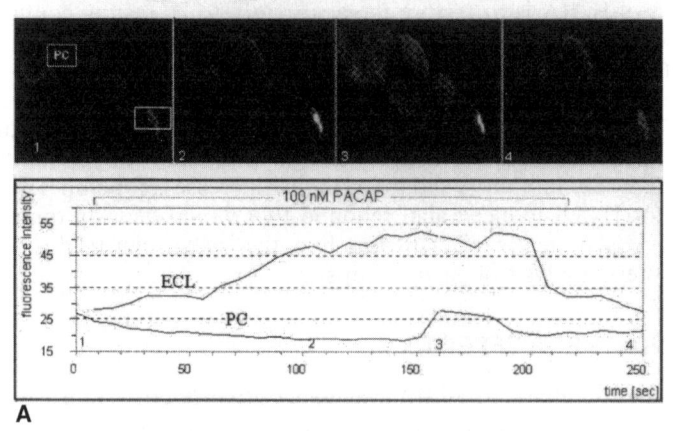

A

Ca^{2+}- signaling with 100 nM PACAP + 100 μM ranitidine

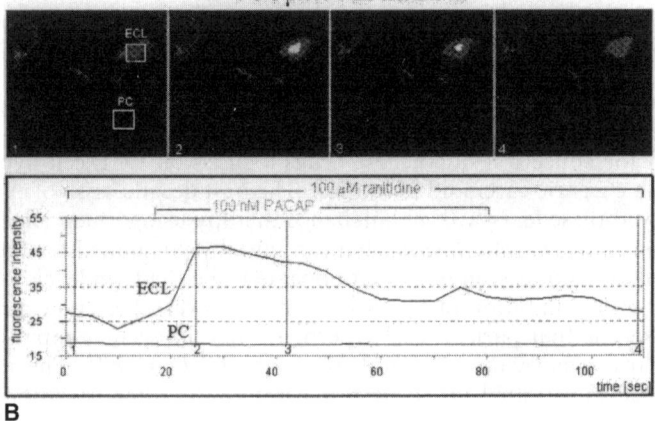

B

Figure 2. **A**: PACAP stimulates ECL cell and adjacent parietal cell calcium signalling. In the relevant image the large increase in intracellular calcium is followed by a change of calcium in the adjacent parietal cells. **B**: Ranitidine ablates the effect of PACAP on parietal cells leaving effects on ECL cells intact, as shown in the figure.

At this 10-fold higher concentration of gastrin, all parietal cells show a calcium signal that is insensitive to H_2RAs and also to somatostatin, a potent inhibitor of cAMP-induced acid secretion. Hence there is a secondary action of gastrin on parietal cells that induces a CCK-B receptor response in the cell calcium pathway. This second, low-affinity response may be the basis for direct gastrin trophism on fundic mucosa, which may be of relevance in the apparent acid hypersecretion that occurs even after short-term PPI treatment (Figure 3C).

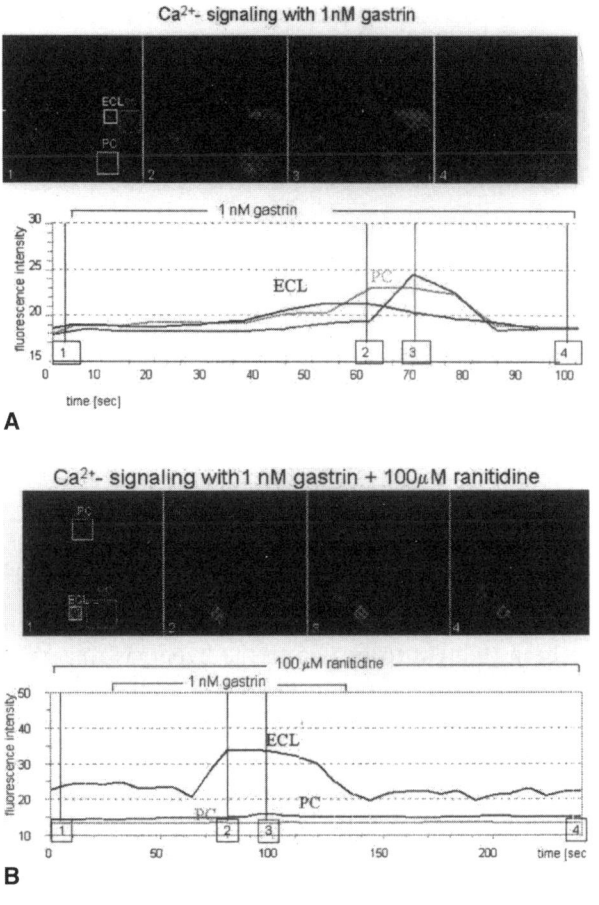

Figure 3. A: The effect of 1 nM gastrin on intracellular calcium of ECL and parietal cells of rabbit gastric gland. The gastric glands were loaded with Fluo-4 AM and visualized using a Zeiss confocal microscope. The trace below corresponds to the images above, with the number at a given time point on the image and the graph. Both ECL cells and adjacent parietal cells respond. **B**: The effect of 1 nM gastrin in the presence of 100 μM ranitidine, showing that the ECL cell response persists but that the parietal cell response is inhibited. **C**: The effect of 10 nM gastrin on calcium signalling in parietal and ECL cells in the presence of 100 μM ranitidine (or 100 nM somatostatin). This shows that, at this concentration of gastrin, all parietal cells respond with an elevation of intracellular calcium that is insensitive to H_2RA and somatostatin. This effect is therefore not directly related to the acid-secretory response in this *in-vitro* model of mammalian acid secretion.

PPIs AND ACID REBOUND

Some compelling evidence has been presented by McColl *et al.* that omeprazole treatment can result, relatively rapidly, in acid rebound after stopping treatment, as has also been found for H_2RA[12]. This somewhat surprising result needs an explanation, and one must wait to see of there are clinical

Ca²⁺- signaling with 10 nM gastrin + 100μM ranitidine

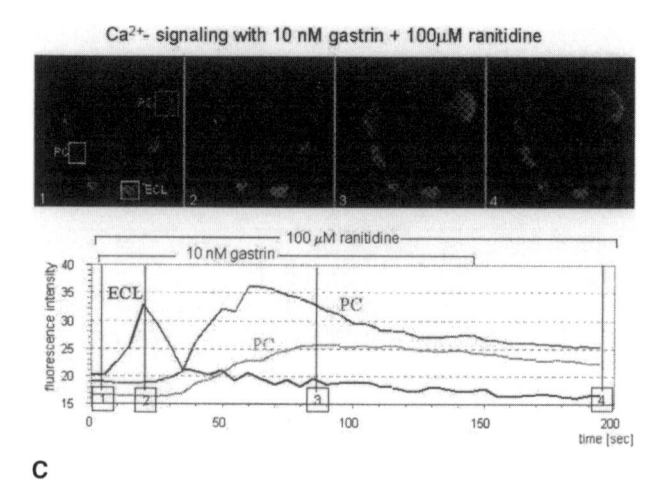

Figure 3. (*Continued.*)

consequences. Here we shall again consider a variety of hypotheses that are testable in the human stomach.

So far, most of the effects of PPIs outside direct inhibition of the H,K-ATPase have been thought to be due to the hypergastrinaemia that results from PPI acid suppression and loss of acid feedback inhibition of gastrin release stimulated by aromatic amino acids. It still seems most likely that endocrine/neurocrine changes in the stomach must account for any finding outside of the covalent inhibition of the acid pump, although there are always surprises until one understands the logic of biology.

A possible effect of PPI therapy could be a change in the half-life of the ATPase. This could either be decreased due to covalent derivatization or be increased. The effect of PPIs does not seem to extend to changing the morphological status of the pump and no change in half-life was detected[9]. Hence acid rebound after short-term treatment is not likely due to changes in H,K-ATPase levels in individual parietal cells. Another explanation should be sought, perhaps related to the ontogeny of the parietal cell.

At any given time the fundic mucosa contains a variety of cell types in the parietal cell axis, stem cells, pre-progenitor cells, parietal progenitor cells and pre-parietal cells, and then young and mature parietal cells. It is not known at which stage gastrin acts as a trophic agent, and it is possible that trophic effects and the rapidity of the response of the gastric mucosa to trophic actions of gastrin depend on which cell class is affected. Stimulation of stem cells and/or pre-progenitor cells will result in both parietal and chief cell hyperplasia. Stimulation of committed parietal progenitor cells will result in selective hyperplasia of the parietal cell, but this may be relatively slow compared to the onset of acid hypersecretion described elsewhere in this volume. Stimulation of pre-parietal cells could result in a quite rapid increase of acid secretory capacity since the time taken for a pre-parietal cell to become a parietal cell may be quite short as compared to the time

GASTRIC EPITHELIAL CELL HYPERPLASIA

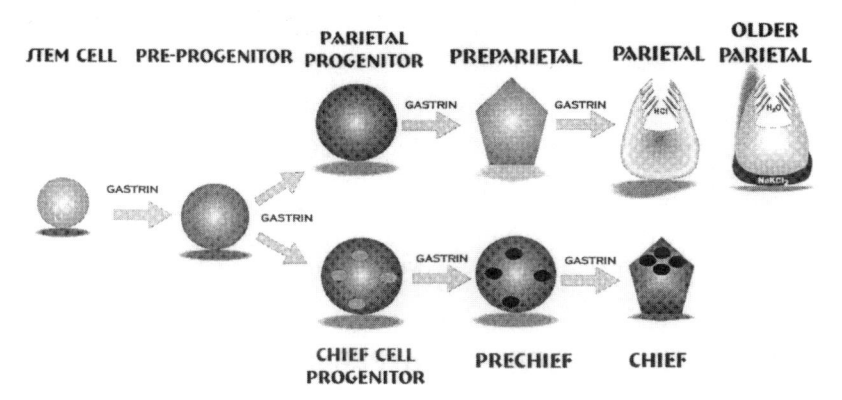

Figure 4. A simplified diagram of the development of gastric fundic epithelial cells with possible sites of action of gastrin on cell growth and differentiation. It seems most likely that a major action of gastrin is on pre-parietal cells in order to explain the hypersection after short-term PPI treatment.

taken for a progenitor cell to commit to a parietal cell lineage and form a parietal cell. This is shown diagrammatically in Figure 4.

Hence, the development of an increased secretory capacity occurs more quickly than that expected from the half-life of parietal cells if there is a significant number of pre-parietal or even parietal progenitor cells at the time of initiation of hypergastrinaemia.

The half-life of the parietal cell is between 90 and 120 days; hence the decay of a larger parietal cell mass after effective hypergastrinaemia will take the same time. If there is a higher than normal acid secretion due to hypergastrinaemia or some other hormonal disturbance (e.g. increased PACAP release from gastric nerves with stimulation of ECL cell growth), about four half-lives of parietal cells will have to pass for acid secretion to normalize. This will be discussed later when considering the effects of *H. pylori* eradication.

Young and old parietal cells are also different. In the deeper part of the gland, parietal cells express the $NaKCl_2$ co-transporter, as if these cells could secrete water in the absence of acid secretion[13]. This could result in a lower concentration of HCl secreted by these cells as compared to the younger, more superficial cells. If gastrin delays the transition of young to older parietal cells, then again, a hypersecretory state could result.

The loss of parietal cells is more likely to be apoptotic as compared to being necrotic. If parietal cell apoptosis is delayed, again the ability of the mucosa to secrete acid will increase. Treatment of rabbits for 3 months or more with omeprazole resulted in an increase in parietal cell mass as well as in H,K-ATPase and pepsinogen levels[14]. Interestingly, the ratio between the ATPase originating from parietal cells and pepsinogen originating in chief cells remained constant. With recent histological evidence for parietal cell hyperplasia in humans following PPI therapy, it is not known whether there is equivalent hyperplasia of chief cells. Prolonged treatment with PPIs would be expected to result in an increased acid-secretory capacity by trophic action on either progenitor or stem cells. Although this is unlikely to account for acid rebound after a short time, given the half-life of the parietal cell it may account for increased secretory capacity after long-term therapy.

The significance of an increase in acid-secretory capacity is not clear, in that there are few studies comparing GERD symptoms after cessation of PPI therapy. One might suppose that at least the frequency of heartburn might increase, but since these patients are in any case on maintenance rather than on demand therapy, it will be difficult to carry out decisive studies.

H. PYLORI ERADICATION AND HYPERSECRETION

Infection of the stomach by *H. pylori* occurs with either antral or fundic dominance, and with often different clinical sequelae. The former predisposes to duodenal ulcer, the latter to atrophic gastritis. When atrophy sets in, the risk of intestinal metaplasia is greater and this also multiplies the risk of gastric cancer. However, it is often considered that some *H. pylori* strains may be commensal, since only $\sim 20\%$ of infections result in symptoms or disease. Another argument is that commensal strains could actually benefit the host by protecting against gastro-oesophageal disease. This is based on the following considerations.

H. pylori synthesize a large amount of urease, up to 15% of their protein. Gastric urea concentration is ~ 1 mM. The presence of urea in the gastric juice is dependent on uncatalysed diffusion from the blood across the epithelium. At pH 5.5 or less there is maximal activity of intra-bacterial urease due to UreI activation. This will provide a sink for urea inside the organism, allowing efficient utilization of gastric urea. Bacterial urease can produce 10 μmol NH_3 per minute per milligram of bacterial protein. The rate of urea entry into gastric juice may be sufficient to maintain saturation of intra-bacterial urease. Depending on the intensity of the infection, relatively large amounts of NH_3 could be produced. With 1 mg bacterial protein in the stomach (a large number of bacteria), 0.6 mmol NH_3 would be produced per hour. This is insufficient to affect the pH of gastric contents with about 15 mmol of HCl produced per hour by the human stomach in relation to meals. Night-time acid secretion is much less, but still sufficient to overwhelm the ammonia production by *H. pylori*.

However, with treatment with PPIs, acid secretion is drastically reduced. On once-daily dosage there is about 70% inhibition of the acid-secretory capacity and on twice-daily dosage there is about 80% inhibition of acid secretion. At this point, although night-time pH is less affected by PPIs than daytime pH, acid production is sufficiently low so that the magnitude of NH_3 production under the highly acidic conditions at night may be sufficient to affect night-time intragastric pH. Data have been presented to show that the pH at night is about 1 unit higher in the presence as compared to the absence of *H. pylori* during PPI treatment[15].

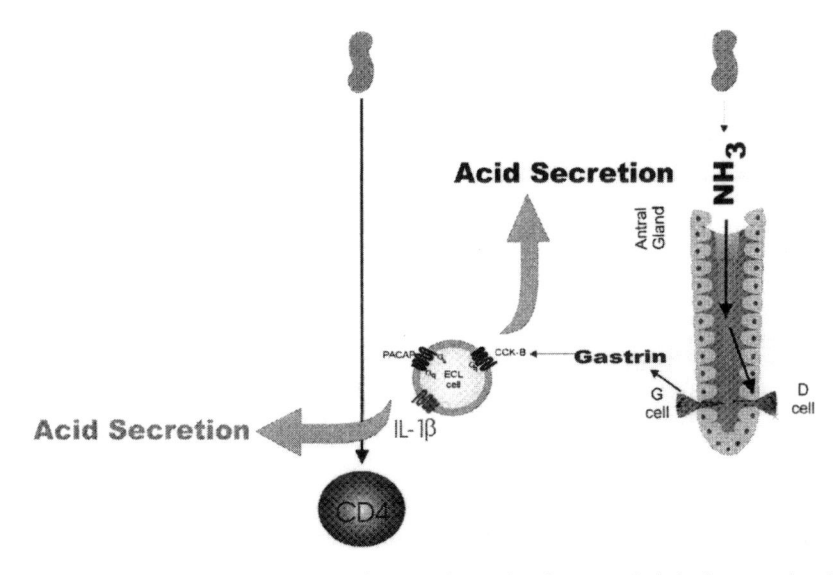

Figure 5. This diagram illustrates the paradox whereby antral infection results in NH_3-dependent hypergastrinaemia and increased acid secretion (although perhaps effective night-time neutralization during PPI therapy), whereas fundic infection elevates IL-1β with a decrease in acid secretion due to inhibition of ECL cell function.

Daytime acidity during PPI treatment might also be affected by the presence of *H. pylori* infection, but this is unlikely to be related to the ammonia-generating ability given the amount of acid secreted, even with treatment by PPIs. Hence, if this is found to be the case, and there are publications claiming this, it must be accounted for by an effect of *H. pylori* on the gastric response to stimulation, not on neutralization of acid secretion.

In the first case one might anticipate worsening of night-time GERD, and in the second case a worsening of ambulatory GERD during PPI treatment when *H. pylori* is eradicated. The situation is also complicated by the different consequences of antral as compared to fundic infection.

Antral infection results in a tendency towards hypersecretion and, if associated with GERD, eradication will reduce the secretory load. Fundic infection results in a tendency for hyposecretion, especially when gastric atrophy sets in. But even before that, production of IL-1β has resulted in inhibition of ECL cell function, in particular its response to hypergastrinaemia. Perhaps eradication here might restore some of the secretory capacity of the stomach. In both sites of infection it is easy to see how acid control by PPIs might be worsened. However, it is easier to treat acid hypersecretion than the risk of gastric cancer or peptic ulcer disease, hence the presence of GERD associated with acid hyposecretion due to *H. pylori* is insufficient grounds to withhold eradication treatment; not until at least the basis for pathogenicity of the organism is fully understood and available on a routine screening basis. Some of these aspects of *H. pylori* effects on acid secretion are illustrated in Figure 5.

References

1. Black JW, Duncan WAM, Durant CJ et al. Definition and antagonism of histamine H2-receptors. Nature. 1972;236:385–7.
2. Sachs G, Shin JM, Briving C et al. The pharmacology of the gastric acid pump: the H^+,K^+ ATPase. Annu Rev Pharmacol Toxicol. 1995;35:277–305.
3. Warren JR, Marshall B. Unidentified curved bacilli on gastric epithelium in active chronic gastritis. Lancet. 1983;1:1273–5.
4. Labenz J, Stolte M, Domian et al. High-dose omeprazole plus amoxicillin or clarithromycin cures Helicobacter pylori infection in duodenal ulcer disease. Digestion. 1995;56:14–20.
5. Yanagisawa K, Yang H, Walsh JH, Tache Y. Role of acetylcholine, histamine and gastrin in the acid response to intracisternal injection of the TRH analog, RX 77368, in the rat. Regul Peptides. 1990;27:161–70.
6. Zeng N, Athmann C, Kang T et al. Role of PACAP in regulation of ECL cell function and acid secretion. J Clin Inv. 1999;194:1383–91.
7. Mungan Z, Ozmen V, Ertan A, Arimura A. Effect of PACAP on gastric acid secretion in rats. Peptides. 1995;16:1051–6.
8. Nwokolo CU, Smith JT, Gavey C, Sawyer A, Pounder RE. Tolerance during 29 days of conventional dosing with cimetidine, nizatidine, famotidine or ranitidine. Aliment Pharmacol Ther. 1990;4(Suppl. 1):29–45.
9. Gedda K, Scott D, Besancon M et al. Turnover of the gastric H^+,K^+-adenosine triphosphatase alpha subunit and its effect on inhibition of rat gastric acid secretion. Gastroenterology. 1995;109:1134–41.
10. Howden CW, Burget DW, Hunt RH. Appropriate acid suppression for optimal healing of duodenal ulcer and gastro-oesophageal reflux disease. Scand J Gastroenterol Suppl. 1994;201:79–82.
11. Driman DK, Wright C, Tougas G, Riddell RH. Omeprazole produces parietal cell hypertrophy and hyperplasia in humans. Dig Dis Sci. 1996;41:2039–47.
12. Tytgat GN. Possibilities and shortcomings of maintenance therapy in gastroesophageal reflux disease. Dig Surg. 1999;16:1–6.
13. McDaniel N, Lytle C. Parietal cells express high levels of Na–K–2Cl cotransporter on migrating into the gastric gland neck. Am J Phys. 1999;276:G1273–8.
14. Larsson H, Carlsson E, Ryberg B, Fryklund J, Wallmark B. Rat parietal cell function after prolonged inhibition of gastric acid secretion. Am J Phys. 1988;254:G33–9.
15. Haruma K, Mihara M, Okamoto E et al. Eradication of Helicobacter pylori increases gastric acidity in patients with atrophic gastritis of the corpus – evaluation of 24-h pH monitoring. Aliment Pharmacol Ther. 1999;13:155–62.

Section VIII
Helicobacter pylori, Dyspepsia and NSAIDs

43
Current concepts of dyspepsia: the role of the nervous system

P. BERCIK and S. M. COLLINS

INTRODUCTION

Dyspepsia is a term which indicates symptoms referable to the upper gastrointestinal tract. It has recently been defined broadly as 'pain or discomfort centered in the upper abdomen'[1]. Dyspepsia encompasses symptoms such as heartburn, acid regurgitation, excessive burping or belching, abdominal bloating, nausea, and fullness or early satiety. Uninvestigated dyspepsia is considered when no underlying cause for the symptoms has yet been sought. The most common organic causes of dyspepsia are gastro-oesophageal reflux disease (GERD), peptic ulcer disease, biliary disease and dyspepsia associated with medications such as non-steroidal anti-inflammatory drugs (NSAIDs). When no underlying cause can be found, a diagnosis of functional dyspepsia, or non-ulcer dyspepsia, is considered. Dyspepsia has been classified according to the main symptoms as ulcer-like, reflux-like, dysmotility-like and non-specific. This division into symptom-based groups has been criticized, as it has low predictive value for identifying the causes of dyspepsia and the pathophysiological mechanisms involved[2].

This chapter will review the main pathophysiological processes that underlie dyspepsia in the absence of an organic cause: gastrointestinal dysmotility, gastroduodenal visceral sensation and psychological factors.

PATHOPHYSIOLOGY OF FUNCTIONAL DYSPEPSIA

Several theories have been put forward in an attempt to explain symptom generation in functional dyspepsia. Motility disorders, visceral hypersensitivity, psychological factors and, more recently, the role of chronic *Helicobacter pylori* gastritis have been considered. Each of these processes involves the enteric nervous system.

Altered gastric and duodenal motor function

Gastrointestinal motility is controlled by complex interactions between the myogenic system, pacemaker system (ICC), neural system and hormonal factors. Coordinated motility is a result of synchronized activity between these factors. An imbalance between single factors may result in dysmotility and, in turn, in generation of dyspeptic symptoms.

Numerous studies have shown abnormal gastric motility and gastric emptying in patients with functional dyspepsia[3-6]. However, in a recent meta-analysis only about 37% of patients with functional dyspepsia had delayed gastric emptying of solid food as measured by scintigraphy. On average, patients with functional dyspepsia had 1.5 times slower gastric emptying than controls[7]. Although postprandial fullness and vomiting may be independently associated with delayed gastric emptying[8], the predictive value of these symptoms for identifying impaired gastric emptying has been challenged[9]. Delayed gastric emptying may be a consequence of antral dysmotility, either as a result of abnormal gastric slow wave activity, weak antral contractions or antro-pyloro-duodenal dyscoordination. It has been shown that gastric dysrhythmias are more frequently present in patients with functional dyspepsia than in controls[10]. Also, patients with functional dyspepsia have larger fasting and postprandial antral 'areas' detected by ultrasonography, and reduced antral motility. It has been hypothesized that this can be a consequence of low vagal tone, since vagotomy weakens antral motility[11,12]. Antral dysmotility may result in disordered intragastric distribution of the meal, with accumulation of gastric contents in the distended antrum rather than in the corpus[13]. Recently, attention has been focused on impaired gastric relaxation as a possible cause of functional dyspepsia. In a recent report 40% of patients with functional dyspepsia had impaired gastric accommodation to a meal, which was associated with early satiety, but not with delayed gastric emptying[14].

Small intestinal abnormalities may also contribute to symptom generation in functional dyspepsia. Patients with functional dyspepsia have a lower frequency of migrating motor complex (MMC) cycles, higher incidence of retrograde contractions and non-propagating phase III of MMC than asymptomatic subjects[15]. In fasting patients with functional dyspepsia there is also a decreased clearance of exogenous acid from the duodenal bulb, probably due to decreased duodenal motor activity[16].

Abnormal mechano- and chemo-sensitivity

Symptom generation in patients with functional dyspepsia may originate from altered mechanisms at the brain–gut axis in the process of gastric accommodation to a meal. Mearin *et al.* have measured sensory responses to gastric accommodation and cold stress in patients with dyspepsia and in healthy controls. Gastric compliance was similar in patients and in healthy controls, but isobaric distension induced more upper abdominal discomfort in dyspeptic patients. Altered perception seemed to be limited to the stomach, because cold stress results, as well as autonomic responses, were similar in both groups. The authors concluded that abnormal afferent sensory pathways are a major mechanism in functional dyspepsia[17]. Gastric hypersensitivity in functional dyspepsia, with normal duodenal and somatic sensitivity, has also been suggested by others[18,19]. The latter study found that gastric hypersensitivity was accompanied by a defective gastric relaxation in response to duodenal distension[19]. Gastric wall tension, and not intragastric volume, determines the perception of gastric distension at least below nociceptive stimuli[20]. This suggests that gastric hypersensitivity is mediated by lower threshold of tension receptors present in the gastric wall. The other possibility is that abnormal gastric sensory function in dyspepsia may result from disturbed vagal function. This was suggested in studies showing that a lower sensory and pain threshold for gastric distension was associated with a diminished pancreatic polypeptide (PP) response to insulin-induced hypoglycaemia[21,22]. In accordance with these findings, some patients with functional dyspepsia have a reduced release of PP after sham feeding, indicating impaired cholinergic vagal function[23].

Sensory function of the duodenum may be impaired in some patients with dyspepsia. It has been reported that patients with irritable bowel syndrome (IBS) and functional dyspepsia have a decreased sensitivity to duodenal distension[24]. Mechano-sensitivity is not the only component of the sensory system which seems to be impaired in patients with dyspepsia. Nausea is induced in dyspeptic patients, but not in healthy volunteers, when acid is perfused into the duodenum[16]. Also, dyspeptic patients have increased sensitivity to intraduodenal lipid. In contrast to controls, lipid sensitizes their stomachs to distension[25]. Sensitization to distension seems to be specific to lipids and not to glucose in patients with functional dyspepsia[26].

Mechanisms of visceral hypersensitivity

Visceral hypersensitivity found in patients with functional dyspepsia can be explained by one or more of the following mechanisms. First, patients with IBS and patients with functional dyspepsia often have overlapping symptoms and may, therefore, share similar pathophysiological mechanisms. Patients with IBS have hypervigilance for visceral stimuli – such as rectal distension, which manifests as a lower discomfort threshold, together with rectal hypersensitivity. It has been proposed that hypervigilance, or the anticipation of discomfort by patients, contributes to the reporting of discomfort following stepwise increases in rectal distension[27].

Second, peripheral and central mechanisms have been proposed to underlie the development of hyperalgesia. Central mechanisms may involve the central processing of pain signals[28] or changes in descending spinal pathways that modulate afferent signals. Peripheral sensitization involves the recruitment of normally silent pain fibres by chemicals such as 5-HT or mediators released from inflammatory cells. Inflammation is invariably used in animal models to predictably induce hyperalgesia; for a review of these processes see Mayer and Gebhart[29]. Briefly, inflammation releases many active substances such as ions, amines, kinins, cytokines, prostanoids and growth factors, which can either directly activate peripheral nerve endings or, more probably, induce functional and structural alterations in sensory neurons. This includes early post-translational changes in the terminals of sensory neurons (peripheral sensitization), which result in increased sensitivity and lower threshold. The mechanisms involved include an increase in inward currents and phosphorylation of membrane-bound receptors/ion channels. Excitability of dorsal horn neurons is also affected by C fibre activity, which results in increased responsiveness to low- and high-intensity stimuli (central sensitization). These mechanisms alter basal sensitivity to painful and to, normally non-painful stimuli. In addition, there are later and long-lasting transcription-dependent changes in effector genes in the dorsal root ganglia and dorsal horn neurons. This process is a consequence of activity-dependent changes in neurons, together with production of specific molecules that initiate particular signal-transduction pathways. The pathways phosphorylate membrane proteins, thus changing their function, and activate transcription factors, altering gene expression. This results in phenotype alteration of low-threshold Aβ fibres which acquire the neurochemical features of C fibres (progressive tactile hypersensitivity)[30]. It has been shown that inflammation increases, in a neural growth factor-dependent manner, expression of substance P in C fibres, but also induces *de-novo* expression of this neurokinin in some A fibres[31].

Thirdly, increased sensitivity of vagal afferents to mechanical or chemical stimuli may result in altered effector responses and produce abnormal gastric wall contraction, resulting in changes in motility or wall compliance. Patients with functional dyspepsia have an altered duodenal sensory system, and this may result in defective gastric accommodation and hypersensitivity.

Since inflammatory processes can induce visceral hypersensitivity, the possible role of *H. pylori*-induced gastritis has long been suspected as a basis for functional dyspepsia. Clinical studies on the impact of *H. pylori* eradication on symptoms in functional dyspepsia have not generated a clear vision of the role of this infection. Essentially, short-term follow-up studies indicate no benefit. Whatever benefit results from eradication is only seen in long-term follow-up. At the end of this chapter we provide some insights from an animal model of *H. pylori* infection that have a bearing on this controversial topic.

Psychological factors, effect of stress, autonomic imbalance

There is evidence that psychological factors are associated with functional dyspepsia. In a case–control study by Talley *et al.*, patients with functional dyspepsia were more likely to be anxious, neurotic and depressed than controls[32]. This was confirmed in another study in which somatic symptoms and psychological measures were compared between 100 patients with dyspepsia, 100 patients with ulcer disease and 100 healthy controls. Patients with dyspepsia had higher levels of state–trait anxiety, general psychopathology, depression, a lower level of functioning and more somatic complaints from different organ systems than patients with ulcer disease or controls[33]. The importance of psychological factors in the management of dyspepsia is illustrated by a study by Mearin *et al.* in which placebo treatment for 8 weeks improved symptoms in 80% of patients with functional dyspepsia. Interestingly, clinical improvement was accompanied by an increased number of phase III of the MMC starting in the gastric antrum, and by an improved antral motility index in a subset of patients who had antral hypomotility. The changes in gastric motility, however, were independent of detectable changes in hypersensitivity to gastric distension[34].

Autonomic imbalance could also be involved in the pathogenesis of dyspepsia. In patients with functional dyspepsia there is lower vagal tone and higher sympathetic tone both before and after acute mental stress[35].

Chronic *H. pylori* infection

H. pylori is the most important cause of peptic ulcers, and plays an aetiological role in gastric cancer, but its role in dyspepsia in the absence of ulcers is unclear[36,37]. Given the spectrum of upper gastrointestinal disease attributable to *H. pylori* it is clearly important to know if a patient with frequent upper gastrointestinal symptoms has a *H. pylori* infection. The presence of *H. pylori* infection increases the likelihood that organic disease will be present[38]; however, its role in functional dyspepsia remains highly controversial.

Data from meta-analysis studies support a role of *H. pylori* in functional dyspepsia. A recent study has shown that the summary odds ratio for *H. pylori* infection in patients with functional dyspepsia is 1.6 (1.4–1.8). Moreover, the odds ratio for improvement of symptoms after eradication therapy is 1.9 (1.3–2.6)[39]. There are, on the other hand, numerous studies with conflicting results. Studies investigating the possible pathophysiological mechanisms underlying functional dyspepsia have revealed a number of functional changes, which might be related to *H. pylori* infection. However, large, prospective studies investigating symptom relief after cure of *H. pylori* infection have failed to show a consistent association between *H. pylori* and the presence of dyspeptic symptoms.

Abnormal gastric emptying is considered one of the possible mechanisms that lead to dyspeptic symptoms. Is there clinical evidence for *H. pylori*-induced changes in gastric emptying? A study in *H. pylori*-positive and *H. pylori*-negative patients with dyspepsia showed no difference in gastric emptying rates between groups; however, eradication of the infection improved symptoms and accelerated gastric emptying in seven out of 11 patients, who cleared the infection[40]. Similarly, perturbed (either rapid or delayed) gastric emptying and dyspeptic symptoms in *H. pylori*-positive patients with functional dyspepsia normalized after eradication therapy. Interestingly, *H. pylori* eradication therapy did not affect gastric emptying in patients who had a pre-treatment gastric emptying within normal parameters[41]. Others have shown that, in patients with functional dyspepsia and *H. pylori* infection, antral motility increases and the antral diameter decreases together with normalization of electric control activity after eradication of the infection[42]. There are, however, some negative reports that show that eradication treatment does not affect gastric emptying of solids in patients with functional dyspepsia[43–45].

Sensory nerves may also be affected by chronic *H. pylori* infection. A study by Thumshirn *et al.* have shown that *H. pylori* infection increases postprandial gastric sensation in patients with functional dyspepsia but does not influence gastric accommodation[46]. Another study has found that patients with functional dyspepsia and high anti-*H. pylori* titres have a lower threshold for first perception in response to duodenal distension when compared with patients with low or no anti-*H. pylori* titres. However, no difference was found between *H. pylori*-positive and *H. pylori*-negative patients[47]. Therefore, it is possible that the degree of immune response examined histologically[48] or by levels of anti-*H. pylori* antibody titres[47], may be an important factor in determining the degree of functional changes. Not all studies support the hypothesis that chronic *H. pylori* infection affects sensory nerves contributing to the generation of symptoms in functional dyspepsia. Two studies have found no association between *H. pylori* infection and gastric hypersensitivity to distension in patients with functional dyspepsia[43,45].

It is clear that clinical studies investigating the role of chronic *H. pylori* infection and dyspepsia have produced conflicting data. Functional dyspepsia is a multifactorial symptom complex rather than a specific disease entity[49]. One explanation for the discrepancy between studies is that *H. pylori* is one of many causes of dyspepsia, and the presence of an *H. pylori* infection in a given patient does not exclude the presence of other causes of dyspepsia, that will remain after antimicrobial therapy. Other factors such as host response to the infection, degree and distribution of gastritis and difference in virulence of *H. pylori* strains may also contribute in preventing us reaching a definite conclusion.

There are also conflicting data arising from trials designed to investigate symptomatic benefit after cure of the *H. pylori* infection. In a multicentre, double-blind study, 328 patients, in whom GERD or a history of peptic ulcer disease was excluded, were randomly assigned either to eradication therapy or to omeprazole treatment for 1 week. In the omeprazole-treated group 20.7% of patients were symptom-free or with minimal symptoms 12 months after treatment. In the group receiving a combination of antibiotics and omeprazole 27.4% of patients were symptom-free, but not statistically different from those who had not received eradication therapy. Gastritis was healed in 3.0% and in 75.0% of patients, respectively[50]. Conversely, a parallel randomized placebo-controlled study, performed in the UK, showed that eradication treatment was more likely to resolve symptoms 12 months after treatment. The number of patients in whom the treatment was successful in the latter study was unusually low (21% in the eradication treatment group vs. 7% in the omeprazole group)[51]. Another randomized placebo-controlled study, performed by Talley *et al.*, showed no evidence of symptom improvement 12 months after eradication of *H. pylori* infection in patients with functional dyspepsia when compared with a placebo-treated group[52]. A multicentre, randomized, double-blind, placebo-controlled study by Talley *et al.* showed a significant association between gastritis scores and treatment success. In this study 32% of patients with mild or no gastritis were free of symptoms vs. 17% of patients who had persistent gastritis[48].

The majority of the above studies have been performed in patients with investigated dyspepsia, and studies investigating neuromuscular or sensory function in asymptomatic subjects with *H. pylori* infection are lacking. A detailed study comparing gastric and vagal function in eight *H. pylori*-positive and eight *H. pylori*-negative asymptomatic volunteers showed lower gastric accommodation in response to meal ingestion in infected subjects. Gastric emptying, gastric tone and phasic contraction, perception and vagal functions were similar between the two groups[53]. Clearly, there is a need for studies investigating the pathophysiological mechanisms of *H. pylori* in dyspepsia. Such studies should ideally control for confounding factors. A more feasible approach would be to develop an animal model for *H. pylori*-induced neuromuscular and sensory changes. To date, data on the effect of *H. pylori* infection on motor activity in animal models or in healthy volunteers, are sparse. One study in rats has shown that *H. pylori* lipopolysaccharide decreases, in a dose-dependent manner, gastric emptying of liquids *in vivo*[54].

Evidence of neural dysfunction in a mouse model of *H. pylori*-induced gastritis

Female Balb/c mice were infected with the Sydney strain of *H. pylori* (load of 10^9 bacteria per mouse) on days 1, 3 and 5. *In vitro*: mice were sacrificed at 2 weeks (acute infection) and 3–6 months post-infection (chronic infection) and compared to their relative controls. The antral full muscle strips were suspended in a muscle bath and evaluated for longitudinal muscle contractility after pharmacological stimulation (carbachol 10^5 M, KCl 50 mM) and electrical field stimulation (EFS) (at nerve or muscle parameters). Acetylcholine release from the strips was measured after preloading the tissue with [^{3}H]choline in response to EFS and KCl stimulation. The amount of acetylcholine released was expressed as a percentage of total choline uptake by the tissue. *In vivo*, a series of experiments was performed to determine gastric emptying and antroduodenal motility in mice. Mice were gavaged intragastrically with barium and fluoroscoped for 4 min. Video images were recorded and digitized. The frequency and velocity of propagation of gastric and duodenal contraction were measured, as described elsewhere[55]. Gastric emptying was measured as gastric surface area multiplied by mean optical density of contrast media in the stomach.

Muscle contractility, as evaluated by carbachol and KCl, tended to be higher during acute infection, but this difference did not reach statistical significance. During chronic infection, muscle contractility was not affected when compared to controls. In contrast to pharmacological stimulation, contractility assessed by EFS (muscle parameters) was increased during acute infection. During chronic infection, muscle function was similar to controls. When applying nerve stimulation by EFS, muscle relaxation was induced. This suggests that antral muscle is under physiological neural inhibitory control. This inhibitory control was significantly enhanced during chronic *H. pylori* infection. Acetylcholine (ACh) release by EFS was lower during chronic infection, which is in accordance with the finding of increased neural inhibition. Stimulating release with KCl gives us information about the total releasable pool of the neurotransmitter in the tissue. During chronic infection, increased amounts of ACh were released, likely as a result of a compensatory mechanism. These *in-vitro* data thus show that chronic *H. pylori* infection induces changes in the neural circuitry of the stomach[56]. However, the question remains to what extent these changes are reflected *in vivo*.

In-vivo experiments have shown that mice with chronic *H. pylori* infection had a larger gastric surface area, which means the stomach was more distended, when compared to control animals. This was associated with delayed gastric emptying in infected animals. However, we have not observed any differences with respect to the frequency or velocity of gastric or duodenal contractions. These results together suggest that chronic *H. pylori* infection delays gastric emptying in mice, probably as a result of impaired neural circuitry[57]. This model of infection-induced changes in gastric neuromuscular function may be useful in our understanding of putative mechanisms involved in the pathogenesis of functional dyspepsia.

The role of the nervous system in dyspepsia

Functional dyspepsia is heterogeneous not only in terms of its clinical presentation but also in terms of its pathogenesis and pathophysiology. The authors believe that *H. pylori* infection is a factor in the pathogenesis of at least a subset of patients with functional dyspepsia. Whether this variability reflects properties of the bacterium or in the host response remains to be determined. The heterogeneity in the pathophysiology of functional dyspepsia is evident. Some patients have demonstrable motor activity whereas others have evidence of visceral hyperalgesia to mechanical or chemical stimuli. These two processes are clearly not mutually exclusive; altered sensory input will alter motility and altered gastric wall tone will influence mechanoreceptor activity. In addition, changes in the distribution and emptying of gastric contents may have effects on chemoreceptor responses. The common factor in each of these processes is the enteric nervous system, and it is the study of this system that will ultimately yield the most important information on the underlying basis for symptom generation in dyspepsia.

References

1. Talley NJ, Stanghellini V, Heading R, Koch KL, Malagelada JR, Tytgat GNJ. Functional gastroduodenal disorders: a working team report for the Rome II consensus on functional gastrointestinal disorders. Gut. 1999;45(Suppl. 2):II37–42.
2. Talley NJ, Weaver AL, Tesmer DL, Zinsmeister A. Lack of discriminant value of dyspepsia subgroups in patients referred for upper endoscopy. Gastroenterology. 1993;105:1378–86.
3. Rees WDW, Miller LJ, Malagelada JR. Dyspepsia, antral motor dysfunction, and gastric stasis of solids. Gastroenterology. 1980;78:360–5.
4. Malagelada JR, Stanghelini V. Manometric evaluation of functional upper gut symptoms. Gastroenterology. 1985;88:1223–31.
5. Camilleri M, Malagelada JR, Kao PC, Zinsmeister AR. Gastric and autonomic responses to stress in functional dyspepsia. Dig Dis Sci. 1986;31:1169–77.
6. Waldron B, Cullen PT, Kumar R *et al.* Evidence of hypomotility in non-ulcer dyspepsia: a prospective multifactorial study. Gut. 1991;32:246–51.
7. Quartero AO, de Witt NJ, Lodders AC, Numans ME, Smout AJPM, Hoes AW. Disturbed solid-phase gastric emptying in functional dyspepsia. A meta-analysis. Dig Dis Sci. 1998;43:2028–33.
8. Stanghelini V, Tosetti C, Paternico A *et al.* Risk indicators of delayed gastric emptying of solids in patients with functional dyspepsia. Gastroenterology. 1996;110:1036–42.
9. Talley NJ, Shuter B, McCrudden G, Jones M, Hoschl R, Piper DW. Lack of association between gastric emptying of solids and symptoms in non-ulcer dyspepsia. J Clin Gastroenterol. 1989;11:625–30.

10. Geldof H, van der Schee EJ, van Blankenstein M, Grashuis JL. Electrogastrographic study of gastric myoelectrical activity in patients with unexplained nausea and vomiting. Gut. 1986;27:799–808.
11. Hveem K, Hausken T, Svebak S, Berstad A. Gastric antral motility in functional dyspepsia. Effect of mental stress and cisapride. Scand J Gastroenterol. 1996;31:452–7.
12. Hausken T, Svebak S, Wilhemsen I et al. Low vagal tone and antral dysmotility in patients with functional dyspepsia. Psychosom Med. 1993;55:12–22.
13. Troncon LE, Bennet RJ, Ahluwalia NK, Thompson DG. Abnormal intragastric distribution of food in functional dyspepsia patients. Gut. 1994;35:327–32.
14. Tack J, Piessevaux H, Coulie B, Caenepeel P, Janssens J. Role of impaired gastric accommodation to a meal in functional dyspepsia. Gastroenterology. 1998;115:1346–52.
15. Jebbink HJA, vanBerge-Henegouwen GP, Akkermans LMA, Smout AJPM. Small intestinal motor abnormalities in patients with functional dyspepsia demonstrated by ambulatory manometry. Gut. 1996;38:694–700.
16. Samsom M, Verhagen MAMT, vanBerge Henegouwen GP, Smout AJPM. Abnormal clearance of exogenous acid and increased acid sensitivity of the proximal duodenum in dyspeptic patients. Gastroenterology. 1999;116:515–20.
17. Mearin F, Cucala M, Aspiroz F, Malagelada JR. The origin of symptoms on the brain–gut axis in functional dyspepsia. Gastroenterology. 1991;101:999–1006.
18. Lemann M, Dederding JP, Flourie B et al. Abnormal perception of visceral pain in response to gastric distension in chronic idiopathic dyspepsia. The irritable stomach syndrome. Dig Dis Sci. 1991;36:1249–54.
19. Coffin B, Aspiroz F, Guarner F, Malagelada JR. Selective gastric hypersensitivity and reflex hypoactivity in functional dyspepsia. Gastroenterology. 1994;107:1345–51.
20. Distrutti E, Aspiroz F, Soldevilla A, Malagelada JR. Gastric wall tension determines perception of of gastric distension. Gastroenterology. 1999;116:1035–42.
21. Holtmann G, Goebell H, Jockenhoevel F, Talley NJ. Altered vagal and intestinal mechanosensory function in chronic unexplained dyspepsia. Gut. 1998;24:501–6.
22. Klatt S, Pieramico O, Guether B, Glassbrenner B, Beckh K, Adler G. Gastric hypersensitivity in non-ulcer dyspepsia. An inconsistent finding. Dig Dis Sci. 1997;24:720–3.
23. Greydanus MP, Vassallo M, Camilleri M et al. Neurohormonal factors in functional dyspepsia: insights on pathophysiological mechanisms. Gatroenterology. 1991;110:1311–18.
24. Holtmann G, Goebell H, Talley NJ. Functional dyspepsia and irritable bowel syndrome: is there a common pathophysiological basis? Am J Gastroenterol. 1997;92:954–9.
25. Barbera R, Feinle C, Read NW. Abnormal sensitivity to duodenal lipid infusion in patients with functional dyspepsia. Eur J Gastroentererol Hepatol. 1995;7:1051–7.
26. Barbera R, Feinle C, Read NW. Nutrient-specific modulation of gastric mechanosensitivity in patients with functional dyspepsia. Dig Dis Sci. 1995;40:1636–41.
27. Naliboff BD, Munakata J, Fullerton S et al. Evidence for two distinct perceptual alterations in irritable bowel syndrome. Gut. 1997;41:505–12.
28. Silverman DH, Munakata JA, Ennes H, Mandelkern MA, Hoh CK, Mayer EA. Regional cerebral activity in normal and pathological perception of visceral pain. Gastroenterology. 1997;112:64–72.
29. Mayer EA, Gebhart GF. Basic and clinical aspects of visceral hyperalgesia. Gastroenterology. 1994,107.271–93.
30. Woolf CJ, Costigan M. Transcriptional and posttranslational plasticity and the generation of inflammatory pain. Proc Natl Acad Sci USA. 1999;96:7723–30.
31. Nicholas RS, Winter J, Wren P, Bergmann R, Woolf CJ. Peripheral inflammation increases the capsaicin sensitivity of dorsal root ganglion neurons in a nerve growth factor-dependent manner. Neuroscience. 1999;91:1425–33.
32. Talley NJ, Fung LH, Gilligan IJ, McNeil D, Piper DW. Association of anxiety, neuroticism, and depression with dyspepsia of unknown cause. A case control study. Gastroenterology. 1986;90:886–92.
33. Haug TT, Svebak S, Wilhelmsen I, Berstad A, Ursin H. Psychological factors and somatic symptoms in functional dyspepsia. A comparison with duodenal ulcer and healthy controls. J Psychosom Res. 1994;38:281–91.
34. Mearin F, Balboa A, Zarate N, Cucala M, Malagelada JR. Placebo in functional dyspepsia: symptomatic, gastrointestinal motor, and gastric sensorial responses. Am J Gastroenterol. 1999;94:116–25.

35. Hweem K, Svebak S, Hausken T, Berstad A. Effect of mental stress and cisapride on autonomic nerve functions in functional dyspepsia. Scand J Gastroenterol. 1998;33:123–7.
36. Veldhuyzen van Zanten SJO. The role of *H. pylori* in NUD? Scand J Gastroenterol. 1997;11:63–9.
37. Talley NJ, Hunt RH. What role does *Helicobacter pylori* play in dyspepsia and non-ulcer dyspepsia? Arguments for and against *H. pylori* being associated with dyspeptic symptoms. Gastroenterology. 1997;113:S67–77.
38. McColl KEL, El-Nujumi A, Murray L et al. The *H. pylori* breath test: a surrogate marker for peptic ulcer disease in dyspeptic patients. Gut. 1997;40:302–6.
39. Jaakkimainen RL, Boyle E, Tudiver F. Is *Helicobacter pylori* associated with non-ulcer dyspepsia and will eradication improve symptoms? A meta-analysis. Br Med J. 1999;319:1040–4.
40. Murakami K, Fujioka T, Shiota K et al. Influence of *Helicobacter pylori* infection and the effects of its eradication on gastric emptying in non-ulcerative gastritis. Eur J Gastroenterol Hepatol. 1995;S1:S93–7.
41. Miyaji H, Azuma T, Ito S et al. The effect of *Helicobacter pylori* eradication therapy on gastric antral myoelectrical activity and gastric emptying in patients with non-ulcer dyspepsia. Aliment Pharmacol Ther. 1999;13:1473–80.
42. Thor P, Lorens K, Tabor S, Herman R, Konturek JW, Konturek SJ. Dysfunction in gastric myoelectrical and motor activity in *Helicobacter pylori*-positive gastritis patients with non-ulcer dyspepsia. J Physiol Pharmacol. 1996;47:469–76.
43. Mearin F, de Ribot X, Balboa A et al. Does *Helicobacter pylori* infection increase gastric sensitivity in functional dyspepsia? Gut. 1995;37:47–51.
44. Parente F, Imbesi V, Maconi G et al. Effects of *Helicobacter pylori* eradication on gastric function indices in functional dyspepsia. Scand J Gastroenterol. 1998;33:461–7.
45. Rhee PL, Kim YH, Son HJ et al. Lack of association of *Helicobacter pylori* infection with gastric hypersensitivity or delayed gastric emptying in functional dyspepsia. Am J Gastroenterol. 1999;94:3165–9.
46. Thumshirn M, Camilleri M, Saslow SB, Williams DE, Burton DD, Hanson RB. Gastric accommodation in non-ulcer dyspepsia and the roles of *Helicobacter pylori* infection and vagal function. Gut. 1999;44:55–64.
47. Holtmann G, Talley NJ, Goebel H. Association between *H. pylori*, duodenal mechanosensory thresholds, and small intestinal motility in chronic unexplained dyspepsia. Dig Dis Sci. 1996;41:1285–91.
48. Talley NJ, Janssens J, Lauritsen K, Racz I, Bolling-Sternevald E. Eradication of *Helicobacter pylori* in functional dyspepsia: randomised double blind placebo controlled trial with 12 months' follow up. The Optimal Regimen Cures *Helicobacter* Induced Dyspepsia (ORCHID) Study Group. Br Med. J. 1999;318:833–7.
49. Armstrong D. *Helicobacter* infection and dyspepsia. Scand J Gastroenterol. Suppl. 1996;215:38–47.
50. Blum AL, Talley NJ, O'Morrain C et al. Lack of effect of treating *Helicobacter pylori* infection in patients with non-ulcer dyspepsia. Omeprazole plus Clarithromycin and Amoxicillin Effect One Year after Treatment (OCAY) Study Group. N Engl J Med. 1998;339:1875–81.
51. McColl K, Murray L, El-Omar E et al. Symptomatic benefit from eradicating *Helicobacter pylori* infection in patients with non-ulcer dyspepsia. N Engl J Med. 1998;339:1869–74.
52. Talley NJ, Vakil N, Ballard ED 2nd, Fenerty MB. Absence of benefit of eradicating *Helicobacter pylori* in patients with non-ulcer dyspepsia. N Engl J Med. 1999;341:1106–11.
53. Saslow SB, Thurmshirn M, Camilleri M et al. Influence of *H. pylori* infection on gastric motor and sensory function in asymptomatic volunteers. Dig Dis Sci. 1998;43:258–64.
54. Okumura T, Shoji E, Takahashi N et al. Delayed gastric emptying by *Helicobacter pylori* lipopolysaccharide in conscious rats. Dig Dis Sci. 1998;43:90–4.
55. Bercik P, Bouley L, Dutoit P, Blum AL, Kucera P. Quantitative analysis of intestinal motor patterns: spatio-temporal organisation of non-neural pacemaker sites in the rat ileum. Gastroenterology. 2000 (In press).
56. Bercik P, Blennerhassett P, Collins SM. *Helicobacter pylori* infection induces *in vitro* evidence of neural dysfunction in the murine gastric antrum. Gastroenterology. 2000;118:A3996 (abstract).
57. Bercik P, Blennerhassett P, Verdu EF, Collins SM. *Helicobacter pylori* infection delays gastric emptying in mice. Gastroenterology. 2000;118:A865 (abstract).

44
How to explain outcome differences in dyspepsia studies

M. B. FENNERTY and L. A. LAINE

INTRODUCTION

Dyspepsia, defined as discomfort in the upper abdomen, is a widely prevalent clinical symptom[1]. With the establishment of *Helicobacter pylori* infection as a major aetiological factor in peptic ulcer disease, which is one of the many causes of symptoms of dyspepsia, it was not surprising that investigation into the association between *H. pylori* infection and non-ulcer dyspepsia (NUD) was also undertaken. Epidemiological studies demonstrated a modest relationship between *H. pylori* and NUD that then resulted in numerous early clinical treatment trials. These early trial results were largely uninterpretable because of serious methodological deficiencies. They were either non-randomized, non-blinded, used inappropriate controls, had too small a sample size, had inappropriate study populations or did not use validated dyspepsia instrument measures, etc.[2]. However, more recently there have been a number of large, well-designed, randomized, placebo-controlled trials using validated instruments with adequate observation periods assessing the response of NUD to the treatment of *H. pylori* infection[3-6]. Unfortunately, these trials have reached discordant conclusions. There are a number of possible explanations for these different outcomes and this discussion will highlight differences in these trials that may explain their discordant results.

TRIALS OF *H. PYLORI* THERAPY IN PATIENTS WITH DYSPEPSIA

Dyspepsia has been a difficult clinical syndrome to investigate because of a number of problems. First and foremost is defining the symptom complex itself, and nearly as important is difficulty in measuring symptom response. Additionally, there were no clinical trials on which to base clinical decisions regarding the treatment of *H. pylori* infection in a patient with dyspepsia. Because of this absence of data from clinical trials, decision analytical models were used to investigate whether there might be a benefit of a 'test-and-treat' strategy in a dyspeptic population[7,8]. These models suggested that this approach was cost-effective if the baseline prevalence of ulcer disease was 5–10% or more in the dyspeptic population. While suggestive of a potential benefit of such a strategy these studies did not conclusively resolve the issue of whether *H. pylori* eradication was effective in resolving dyspeptic symptoms.

In 1991 a working group of experts defined dyspepsia as pain or discomfort centred in the upper abdomen[9]. This discomfort could or could not be related to meals, and specifically symptoms of reflux disease were excluded. These specific criteria defining dyspepsia now allowed for an objective means of enrolling patients in clinical trials. Following this, a number of instruments measuring dyspepsia were developed and validated. The setting was now established for well-designed trials of therapy to be implemented.

Surprisingly, there is still little data from randomized, controlled trials of *H. pylori* eradication treatment and outcomes of dyspepsia. Recently, Moayyedi and colleagues reported the results of a randomized, controlled trial of a community-based screening and treatment programme for *H. pylori* infection and the effect on dyspeptic symptoms over time[10]. Patients in this trial had to be between the ages of 40 and 49 years and were drawn from 36 general practice sites. A urea breath test was used to confirm the diagnosis of *H. pylori* infection and then patients were randomized to treatment with 7 days of a proton pump inhibitor based triple therapy regimen vs. placebo. A validated dyspepsia questionnaire was used to assess response and patients were followed for up to 2 years. Of the 8429 patients recruited, 28% were *H. pylori*-positive; 43% of these patients infected with *H. pylori* had dyspepsia. At conclusion 1751 patients were evaluable at the end of 2 years, and 74% were cured of *H. pylori* infection with active treatment versus only 5% of the placebo-treated subjects. By intention-to-treat analysis there was a clinically significant improvement in the resolution of dyspepsia in the actively treated group. The screening and treatment strategy for dyspepsia resulted in a 5% reduction in dyspepsia over a 2-year period of follow-up. Interestingly, this finding reflects very closely the results predicted by the decision analytical models previously published. While the therapeutic gain is small, the benefit may render this strategy cost-effective. Full analysis of this study, and hopefully other such studies, is needed in order to determine whether treatment of *H. pylori* infection is beneficial in patients with dyspepsia.

TRIALS OF *H. PYLORI* THERAPY IN NUD

The resolution of dyspepsia related to ulcer disease is not surprising to investigators or practitioners. However, the majority of patients with dyspepsia do not have ulcer disease and suffer from NUD. As has been seen in patients with dyspepsia, there is also epidemiological evidence suggesting an increased prevalence of *H. pylori* infection, in those with NUD. Unlike the absence of data available from trials of therapy in patients with dyspepsia, there are now a number of well-designed, randomized, placebo-controlled trials with adequate follow-up using validated instruments on which to base an evidence-based approach to this clinical problem of NUD. However, these studies investigating the treatment of *H. pylori* infection in patients with NUD have produced conflicting results. There are a number of possible explanations for these discrepancies.

The four recent trials represent the highest-quality studies performed to evaluate outcomes of treatment of *H. pylori* infection in patients with NUD[3-6]. The first trial, the UK MRC trial, enrolled 318 NUD patients to either proton pump inhibitor-based triple therapy vs. placebo[6]. Patients were then followed for 1 year using a validated dyspepsia instrument measure (the Glasgow Dyspepsia Severity Scale or GDSS). At the end of 1 year, 21% of patients in the treatment arm had resolution of dyspeptic symptoms compared with only 7% of patients in the placebo arm ($p < 0.001$). Reported concurrently was the result of an international study which enrolled 348 patients from a number of sites throughout Europe, Canada and South Africa[5]. This trial also used a similar treatment strategy with a proton pump inhibitor-based triple therapy compared with placebo. These investigators also followed patients for 1 year using a validated dyspepsia instrument (the Gastrointestinal Symptom Rating Scale, or GSRS). Symptom resolution in this study was 27% in the treatment arm and 21% in the placebo arm, a difference that was not statistically significant. This was followed by a very similar international study, the Orchid study, which also followed patients for 1 year following treatment with a proton pump inhibitor-based triple therapy compared with placebo[4]. In this trial of 278 patients a response was seen in 24% in the treatment arm and 22% in the placebo arm, a result that was not significant. Most recently a multi-centre US study involving 337 patients was reported[3]. Like the above three studies, patients with NUD were randomized to a proton pump inhibitor-based triple therapy compared with placebo, and followed for 1 year using a validated dyspepsia instrument, in this case the GSRS as well. Treatment benefit was seen in 48% of actively treated patients, and 50% of placebo-treated patients.

Recently, Laine *et al.* performed a meta-analysis of the literature involving the *H. pylori* eradication treatment effect on the symptoms of NUD[11]. Seven trials meeting predefined criteria were identified. The common odds ratio for treatment success with *H. pylori* eradication therapy compared with control was 1.2 (95% CI 0.98–1.6; $p = 0.08$). However, there was statistically significant heterogeneity between the studies, and when the one study that resulted in this heterogeneity was excluded from the analysis, the odds ratio was 0.8 (95% CI 0.6–1.1; $p = 0.3$).

IS THERE AN EXPLANATION FOR THESE DISCORDANT RESULTS?

All of the above studies, while being well-designed trials, have methodological differences. A critical appraisal of the studies reveals that there are some differences that are substantial and may, in part, explain the discordant results. While the length of follow-up in these four studies is all for 1 year, many of the earlier trials had used much shorter observation periods that may have confounded their results. This is not an issue in these four trials. Differences in these studies did, however, include definition of resolution of symptoms, differences in the instrument scoring systems used, and differences in the populations studied.

One possible explanation of the discordant results lies in the definition of the resolution of symptoms used in the trials. In the study with a positive treatment effect reported by McColl *et al.*, a scoring system of 0–20 with the GDSS was used. Resolution of symptoms was defined as a score of 0–1. The other three trials that did not demonstrate a treatment effect used a scale of 0–6 in two of the studies (Talley and Blum), and 0–3 in another study (Talley). As in the McColl study, these three trials required a symptom score of 0–1 to meet the definition of resolution of symptoms. Thus, patients in the McColl trial needed to show a proportionally much greater improvement of symptoms to be considered as having symptom resolution compared to patients in the other three trials. This difference in the symptom scales used in these studies may, in part, explain the differences in trial results as the symptom response between control and active treatment groups may be less apparent in trials using a smaller symptom scale.

Another possible explanation of the discordance in trial results may lie in the differences in the instruments used to measure symptoms. In these four studies one used the GDSS and the other three the GSRS. Not only do these instruments have different scales, as discussed above, the GDSS includes in its score frequency of symptoms, effect on normal activities, time off work, consultations with physicians, physician office visits, home visits, testing, and whether the patient is using medications for dyspepsia either over the counter or by prescription. The GSRS measures other dimensions including abdominal pain, reflux indigestion, diarrhoea and constipation. Within a given dimension a seven-point Likert scale is used, and a patient can score between 0 and 6. These different instruments may measure different aspects of dyspepsia, resulting in differences in outcomes of treatment trials, which may also explain differences in the results between these studies.

Another explanation of the discordant results between these four studies may lie in the populations studied. Each of the three negative trials were multicentre and/or multinational studies. The one trial demonstrating treatment success was from a single setting and, furthermore, one-third of the patients in this trial had a predominant symptom of substernal pain or reflux. Some have also postulated that the background prevalence of ulcer disease may be higher in this population, further contributing to a beneficial treatment effect. Whether differences in populations studied account for the differences in outcomes is not known, but is another potential explanation for the discordant results.

CONCLUSIONS

The predominance of evidence suggests that there is no, or little, *H. pylori* eradication treatment effect in patients with dyspepsia, or NUD. Whether specific populations or NUD subtypes benefit from *H. pylori* eradication remains unclear, and cannot be answered based on the available evidence.

Differences in trial design, even though the trials are of high quality, can in part explain the discordant results leading to the above conclusions. Future trials of *H. pylori* eradication therapy in patients with dyspepsia or NUD will need to keep these, and other possible confounders, in mind during trial design and analysis, in order to be able to evaluate the data correctly.

References

1. Talley NJ, Silverstein MD, Agreus L et al. AGA technical review: evaluation of dyspepsia. Gastroenterology. 1997;114:582–95.
2. Talley NJ. A critique of therapeutic trials in *Helicobacter pylori*-positive functional dyspepsia. Gastroenterology. 1994;106:1174–83.
3. Talley NJ, Vakil N, Ballard ED, Fennerty MB. Absence of benefit of eradicating *Helicobacter pylori* in patients with nonulcer dyspepsia. N Engl J Med. 1999;341:1106–11.
4. Talley NJ, Janssens J, Lauritsen K et al. Eradication of *Helicobacter pylori* in functional dyspepsia: randomised double-blind placebo controlled trial with 12 months follow-up. Br Med J. 1999;318:833–7.
5. Blum AL, Talley NJ, O'Morain C et al. Lack of effect of treating *Helicobacter pylori* infection in patients with nonulcer dyspepsia. N Engl J Med. 1998;339:1875–81.
6. McColl K, Murray L, El-Omar E et al. Symptomatic benefit from eradicating *Helicobacter pylori* infection in patients with nonulcer dyspepsia. N Engl J Med. 1998;339:1869–74.
7. Fendrick AM, Chernew M, Hirth R, Bloom B. Alternative management strategies for patients with suspected peptic ulcer disease. Ann Intern Med. 1995;155:922–8.
8. Ofman JJ, Etchason J, Fullerton S et al. Management strategies for *Helicobacter pylori*-seropositive patients with dyspepsia: clinical and economic consequences. Ann Intern Med. 1997;126:280–91.
9. Talley NJ, Colin-Jones D, Kock KL et al. Functional dyspepsia: a classification with guidelines for diagnosis and management. Gastroenterol Int. 1991;4:145–60.
10. Moayyedi P, Feltbower R, Brown J et al. *H. pylori* screening and treatment reduces dyspepsia in the community. Gastroenterology. 1999;116:A81 (abstract).
11. Laine LA, Schoenfeld P, Fennerty MB. *H. pylori* therapy is not effective for treatment of nonulcer dyspepsia: meta-analysis of randomized controlled trials. Gastroenterology. 2000;118 (In press).

45
Helicobacter pylori eradication for dyspepsia is clinically useful

D. McNAMARA and C. O'MORAIN

INTRODUCTION

Dyspepsia, defined as persistent or recurrent pain or discomfort centred in the upper abdomen, is a common condition[1]. It affects 20–40% of the population with an annual prevalence of 25% in the Western world[2–6]. It is a considerable financial burden on the health-care system, accounting for 2–3% of all general practice consultations and representing the third most common presenting complaint[7,8]. It is a chronic recurring condition and as such is responsible for a considerable proportion of over-the-counter medication consumption and work-days lost.

Previously, management involved a trial of acid-suppressants and reassurance with subsequent investigation for treatment failures[9]. The discovery of *Helicobacter pylori* and its causal association with the development of gastritis and peptic ulcer disease has revolutionized our management of these conditions, with successful eradication resulting in healing and prevention of ulcer recurrence[10–15]. The spectrum of conditions associated with this infection has expanded to include gastric cancer, mucosal-associated lymphoid tissue lymphoma (MALT) and non-ulcer dyspepsia, as well as several extra-intestinal diseases[16–18]. The association of *H. pylori* infection with these conditions led to trials of eradication therapy. The weight of evidence to date to support active treatment varies for each condition.

It is universally accepted that *H. pylori* should be sought and eradicated in patients with peptic ulcer disease, early gastric cancer and those with MALT lymphoma. This necessitates investigation by means of endoscopy of all suspected cases, namely patients with dyspepsia, as it has been shown that symptoms are a poor predictor of underlying pathology. However, the majority of patients who present with dyspepsia will not have a peptic ulcer or gastric cancer. Non-ulcer dyspepsia is the most commonly diagnosed condition following endoscopy, even in those who are found to be *H. pylori*-positive[19]. Debate centres on the efficacy of *H. pylori* eradication in patients with non-ulcer dyspepsia, and whether eradication of the bacterium may in some situations be detrimental. In such cases *H. pylori* infection has been suggested to be an innocent bystander!

The advent of effective and economical non-invasive diagnostic tools, urea breath testing (UBT), serology and stool testing, has allowed the primary-care physician to test for, and thus treat, this infection. Non-invasive testing has negated the need for endoscopy unless alarm symptoms are present or the individual is at greater risk of gastric cancer; those >45 years of age.

The question thus arose whether *H. pylori* infection should be diagnosed at a primary-care level and, if documented, whether to treat or to refer for a subsequent endoscopy to establish an additional diagnosis such as peptic ulcer disease, gastro-oesophageal reflux or non-ulcer dyspepsia, and treat selectively based on these diagnoses. These are important and controversial issues.

Recently, both in Europe and Canada, the broader role of *H. pylori* infection as a gastroduodenal pathogen and a public health-care issue was considered and consensus guidelines published[20,21]. Similarly in America a position statement regarding *H. pylori* infection and dyspepsia was issued[22]. While in agreement over many issues they differed considerably in their recommendations to primary health-care physicians and over the central issues of dyspepsia and gastric cancer. Interpretation of available evidence to date may account for the apparent discrepancies, as well as different health-care structures. However, there is a need for consensus, as without consistent guidelines different management practices may develop together with individual practitioners determining the relative advantages and disadvantages of treatment in any one case. Such a situation is less than ideal, particularly in a general practice setting where new evidence is not readily to hand.

The weight of evidence to show a treatment advantage is such that *H. pylori* eradication should be considered in all infected dyspeptic patients who present to their practitioner both to alleviate symptoms and to prevent the long-term sequelae of infection.

HELICOBACTER PYLORI INFECTION AND DYSPEPSIA

H. pylori infection is common, affecting 15–30% of the adult population in the developed world[23]. It is responsible for 90% of duodenal ulcers and 70% of gastric ulcers. *H. pylori* colonization of the gastric mucosa confers a 1:6 and 1:100 lifetime risk of developing a peptic ulcer and gastric cancer, respectively[24,25]. The majority of infected individuals are asymptomatic.

Dyspepsia as a symptom may result from a variety of disease entities. In subjects who develop dyspepsia previous endoscopic studies have reported that 15–20% will have a peptic ulcer, 5–15% gastro-oesophageal reflux, <2% gastric cancer and the majority (60%) non-ulcer dyspepsia (NUD)[26–31]. These studies did not take into account the prevalence of *H. pylori* infection. More recently investigators have examined specifically the role of *H. pylori* in dyspepsia. There is evidence to suggest that *H. pylori* infection precedes the development of dyspepsia. Rosenstock *et al.* investigated a group of asymptomatic individuals and assessed their *H. pylori* status using validated serology. During a 5-year follow-up symptoms were assessed regularly. Results revealed that being *H. pylori*-positive conferred a significantly increased risk of subsequent dyspepsia development. The estimated 1-year prevalence was 13%, and lifetime prevalence 17%[32]. This study confirmed previous work by Parsonett *et al.*, which showed that *H. pylori* infection preceded the onset of dyspepsia in a cohort of epidemiologists[33].

The majority will accept that *H. pylori* is the causal factor responsible for chronic active gastritis, peptic ulcer disease and gastric cancer. However, as shown from these studies, most patients with dyspepsia do not have these conditions. NUD is the most commonly diagnosed condition in investigated patients with dyspepsia, and as shown in these studies *H. pylori* infection is responsible for symptom development and therefore it must have some causal role in NUD. There have been numerous association studies investigating the role of *H. pylori* infection in NUD. *H. pylori* infection is more common in these patients than in asymptomatic controls. A recent meta-analysis of 23 studies reported a summary odds ratio for *H. pylori* and NUD of 1.6[34]. Evidence to date, therefore, confirms an association between *H. pylori* infection and dyspepsia, and links infection with the majority of underlying disease entities.

There is evidence to show that dyspeptic patients with *H. pylori* infection differ from non-infected subjects with regard to the underlying endoscopic diagnosis. McColl *et al.* investigated 318 dyspeptic patients and found a peptic ulcer in 53% of *H. pylori*-positive and only 4% of negative subjects. NUD occurred in 33% and 79% of positive and negative subjects, respectively. The prevalence of gastro-oesophageal reflux disease did not differ significantly based on *H. pylori* status[35]. Thus, *H. pylori* infection may be taken as a risk factor for significant underlying pathology in patients with dyspepsia.

HELICOBACTER PYLORI TREATMENT AND DYSPEPSIA

To date there are few studies which have examined the role of *H. pylori* eradication in patients with non-investigated dyspepsia, a 'test-and-treat' strategy. The evidence from published work suggests that *H. pylori* eradication is of benefit in patients with dyspepsia. Heaney *et al.*, in a prospective randomized study of young dyspeptic patients, demonstrated that symptom scores decreased to similar levels in *H. pylori*-positive subjects who received empirical eradication compared to those who underwent endoscopy and selective treatment based on diagnosis[36]. Slade *et al.* reported similar findings, when studying both a test-and-treat approach and empirical therapy, rather than endoscopy, for seronegative patients with dyspepsia[37]. Moayyedi *et al.* found that the overall symptom reduction was greater in patients who underwent non-invasive *H. pylori* testing and eradication compared to traditional endoscopy and selective treatment. In addition, there was a reduction in the number of general practice consultations and consumption of H_2-receptor antagonists, but not proton pump inhibitors in the test-and-treat group. Unfortunately, the retrospective design of this study limits its interpretation[38].

These studies were all undertaken in secondary care centres, and critics have suggested that this management strategy would not be as effective in primary care. A recent study by Jones et al., undertaken in primary care, found that a test-and-treat strategy for all young H. pylori-positive subjects was not only clinically effective but also cost-effective, reporting an average saving of £200 sterling per patient[39]. Similarly, research by a group in The Netherlands has shown that H. pylori screening and treatment of positive subjects confers both symptomatic, and quality-of-life score improvements, as well as reducing health-care costs in patients with chronic dyspepsia requiring acid-suppression therapy in a general practice setting[40].

Despite this evidence to support H. pylori eradication in young dyspeptic patients the issue is still hotly debated. More studies are required. However, there is a wealth of evidence to show that H. pylori eradication is of benefit for the likely underlying conditions, other than GERD, in patients with dyspepsia. It is universally accepted that H. pylori infection should be treated in patients with peptic ulcer disease. In addition, there is strong supportive evidence to show that H. pylori eradication is of benefit, at least to a subset of patients, with NUD. The debate centres on whether one believes H. pylori infection is effective in NUD.

Numerous eradication trials in NUD have been performed, and to date three meta-analyses have been published. The first by Laheij et al. reviewed 10 studies and found a significant improvement in symptoms for those who received H. pylori eradication and those who remained positive. In all, 73% of successfully treated patients, compared to 45% of those who remained positive, reported symptom improvement[41]. Talley et al., in their meta-analysis, found a significant association between H. pylori infection and NUD (odds ratio of 2.3), but failed to demonstrate any treatment advantage[42]. More recently, Jaakkimainen et al. reported a summary odds ratio for improvement in dyspeptic symptoms in patients with NUD, in whom H. pylori infection was eradicated, of 1.9. This review considered only five studies, citing methodological flaws in the remainder[34]. It would appear from available evidence that H. pylori eradication is of benefit in the long-term management of NUD. This adds additional supportive evidence to promote active H. pylori treatment in subjects who present with dyspepsia.

To be cost-effective any management strategy must be clinically effective. H. pylori testing and subsequent treatment has been examined as to whether it is cost-effective compared to the traditional dyspepsia management strategies of either empirical acid-suppression therapy or endoscopy and subsequent tailored treatments. The studies mentioned previously, in addition to others, have in general found that endoscopy can be avoided in up to 37% of patients managed effectively employing a test-and-treat policy[43].

CONCLUSION

The question asked is whether H. pylori eradication for dyspepsia is clinically useful. The answer is yes! Dyspepsia is a common condition and is responsible for significant morbidity, and indeed mortality. The probable underlying diagnoses in uninvestigated patients are known. Gastric cancer is extremely uncommon in subjects over the age of 45 years and the majority of young *H. pylori*-positive sufferers will have either a peptic ulcer or NUD. Treatment of *H. pylori* infection is of benefit for the majority of probable underlying diagnoses, apart from GERD. However, in patients with GERD there is a body of evidence to support treatment of *H. pylori* infection to prevent the accelerated development of gastric atrophy, in positive patients who require long-term acid suppression[44].

In addition to conferring symptomatic benefit, *H. pylori* treatment, when employed as part of a test-and-treat policy, is also financially superior in comparison with traditional management strategies, as a result of a reduction in the number of endoscopies undertaken, medication consumption and work-days lost.

Lastly *H. pylori* infection is causally associated with the development of both gastric cancer and peptic ulcer. Active treatment of dyspeptic patients will not only treat the current problem, but also prevent the development of these serious sequelae of infection.

References:

1. Talley NJ, Calis-Jones D, Koch KJ et al. Functional dyspepsia: a classification with guidelines for diagnosis and management. Gastroenterol Int. 1991;4:145–60.
2. Jones R, Lydeard SE, Hobbs FD et al. Dyspepsia in England and Scotland. Gut. 1990; 31:401–5.,
3. Drossman DA, Li Z, Andreyzi E et al. Householder survey of functional gastrointestinal disorders: prevalence, sociodemography and health impact. Dig Dis Sci. 1993;38:1569–80.
4. Holtman G, Goebell H, Talley NJ. Dyspepsia in consulters and non consulters: prevalence, health care seeking behavior and risk factors. Eur J Gastroenterol Hepatol. 1994;6:917–24.
5. Johnson R, Straune B, Forde OH. Peptic ulcer and non-ulcer dyspepsia: a disease and a disorder. Scand J Prim Health Care. 1988;23:40–3.
6. Gasburini M, Bassoti G, Bacci G et al. Functional gut and health care seeking behaviour in an Italian non-patient population. Recent Prog Med. 1989;80:241–4.
7. Jones R, Lydeard S. Dyspepsia in the community: a follow up study. Br J Clin Pract. 1992;46:59–97.
8. Knill-Jones RP. Geographical differences in the prevalence of dyspepsia. Scand J Gastroenterol. 1991;26(Suppl. 182):17–24.
9. Health and Public Policy Committee. Endoscopy in the evaluation of dyspepsia. Am Intern Med. 1985;102:266–9.
10. Soll AH. Consensus Conference. Medical treatment of peptic ulcer disease: practice guidelines. Practice Parameters Committee of the American College of Gastroenterology. J Am Med Assoc. 1996;275:622–9.
11. Graham DY. Treatment of peptic ulcers caused by *Helicobacter pylori*. N Engl J Med 1993;328:449–50.
12. NIH Consensus Conference. *Helicobacter pylori* in peptic ulcer disease NIH consensus development panel. J Am Med Assoc. 1994;272:65–9.
13. Glise H. Epidemiology in peptic ulcer disease: current status and future aspects. Scand J Gastroenterol. 1990;175:13–18.
14. Coghlan JG, Gilligan DH, Humphries H et al. *Campylobacter* and recurrence of duodenal ulcers: a 12 month follow up study. Lancet. 1987;2:1109–11.
15. Hopkins RJ, Giardi LS, Turney EA. The relationship between *Helicobacter pylori* eradication and reduced duodenal and gastric ulcer recurrance: a review. Gastroenterology. 1996;110:1244–52.
16. The Eurogast Study Group. An international association between *Helicobacter pylori* infection and gastric cancer. Lancet. 1993;341:1359–62.

17. Wotherspoon DC, Dogliosi C, Diss TC et al. Regression of primary low grade B-cell gastric lymphoma of mucosal associated lymphoid tissue type after eradication of *Helicobacter pylori*. Lancet. 1993;342:575–7.
18. Armstrong D. *Helicobacter pylori* infection and dyspepsia. Scand J Gastroenterol. 1996;31:38–47.
19. Talley NJ, Weaver AL, Tesmer DL et al. Lack of discriminant value of dyspepsia subgroups in patients referred for upper endoscopy. Gastroenterol. 1993;105:1378–86.
20. European *Helicobacter pylori* Study Group. Current European concepts in the management of *Helicobacter pylori* infection. Maastricht Consensus Report. Gut. 1997;41:8–31.
21. Hunt R, Thompson A. Canadian *Helicobacter pylori* consensus conference. Can J Gastroenterology. 1998;12:31–41.
22. American Gastroenterology Association. American Gastroenterology Association medical position statement: evaluation of dyspepsia. Gastroenterology. 1998;114:579–81.
23. Dooley CP, Cohen H, Fitzgibbons PL et al. Prevalence of *Helicobacter pylori* infection and histological gastritis in asymptomatic persons. N Eng J Med. 1989;321:1562–6.
24. Graham DY. Can therapy be denied for *Helicobacter pylori* infection. Gastroenterology. 1997;133:5173–7.
25. Cancer Statistics Review, 1973–1992; Tables and Graphics. Bethesda, MD: NCI; 1995, NIH publications No. 96-2789.
26. Barnes RJ, Gear MW, Nicol A et al. Study of dyspepsia in general practice as assessed by endoscopy and radiology. Br Med J. 1975;4:214–16.
27. Johannesson T, Peterson H, Kleneland PM et al. The predictive value of history in dyspepsia. Scand J Gastroenterol. 1990;25:689–97.
28. Mansi C, Mela GS, Pasini D et al. Patterns of dyspepsia in patients with no clinical evidence of organic disease. Dig Dis Sci. 1990;35:1452–8.
29. Heikkinen M, Pikkarainen P, Takula J et al. Aetiology of dyspepsia. Four hundred unselected consecutive patients in general practice. Scand J Gastroenterol. 1995;30:519–23.
30. Ayoola EA, al-Rashed RS, al-Mofleh IA et al. Diagnostic yield of upper gastrointestinal endoscopy in relation to age and gender: a study of 10,112 Saudi patients. Hepatogastroenterology. 1996;43:405–15.
31. Bytzer P, Schaffalitzky de Muckadell OB. Prediction of major pathological conditions in dyspeptic patients referred for endoscopy: a prospective validation study of a scoring symptoms. Scand J Gastroenterol. 1992;27:987–92.
32. Rosenstock S, Kay L, Rosenstock C et al. Relation between *Helicobacter pylori* infection and gastrointestinal syndromes. Gut. 1997;41:169–76.
33. Parsonnet J, Blaser MJ, Perez-Perez GI et al. Symptoms and factors of *Helicobacter pylori* infection in a cohort of epidemiologists. Gastroenterology. 1992;102:41–6.
34. Jaakikimainen LR, Boyle E, Tudiver F. Is *Helicobacter pylori* associated with non-ulcer dyspepsia and will eradication improve symptoms? A meta-analysis. Br Med J. 1999;319:1040–104.
35. McColl KEL, el-Nujiumi A, Murray L, et al. The *Helicobacter pylori* breath test: a surrogate marker for peptic ulcer disease in dyspeptic patients. Gut. 1997;40:301–6.
36. Heaney A, Collins JS, Watson RG et al. A prospective randomised trial of a test and treat policy versus endoscopy based management in young *Helicobacter pylori* positive patients with ulcer like dyspepsia referred to a hospital clinic. Gut. 1999;45:186–90.
37. Slade PE, Davidson AR, Steel A et al. Reducing endoscopy workload: does serological testing for *Helicobacter pylori* help? Eur J Gastroenterol Hepatol. 1999;11;857–62
38. Moayyedi P, Zillen A, Clough M et al. The effectiveness of screening and treating *Helicobacter pylori* in the management of dyspepsia. Eur J Gastroenterol Hepatol. 1999;11:1245–50.
39. Jones R, Tait C, Sladen G et al. A trial of a test and treat strategy for Helicobacter pylori positive dyspeptic patients in general practice. Int J Clin Pract. 1999;53:413–16.
40. Joosen EAM, Reininga JHA, Manders JMW et al. Costs and benefits of a test and treat strategy in *Helicobacter pylori* infected subjects; a prospective intervention study in general practice. In Press Eur J Gastroenterol Hepatol. 1999 (In press).
41. Laheij RJ, Jansen JB, Van der Lisdonk EH et al. Review article: Symptom improvement through eradication of *Helicobacter pylori* in patients with non-ulcer dyspepsia. Aliment Pharmacol Ther. 1996;10:843–50.

42. Talley NJ, Xia HH. *Helicobacter pylori* infection and non ulcer dyspepsia. Br Med Bull. 1998;54:63–9.
43. Breslin NP, Lee J, Buckley M *et al.* Screening for *Helicobacter pylori* in young dyspeptic patients referred for investigation – endoscopy for those who test negative. Aliment Pharmacol Ther. 1998;12:577–82.
44. Kuipers EJ, Klinkenberg-Knol EC. *Helicobacter pylori*, acid, and omeprazole revisited: bacterial eradication and rebound hypersecretion. Gastroenterology. 1999;116:479–83.

46
Dyspepsia is no indication for *Helicobacter pylori* eradication

S. J. O. VELDHUYZEN VAN ZANTEN

INTRODUCTION

Many questions regarding the potential role of *Helicobacter pylori* infection in dyspepsia are unresolved. As a result of the ongoing debate among gastroenterologists on this topic, primary-care physicians are even more confused. Although discussions about the advantages and disadvantages of *H. pylori* treatment in infected patients with dyspepsia need to continue, the more important issue is that primary-care physicians receive a clear message from the gastroenterology community. In discussions of dyspepsia the terminology used needs to be clearly defined. Recently, the Rome working party on Functional Gastrointestinal Disorders has updated the definitions for dyspepsia and other functional GI disorders[1].

DYSPEPSIA DEFINITIONS

In the Rome II working party report it has been reaffirmed that dyspepsia should be defined as a syndrome which has, as its cardinal symptom, epigastric pain or discomfort. Importantly, symptoms of heartburn are excluded from this definition, as it is felt that this is indicative of gastro-oesophageal reflux disease (GERD) and, therefore, should not come under the heading of dyspepsia. The important shortcoming of this definition is that it does not fit with the conceptual framework that is used in primary care. Family physicians consider symptoms of GERD such as heartburn and acid regurgitation to be part of the symptom complex of dyspepsia. Insisting on the Rome II definition will confuse family physicians. Recently, the Canadian Dyspepsia Working group amended the Rome definition of dyspepsia and include GERD symptoms in their definition[2].

The other important issue in discussion of this topic is to make a distinction between *uninvestigated dyspepsia* and *investigated dyspepsia*. Usually the investigation of choice is upper endoscopy. Patients are diagnosed as having functional dyspepsia only if they have a normal endoscopy. In the

Table 1. Results of four functional dyspepsia studies

		Response rate (%)	
	Study	Active	Control
OCAY[3]	Blum et al.	27	21
Orchid[4]	Talley et al.	24	22
USA study[6]	Talley et al.	28	23
UK-MRC[5]	McColl et al.	21	7

literature, what constitutes a normal endoscopy is poorly defined. For example, most studies do not make clear whether the patients were taking acid-suppressive therapy or had taken such medications in the past. In functional dyspepsia trials it is not unusual to require discontinuation of these medications prior to inclusion in the study. It would be important to know whether patients were responders to acid-suppressive therapy if they took these medications in the past. A common time frame for discontinuation of acid-suppressive therapy is 4 weeks prior to inclusion in a study. However, based on relapse data from studies of oesophagitis and also duodenal and gastric ulcers it is clear that it may take much longer than 4 weeks for symptoms or endoscopic abnormalities to recur.

DOES CURE OF THE INFECTION LEAD TO A SUSTAINED IMPROVEMENT IN SYMPTOMS IN FUNCTIONAL DYSPEPSIA?

Currently, there is a lively debate about the four pivotal *functional dyspepsia* studies which have been published in the past 2 years. These include the OCAY, ORCHID, and UK-MRC trials, and the USA study by Talley et al.[3-6]. The OCAY and ORCHID studies used an identical outcome measure, a seven-point Likert scale to assess the severity of epigastric pain. In the USA study by Talley et al. results are reported on a four-point scale. When the main outcome measure is reported as the proportion of patients who have rated their severity of epigastric pain as none the results are virtually identical to the OCAY and ORCHID studies (Table 1). The results are remarkably consistent, showing a response rate in the active treatment group between 24% and 28%, and in the placebo group between 21% and 23%. In contrast, the UK-MRC trial showed a highly significant benefit in favour of *H. pylori* eradication. In this study 21% of patients were responders in the active treatment group compared to 7% in the placebo.

A circular argument is currently being played out in the literature, which either states that the development of ulcers after 12 months in the OCAY, ORCHID and USA study was surprisingly low, or alternatively that it was inappropriately high in the UK-MRC study[7-9]. It is clear that the most likely explanation for the positive outcome in the UK-MRC, study and negative results in the other three studies, is the background prevalence of peptic ulcer disease in the population where the studies were carried out. This is known to be high in countries such as Scotland and Ireland[10,11], and probably many less developed countries, but much lower in the USA, Canada, Scandinavia and several Western European countries.

The background prevalence of peptic ulcer disease, therefore, is one of the determining factors as to whether all patients with *endoscopy-investigated (functional)* dyspepsia should be treated. Strictly limiting this decision to improvement in symptoms will be dictated by the ulcer prevalence in the population under consideration. However, there is consensus that patients should be offered treatment if they are known to H. pylori infected[12,13]. In reality many gastroenterologists will now routinely biopsy for H. pylori if gastroscopy is performed. This practice is undoubtedly driven both by knowledge about the established link between H. pylori infection and gastric cancer, and by a desire by many patients to know their H. pylori status.

TREATMENT OF UNINVESTIGATED DYSPEPSIA

A discussion about which non-invasive test to use is beyond the scope of this chapter. Given the superior test operating characteristics the urea breath test[14], or perhaps the stool antigen test[15,16], is preferred over serology[17], but these tests are not widely available in most countries. A non-invasive test-and-treat strategy is advocated in the younger population, i.e. patients less than 45–50 years of age. In this age group, serology can have a substantial rate of false-positive results[14,17]. This would negatively affect the overall effectiveness of a test-and-treat strategy.

There is evidence that a non-invasive test-and-treat strategy in uninvestigated dyspeptic patients will lead to a decrease in investigations and referrals[18–21]. Recently the CADET H. pylori study was completed in Canada, in which 348 patients were randomized in primary care following a positive urea breath test for H. pylori infection to treatment with either omeprazole, clarithromycin and metronidazole for 7 days or omeprazole and placebo antibiotics for 7 days[22]. Patients were followed for 12 months and were defined as responders if they had no or minimal symptoms in the final month of a 12-month follow-up. The success rate in the OCM group was 50% compared to 36% in controls ($p < 0.005$), a significant difference. This is one of the first test-and-treat trials reported to date which was carried out in primary care. If other studies done in primary care support these findings it is likely that the non-invasive test-and-treat strategy in uninvestigated dyspepsia will indeed be evidence-based.

ARGUMENTS AGAINST TREATMENT FOR DYSPEPSIA

Several arguments as to why dyspepsia should not be an indication for treatment can be put forward (Table 2). A compelling argument against treating all patients with dyspepsia, at least in Western countries is the spontaneous decrease of H. pylori prevalence[23] (see also Chapter 5 in this volume). This is best explained by a lower acquisition rate of the infection during childhood. Since most of the test-and-treat strategies for H. pylori infection are targeted at the younger population (< 50 years of age) the yield of this strategy is likely to be modest at best, and costs will be relatively high.

Table 2. Arguments against treatment of *H. pylori* positive dyspepsia

---
The prevalence of *H. pylori* infection is spontaneously decreasing.

Widespread use of antibiotics will lead to selection of antibiotic resistance, not only in *Helicobacter* organisms but also in other organisms, even organisms which by themselves are not pathogenic.

Cost and frequency of side-effects.

Does not lead to a marked decrease in the need of further acid-suppressive therapy.

Eradication of *H. pylori* leads to less adequate intragastric control of pH. As a result there may be an increased need for higher doses of medications in patients with GERD, to control symptoms.

A second reason is that widespread use of antibiotics will lead to selection of antibiotic-resistant strains. This will occur not only in *H. pylori*, but also in other organisms, even those which by themselves are not pathogenic[24]. Evidence is convincing that widespread use of antibiotics does lead to an increase in antibiotic resistance in multiple organisms.

A third issue is cost. With regard to costs, it is unlikely that any health-care system would be able to afford to identify and treat all patients irrespective of whether or not they have dyspepsia symptoms. Although the prevalence of the infection is decreasing, many individuals currently are still infected, meaning that large numbers of patients would require testing and treatment. The fourth argument against treating is that *H. pylori* treatment does not lead to a marked decrease in the need of further acid-suppressive therapy in patients who have been taking these medications[25]. GERD as a diagnosis is a more likely explanation than peptic ulcer as to why patients require ongoing acid-suppressive therapy. Originally it was the hope that, by eradicating the *H. pylori*-associated ulcers many patients taking maintenance acid-suppressive therapy could be taken off these medications for the rest of their lives. Increasingly, it is clear that many patients either have concomitant ulcer disease and GERD, or more likely have reflux disease as their dominant problem[26,27].

In practice, a common scenario seen in primary care is a patient in whom a non-invasive *H. pylori* test is performed because of dyspepsia. If the test is positive the patient is treated with first-line eradication therapy, which in most countries consists of a twice-daily proton-pump inhibitor with two antibiotics. Often the patient, despite the potential for side-effects of the medication, quickly feels much better. In the weeks or months following treatment patients may experience a recurrence of their symptoms. Most commonly, in this scenario, patients had GERD as their underlying problem and the real reason for the symptomatic improvement has been the profound acid suppression with a twice-daily proton-pump inhibitor. To date, there is no convincing evidence that eradication of *H. pylori* either increases the risk of developing GERD or that this risk is increased following successful eradication of the infection[28-30]. The fifth argument is that there is compelling evidence that eradication of *H. pylori* leads to less adequate intragastric

Table 3. Canadian Dyspepsia Working Group clinical management tool for uninvestigated dyspepsia: five diagnostic steps

Are dyspepsia symptoms originating in upper gastrointestinal-tract?
Are alarm symptoms present and/or is patient > 50 years of age
Is patient taking NSAIDs or aspirin-containing drugs?
Does patient have heartburn as a dominant symptom?
Perform a non-invasive *Helicobacter* test.

control of pH. As a result there may be a need for higher doses of antisecretory medications in patients with GERD, to control symptoms[31,32].

CLEAR MESSAGE NEEDED FOR PRIMARY-CARE PHYSICIANS

A clear message to all family physicians about the indications for eradication of *H. pylori* in dyspepsia is needed. In Canada, a five-step management tool for family physicians has been suggested by the Canadian Dyspepsia Working Group (CanDys)[2]. The five key steps in the algorithm for the management of patients with previously uninvestigated dyspepsia are listed in Table 3. The first is to make sure that symptoms arise from the upper gastrointestinal tract. Every year, some patients who are labelled as having dyspepsia turn out to have serious heart disease, with sometimes fatal consequences. The second point is to evaluate patients for the presence of alarm symptoms. These include vomiting, evidence of bleeding, abdominal mass and dysphagia. In addition to that, age is often used as a cut-off for a decision as to whether to investigate. In most Western countries the age can range from 50 to 55 years, but may depend on the local population[33]. The third issue is whether patients are taking conventional NSAIDs or aspirin. For both, there is good evidence that they can increase the frequency of dyspepsia, and this requires separate treatment[34]. Perhaps the most important step in the work-up is to determine whether heartburn is the dominant symptom about which patients are complaining. The sensitivity of heartburn as a symptom can be increased by describing the symptoms as a burning sensation rising in the chest from the upper abdomen[35]. Such patients can confidently be diagnosed with GERD, and should be treated with acid-suppressive therapy. The fifth and final step in the work-up is to order a non-invasive *H. pylori* test. Given the better test operating characteristics the urea breath test is preferred, but this could also be a validated serological test[14]. This five-step approach is supported with different evidence-based management schemes for each of the key steps. Following this approach will make the diagnosis and treatment of dyspepsia patients explicit, and lead to a more rational use of *H. pylori* eradication treatment[2].

CONCLUSION

In the debate about dyspepsia the most important issue is the delivery of a clear message to primary care. The benefit of *H. pylori* eradication treatment and functional dyspepsia depends on the ulcer prevalence in the population that is being treated. Patients who have definite GERD should be treated for their reflux disease with antisecretory therapy and not ruotinely be investigated for *H. pylori* infection. There is increasing evidence for the benefit of a non-invasive *H. pylori* test-and-treat strategy in uninvestigated dyspepsia patients and in patients who do not have heartburn as their dominant symptom.

Acknowledgements

Dr Veldhuyzen van Zanten is the recipient of a Nova Scotia Clinical Scholar Award.

References

1. Talley NJ, Stanghellini V, Heading RC, Koch KL, Malagelada JR, Tytgat GN. Functional gastroduodenal disorders. Gut. 1999;45(Suppl. II):1137–41.
2. Veldhuyzen van Zanten SJO, Flook N, Chiba N et al. Canadian Dyspepsia Working Group. Can Med Assoc J. 2000;162(Suppl. 12):513–23.
3. Blum AL, Talley NJ, O'Morain CA et al. Lack of effect of treating *Helicobacter pylori* infection in patients with nonulcer dyspepsia. N Engl J Med. 1998;339:1875–81.
4. Talley NJ, Janssens J, Lauritsen K, Racz J, Bolling-Sternevald E. Long-term follow-up of patients with non-ulcer dyspepsia after *Helicobacter pylori* eradication. A randomized double-blind placebo-controlled trial. Br Med J. 1999;318:833–7.
5. McColl K, Murray L, El-Omar E et al. Symptomatic benefit from eradicating *Helicobacter pylori* infection in patients with nonulcer dyspepsia. N Engl J Med. 1998;339:1869–74.
6. Talley NJ, Vakil N, Ballard ED, Fennerty MB. Absence of benefit of eradicating *Helicobacter pylori* in patients with nonulcer dyspepsia. N Engl J Med. 1999;341:1106–11.
7. McColl KEL, Gillen D, Dickson AS. Eradication of *Helicobacter pylori* in functional dyspepsia. Br Med J. 2000;320:311–2.
8. Leiber, CS. *Helicobacter pylori* and nonulcer dyspepsia. N Engl J Med. 1999;349:1508–12.
9. McColl KEL. Absence of benefit of eradicating *Helicobacter pylori* in patients with nonulcer dyspepsia. N Engl J Med. 1999;342:589–90.
10. McColl KEL, El-Nujumi A, Murray L et al. The *Helicobacter pylori* breath test: a surrogate marker for peptic ulcer disease in dyspeptic patients. Gut. 1997;40:302–6.
11. McGillvary J, Buckley MJM, Beattie S, Hamilton H, O'Morain CA. Eradication of *Helicobacter pylori* affects symptoms in non-ulcer dyspepsia. Scand J Gastroenterol. 1997; 32:535–40.
12. Malfertheiner P, Mégraud F, O'Morain C. Current European concepts in the management of *Helicobacter pylori* infection. The Maastricht Consensus Report. Gut. 1997;41:8–13.
13. Hunt RH, Fallone CA, Thomson ABR, Canadian Helicobacter Study Group. Canadian *Helicobacter pylori* Consensus Conference update: infections in adults. Can J Gastroenterol. 1999;13:213–17.
14. Chiba N, Veldhuyzen van Zanten SJO. C-Urea breath tests are the non-invasive method of choice for *Helicobacter pylori* detection. Can J Gastroenterol. 1999;13:681–3.
15. Vaira D, Malfertheiner P, Megraud F et al. Diagnosis of *Helicobacter pylori* infection with a new non-invasive antigen-b assay. HpSA European study group. Lancet. 1999;354:30–3.
16. Veldhuyzen van Zanten SJO, Bleau BL, Best LM, Hutchison D, Blevins J, Thee D. Use of the *Helicobacter pylori* stool antigen test (HPSAT) for detection of *Helicobacter pylori*. Gut. 1998;43(Suppl. 2):A19(06/164).
17. Loy, CT, Irwig LM, Katelaris PH, Talley NJ. Do commercial serology kits for *Helicobacter pylori* infection differ in accuracy? A meta-analysis. Gastroenterology 1996;91:1138–44.
18. Heaney A, Collins JS, Watson RG, McFarland RJ, Bamford KB, Tham TC. A prospective randomised trial of a 'test and treat' policy versus endoscopy-based management in young *Helicobacter pylori* positive patients with ulcer-like dyspepsia, referred to a hospital clinic. Gut. 1999;24:186–90.
19. Jones R, Tait C, Sladen G, Weston-Baker J. A trial of a test-and-treat strategy for *Helicobacter pylori* positive dyspeptic patients in general practice. Int J Clin Pract. 1999;53:413–6.

20. Lassen AT, Pedersen FM, Bytzer P, Schaffalitzky de Muckadell OB. *H. pylori* 'test and treat' or prompt endoscopy for dyspeptic patients in primary care. A randomized controlled trial of two management strategies: one year follow-up. Gastroenterology. 1998;114:A196 (abstract G0803).
21. Moayyedi P, Mason J, Zilles A, Axon ATR, Chalmers DM, Drummond MF. Screening and treating for *H. pylori* – is it cost-effective in clinical practice? Digestion. 1998;59(Suppl. 3):10.
22. Chiba N, Veldhuyzen van Zanten SJO, Sinclair P, Ferguson RA, Escobedo SR. The CADET-Hp Study Group. Beneficial effect of *H. pylori* eradication therapy on long term symptom relief in primary care patients with uninvestigated dyspepsia: the CADET-Hp study. Gastroenterology. 2000;118(Suppl. 2):A2390.
23. Parsonnet J. The incidence of *Helicobacter pylori* infection. Aliment Pharmacol Ther. 1995;9(Suppl. 2):45–51.
24. Amyes SGB. The rise in bacterial resistance. Br Med J. 2000;320:199–200.
25. Tan AC, Hartog GD, Mulder CJ. Eradication of *Helicobacter pylori* does not decrease the long-term use of acid-suppressive medication. Ailment Pharmacol Ther. 1999;13:1519–22.
26. McColl KEL, Dickson A, El-Nujumi A, El-Omar E, Kelman A. Symptomatic benefit 1–3 years after *H. pylori* eradication in ulcer patients: impact of gastroesophageal reflux disease. Am J Gastroenterol. 2000;95:101–5.
27. Boyd EJ. The prevalence of esophagitis in patients with duodenal ulcer or ulcer-like dyspepsia. Am J Gastroenterol. 1996;91:1539–43.
28. Labenz J, Malfertheiner P. *Helicobacter pylori* in gastro-oesophageal reflux disease: causal agent, independent or protective factor? Gut. 1997;41:277–80.
29. Tefera S, Hatlebakk JG, Berstad A. The effect of *Helicobacter pylori* eradication on gastro-oesophageal reflux. Aliment Pharmacol Ther. 1999;13:915–20.
30. O'Connor HJ. Review article: *Helicobacter pylori* and gastro-oesophageal reflux disease – clinical implications and management. Aliment Pharmacol Ther. 1999;13:117–27.
31. Verdu EF, Armstrong D, Fraser R *et al.* Effect of *Helicobacter pylori* status on intragastric pH during treatment with omeprazole. Gut. 1995;36:539–43.
32. Healey Z, Calam J. Inhibiting acid and *Helicobacter pylori*? Gut. 1997;41:125–6.
33. Veldhuyzen van Zanten SJO. Can the age limit for endoscopy be increased in dyspepsia patients who do not have alarm symptoms? Am J Gastroenterol. 1999;94:9–11.
34. Ofman JJ, MacLean C, Morton S, Straus W, Shekelle P. The risk of dyspepsia and serious gastrointestinal complications from NSAIDs; a meta-analysis. Gastroenterology. 1999; 116:A270 (abstract).
35. Carlsson R, dent J, Bolling-Sternevald E *et al.* The usefulness of a structured questionnaire in the assessment of symptomatic gastroesophageal reflux disease. Scand J Gastroenterol. 1998;33:1023–9.

47
Role of *Helicobacter pylori* infection in NSAID-associated gastropathy

J.-Q. HUANG, R. LAD and R. H. HUNT

INTRODUCTION

Helicobacter pylori infection and the use of non-steroidal anti-inflammatory drugs (NSAIDs) are the two most important risk factors for peptic ulcer disease[1]. The population-attributable risk associated with peptic ulcer is estimated at 48% for *H. pylori* infection and 24% for NSAID use, respectively[2]. Results from numerous randomized controlled clinical trials have shown that eradication of *H. pylori* infection cures most peptic ulcers and virtually eliminates ulcer recurrence[3,4]. Although the management of NSAID-related peptic ulcer is more difficult than that of *H. pylori*-associated ulcers, the simplest and most effective treatment is to discontinue the NSAIDs[5], suggesting a strong causal relationship between NSAID use and peptic ulcer disease.

Despite progress in our understanding of the role of *H. pylori* infection and NSAIDs in ulcer development, the interactions between these two risk factors remain poorly understood and highly controversial. The results from epidemiological studies and clinical trials examining the relationship between *H. pylori* infection and NSAID-associated gastropathy have been conflicting[6,7]. Some studies have found that the occurrence of peptic ulcer is increased in *H. pylori*-infected NSAID takers[8–10], whereas others showed a reduction in the prevalence of peptic ulcer disease when *H. pylori* infection and NSAID use coexist[11,12]. These discrepant results may reflect a complex relationship between *H. pylori* infection and NSAID-associated gastropathy. Four possible scenarios should be considered with respect to *H. pylori* infection and NSAID-associated gastropathy; they comprise lack of interaction, additive, synergistic or antagonistic effects between the two risk factors. This chapter reviews systematically the current evidence on the relationship between *H. pylori* infection and NSAID-associated gastropathy, examines the totality of the evidence and discusses several methodological issues that may explain some of the disagreements among studies.

MECHANISMS LEADING TO GASTRODUODENAL MUCOSAL DAMAGE

Although *H. pylori* infection and NSAIDs cause gastroduodenal mucosal damage through different mechanisms, they share certain important pathways leading to mucosal ulceration. For example, *H. pylori*-related mucosal damage mainly involves the inflammatory cascade of cytokines and neutrophils, whereas NSAIDs inhibit the synthesis of prostaglandins in the gastric mucosa resulting in gastric epithelial cell damage. However, both *H. pylori* and NSAIDs increase paracellular gastric mucosal permeability and expose the weakened mucosa to acid, pepsin and other exogenous aggressive factors[13].

H. pylori has extensive interactions with the gastric epithelium throughout the entire process of colonization and survival. The bacteria produce a large number of enzymes, including urease, proteolytic enzymes, antioxidant and metabolic enzymes, lipase and phospholipase A_2 etc., which can degrade mucus glycoproteins and damage gastric surface epithelial cells[14]. Furthermore, *H. pylori* infection initiates an inflammatory cascade with the release of proinflammatory cytokines which, in turn, also induce mucosal damage[15].

The inhibition of mucosal prostaglandins by NSAIDs results in decreased secretion of mucus and bicarbonate from the gastric epithelial cells, reduction of mucosal blood flow and retardation of the speed of cell restitution[1]. Moreover, use of NSAIDs significantly reduces the ability of prostaglandins to exert anti-inflammatory and anti-ulcerogenic effects in the gastrointestinal tract, leading to the infiltration of neutrophils in the gastric mucosa and subsequent mucosal injury[16].

In long-term NSAID users, *H. pylori* infection and neutrophil infiltration in the gastric mucosa significantly increased the prevalence of peptic ulceration compared to those without the infection and neutrophil infiltration in the gastric mucosa[17]. This suggests a possible interaction on gastric mucosa damage between *H. pylori* infection and NSAID use.

EPIDEMIOLOGICAL STUDIES

The results from epidemiological studies have been conflicting with respect to whether NSAID takers who are infected with *H. pylori* infection are prone to the development of peptic ulcer compared to those without the infection[6,7,18,19]. The confusion may arise from the considerable heterogeneity in the patient and control populations and the different criteria used for outcome measurement. For example, most early cross-sectional studies examining the prevalence of peptic ulcer in NSAID takers included patients with different background history of NSAID use and different diagnostic methods for *H. pylori* infection, and thus generated conflicting results[7,18,19]. We systematically reviewed the literature of epidemiological studies to explore if any interaction between *H. pylori* infection and use of NSAIDs exists, and to assess the magnitude of the effect, if any, on the development of peptic ulcer or its complications.

Prevalence of *H. pylori* infection and peptic ulcer in NSAID takers

Overall analysis

There were a total of 17 studies published in full articles in the literature up to February 2000 that provided data on the prevalence of *H. pylori* infection and/or occurrence of peptic ulcer in NSAID takers[8–12,20–31]. Overall, *H. pylori* infection was diagnosed in 49.7% of the cases (842/1694). Sixteen studies had information on the occurrence of peptic ulcer, and provided an overall rate of peptic ulcer at 33.2% (545/1640), irrespective of *H. pylori* status[8–12,20–24,26–31]. When *H. pylori* status was taken into account, peptic ulcer was diagnosed in 41.4% (344/831) of the cases infected with *H. pylori* compared to 24.8% (201/809) of those without the infection, yielding a summary odds ratio at 2.14 (95% CI 1.73–2.64) with the Mantel–Haenszel method. The result suggests that *H. pylori* infection increases the likelihood of developing peptic ulcer by 2-fold in NSAID takers compared to those without the infection.

Twelve studies had raw data on the site of ulcer[8,10–12,21,23,24,26–29,31]. Overall, gastric ulcer was found in 19.1% (225/1181) of the cases and duodenal ulcer in 12.5% (148/1181). When studies were analysed by *H. pylori* status of the cases, gastric ulcer was diagnosed in 20.4% (117/573) of the *H. pylori*-positive cases compared to 17.8% (108/608) of those without the infection, giving a summary odds ratio of 1.18 (95% CI 0.89–1.59). However, duodenal ulcer was found to be significantly more common in *H. pylori*-positive NSAID takers than in those without the infection (16.8% vs. 8.6%). There was a significant difference in the duodenal ulcer rates between these two groups, yielding a pooled odds ratio of 2.15 (95% CI 1.5–3.08).

Case-control studies

Five studies compared the prevalence of *H. pylori* infection and peptic ulcer in NSAID takers with non-NSAID takers[8–12]. The characteristics of the five studies are tabulated in Table 1. Overall, *H. pylori* infection was diagnosed in 44% (242/550) of the cases and 52.8% (344/651) of the controls. There was a significant difference in the prevalence of *H. pylori* infection between the two groups ($\chi^2 = 9.32$, d.f. $= 1$, $p = 0.0023$). However, peptic ulcer was significantly more commonly seen in NSAID takers ($n = 550$) than in non-NSAID takers ($n = 651$) (36.2% vs. 15.8%, OR 3.02, 95% CI 2.29–3.96), irrespective of *H. pylori* infection.

When *H. pylori* status was taken into account, in NSAID takers, peptic ulcer was found in 49.2% (119/242) of those infected with *H. pylori* and 26% (80/308) of those without the infection, yielding a pooled odds ratio of 2.76 (95% CI 1.93–3.94). In non-NSAID takers, peptic ulcer was diagnosed in 25% (86/344) of *H. pylori*-infected subjects and 5.5% (17/307) of those without the infection, giving an odds ratio of 5.69 (95% CI 3.29–9.82).

Use of NSAIDs also significantly increased the likelihood of developing peptic ulcer by 2.9-fold (95% CI 2.04–4.12) in *H. pylori*-infected subjects and by 5.99-fold (95% CI 3.45–10.38) in *H. pylori*-negative subjects. However, when the comparison was made between *H. pylori*-infected NSAID

Table 1. Case-control studies examining the relationship between *H. pylori* infection and NSAID-associated peptic ulcer disease (PUD)

Reference	Cases	Control	PUD in cases (%)		PUD in controls (%)	
			H. pylori-positive	H. pylori-positive	H. pylori-positive	H. pylori-negative
8	Chronic NSAID takers with RA	Dyspeptic non-NSAID takers	17/35 (48.6%)	16/61 (26.2%)	6/34 (17.6)	0/62 (0%)
11	Patients with RA taking NSAIDs >1 month	Non-NSAID takers without RA	3/26 (11.5%)	4/59 (6.8%)	11/59 (18.6%)	0/41 (0%)
9*	Patients with ischaemic heart disease taking aspirin >4 weeks	Patients with ischaemic heart disease, but not taking aspirin	49/65 (75.4%)	11/31 (35.5%)	18/38 (47.4%)	15/42 (35.7%)
10	NSAID takers with gastrointestinal symptoms	Non-NSAID takers with gastrointestinal symptoms	23/60 (38.3%)	8/39 (20.5%)	37/191 (19.4%)	2/140 (1.4%)
12	Patients with RA taking NSAIDs >4 weeks	RA patients not taking NSAIDs >4 weeks	27/56 (48.2%)	41/118 (34.7%)	14/22 (63.6%)	0/22 (0%)

RA = rheumatoid arthritis.
*Including patients with gastric or duodenal erosions of more than 4.

takers and *H. pylori*-negative non-NSAID takers, there was a highly statistical difference in the prevalence of peptic ulcer between these two groups, with an odds ratio of 16.5 (95% CI 9.53–28.57). These results suggest that *H. pylori* infection and NSAIDs are independent risk factors for peptic ulcer disease. There is an additive or probably synergistic effect between *H. pylori* infection and NSAID use on the development of peptic ulcer.

When studies were stratified by the site of ulcer, in NSAID takers *H. pylori* infection did not increase the risk for gastric ulcer compared to non-infected NSAID takers (OR 1.09, 95% CI 0.7–1.7). However, *H. pylori* infection increased the risk for duodenal ulcer by 3.98-fold (95% CI 1.91–8.3) compared to non-infected NSAID takers.

Among *H. pylori*-infected subjects the use of NSAIDs increased the risk for gastric ulcer by 4.59-fold (95% CI 2.6–8.1), but had no impact on the risk of duodenal ulcer (OR 0.88, 95% CI 0.52–1.49). In subjects without the infection the use of NSAIDs increased the risk for gastric ulcer by 38.7-fold (95% CI 9.39–159.55) and for duodenal ulcer by 21.9-fold (95% CI 1.29–373.04).

These results suggest that, in *H. pylori*-infected NSAID takers, *H. pylori* infection increased the risk of duodenal ulcer, but not the risk for gastric ulcer. However, when *H. pylori* infection was absent, use of NSAIDs increased the risk for both gastric and duodenal ulcer.

H. pylori infection and use of NSAIDs in bleeding peptic ulcer

We have found nine studies published in full in English in the literature up to February 2000 that examined the role of *H. pylori* infection and NSAIDs in peptic ulcer bleeding[32–40]. These studies assessed the prevalence of *H. pylori* infection and use of NSAIDs in patients with bleeding peptic ulcer and compared them with non-bleeding controls. *H. pylori* infection was diagnosed in 73.6% (657/893) of the cases and 67.3% (674/1002) of the controls, yielding a pooled odds ratio of 1.4 (95% CI 1.1–1.7). Sixty-seven per cent (523/787) of the cases and 37.5% (366/975) of the controls reported recent use of NSAIDs prior to the onset of ulcer bleeding. There was a significant difference in the prevalence of use of NSAIDs between the cases and controls, giving an odds ratio of 3.3 (95% CI 2.71–4.01). When both *H. pylori* infection and use of NSAIDs were taken into account, the presence of these two risk factors was significantly more commonly seen in the cases than in the controls (59.7% vs. 24.8%, OR 4.5, 95% CI 3.1–6.5). These results suggest that *H. pylori* infection and use of NSAIDs are both related to peptic ulcer bleeding. However, use of NSAIDs may play a more important role than *H. pylori* infection in the development of ulcer bleeding.

DISCUSSION

Previous studies have shown that *H. pylori* infection or use of NSAIDs confers to 3–4-fold increased risk for peptic ulcer[2,41,42]. However, it is not known if the magnitude of the risk reported in these studies was for individual or combined contribution of *H. pylori* infection and/or NSAIDs to the development of peptic ulcer disease.

We have found, in this systematic review, that one-third of chronic NSAID takers had gastric and/or duodenal ulcer, irrespective of *H. pylori* status and study design. *H. pylori* infection increased the magnitude of risk for peptic ulcer by 2-fold. However, the increase in ulcer risk was seen only in patients with duodenal ulcer, but not in patients with gastric ulcer, while no difference in the prevalence of gastric ulcer was seen between *H. pylori*-positive and *H. pylori*-negative NSAID takers. The results suggest that *H. pylori* infection plays a more important role in the formation of duodenal ulcer in NSAID takers, but has less impact on gastric ulcer. In other words, NSAID-associated gastric ulcer is not related to *H. pylori* infection, whereas *H. pylori* infection increases the risk of duodenal ulcer associated with NSAIDs.

In studies in which a control group of non-NSAID takers was available, the risk of peptic ulcer was increased by 3-fold compared to non-NSAID takers, irrespective of *H. pylori* status. *H. pylori* infection increased the risk for peptic ulcer by 3- and 6-fold in NSAID takers and non-NSAID takers, respectively. Furthermore, the magnitude of risk multiplied when *H. pylori*-infected NSAID takers were compared with *H. pylori*-negative non-NSAID takers, suggesting a possible synergism between these two risk factors. *H. pylori* infection did not increase the risk of gastric ulcer in NSAID takers, whereas in *H. pylori*-infected patients the use of NSAIDs increased the risk for gastric ulcer by 4.6-fold, but had no effect on the risk of duodenal ulcer. These results further confirm that gastric ulcer is predominantly related to NSAID use, and duodenal ulcer is, to a large extent, associated with *H. pylori* infection.

There has been debate over the clinical importance of endoscopically detected gastric and/or duodenal ulcers associated with NSAID use, because of a poor relationship between endoscopically observed gastroduodenal mucosal lesions and symptoms[5,43]. However, previous studies have not taken *H. pylori* infection into consideration[42]; therefore it is not known if any relationship exists between endoscopically observed ulcers and symptoms in patients infected with *H. pylori*. Thus, results from studies of patients with complicated ulcer may provide more important and clinically relevant information on the interaction between *H. pylori* infection and NSAIDs. In this systematic review we have found that both *H. pylori* infection (OR 1.4) and NSAID use (OR 3.3) were significantly more prevalent in patients with bleeding peptic ulcer than in their non-bleeding controls. When the two risk factors coexisted the magnitude of the risk was additive (OR 4.5), suggesting that both *H. pylori* infection and NSAID use contribute to peptic ulcer bleeding, while NSAIDs play a major role based on the magnitude of the risk ratio.

The best approach to assess the role of *H. pylori* infection in NSAID-associated gastropathy is through randomized controlled clinical trials. If eradication of the infection can affect the incidence of peptic ulcer in patients taking conventional NSAIDs, this would provide the best evidence for any interactions between the two risk factors. To date, five studies have been published[20,44-47]. Unfortunately they provide further confusion, rather than answers, because of the vast heterogeneity in the patient population and in outcome measurement. These studies have recently been the subject of a comprehensive review by Chan and Sung[7]; examples are the studies by Chan et al.[44] and Hawkey et al.[47]. In the Chan study, an NSAID-naive population was included. An ulcer was defined as being 5 mm in size. However, the study by Hawkey et al. included *H. pylori*-infected chronic NSAID users with a mixed diagnosis of peptic ulcer and dyspepsia, and an endoscopic ulcer was defined as one of 3 mm or greater[47]. Furthermore, the baseline characteristics between the two groups were unbalanced, and the authors did not analyse the results by final *H. pylori* status, leaving the question of any interactions between *H. pylori* infection and NSAID use unanswered. Because of the limited number of published interventional studies available, and the above examples of heterogeneity, a meta-analysis was not performed for these studies. Future evaluation of the relationship of NSAIDs to *H. pylori* is warranted when new studies become available.

As with meta-analysis in general, methodological flaws of individual studies cannot be corrected by our meta-analysis, or indeed accounted for. Although a formal test for heterogeneity was not performed, the differences in patient and control populations and definition of ulcer size may limit the explanation of the current analysis. Nevertheless, we believe that meta-analysis is a useful tool for systematically assessing the totality of evidence in the literature and providing directions for future studies.

In conclusion, *H. pylori* infection or NSAID use independently increases the risk of peptic ulcer disease and ulcer bleeding. There is a synergism on the formation of peptic ulcer between *H. pylori* infection and NSAID use, based on the magnitude of the risk ratio. *H. pylori* infection increases the risk of duodenal ulcer, but has no impact on the risk of gastric ulcer in NSAID takers. However, NSAID use increases the risk for both gastric and duodenal ulcer in *H. pylori*-negative subjects. Both gastric and duodenal ulcers are seldom seen in *H. pylori*-negative non-NSAID takers.

Acknowledgements

We thank Drs P. Ekstrom (Sweden), J.-P. Kuyvenhoven (The Netherlands), M. Voutilainen (Finland) and C. Y. Wu (China) for their generosity in providing us with the raw data of their study.

References

1. Huang JQ, Hunt RH. The management of acute gastric and duodenal ulcer. In: Wolf MM, editor. Therapy of Digestive Disorders: a Companion to Sleisenger and Fordtran's Gastrointestinal and Liver Disease. Philadelphia, PA: Saunders; 2000:113–26.
2. Kurata JH, Nogawa AN. Meta-analysis of risk factors for peptic ulcer: nonsteroidal anti-inflammatory drugs, *Helicobacter pylori*, and smoking. J Clin Gastroenterol. 1997;241:2–17.
3. Penston JG. Review article: Clinical aspects of *Helicobacter pylori* eradication therapy in peptic ulcer disease. Aliment Pharmacol Ther. 1996;10:469–86.
4. Huang JQ, Chen Y, Wilkinson J, Hunt RH. Does initial choice of *Helicobacter pylori* (HP) treatment regimen influence the recurrence rate of duodenal ulcer (DU)? A meta-analysis. Am J Gastroenterol. 1996;91:1914 (abstract 125).
5. Huang JQ, Hunt RH. A clinician's view of strategies for preventing NSAID-induced gastrointestinal ulcers. Inflammopharmacology. 1996;4:17–30.
6. Fennerty MB. The *Helicobacter pylori*-non-steroidal anti-inflammatory drug interaction: consensus at last? In: Hunt RH, Tytgat GNJ editors. *Helicobacter pylori*: Basic Mechanisms to Clinical Cure 1998. Lancaster: Kluwer; 1998;260–6.

7. Chan FKL, Sung JJY. How does *Helicobacter pylori* infection interact with non-steroidal anti-inflammatory drugs? Baillière's Clin Gastroenterol. 2000;14:161–72.
8. Voutilainen M, Sokka T, Juhola M, Farkkila M, Hannonen P. Nonsteroidal anti-inflammatory drug-associated upper gastrointestinal lesions in rheumatoid arthritis patients. Relationships to gastric histology, *Helicobacter pylori* infection, and other risk factors for peptic ulcer. Scand J Gastroenterol. 1998;33:811–16.
9. Kordecki H, Kurowski M, Kosik R, Pilecka D. Is *Helicobacter pylori* infection a risk or protective factor for mucosal lesions development in patients chronically treated with acetylsalicylic acid? J Physiol Pharmacol. 1997;48(Suppl. 4):85–91.
10. Shallcross TM, Rathbone BJ, Wyatt JI, Heatley RV. *Helicobacter pylori* associated chronic gastritis and peptic ulceration in patients taking non-steroidal anti-inflammatory drugs. Aliment Pharmacol Ther. 1990;4:515–22.
11. Caselli M, Pazzi P, LaCorte R, Aleotti A, Trevisani L, Stabellini G. *Campylobacter*-like organisms, nonsteroidal anti-inflammatory drugs and gastric lesions in patients with rheumatoid arthritis. Digestion. 1989;44:101–4.
12. Taha AS, Nakshabendi I, Lee FD, Sturrock RD, Russell RI. Chemical gastritis and *Helicobacter pylori* related gastritis in patients receiving non-steroidal anti-inflammatory drugs: comparison and correlation with peptic ulceration. J Clin Pathol. 1992;45:135–9.
13. Hawkey CJ. Are NSAIDs and *Helicobacter pylori* separate risk factors? In: Hunt RH, Tytgat GNJ editors. *Helicobacter pylori*: Basic Mechanisms to Clinical Cure 1996. Lancaster: Kluwer; 1996:312–23.
14. Nilius M, Malfertheiner P. *Helicobacter pylori* enzymes. Aliment Pharmacol Ther. 1996;10(Suppl. 1):65–71.
15. Ernst PB, Crowe SE, Reyes VE. How does *Helicobacter pylori* cause mucosal damage? The inflammatory response. Gastroenterology. 1997;113:S35–42.
16. Wallace JL, Tigley AW. Review article: New insights into prostaglandins and mucosal defence. Aliment Pharmacol Ther. 1995;9:227–35.
17. Taha AS, Dahill S, Morran C et al. Neutrophils, *Helicobacter pylori*, and nonsteroidal anti-inflammatory drug ulcers. Gastroenterology. 1999;116:254–8.
18. Veldhuyzen van Zanten SJO. *H. pylori* and NSAIDs: a meta-analysis on interactions of acute gastroduodenal injury, gastric and duodenal ulcers and upper gastrointestinal symptoms. In: Hunt RH, Tytgat GNJ editors. *Helicobacter pylori*: Basic Mechanisms to Clinical Cure. Lancaster: Kluwer; 1994:449–57.
19. McCarthy DM. *Helicobacter pylori* and non-steroidal anti-inflammatory drugs: does infection affect the outcome of NSAID therapy? Yale J Biol Med. 1998;71:101–11.
20. Bianchi Porro G, Parente F, Imbesi V, Montrone F, Caruso I. Role of *Helicobacter pylori* in ulcer healing and recurrence of gastric and duodenal ulcers in longterm NSAID users. Response to omeprazole dual therapy. Gut. 1996;39:22–6.
21. Graham DY, Lidsky MD, Cox AM et al. Long-term nonsteroidal antiinflammatory drug use and *Helicobacter pylori* infection. Gastroenterology. 1991;100:1653–7.
22. Hudson N, Balsitis M, Filipowicz F, Hawkey CJ. Effect of *Helicobacter pylori* colonisation on gastric mucosal eicosanoid synthesis in patients taking non-steroidal anti-inflammatory drugs. Gut. 1993;34:748–51.
23. Kim JG, Graham DY. *Helicobacter pylori* infection and development of gastric or duodenal ulcer in arthritic patients receiving chronic NSAID therapy. The Misoprostol Study Group. Am J Gastroenterol. 1994;89:203–7.
24. Li EK, Sung JJ, Suen R et al. *Helicobacter pylori* infection increases the risk of peptic ulcers in chronic users of non-steroidal anti-inflammatory drugs. Scand J Rheumatol. 1996;25:42–6.
25. Loeb DS, Talley NJ, Ahlquist DA, Carpenter HA, Zinsmeister AR. Long-term nonsteroidal anti-inflammatory drug use and gastroduodenal injury: the role of *Helicobacter pylori*. Gastroenterology. 1992;102:1899–905.
26. Mizokami Y, Tamura K, Fukuda Y, Yamamoto I, Shimoyama T. Non-steroidal anti-inflammatory drugs associated with gastroduodenal injury and *Helicobacter pylori*. Eur J Gastroenterol Hepatol. 1994;6(Suppl. 1):S109–12.
27. Pilotto A, Franceschi M, Leandro G, Di Mario F, Valerio G. The effect of *Helicobacter pylori* infection on NSAID-related gastroduodenal damage in the elderly. Eur J Gastroenterol Hepatol. 1997;9:951–6.

28. Santucci L, Fiorucci S, Patoia L, Di Matteo FM, Brunori PM, Morelli A. Severe gastric mucosal damage induced by NSAIDs in healthy subjects is associated with *Helicobacter pylori* infection and high levels of serum pepsinogens. Dig Dis Sci. 1995;40:2074–80.
29. Taha AS, Angerson W, Nakshabendi I *et al*. Gastric and duodenal mucosal blood flow in patients receiving non-steroidal anti-inflammatory drugs – influence of age, smoking, ulceration and *Helicobacter pylori*. Aliment Pharmacol Ther. 1993;7:41–5.
30. Upadhyay R, Howatson A, McKinlay A, Danesh BJZ, Sturrock RD, Russell RI. *Campylobacter pylori* associated gastritis in patients with rheumatoid arthritis taking non-steroidal anti-inflammatory drugs. Br J Rheumatol. 1988;27:113–16.
31. Vcev A, Ivandic A, Vceva A *et al*. Infection with *Helicobacter pylori* and long-term use of non-steroidal antiinflammatory drugs. Acta Med Croatica. 1998;52:27–31.
32. Wu CY, Poon SK, Chen GH, Chang CS, Yeh HZ. Interaction between *Helicobacter pylori* and non-steroidal anti-inflammatory drugs in peptic ulcer bleeding. Scand J Gastroenterol. 1999;34:234–7.
33. Ng TM, Fock KM, Khor JL *et al*. Non-steroidal anti-inflammatory drugs, *Helicobacter pylori* and bleeding gastric ulcer. Aliment Pharmacol Ther. 2000;14:203–9.
34. Pilotto A, Leandro G, Di Mario F, Franceschi M, Bozzola L, Valerio G. Role of *Helicobacter pylori* infection on upper gastrointestinal bleeding in the elderly: a case–control study. Dig Dis Sci. 1997;42:586–91.
35. Santolaria S, Lanas A, Benito R, Perez-Aisa MF, Montoro M, Sainz R. *Helicobacter pylori* infection is a protective factor for bleeding gastric ulcers but not for bleeding duodenal ulcers in NSAID users. Aliment Pharmacol Ther. 1999;13:1511–18.
36. Aalykke C, Lauritsen JM, Hallas J, Reinholdt S, Krogfelt K, Lauritsen K. *Helicobacter pylori* and risk of ulcer bleeding among users of nonsteroidal anti-inflammatory drugs: a case-control study. Gastroenterology. 1999;116:1305–9.
37. al-Assi MT, Genta RM, Karttunen TJ, Graham DY. Ulcer site and complications: relation to *Helicobacter pylori* infection and NSAID use. Endoscopy. 1996;28:229–33.
38. Cullen DJ, Hawkey GM, Greenwood DC *et al*. Peptic ulcer bleeding in the elderly: relative roles of *Helicobacter pylori* and non-steroidal anti-inflammatory drugs. Gut. 1997;41:459–62.
39. Henriksson AE, Edman AC, Nilsson I, Bergqvist D, Wadstrom T. *Helicobacter pylori* and the relation to other risk factors in patients with acute bleeding peptic ulcer. Scand J Gastroenterol. 1998;33:1030–3.
40. Labenz J, Peitz U, Kohl H *et al*. *Helicobacter pylori* increases the risk of peptic ulcer bleeding: a case–control study. Ital J Gastroenterol Hepatol. 1999;31:110–15.
41. Nomura A, Stemmermann GN, Chyou PH, Perez-Perez GI, Blaser MJ. *Helicobacter pylori* infection and the risk for duodenal and gastric ulceration. Ann Intern Med. 1994;120:977–81.
42. Hawkey CJ. Non-steroidal anti-inflammatory drugs and peptic ulcers. Br Med J. 1990;300:278–84.
43. Hunt RH. NSAID-induced gastric ulcers: exploring the silent dilemma. Can J Gastroenterol. 1990;4:89–90.
44. Chan FKL, Sung JJY, Chung SCS *et al*. Randomized trial of eradication of *Helicobacter pylori* before non-steroidal anti-inflammatory drug therapy to prevent peptic ulcers. Lancet. 1997;350:975–9.
45. Chan FK, Sung JJ, Suen R *et al*. Does eradication of *Helicobacter pylori* impair healing of nonsteroidal anti-inflammatory drug associated bleeding peptic ulcers? A prospective randomized study. Aliment Pharmacol Ther. 199812:1201–5.
46. Chan FKL, Sung JY, Suen R *et al*. Eradication of *H. pylori* versus maintenance acid suppression to prevent recurrent ulcer haemorrhage in high-risk NSAID users: a prospective randomized study. Gastroenterology. 1998;114:A87.
47. Hawkey CJ, Tulassay Z, Szczepanski L *et al*. Randomised controlled trial of Helicobacter pylori eradication in patients on non-steroidal anti-inflammatory drugs: HELP NSAIDs study. *Helicobacter* eradication for lesion prevention. Lancet. 1998;352:1016–21.

48
Role of *Helicobacter pylori* in NSAID gastrophy: can *H. pylori* infection be beneficial?

D. Y. GRAHAM

INTRODUCTION

Helicobacter pylori infection is a serious, destructive, transmissible, infectious disease that causes progressive damage to the stomach. The infection may remain latent or present symptomatically as peptic ulcer disease or as gastric cancer. *H. pylori* infection and use of nonsteroidal anti-inflammatory drugs are the two most common causes of peptic ulcer disease, and together are responsible for considerable morbidity and mortality. For example, the FDA estimated the risk of a serious gastrointestinal complication among chronic NSAID users to be in the range of 2–4% per year[1]. The proportion of chronic NSAID users that develop endoscopic ulcers is much higher, and the model of endoscopic examination of the upper gastrointestinal tract in chronic NSAID users has been the focus of much research and debate.

It is unclear whether the presence or absence of an *H. pylori* infection has an interaction with clinical ulcer complications or with endoscopic ulcers among NSAID users. It is reasonable to ask whether, if an *H. pylori* infection were present, one could expect to identify the effect. It is also important to know if the proportion of *H. pylori*-infected individuals in the study might be responsible for some of the differences reported in different trials. The risk of developing a new ulcer in an *H. pylori*-infected individual is low. For the purposes of this analysis we will use estimates of 0.5–1% per year for development of an ulcer in a patient with a latent *H. pylori* infection. In contrast, a patient with a prior *H. pylori* ulcer has a very high risk of developing a recurrence over 1 year of follow-up. Here we will use a conservative range of 50–80% per year. If ulcer complications were our endpoint, as it would likely be if we were doing a prospective study of a new drug to prevent ulcer complications, we would use rates of 1–2% per year for an ulcer complication among those with prior *H. pylori* ulcers who had not previously experienced an ulcer complication, and at least 12% for those who had.

We will now use those estimates in a model study consisting of 500 chronic NSAID users in which, over the study period of 1 year, 30% develop endoscopic ulcers. If we plug the estimates above into the results of this typical ulcer prevention trial how many ulcers might be due to *H. pylori*? In the subgroup with *H. pylori* infection we would expect approximately 0.5–1% to develop new *H. pylori*-associated ulcers. Thus, even if all 500 had *H. pylori* infection, we would experience, at the most, five ulcers that were not attributable to the NSAIDs. It is obvious that any contribution from latent *H. pylori* infection would be invisible unless there was an *H. pylori*–NSAID interaction that increased the proportion who developed ulcers; see more about that below. In contrast, if the proportion entered with a prior *H. pylori* ulcer were high it would have a major impact on outcome because at least 50% of them would be expected to experience an ulcer recurrence during the study. Thus, it is clear that one could perform a study in which the outcome in any treatment arm would be greatly influenced by the proportion of patients with prior *H. pylori* ulcers who entered into the study. For example, a comparison of an antisecretory drug, such as an H_2-receptor antagonist proven to reduce the rate of recurrence of *H. pylori* ulcers, versus placebo would be subject to a major bias against placebo that was proportional to the number of patients with prior *H. pylori* ulcers in the placebo group. Consider our study of 500 individuals. If in that study the proportion with prior *H. pylori* ulcers was 10%, and they were randomly distributed between groups. If the H_2-receptor antagonist therapy was 80% effective in preventing *H. pylori* ulcer recurrences, there would be 25 patients per group with a prior *H. pylori* ulcer and, as one would expect, a 50–80% recurrence rate, there would be between 12 and 20 ulcers in those receiving placebo compared to two to four recurrent *H. pylori* ulcers among those receiving the H_2-receptor antagonist (about a 5-fold difference). These 'real' ulcers would be added to the endoscopic ulcers occurring in the two groups. If the H_2-receptor antagonists had a minor effect on NSAID ulcers (e.g. a reduction in the number of ulcers to 60 from the expected 75) and the placebo yielded the expected 75 ulcers, the comparison would be not statistically significant (i.e. 24% vs. 30%; $p = 0.104$). When we added the 20 *H. pylori* ulcers to the NSAID ulcers in the placebo group and four *H. pylori* ulcers to the H_2-receptor antagonists group we would now have a significant difference (64/250 or 25.6% vs. 95/250 or 38% for H_2-receptor antagonists vs. placebo; $p < 0.001$). We would falsely conclude that the H_2-receptor antagonist was superior to placebo. This scenario has probably not been missed by the pharmaceutical companies designing marketing comparisons of antisecretory drugs among chronic NSAID users. We can conclude that if there were no interaction between *H. pylori* and NSAIDs, and the comparison drug has anti-ulcer effects, it becomes critical to exclude all those with a history of an *H. pylori* ulcer or with an ulcer complication from the study, or to keep track of them separately.

H. PYLORI INFECTION AS A PROTECTIVE OR AGGRAVATING FACTOR IN NSAID USERS

The calculations are different if the presence of *H. pylori* infection either markedly increased (aggravating) or reduced (protective) the prevalence of

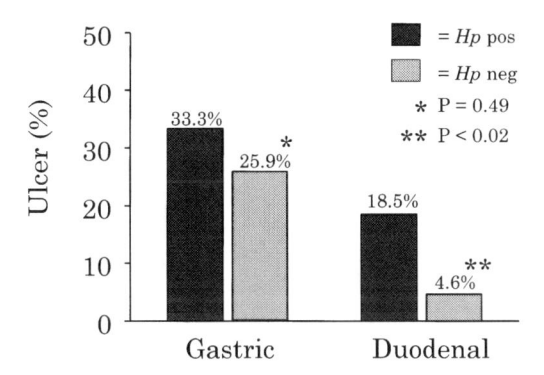

Figure 1. Proportion with ulcers in the placebo group of the OMNIUM study[5]. Data in relation to *H. pylori* status kindly provided by Jorgen Naesdal, AstraZeneca, Molndal, Sweden.

ulcers among NSAID users. There are data available to address this question. The presence of *H. pylori* infection is associated with a marked increase in the proportion with duodenal ulcers seen in endoscopic ulcer prevention trials, and possibly with a modest increase in gastric ulcers[2-5]. Figure 1 shows the results in the placebo group of the OMNIUM study. The presence of *H. pylori* infection was associated with a modest, and not significant, increase in gastric ulcers and a marked and significant increase in duodenal ulcers. As noted above, this study had a design bias because the proton pump inhibitor was known to have anti-ulcer effects in duodenal ulcer whereas the non-antisecretory dose of misoprostol would not. This produced a bias in favour of the proton pump inhibitor for the prevention of ulcer relapse.

The presence of an *H. pylori* infection also proved to have an important effect on the effectiveness of a proton pump inhibitor for ulcer healing[6-8]. The effectiveness of a proton pump inhibitor in the prevention of gastric ulcer was markedly reduced in the absence of *H. pylori* infection to the point where 20 g of omeprazole was not superior to 300 mg of ranitidine which had previously been ineffective for this indication[9-13]. Omeprazole was also inferior $(p < 0.05)$ to the subtherapeutic dose of misoprostol used in the trial (Figure 2). Overall, there are strong data from prospective endoscopic studies in chronic NSAID users suggesting that *H. pylori* infection does not play a protective role in the prevention of NSAID ulcers. Failure to present the data stratified by *H. pylori* status resulted in the ASTRONAUT and OMNIUM studies drawing an erroneous conclusion regarding the estimate of the effectiveness of omeprazole for either ulcer therapy or prevention[5,14].

PROTECTIVE ROLE OF *H. PYLORI* INFECTIONS

It is possible that *H. pylori* infection does have a protective role against NSAID damage? We performed a prospective study in volunteers receiving naproxen, in which we evaluated whether mucosal damage (or protection) could be correlated with the levels of mucosal nitric oxide or interleukin-8

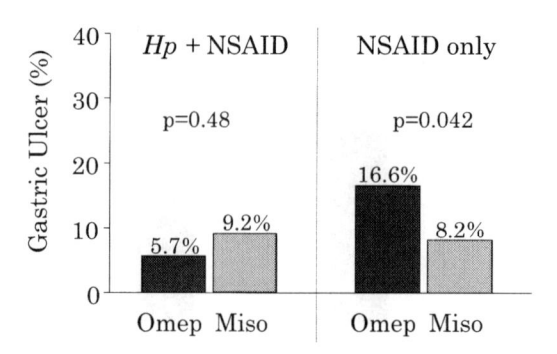

Figure 2. Results of gastric development with co-therapy with 20 mg of omeprazole or 400 µg of misoprostol is shown in relation to H. pylori status.

(IL-8), histological parameters including the density of *H. pylori*, polymorphonuclear cells, mononuclear cells, or with luminal pH. Only those with high intraluminal pH and severe corpus gastritis were protected[15]. In this instance, *H. pylori* was acting as a biological antisecretory agent[16]. These results are also consistent with the clinical observations that cure of *H. pylori* infection slows the healing of endoscopic ulcers in those who continue to take NSAIDs. It is well established that cure of *H. pylori* infection reduces the effectiveness of proton pump inhibitor therapy due to the loss of ammonia from the hydrolysis of urea by *H. pylori* urease, and by an increase in the ability of the corpus to make acid following healing of the gastritis, which acts to inhibit acid secretion[9,12,17–19].

The slight reduction in the rate of gastric ulcer healing following cure of *H. pylori* infection is of no clinical significance for two reasons. First, the prudent physician would discontinue NSAIDs while healing the ulcer and use an alternative therapy such as acetaminophen or low-dose corticosteroids for those few patients who 'required' NSAIDs during the period of ulcer healing[13,20]. Moreover, the difference is one of a few days or weeks which should not be made a major issue since it is not a critical concern. Thus, any difference in healing rates is academic and not clinically important.

EFFECT OF ERADICATION OF *H. PYLORI* ON RECURRENCE OF ULCER COMPLICATIONS IN NSAID ULCERS

As a general rule one should expect the results of clinical trials to reflect what is seen in clinical practice. The clinical trials have produced few, if any, surprises. For example, as part of our studies of *H. pylori* eradication we observed individuals with large gastric ulcers that had been present for more than 1 year. Cure of *H. pylori* led to rapid healing of the ulcers and the ulcer did not recur over the 2 years of observation, despite the patient continuing to take NSAIDs daily. These were clearly *H. pylori* ulcers in NSAID users. In contrast, we also saw patients whose ulcer healed following cure of the *H. pylori* infection and discontinuation of the NSAID. Within a few days (always less than 2 weeks following documented ulcer healing) after the patient restarted NSAID therapy the ulcer recurred and the patient presented with a very large recurrent ulcer, often with bleeding. We considered these to be NSAID ulcers in patients with incidental *H. pylori* infection. We have also had several patients with large chronic true NSAID ulcers (i.e. no *H. pylori* infection) that required more than 6 months of continuous high-dose proton pump inhibitor therapy to heal, and these recurred within a week of restarting NSAID therapy. At operation, no special histological features of these ulcers was evident, and after the ulcer was removed the NSAIDs could be used again without recurrent ulceration. It is clear that the clinical trials with endoscopic ulcers do not mirror the clinical situation, in part because most endoscopic 'ulcers' are actually erosions and do not carry the same risks associated with actual ulcers.

EXPECTATIONS OF CLINICAL TRIALS FOR PREVENTION OF RECURRENT ULCER COMPLICATIONS IN NSAID USERS

Based on clinical experience one should expect that cure of *H. pylori* infection in patients with complicated NSAID ulcers (e.g. with bleeding) would not be expected to reduce the rate of ulcer recurrence or rebleeding in those with NSAID ulcers. In contrast, there is very good evidence that eradication of *H. pylori* in complicated *H. pylori* ulcers will markedly reduce or eliminate rebleeding. This is one of those classical 'apples and oranges' issues, as it is impossible to prospectively decide in an *H. pylori*-infected individual whether the complicated ulcer is an apple (e.g. an *H. pylori* ulcer) or an orange (an NSAID ulcer). Nevertheless, the clinical trials that have been done are consistent with the fact that complicated NSAID ulcers are not responsive to *H. pylori* eradication, and that restarting NSAIDs is often associated with recurrence despite use of drugs such as misoprostol that are effective in the prevention of ulcers seen at endoscopy. The large MUCOSA trial showed that misoprostol was effective for the prevention of life-threatening ulcer complications among NSAID users[21]. These results supported the hypothesis that results of ulcer prevention studies could be used to predict efficacy in preventing ulcer complications. However, there was not a one-to-one correlation: the benefit in terms of prevention of the ulcer complications was less than predicted (approximately 40% reduction of ulcer complications compared to more than 80% protection against the development of ulcers). Unfortunately, *H. pylori* status was not assessed in the MUCOSA trial, and it is possible that there were marked differences in outcome based on whether or not *H. pylori* infection complicated the problem of NSAID use. Subsequent studies will be required to address this question.

CAN *H. PYLORI* INFECTION BE RELIED UPON TO PROTECT AGAINST NSAID ULCERS?

Complicated NSAID ulcers are different from endoscopic ulcers, which are frequently only erosions. We found that those with severe corpus gastritis were 'protected', at least partially, against endoscopic damage associated with NSAID use. This is consistent with the protection seen with antisecretory therapy. Thus, if one could prospectively identify those with severe pangastritis, preferably with achlorhydria, they could reasonably be considered to have some protection against endoscopic NSAID ulcers. Serum pepsinogen levels have been used to identify such patients in gastric cancer screening protocols, because the phenotype of protection is the same as that at highest risk of *H. pylori*-related gastric cancer. Thus, those with some protection against NSAID damage are also those whom we would like to identify in order to cure the infection.

ARE SOME *H. PYLORI* INFECTIONS 'GOOD'?

Should we search for *H. pylori* infection in NSAID users knowing that *H. pylori* infection is a serious transmissible disease and, once diagnosed, must be cured? The answer is probably 'yes'. As noted above, *H. pylori* infection is a serious, destructive, infectious disease that causes progressive damage to the stomach. It can be latent but it is never good for the individual, and is transmissible to others. Those that wish to 'save' *H. pylori* appear to be seeking immortality based on how the future will view that perspective, a concept based on the quote from John Kenneth Galbraith, 'immortality can always be assured by spectacular error'.

References

1. Rauws EJ, Tytgat GN. *Helicobacter pylori* in duodenal and gastric ulcer disease. Baillieres Clin Gastroenterol. 1995;9:529–47.
2. Taha AS, Hudson N, Hawkey CJ et al. Famotidine for the prevention of gastric and duodenal ulcers caused by nonsteroidal antiinflammatory drugs. N Engl J Med. 1996;334:1435–9.
3. Hudson N, Taha AS, Russell RI et al. Famotidine for healing and maintenance in nonsteroidal anti-inflammatory drug associated gastro-duodenal ulceration. Gastroenterology. 1997;112:1817–22.
4. Taha AS, Dahill S, Morran C et al. Neutrophils, *Helicobacter pylori*, and nonsteroidal anti-inflammatory drug ulcers. Gastroenterology. 1999;116:254–8.
5. Hawkey CJ, Karrasch JA, Szczenpanski L et al. Omeprazole compared with misoprostol for ulcers associated with nonsteroidal antiinflammatory drugs. Omeprazole versus Misoprostol for NSAID-induced Ulcer Management (OMNIUM) Study Group. N Engl J Med. 1998;338:727–34.
6. Hawkey CJ, Tulassay Z, Szczepanski L et al. Randomised controlled trial of *Helicobacter pylori* eradication in patients on non-steroidal anti-inflammatory drugs: HELP NSAIDs study. Helicobacter Eradication for Lesion Prevention. Lancet. 1998;352:1016–21.
7. Chan FK, Sung JJ, Suen R et al. Does eradication of *Helicobacter pylori* impair healing of nonsteroidal anti-inflammatory drug associated bleeding peptic ulcers? A prospective randomized study. Aliment Pharmacol Ther. 1998;12:1201–5.
8. Bianchi Porro G, Parente F, Imbesi V, Montrone F, Caruso I. Role of *Helicobacter pylori* in ulcer healing and recurrence of gastric and duodenal ulcers in long term NSAID users. Response to omeprazole dual therapy. Gut. 1996;39:22–6.
9. Gutierrez O, Melo M, Segura AM, Angel A, Genta RM, Graham DY. Cure of *Helicobacter pylori* infection improves gastric acid secretion in patients with corpus gastritis. Scand J Gastroenterol. 1997;32:664–8.
10. El-Omar EM, Oien K, El-Nujumi A et al. *Helicobacter pylori* infection and chronic gastric acid hyposecretion. Gastroenterology. 1997;113:15–24.
11. Miehlke S, Hackelsberger A, Meining A et al. Severe expression of corpus gastritis is characteristic in gastric cancer patients infected with *Helicobacter pylori*. Br J Cancer. 1998;78:263–6.

12. Labenz J, Tillenburg B, Peitz U et al. Helicobacter pylori augments the pH-increasing effect of omeprazole in patients with duodenal ulcer. Gastroenterology. 1996;110:725–32.
13. Graham DY. NSAID ulcers: prevalence and prevention. Mod Rheumatol. 2000;10:2–7.
14. Yeomans ND, Tulassay Z, Juhasz et al. A comparison of omeprazole with ranitidine for ulcers associated with nonsteroidal antiinflammatory drugs. Acid Suppression Trial: Ranitidine versus Omeprazole for NSAID-associated Ulcer Treatment (ASTRONAUT) Study Group. N Engl J Med. 1998;338:719–26.
15. Shiotani A, Yamoaka Y, El-Zimaity H, Saeed A, Graham DY. Interaction between *H. pylori* and NSAIDs: predictive value of density of PMNs, mucosal IL-8 or mucosal and gastric juice nitrite levels. Gastroenterology 2000;118 (In press) (abstract).
16. Graham DY, Yamoaka Y. *H. pylori* and *cagA*: relationships with gastric cancer, duodenal ulcer, and reflux esophagitis and its complications. Helicobacter. 1998;3:145–51.
17. Verdu EF, Armstrong D, Idstrom JP et al. Intragastric pH during treatment with omeprazole: role of *Helicobacter pylori* and *H. pylori*-associated gastritis. Scand J Gastroenterol. 1996;31:1151–6.
18. Labenz J, Tillenburg B, Peitz U et al. Efficacy of omeprazole one year after cure of *Helicobacter pylori* infection in duodenal ulcer patients. Am J Gastroenterol. 1997;92:576–81.
19. Verdu EF, Fraser R, Armstrong D, Blum AL. Effects of omeprazole and lansoprazole on 24-hour intragastric pH in *Helicobacter pylori*-positive volunteers. Scand J Gastroenterol 1994;29:1065–9.
20. Graham DY. Nonsteroidal anti-inflammatory drugs, *Helicobacter pylori*, and ulcers: where we stand. Am J Gastroenterol. 1996;91:2080–6.
21. Silverstein FE, Graham DY, Senior JR et al. Misoprostol reduces serious gastrointestinal complications in patients with rheumatoid arthritis receiving nonsteroidal anti-inflammatory drugs. A randomized, double-blind, placebo-controlled trial. Ann Intern Med. 1995;123:241–9.

49
Helicobacter pylori and non-steroidal anti-inflammatory drugs

C. J. HAWKEY

Imagine you admit a patient with a bleeding gastric ulcer. The patient is not taking aspirin or non-aspirin non-steroidal anti-inflammatory drugs (NSAIDs). What do you do to prevent further ulceration and ulcer complications? Probably, all would seek to eradicate the causative *Helicobacter pylori*, as this is logical, intellectually coherent and supported by pragmatic experience. You know that *H. pylori* eradication on its own will lead to ulcer healing but the patient has had a bleed and you want him/her to be safe so, in addition, you give an ulcer-healing agent, at least until ulcer healing has occurred.

Unfortunately, the patient's strain of *H. pylori* is highly resistant and four attempts at eradication, including determination of antibiotic sensitivities, are unsuccessful. What would you do now? You would probably seek to interrupt the pathogenic processes by which *H. pylori* causes ulceration by administration of an acid-suppressing drug. This is logical, intellectually coherent and supported by pragmatic evidence showing that this reduces recurrence of gastric ulcer and its complications.

Imagine now that the patient *is* taking NSAIDs and is not infected with *H. pylori*. I imagine you would employ the same principles – stop the offending agent (NSAID) if possible and, if this is not possible, use an effective agent (misoprostol or a proton pump inhibitor) to interrupt the pathological processes leading to NSAID ulceration. This is logical, intellectually coherent and supported by pragmatic evidence.

Now imagine that the patient with the bleeding gastric ulcer, who is taking NSAIDs, is infected with *H. pylori*. Here logic fails because it is impossible to say whether the ulcer is due to the NSAID or due to the *H. pylori*. Consequently, it is best to be guided by pragmatic evidence. Unfortunately, much thinking in this area is driven by (often rather flawed) logic, perhaps motivated by a desire to retain the attractive but simplistic intellectual coherence of believing that all *H. pylori* infections are bad and should be eradicated.

One problem in this area is that much of the early pioneering work on the prevention of NSAID injury by Graham and others did not define *H. pylori* status in these seminal studies, even though it was possible to do this at the time they were conducted. Graham did, however, find that 'non-steroidal anti-inflammatory drug-induced mucosal injury ... was more frequent in those without infection than with infection'[1] and stated that '*H. pylori* does not confer increased risk of ulcerations in arthritics receiving NSAIDs chronically'[2]. More recent studies that have investigated the issue directly have confirmed Dr Graham's assertion that there is little or no net harm from *H. pylori* in unselected NSAID users, but has shown that the interaction varies with different patient subgroups, with some clearly being protected by concurrent *H. pylori* infection.

Assessment of *H. pylori* infection and NSAIDs can be broken down into a number of questions:

1. *Can NSAID ulcer healing be achieved in the presence of* H. pylori *infection?*

Trials in which *H. pylori* status has been defined have shown that, far from being retarded, healing of gastric ulcers by acid suppression in patients continuing to take NSAIDs is faster in *H. pylori*-infected individuals[3–6].

2. *What does eradication of* H. pylori *infection do to ulcer healing in patients with gastric ulcers who continue to take NSAIDs?*

Three studies have addressed this issue[7–9]. None of them has shown acceleration of healing, two have shown non-significant retardation and another showed highly significant retardation of ulcer healing by *H. pylori* eradication in NSAID users treated with proton pump inhibitors (PPIs). The average retardation of ulcer healing over 8 weeks was 18%. Data from naturally uninfected subjects and those who have undergone eradication therapy are coherent in showing numerical or significant worsening of healing compared to infected patients when treated with acid suppression.

This beneficial impact of *H. pylori* infection on ulcer healing is hardly surprising given that, in terms of intragastric hydrogen ion concentration, H_2-receptor antagonists and PPIs are some 100-fold more effective in the presence of *H. pylori* infection that in its absence. This is true for both the comparison between naturally infected and uninfected individuals and after *H. pylori* eradication[10,11].

3. *Does* H. pylori *eradication alone heal ulcers in NSAID users?*

This is implausible, illogical and intellectually incoherent, given everything that is now known, and no-one has thought it ethical or sensible to address this question.

4. *Does* H. pylori *eradication alone prevent gastric ulcer recurrence in NSAID users?*

This question is equally illogical but has been tested and the evidence is consistent in showing that *H. pylori* eradication does not protect such patients. There are three long-term endoscopic studies which show no evidence of any reduction in the rate of gastric ulcer recurrence[7,9,12]. These endoscopic studies are supported by one study using a clinically important endpoint, namely rebleeding following initial presentation of gastric ulcer haemorrhage[13]. Patients who underwent *H. pylori* eradication had a 20% recurrence rate of ulcer bleeding over the next 6 months, compared to 2% seen with omeprazole maintenance treatment. *H. pylori* eradication is thus both illogical and an ineffective strategy for the management of such patients.

5. *Does* H. pylori *eradication further reduce relapse rates when added to maintenance treatment?*

This is a more reasonable question although, from what is known of the relationship between *H. pylori* and acid suppression, it would be surprising if *H. pylori* enhanced the effectiveness of maintenance treatment with acid suppression. Moreover, there are no studies that address this issue directly, so clinical judgements must be made by extension from what occurs in naturally infected and uninfected individuals and with regard to the deleterious effects of *H. pylori* eradication on ulcer healing by acid suppression. Again, the evidence is consistent in showing that protection of patients against gastric ulceration using acid suppression is much more effective in those who are *H. pylori*-infected compared to those who are not[4,5].

No similar relationship with *H. pylori* infection is seen if misoprostol is used for maintenance treatment[4]. Misoprostol appears somewhat more effective in maintaining patients who are not infected with *H. pylori* than in those who are infected. It therefore follows that maintenance treatment with misoprostol is a logically complementary strategy to *H. pylori* eradication. There may, however, be both tolerability and efficacy disadvantages to this approach. The side-effects of misoprostol are well known and, even at a low dose of 400 µg daily, are more common than those seen with a PPI. Moreover, from the efficacy point of view, what little evidence there is suggests that misoprostol is ineffective at preventing recurrence of ulcer bleeding[14] (as opposed to its clear, but modest effectiveness for primary prophylaxis[15]). By contrast, use of a PPI without *H. pylori* eradication has been shown to be highly effective for secondary prevention[13] of ulcer bleeding and also to be well tolerated.

6. *Are there any subgroups in whom* H. pylori *infection may be harmful?*

One interesting intervention study has reported that eradication of *H. pylori* infection with a bismuth-based regime in patients starting NSAIDs for the first time appeared to protect them at 2 months, raising the possibility that *H. pylori* was harmful in this group of patients[16]. These patients were different from those studied in other trials of *H. pylori* eradication. To enter the study they had to have had no more than 1 month's total lifetime NSAID use and no past history of dyspepsia or peptic ulcer. They were therefore probably a group of patients with a virgin gastroduodenal mucosa. This study implies that *H. pylori* infection may accelerate injury in patients with a 'virgin' mucosa when they use NSAIDs for the first time. However, it seems unlikely that the major effect reported in this study would persist for a long time, since epidemiological studies (see below) show that NSAID ulcer complications occur at roughly the same rate in patients who are infected or not with *H. pylori*. Confirmatory studies that are both double-blind and of longer duration will be needed before *H. pylori* eradication can be recommended routinely for patients starting NSAIDs.

7. *Are there other hidden problems from long-term proton pump inhibition in* H. pylori-*positive individuals taking NSAIDs?*

This question has not been investigated directly. In patients not taking NSAIDs there have been concerns that chronic use of PPIs in *H. pylori*-infected patients may accelerate the development of gastric atrophy, and that this may subsequently predispose to gastric cancer. Whether enhanced gastric atrophy occurs or not remains controversial, and there is no evidence for an increased incidence of gastric cancer with long-term use of PPIs. Moreover, in patients who use NSAIDs, the risk of gastric cancer that is associated with *H. pylori* is reduced to about the same extent as *H. pylori* itself increases it. Thus, the risks of gastric cancer with long-term PPI use are theoretical rather than real, and probably do not apply to NSAID users.

CONCLUSIONS FROM THERAPEUTIC STUDIES

From these considerations we can conclude that no therapeutically useful consequence of *H. pylori* eradication can be identified in patients taking NSAIDs who have already experienced a gastric ulcer, and that there is therefore no evidence that *H. pylori* infection causes clinically important harm in these patients. Indeed, it is incontrovertible that *H. pylori* enhances the effectiveness of PPI to an extent that would undoubtedly influence whether a patient has a recurrent life-threatening ulcer bleed or not. In other circumstances, for example the patient starting NSAIDs, there is some evidence for benefit, but it is not sufficiently well established to influence policy. It is irrelevant to the management of patients who have already experienced NSAID complications, where the relationship with *H. pylori* is clearly different.

Returning to the initial dilemma, it can be seen that ulcers occurring in patients taking NSAIDs who are infected with *H. pylori* are neither '*H. pylori* ulcers' nor 'NSAID ulcers'. They behave in a homogeneous way that is different from *H. pylori*-negative NSAID ulcers and from *H. pylori* ulcers in patients not using NSAIDs. They should be regarded as a category in their own right, and their management should be based upon empirical evidence rather than emotion, prejudice or vague assertion.

WHAT IS THE ENDOSCOPIC AND EPIDEMIOLOGICAL EVIDENCE?

Meta-analysis of endoscopic studies shows an approximately 80% increase in the incidence of NSAID-associated ulcers in subjects who are infected with *H. pylori*[17]. This is significant, but small by comparison with the 500–1000% increase caused by the NSAID itself. Endoscopic evidence leads one to predict that *H. pylori* eradication might reduce NSAID-associated ulcer incidence by 8–12%. This has not been shown in clinical studies, but is a sufficiently small effect that this benefit could have been missed. However, the 20% recurrence of life-threatening ulcer bleeding that occurs following *H. pylori* eradication emphasizes that, even if this benefit is there, it is not clinically useful.

Moreover, the picture is complicated because there is a discrepancy between the relatively clear message from endoscopic studies for a small increase and that of epidemiological studies with a balance of evidence if anything favouring a protective effect of *H. pylori*. In seven epidemiological studies[18-24], *H. pylori* was reported to exert a harmful influence in one, a beneficial influence in three and to have a neutral impact in three studies. Since the net effect of *H. pylori* infection in NSAID users is a balance between the harmful and the beneficial effects, it may not be surprising that results vary between different countries where the population susceptibility to *H. pylori* infection and/or *H. pylori* toxicity may vary.

CONCLUSIONS FROM OBSERVATIONAL STUDIES

There is a discrepancy in the results from endoscopic and epidemiological studies. This is seen for influences other than *H. pylori* infection, such as age and past history, which are much bigger risk factors in epidemiological than endoscopic studies of patients taking NSAIDs. The epidemiological studies show clearly that any harmful effect of *H. pylori* infection is very limited, and overall suggest that it is more likely to be protective than harmful in users of non-selective NSAIDs. Thus, there are many outstanding questions, for example about the extent to which prokaryotic and eukaryotic variation may explain differences from different countries. However, these are likely to become relevant because there is no reason to believe that the effect of *H. pylori* infection in patients using COX-2 inhibitors should be different from that seen in patients not using anti-rheumatic drugs, and limited evidence to date supports this view. Thus, the clear evidence that *H. pylori* infection does not have a harmful effect in users of non-selective NSAIDs should now be put into the interesting medical history bin, as it is rapidly ceasing to be an issue of current relevance.

References

1. Graham DY, Lidsky MD, Cox AM et al. Long-term non-steroidal anti-inflammatory drug use and *Helicobacter pylori* infection. Gastroenterology. 1991;100:1653.
2. Kim JG, Graham DY. *Helicobacter pylori* infection and development of gastric or duodenal ulcer in arthritic patients receiving chronic NSAID therapy. The Misoprostol Study Group. Am J Gastroenterol. 1994;89:203.
3. Hudson N, Taha AS, Russell RI et al. Famotidine for healing and maintenance in non-steroidal anti-inflammatory drug-associated gastroduodenal ulceration. Gastroenterology. 1997;112:1819.
4. Hawkey CJ, Karrasch JA, Szczepañski L et al. Omeprazole compared with misoprostol for ulcers associated with nonsteroidal antiinflammatory drugs. N Engl J Med. 1998;338:727.
5. Yeomans ND, Tulassay Z, Juhász L et al. A comparison of omeprazole with ranitidine for ulcers associated with nonsteroidal antiinflammatory drugs. N Engl J Med. 1998;338:719.
6. Cullen D, Bardhan KD, Eisner M et al. Primary gastroduodenal prophylaxis with omeprazole for non-steroidal anti-inflammatory drug users. Aliment Pharmacol Ther. 1998;12:135.

7. Bianchi Porro G, Parente F, Imbesi V et al. Role of *Helicobacter pylori* in ulcer healing and recurrence of gastric and duodenal ulcers in longterm NSAID users. Response to omeprazole dual therapy. Gut. 1996;39:22.
8. Chan FK, Sung JJ, Suen R et al. Does eradication of *Helicobacter pylori* impair healing of nonsteroidal anti-inflammatory drug associated bleeding peptic ulcers? A prospective randomized study. Aliment Pharmacol Ther. 1998;12:1201.
9. Hawkey CJ, Tulassay Z, Szczepanski L et al. Randomised controlled trial of *Helicobacter pylori* eradication in patients on non-steroidal anti-inflammatory drugs: HELP NSAIDs study. Lancet. 1998;352:1016.
10. Labenz J, Tillenburg B, Peitz U et al. Irreversible fall of efficacy of omeprazole after cure of *H. pylori* infection in duodenal ulcer patients. Gastroenterology. 1996;110:A165.
11. Labenz J, Tillenburg B, Peitz U, Verdu E, Stolte M, Borsch G, Blum AL. Effect of curing *Helicobacter pylori* infection on intragastric acidity during treatment with ranitidine in patients with duodenal ulcer. Gut. 1997;41:33–6.
12. Yanaka A, Nakahara A, Tanaka N et al. Eradication of *Helicobacter pylori* does not prevent ulcer relapse in patients with NSAIDs-induced gastric ulcer. Gastroenterology. 1999;116, A362.
13. Chan FKL, Sung JY, Suen R et al. Eradication of *H. pylori* versus maintenance acid suppression to prevent recurrent ulcer hemorrhage in high-risk NSAID users: a prospective randomized study. Gastroenterology. 1998;114:A87.
14. Chan FKL, Sung JYJ, Ching JYL et al. Prospective randomised trial of misoprostol plus naproxen versus nabumetone to prevent recurrent ulcer haemorrhage in high-risk NSAID users. Gastroenterology. 1999;116:A134.
15. Silverstein FE, Graham DY, Senior JR et al. Misoprostol reduces serious gastrointestinal complications in patients with arthritis receiving non steroidal antiinflammatory drugs – a randomised double blind placebo controlled study. Ann Intern Med. 1995;123:241–9.
16. Chan FK, Sung JJ, Chung SC et al. Randomised trial of eradication of *Helicobacter pylori* before non-steroidal anti-inflammatory drug therapy to prevent peptic ulcers. Lancet. 1997;350:975.
17. Huang JQ, Lad RJ, Sridhar S, Sumanac K, Hunt RH. *H. pylori* infection increases the risk of non-steroidal anti-inflammatory drug (NSAID)-induced gastro-duodenal ulceration. Gastroenterology. 1999;116:A192.
18. Cullen DJ, Hawkey GM, Greenwood DC et al. Peptic ulcer bleeding in the elderly: relative roles of *Helicobacter pylori* and non-steroidal anti-inflammatory drugs. Gut. 1997;41:459.
19. Aalykke C, Lauritsen JM, Hallas J et al. *Helicobacter pylori* and risk of ulcer bleeding among users of nonsteroidal anti-inflammatory drugs: a case–control study. Gastroenterology. 1999;116:1305.
20. Labenz J, Peitz U, Köhl H et al. *Helicobacter pylori* increases the risk of peptic ulcer bleeding: a case–control study. Ital J Gastroenterol Hepatol. 1999;31:110.
21. Pilotto A, Leandro G, Di Mario F et al.: Role of *Helicobacter pylori* infection on upper gastrointestinal bleeding in the elderly: a case–control study. Dig Dis Sci. 1997;42:586.
22. Wu CY, Poon SK, Chen GH et al. Interaction between *Helicobacter pylori* and non-steroidal anti-inflammatory drugs in peptic ulcer bleeding. Scand J Gastroenterol. 1999;34:234.
23. Stack WA, Hawkey GM, Atherton JC et al. Interaction of risk factors for peptic ulcer bleeding. Gastroenterology. 1999;116:A97.
24. Santolaria S, Lanas A, Benito R et al. *Helicobacter pylori* infection is a protective factor for bleeding gastric ulcers but is not for bleeding duodenal ulcers in NSAID users. Gastroenterology. 1999;116:A231.

Section IX
Helicobacter pylori and 'Test-and-Treat' Strategies

50
The impact of a test-and-treat strategy for *Helicobacter pylori*: the United States perspective

D. A. PEURA

Dyspepsia can be defined as persistent or recurrent abdominal pain or discomfort centred in the upper abdomen[1]. Pain is easier for a patient to describe and/or localize while discomfort is more subjective and often characterized by symptoms such as fullness, bloating, nausea or satiety. As defined, 10–40%[2–6] of the adult population suffers from dyspepsia, but this frequency varies considerably around the world and even within regional localities. Dyspepsia accounts for almost 50% of gastroenterology consultations and 5% of primary-care physician patient visits[7]. The costs of evaluation and treatment are tremendous, and symptoms have a considerable impact on the quality of life and psychological well-being of those afflicted[6,8–10].

There is no single aetiology for all dyspeptic symptoms. An obvious organic cause such as ulcer disease or gastric cancer is rarely found[7], especially in the United States. However, in areas of the world where prevalence of ulcer and cancer is high, and even in the United States in older individuals or those of any age with associated alarm features (i.e. weight loss, vomiting, signs of bleeding, etc.), serious disease should be excluded. In the end, most patients with dyspepsia have no obvious cause of their symptoms found[7], and economic reality precludes extensive investigation in everyone. Therefore, empirical treatment of symptoms with prokinetics, or more often acid-suppressive agents, H_2-receptor antagonists (H2RAs) or proton pump inhibitors (PPIs) has been suggested as a practical management strategy[7]. The clinical response to such empirical treatment has been reported to be quite variable[11], but data do appear to support the use of PPIs[12]. A report of two recent 8-week US trials suggests that PPIs can totally relieve dyspeptic symptoms and improve quality of life in many patients[13].

The pathogenic role of *Helicobacter pylori* as a cause of dyspeptic symptoms remains controversial[14]. Infectious ulcers do explain recurrent symptoms in some, but up to 60% of patients with dyspepsia are subsequently found to have only *H. pylori*-related gastritis[7]. This prevalence of gastritis

Table 1. Factors impacting feasibility of test-and-treat strategy

Accuracy of non-invasive testing population
   Population prevalence of infection
Impact of treatment on outcome
Likelihood of eliminating symptoms
   Prevalence of ulcer, cancer, NUD and GERD
Cost of endoscopy
   Managed care and Medicare
Need to make a clinical diagnosis

varies considerably around the world and appears to parallel the background population prevalence of infection[7]. Furthermore, the mechanism(s) by which the bacterium could lead to symptoms in the absence of ulcer disease remains conjectural[14]. Clearly, some patients benefit from bacterial eradication but the absolute therapeutic gain is also quite variable and may depend on the likelihood of underlying ulcer disease or gastro-oesophageal reflux[15,16], the latter a condition unlikely to benefit from (in fact, which may worsen after) bacterial cure[17].

Nevertheless, most studies suggest that *H. pylori* gastritis is more frequent in symptomatic individuals than in those without symptoms[18]. While this observation does not definitely implicate *H. pylori* infection as the cause of dyspepsia, it does form the basis for the 'test-and-treat' management strategy. An inexpensive, non-invasive test for infection followed by antibiotics in those testing positive would presumably obviate expensive diagnostic evaluation involving endoscopy in some patients[19]. Furthermore, this approach would cure infectious ulcer disease, thereby eliminating the cost associated with recurrent ulcer symptoms and complications. Cost modelling supports the economics of a test-and-treat management strategy, primarily because endoscopy is so expensive. If endoscopic costs remain at their current level a test-and-treat strategy provides the desired clinical outcome, symptom relief, at the lowest possible price, when the prevalence of *H. pylori*-associated ulcer is at least 10% or symptom response to antibiotics in those without ulcers is at least 8%[20,21].

From the American perspective it is difficult to precisely measure the current impact of any test-and-treat strategy since factors influencing cost and outcomes vary geographically (Table 1). Take for example the accuracy of *H. pylori* testing. In many areas of the United States, prevalence of *H. pylori* infection is quite low (<20%), making the positive predictive value of serology unacceptable (Figure 1). Either a urea breath test or a stool antigen test would be a more appropriate non-invasive diagnostic alternative in this setting. However, most US physicians are not familiar with these tests, they are not readily available clinically even though they are approved and commercially marketed, and complicated reimbursement mechanisms are an obstacle to their use in the office setting.

Another factor is the likelihood that ulcer disease is causing symptoms, the major clinical and economic premise upon which the test-and-treat strategy depends. In most parts of the United States, ulcers account for only a small percentage of dyspeptic symptoms, and quite often these ulcers are

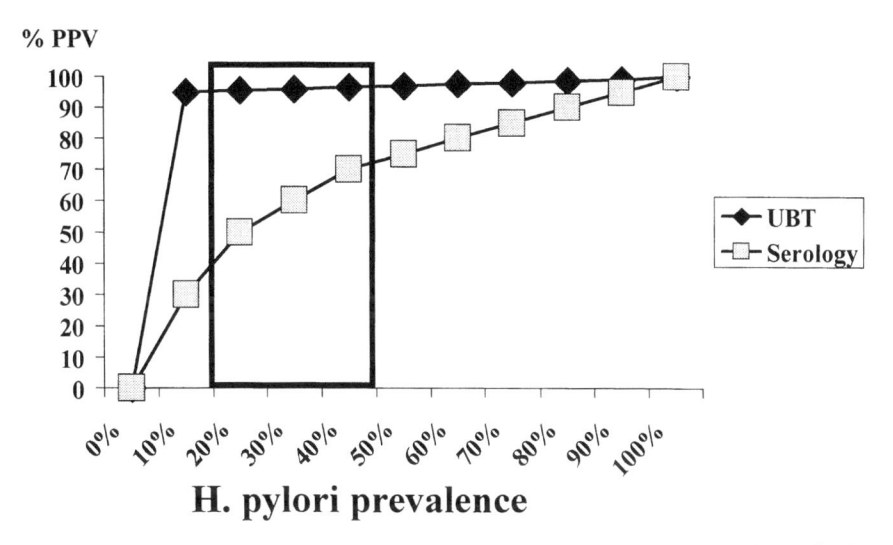

Figure 1. Positive predictive value of test versus *H. pylori* prevalence (adapted from ref. 30)

not infectious[22]. In the United States up to 20% of ulcers recur in spite of *H. pylori* eradication[23] and many patients cured of their infectious ulcer disease continue to have symptoms and will still require some form of treatment[24,25]. Most dyspeptic symptoms in the United States are due to non-ulcer dyspepsia (NUD) or gastro-oesophageal reflux disease (GERD), conditions for which any pathogenic role of *H.* pylori remains controversial. At best curing infection in those with NUD eliminates symptoms in only a few[7,24], if any, while in those with GERD it may actually worsen symptoms and/or make subsequent treatment with acid suppression less effective[17]. The population prevalence of *H. pylori* infection has a major impact on the success of a test-and-treat strategy. Stanghellini *et al.* illustrated this concept using a conservative hypothetical model[26]. For example, they assumed 40% prevalence of peptic ulcer disease in dyspeptic patients and a 90% eradication rate with treatment. Further, they assumed that, following eradication, 30% of those with NUD and 70% of those with peptic ulcer disease had their symptoms permanently cured. If the population prevalence of *H. pylori* infection were 100%, then 40% of those with dyspepsia who underwent testing and treatment would be rendered symptom-free. If the prevalence were 60% then 25% would benefit. However, in an environment such as the United States, where the prevalence of *H. pylori* might be only 20%, success of a test-and-treat approach is at best 9%.

The situation in the United States does not necessarily favour a test-and-treat approach to dyspepsia (Table 2). The prevalence of infection is decreasing and is actually less than 20% in many areas, especially in younger patients who are candidates for empirical management of symptoms. Ulcers are uncommon and often test *H. pylori* negative, and stomach cancer is rare. NUD and GERD, conditions for which *H. pylori* eradication treatment remains controversial at best, are common. Although the cost of endoscopy

Table 2. The American environment

Prevalence of *H. pylori*	Low
Impact of treatment	Low
Ulcer and cancer	Low
NUD and GER	High
Cost of endoscopy	High
but	
Pressure to make diagnosis	Very high

is high, the pressure to make a clinical diagnosis, especially in those with chronic recurrent symptoms that affect quality of life, is very high.

So what is actually done? In reality, whatever the physician and patient want and insurance will allow. Many undergo initial serological testing (more often than not this is negative) and treatment for *H. pylori* infection at the primary-care level[27]. Often the treatment that is prescribed is inappropriate or inadequate[28], so infection may not be cured and organisms may develop antibiotic resistance. Some ulcer disease is cured, a rare cancer may be prevented and, occasionally, symptoms are alleviated[9,27]. More often, however, symptoms persist, recur or actually worsen; so endoscopy is eventually performed[29]. While endoscopy has been delayed, this is not clinically relevant, since results are generally negative and no serious disease has been missed. Patients are prescribed proton pump inhibitors for symptomatic relief; this works in many. Those who do not respond receive other therapies, generally with poor or unpredictable results.

References

1. Talley NJ, Stanghellini V, Heading RC, Koch KL, Malagelada JR, Tytgat GNJ. Functional gastroduodenal disorders. Gut. 1999;45(Suppl. II):II37–42.
2. Talley NJ, Zinsmeister AR, Schleck CD, Melton III LJ. Dyspepsia and dyspepsia subgroups: a population-based study. Gastroenterology. 1992;102:1259–68.
3. Talley NJ, Weaver AL, Zinsmeister AR, Melton III LJ. Onset and disappearance of gastrointestinal symptoms and functional gastrointestinal disorders. Am J Epidemiol. 1992;15:165–77.
4. Drossman DA, Li Z, Andruzzi E *et al.* U.S. householder survey of functional gastrointestinal disorders: prevalence, sociodemography, and health impact. Dig Dis Sci. 1993;38:1569–80.
5. Knill-Jones RP. Geographical differences in the prevalence of dyspepsia. Scand J Gastroenterol. 1991;26(Suppl. 182):17–24.
6. Tougas G, Chen Y, Hwang P, Liu MM, Eggleston A. Prevalence and impact of upper gastrointestinal symptoms in the Canadian population: findings from the DIGEST Study. Am J Gastroenterol. 1999;94:2845–54.
7. Talley NJ, Silverstein MD, Agreus L, Nyren O, Sonnenberg A, Holtmann, G. AGA Technical Review: Evaluation of dyspepsia. Gastroenterology. 1998;114:582–95.
8. Nyren O, Lindberg G, Linstrom E *et al.* Economic costs of functional dyspepsia. PharmacoEconomics. 1992;1:312–24.
9. Heaney A, Colllins JSA, Watson RGP, McFarland RJ, Bamford KB, Tham TCK. A prospective randomised trial of a 'test and treat' policy versus endoscopy based management in young *Helicobacter pylori* positive patients with ulcer-like dyspepsia, referred to a hospital clinic. Gut. 1999;45:186–90.
10. Wilhemlsen I. Quality-of-life in upper gastrointestinal disorders. Scand J Gastroenterol. 1995;30(Suppl. 211):21–5.

11. Veldhuyzen van Zanten SJO, Cleary C, Talley NJ et al. Drug treatment of functional dyspepsia. A systematic analysis of trial methodology with recommendations for design of future trials. Am J Gastroenterol. 1996;91:660–73.
12. Talley NJ, Meineche-Schmidt V, Pare P et al. Efficacy of omeprazole in functional dyspepsia: double-blind, randomized, placebo-controlled trial (the Bond and Opera studies). Aliment Pharmacol Ther. 1998;12:1055–65.
13. Peura D, Kovacs T, Metz D, Gudmundson J, Pilmer B. Low-dose lansoprazole: effective for non-ulcer dyspepsia (NUD). Gastroenterology. 2000;118:A939.
14. Talley NJ, Hunt RH. What role does *Helicobacter pylori* play in dyspepsia and nonulcer dyspepsia? Arguments for and against *H. pylori* being associated with dyspeptic symptoms. Gastroenterology. 1997;113:S67–77.
15. Blum AL, Talley NJ, O'Morain C et al. Lack of effect of treating *Helicobacater pylori* infection in patients with nonulcer dyspepsia. N Engl J Med. 1998;339:1875–9.
16. McColl KEL, Murray L, El-Omar E et al. Symptomatic benefit from eradicating *Helicobacter pylori* infection in patients with nonulcer dyspepsia. N Engl J Med. 1998;339:1869–74.
17. O'Connor HJ. Review article: *Helicobacter pylori* and gastro-oesophageal reflux disease – clinical implications and management. Aliment Pharmacol Ther. 1999;13:117–27.
18. Armstrong D. *Helicobacter pylori* infection and dyspepsia. Scand J Gastroenterol Suppl. 1996;31:38–47.
19. Gisbert JP, Pajares JM. *Helicobacter pylori* 'test-and-treat' strategy for dyspeptic patients. Scand J Gastroenterol. 1999;34:644–52.
20. Sonnenberg A. Cost–benefit analysis of testing for *Helicobacter pylori* in dyspeptic subjects. Am J Gastroenterol. 1996;91:1773–7.
21. Sonnenberg A, Inadomi JM. Economic perspectives in the management of *Helicobacter pylori* infections. Curr Top Microbiol Immunol. 1999;241:237–60.
22. Ciociola AA, McSorley DJ, Turner K, Sykes D, Palmer JBD. *Helicobacter pylori* infection rates in duodenal ulcer patients in the United States may be lower than previously estimated. Am J Gastroenterol. 1999;94:1834–40.
23. Laine L, Hopkins RJ, Girardi LS. Has the impact of *Helicobacter pylori* therapy on ulcer recurrence in the United States been overstated? A meta-analysis of rigorously designed trials. Am J Gastroenterol. 1998;93:1409–15.
24. Tan ACITL, Den Hartog G, Mulder CJJ. Eradication of *Helicobacter pylori* does not decrease the long-term use of acid-suppressive medication. Aliment Pharmacol Ther. 1999;13:1519–22.
25. McColl KE, el-Nujumi A, Murray LS et al. Assessment of symptomatic response as predictor of *Helicobacter pylori* status following eradication therapy in patients with ulcer. Gut. 1998;42:618–22.
26. Stanghellini V, Tosetti C, De Giorgio R, Barbara G, Salvioli B, Corinaldesi R. How should *Helicobacter pylori* negative patients be managed? Gut. 1999;45(Suppl. 1):I32–5.
27. Kearney DJ, Brousal A. Effect of *Helicobacter pylori* treatment on outpatient pharmacy costs. Gastroenterology. 1999;116:A70.
28. Breuer T, Goodman KJ, Malaty HM, Sudhop T, Graham DY. How do clinicians practicing in the U.S. manage *Helicobacter pylori*-related gastrointestinal diseases? A comparison of primary care and specialist physicians. Am J Gastroenterol. 1998;93:553–61.
29. Ladabaum U, Fendrick AM, Scheiman JM. Clinical outcomes of primary care patients undergoing office-based serologic testing for *Helicobacter pylori*. Gastroenterology. 1999;116:A72.
30. Chiba N, Veldhuyzen van Zanten S. ^{13}C-Urea breath tests are the noninvasive method of choice for *Helicobacter pylori* detection. Can J Gastroenterol. 1999;13:681–3.

51
Test-and-treat strategy in dyspepsia – the European perspective

P. MALFERTHEINER

INTRODUCTION

Dyspepsia accounts for around 1–4% of all consultations in general practice according to surveys conducted in some European countries, but it is possible that many more adults suffer from this condition[1–3].

The key question for the investigating physician is 'Does the patient suffer from dyspeptic symptoms because of an underlying organic disease or is it a functional disorder?' If patients are investigated by upper gastrointestinal endoscopy, the most frequently detected organic cause of dyspeptic symptoms, in the absence of heartburn as leading symptom, is peptic ulcer. In at least half of the patients, dyspepsia will be classified as functional after comprehensive diagnostic evaluation[4,5]. The main concern remains gastric cancer, and whether it is still in a curable state.

Gastric cancer is the most frequent malignancy among neoplastic disorders to be considered in the diagnostic evaluation of dyspeptic symptoms, and varies considerbly in its prevalence across European regions[16].

At present, doctors in general practice most often proceed to prescribe empiric therapy for the symptomatic relief of dyspeptic symptoms, especially if patients are young and dyspepsia is a first presentation. In many European countries, however, early referral to the specialist for upper gastrointestinal endoscopy is still advised.

It is generally recommended to proceed to immediate upper gastrointestinal endoscopy in all cases with a family history of gastric cancer, or those in whom empiric symptom-oriented therapy fails, or in those with symptom relapse after transient relief. Early endoscopy is mandatory in all cases with unexplained weight loss and anaemia[7].

The discovery and recognition of *H. pylori* as a key pathogen in peptic ulcer disease has led to the search for this infection in the management of patients with dyspeptic symptoms. The subsequent availability of non-inva-

Table 1. Strategy options for dyspepsia management

1. Empirical therapy targeting main symptom(s).
2. First-line endoscopy.
3. Test for *H. pylori* and treat.
4. Non-invasive *H. pylori* testing followed by endoscopy of *H. pylori*-positives (test and scope).
5. Screen for *H. pylori*-negatives and endoscope *H. pylori*-negatives.
6. Empirical *H. pylori* therapy.

sive tests for the detection of *H. pylori* infection has extended the diagnostic option to physicians in general practice for their first-line management of dyspepsia. The detection of the presence of *H. pylori* would allow the inclusion of patients with dyspeptic symptoms and those suffering from peptic ulcer disease, and if followed by *H. pylori* eradication this would be appropriate therapy. Non-invasive testing for *H. pylori* could alternatively be followed by endoscopy in *H. pylori*-positive patients to define gastroduodenal lesions as a 'test-and-scope strategy'.

The most important progress, however, was achieved by non-invasive testing followed by treatment of *H. pylori*-positives. This strategy has to be seen in the context of different first-line options proposed for dyspepsia management (Table 1), with only options 1 and 2 being important alternatives. Options 4–6 have not found major acceptance (option 6 may even be at risk), and their clinical usefulness was not sufficiently evaluated.

MAASTRICHT GUIDELINES: TEST-AND-TREAT AN ADVISABLE STRATEGY OPTION

Non-invasive *H. pylori* testing and treatment has been considered as an option for the management of young dyspeptic patients since the late 1980s[8], but it was not until the meeting in Maastricht that this strategy was brought to the attention of a much larger circle of general practitioners and specialists in Europe. In the guidelines, reported from Maastricht, 'test-and-treat' is given as an advisable indication for the management of young dyspeptic patients with no alarm symptoms and no NSAID intake. The age cut-off was set at below 45 years of age, while patients over this age should undergo an immediate thorough investigation by endoscopy (Figure 1)[9].

The majority of participants supported this strategy, and one-third of the participants from various countries rejected this option. The test-and-treat strategy was also perceived with varying enthusiasm in various countries in Europe[10]. The rationale for 'test-and-treat' in Europe is that gastric malignancy in most countries is rare in the young age group, who do not present with sinister symptoms. Moreover, patients with peptic ulcer disease included among those who tested *H. pylori*-positive would receive optimal treatment for their disease with eradication treatment. This, in itself, would result in a positive cost benefit and justify the strategy. The cost benefit would become more substantial if, in addition to patients with peptic ulcer disease, a subset of those with functional dyspepsia would also benefit from *H. pylori* eradica-

```
                    ┌─────────────────────────┐
                    │  Dyspeptic patient      │
                    │  First primary care visit│
                    └─────────────────────────┘
                       /                    \
                      /                      \
   ┌──────────────────────┐          ┌──────────────────────────────┐
   │ < 45 years* without  │          │ > 45 years* or with alarm     │
   │   alarm symptoms     │          │   symptoms (irrespective of age)│
   └──────────────────────┘          └──────────────────────────────┘
            │                                      │
   ┌──────────────────────────┐          ┌──────────────────────┐
   │ Review patients history  │          │ Refer to             │
   │ Test for Helicobacter pylori│       │ gastroenterologist   │
   │ - 13C-urea breath test** │          └──────────────────────┘
   │   or                     │
   │ - Laboratory serology    │
   └──────────────────────────┘
            │
   ┌──────────────────────────┐
   │ If H. pylori-positive,   │
   │ treat the infection      │
   └──────────────────────────┘
```

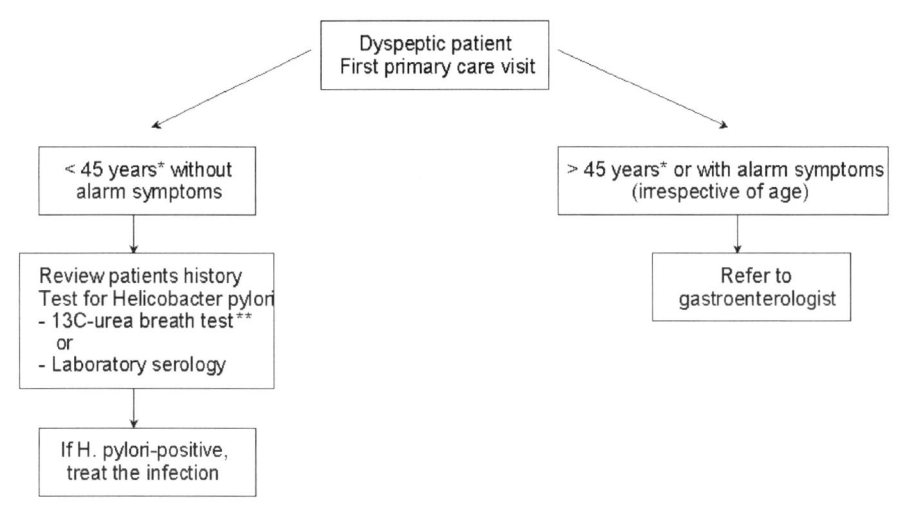

Figure 1. Summary of the recommended approach to the management of dyspeptic patients in the community. *The cut-off value may be below 45 years of age depending on the regional differences in the incidence of gastric malignancy. **H. pylori* stool antigen test is a valid alternative. Published with permission.

tion treatment[11]. The benefit of *H. pylori* eradication therapy in patients with functional dyspepsia remains controversial[12–14], but obviously has an important impact on the test-and-treat strategy.

The major concern expressed against the wide use of a test-and-treat strategy continues to be the missed diagnosis of gastric malignancy at an early stage in some patients. Moreover, by treating an increasing number of infected patients the emergence of antibiotic resistance might become an increasing problem[15].

Important advice given in the guidelines proposed at Maastricht, but often not quoted, is that surveillance in the European regions should be within a tight interdisciplinary network of GPs, gastroenterologists, and microbiologists. It is also recommended that, in areas with a high incidence of gastric cancer in patients below 45 years, this strategy cannot be a primary option.

The network of GPs and specialists should also guarantee control of the therapy. A decrease in therapeutic efficacy of the recommended standard therapies due to the emergence of antibiotic resistance should lead to withdrawal of unsuccessful therapies, and initiation of other appropriate measures.

CONSIDERATIONS AND EVALUATIONS OF TEST-AND-TREAT FROM EUROPEAN STUDIES SINCE MAASTRICHT

The acceptance of the test-and-treat strategy varies among different countries, and while the response from GPs is in favour of this approach, specialists are more reluctant to accept this strategy. The reason for specialists maintaining a sceptical and restrictive attitude is that they are used to dealing with a more selected population of patients than are GPs, and it is their responsibility to make a firm diagnosis based usually on upper gastro-intestinal endoscopy. Contrary to US practice the cost of endoscopy is low in Europe, and this is another argument raised by opponents of the test-and-treat strategy in favour of endoscopy as first-line approach in Europe as compared to the USA[16,17]. A survey conducted in the UK among 26 GPs and 55 gastroenterologists reported that 25% of specialists were willing to accept the test-and-treat strategy while 46% of GPs stated this to be their preferred option[18]. A limiting factor for a broad application of the test-and-treat strategy until recently has been the difficult access for GPs to the ^{13}C-urea breath test (UBT), which has become the gold standard for non-invasive tests[19,20].

The introduction of new equipment and a better price for the stable isotope labelled urea have made the UBT more popular, but despite this the acceptance of the UBT in several Europen countries remains poor. Serology, which was the other method recommended in Maastricht, with a recommendation for local validation, is easily available, but has a lower accuracy than the UBT[21,22]. Whole blood tests, performed in the doctor's office, are not sufficiently accurate for determining the treatment decisions. Recently a novel stool test for the detection of *H. pylori* antigens has been introduced[23], and this may have an important impact on the adoption of the test-and-treat strategy among European GPs.

An important problem in Europe is that regulatory authorities have still not accepted the test-and-treat strategy as equally valid, or even superior to the endoscopy-based management of dyspepsia in the young patient population. Moreover, costs of tests are not reimbursed by most health insurance organizations.

This reluctance of health authorities is reflected by the current attitude to the test-and-treat strategy in general practice. We randomly selected GPs in various European countries and interviewed them through a special questionnaire on the strategy of dealing with dyspepsia at first presentation. Results are shown in Figures 2–4, and confirm the low acceptance of the test-and-treat strategy despite evidence provided for this strategy being equally effective and reliable, with lower health costs, when applied to properly selected patients. Two further important steps need to be taken for better acceptance and implementation of test-and-treat strategies in Europe: (a) large-scale studies in different European regions, (b) acceptance of accurate non-invasive tests such as the UBT and *H. pylori* stool antigen tests with a low price and (c) reimbursement provided by health insurance companies.

TEST-AND-TREAT: THE EVIDENCE FOR IT

Two studies have, to date, been performed strictly according to the European *H. pylori* study group guidelines; including patients below the age of 45 years with no sinister symptoms and taking no NSAIDs. The unequivocal result of these studies was that test-and-treat of *H. pylori*-positive dyspeptic patients

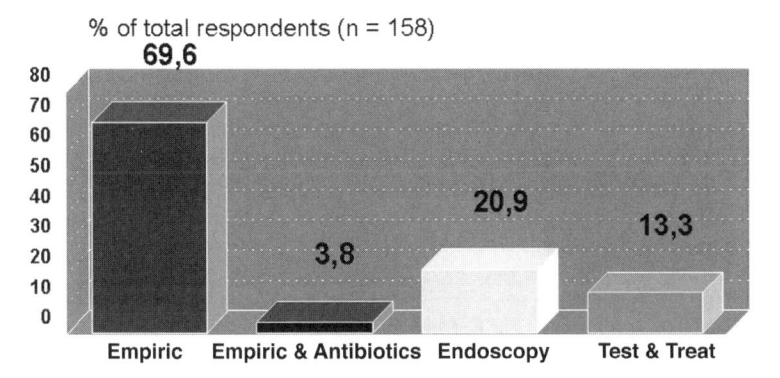

Figure 2. Knowledge about *H. pylori* in primary care in Europe. What do you do in patients with 'first time' dyspepsia?

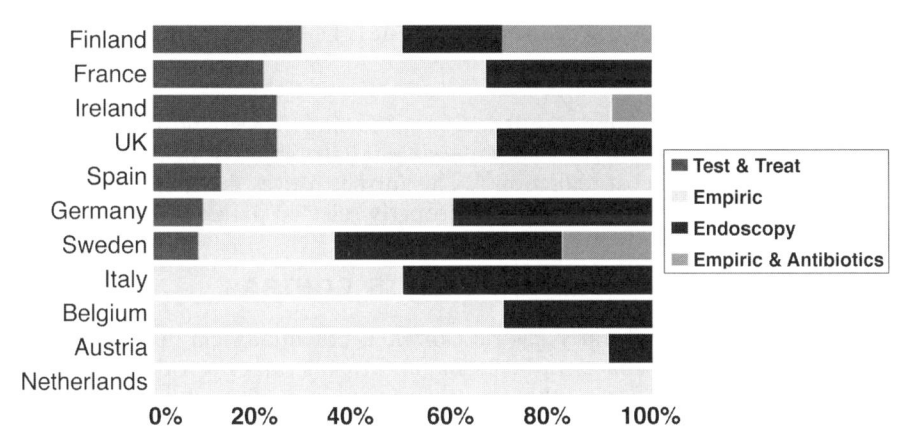

Figure 3. Knowledge about *H. pylori* in primary care in European countries. What do you do in patients with 'first time' dyspepsia?

was as efficient as the endoscopy-based management of patients with dyspepsia[24,25]. Reduction of the endoscopic workload was significant, and in the order of 28–67%. No malignancy was detected during a 1-year follow up in this study.

In a further study including patients up to the age of 50 years, 20 of 190 patients (10.5%) required upper gastrointestinal endoscopy after the test-and-treat strategy because of continuing dyspeptic symptoms[26].

In a large community-based study in the UK a 37% reduction in open-access endoscopy in patients younger than 40 years was observed following the introduction of the UBT as an alternative primary diagnostic tool in this age group[27]. Dyspeptic symptoms, consultation rates and the use of antisecretory drugs was similar in patients on the test-and-treat strategy or managed traditionally based on the endoscopy findings.

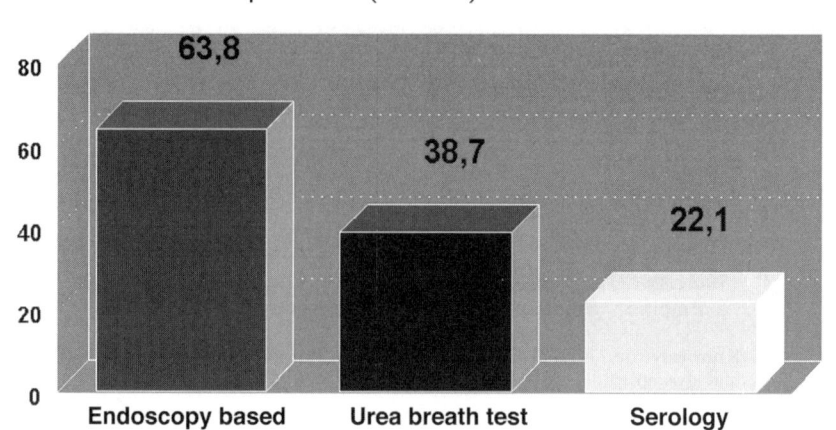

% of total respondents (n = 163)

[Bar chart: Endoscopy based 63.8, Urea breath test 38.7, Serology 22.1]

Figure 4. Knowledge about *H. pylori* in primary care in Europe. Which test do you prefer?

A different and age-independent approach using the test-and-treat strategy for patients on long-term acid suppressants also showed an advantage in health benefit and cost reduction[28]. This further proves the value of the test-and-treat strategy when applied to properly selected patient groups.

TEST-AND-TREAT: THE ARGUMENTS CONTRA

Delayed detection of early gastric cancer, a potentially curable condition, has been the major concern when a test-and-treat strategy is widely practised among GPs. The fact is that gastric cancer in young adults is rare. A prospective series of patients with gastric cancer at the University Hospital in Magdeburg revealed that patients below 45 years of age represent 8% (21 of 311 patients) of the total population of patients with gastric cancer during a 5-year observation period. Most of these patients present with alarm symptoms at their first visit. Based on these observations, a young patient with uncomplicated dyspepsia is unlikely to have a neoplastic gastric disease. Failure of the test-and-treat strategy to relieve symptoms would, in any case, mandate endoscopy in the further management.

In two recent studies an age cut-off was proposed at an older age of 55 years. In both these studies dyspepsia associated with gastric cancer again appeared to be a rare event, and it was exceptional for uncomplicated dyspepsia to be associated with gastric cancer[29,30]. To extrapolate these experiences to all European countries is not justifiable, and the test-and-treat strategy needs to be restricted to those areas with a low prevalence of gastric cancer in young patients.

Another important argument for endoscopy as the first diagnostic approach as opposed to non-invasive testing for *H. pylori*, is that many patients with dyspepsia may have gastro-oesophageal reflux disease. For these patients, it is important to exclude Barrett's mucosa as this group will not require follow-up surveillance, and can be managed by symptom control.

Furthermore, the cost of endoscopy is low in many European countries, and truly competitive with non-invasive testing for *H. pylori* infection. Industrial manufacturers and regulatory health providers need to move forward to make non-invasive testing more accessible.

CONCLUSION

In summary, the test-and-treat strategy is a valid option for first-line management in Europe of patients presenting with dyspepsia.

This strategy is effective, appears to be cost-effective, and is safe provided that caution is exercised by taking a correct and careful clinical history, and when there is a low prevalence of gastric cancer in young adults in the geographical/national region where the physician is practising.

References

1. Jones R, Lydeard S. Dyspepsia in the community: a follow-up study. Br J Clin Pract. 1992;46:95–7.
2. Knill-Jones RP. Geographical differences in the prevalence of dyspepsia. Scand J Gastroenterol. 1991;26:17–24.
3. Jones RH, Lydeard SE, Hobbs FRD et al. Dyspepsia in England and Scotland. Gut. 1999;31:401–5.
4. Agreus L, Talley N. Challenges in managing dyspepsia in general practice. Br Med J. 1997;315:1284–8.
5. Talley NJ. Modern management of dyspepsia. Aust Fam Phys. 1996;25:47–52.
6. Black RJ, Bray F, Ferlay J, Parkin DM. Cancer incidence and mortality in the European Union: cancer registry data and estimates of national incidence for 1990. Eur J Cancer. 1997;33:1075–107.
7. Tytgat G, Hingin APS, Malfertheiner P et al. Decision-making in dyspepsia: controversies in primary and secondary care. Eur J Gastroenterol Hepatol. 1999;11:223–30.
8. Sobala GM. Possible clinical uses of serology of *Helicobacter pylori*. In: Malfertheiner P, Ditschuneit H, editors. *Helicobacter pylori*, Gastritis and Peptic Ulcer. Berlin: Springer Verlag; 1990:147–53.
9. European *Helicobacter pylori* Study Group. Current European concepts in the management of *Helicobacter pylori* infection. The Maastricht Consensus Report. Gut. 1997;41:8–13.
10. Malfertheiner P. The Maastricht recommendations and their impact on general practice. Eur J Gastroenterol Hepatol. 1999;11:263–7
11. Sonnenberg A. Cost–benefit analysis of testing for *Helicobacter pylori* in dyspeptic subjects Am J Gastroenterol. 1996;91:1773–7.
12. Blum AL, Talley NJ, O'Morain C et al. Lack of effect of treating *Helicobacter pylori* infection in patients with nonulcer dyspepsia. Omeprazole plus clarithromycin and amoxicillin effect one year after treatment. (OCAY) Study Group. N Engl J Med. 1998;24,339,26:1875–81.
13. McColl K, Murray L, El-Omar E et al. Symptomatic benefit from eradicating *Helicobacter pylori* infection in patients with nonulcer dyspepsia. N Engl J Med. 1998;24,339,26:1869–74.
14. Talley NJ, Vakil N, Ballard ED, Fennerty MB. Absence of benefit of eradicating *H. pylori* in patients with nonulcer dyspepsia. N Engl J Med. 1999;7,341:1106–11.
15. Megraud F, Doermann HP. Clinical relevance of resistant strains: a review of current data. Gut. 1998;43:S61–5.
16. Silverstein MD, Petterson T, Talley NJ. Initial endoscopy or empirical therapy with or without testing for *Helicobacter pylori* for dyspepsia: a decision analysis. Gastroenterology. 1996;110:72–83.

17. Ofman JJ, Etchason J, Fullerton S et al. Management strategies for *Helicobacter pylori*-seropositive patients with dyspepsia: clinical and economic consequences. Ann Intern Med. 1997;126:280–91.
18. Lim AG, Martin RM, Monteleone M et al. *Helicobacter pylori* serology and the management of young dyspeptics: a UK survey of gastroenterologists and general practitioners with an interest in gastroenterology. Aliment Pharmacol Ther. 1997;11:299–303.
19. Logan RP. Urea breath tests in the management of *Helicobacter pylori* infection. Gut. 1998;41,1:S47–50.
20. Leodolter A, Domingues-Munoz JE, von Arnim U, Kahl S, Peitz U, Malfertheiner P. Validity of a modified ^{13}C-urea breath test for pre- and posttreatment diagnosis of *Helicobacter pylori* infection in the routine clinical setting. Am J Gastroenterol. 1999;94,8:2100–4.
21. Thijs JC, van Zwet AA, Thijs WJ et al. Diagnostic tests for *Helicobacter pylori*: a prospective evaluation of their accuracy, without selecting a single test as the gold standard. Am J Gastroenterol. 1996;91,10:2125–9.
22. Cohen H, Rose S, Lewin DN et al. Accuracy of four commercially available serologic tests, including two office-based tests and a commercially available ^{13}C urea breath test, for diagnosis of *Helicobacter pylori*. Helicobacter. 1999;4,1:49–53.
23. Vaira D, Malfertheiner P, Megraud F et al. Diagnosis of *Helicobacter pylori* infection with a new non-invasive antigen-based assay. Lancet. 1999;354:30–3.
24. Lassen AT, Pedersen FM, Byther P, Schaffalitzky de Muckadell OB. *H. pylori* 'test and treat' or prompt endoscopy for dyspeptic patients in primary care. A randomized controlled trial of two management strategies: one year follow up. Gastroenterology. 1998;114:G0803.
25. Heaney A, Collins JSA, Watson RGP, McFarland RJ, Bamford KB, Tham TCK. A prospective randomised trial of a 'test and treat' policy versus endoscopy based management in young *Helicobacter pylori* positive patients with ulcer-like dyspepsia, referred to a hospital clinic. Gut. 1999;45:186–90.
26. Besherdas K, Oben JA, Beck ER, Vicary FR, Wong VS. What proportion of dyspeptic patients having *H. pylori* breath test subsequently undergo endoscopy? Gut. 2000;46,2:W78.
27. Moayyedi P, Zilles A, Clough A, Hemingbrough E, Chlamers DM, Axon ATR. The effectiveness of screening and treating *Helicobacter pylori* in the management of dyspepsia. Eur J Gastroenterol Hepatol. 1999;11:1245–50.
28. Joosen EAM, Reininga JHA, Manders JMW, ten Ham JC, de Boer WA. Costs and benefits of a test-and-treat strategy in *Helicobacter pylori*-infected subjects: a prospective intervention study in general practice. Eur J Gastroenterol Hepatol. 2000;12:319–25.
29. Christie J, Shepherd NA, Codling BW, Valori RM. Gastric cancer below the age of 55: implications for screening patients with uncomplicated dyspepsia. Gut. 1997;41:513–17.
30. Gillen D, McColl KEL. Does concern about missing malignancy justify endoscopy in uncomplicated dyspepsia in patients aged less than 55? Am J Gastroenterol. 1999;94:75–9.

52
The impact of the 'test-and-treat' strategies for *Helicobacter pylori* infection – an Asian perspective?

J. J. Y. SUNG

Optimal management of dyspepsia is still a controversial subject despite intense investigation. Confusion arises from the poor correlation of symptoms with the underlying condition[1], the uncertain role of *Helicobacter pylori* in causation of dyspepsia, the geographical variation of gastro-esophageal cancer prevalence and the worldwide concern of the cost-effectiveness of endoscopy. So far, most recommendations have been based upon data from Western countries where gastric cancer incidence is low. In Asia, gastric cancer has been reported between five and 80 cases per 100 000 population, varying from different nations and ethnic groups[2]. Although declining in recent decades, gastric cancer is still common in Hong Kong, with an annual age-adjusted incidence[3] of 24 per 100 000. Figures from the Hong Kong Cancer Registry show that about 10% of patients are below the age of 45 years. The use of a 'test-and-treat' strategy in Asia is further complicated by the fact that commercially available diagnostic kits on the market have produced sub-optimal results from local validation studies[4,5]. On the other hand, the urea breath test is not widely available to doctors, especially in the primary-care setting, in most Asian countries[6]. While the 'test-and-treat' approach quickly gained popularity in the West, Asian workers are concerned about missing a diagnosis of malignant disease without proper endoscopic examination.

We have undertaken a prospective study to test the safety of adopting the 'test-and-treat' strategy using *H. pylori* serology as a screening test for dyspepsia. This is a collaborative study involving four regional hospitals in Hong Kong, serving a total population of 2.4 million. The majority of these patients were referred from primary-care physicians because of upper abdominal discomfort. Consecutive patients were recruited into the study if their symptoms of dyspepsia had lasted for over 4 weeks. Patients with predominant symptoms of acid regurgitation, heartburn or diarrhoea were excluded.

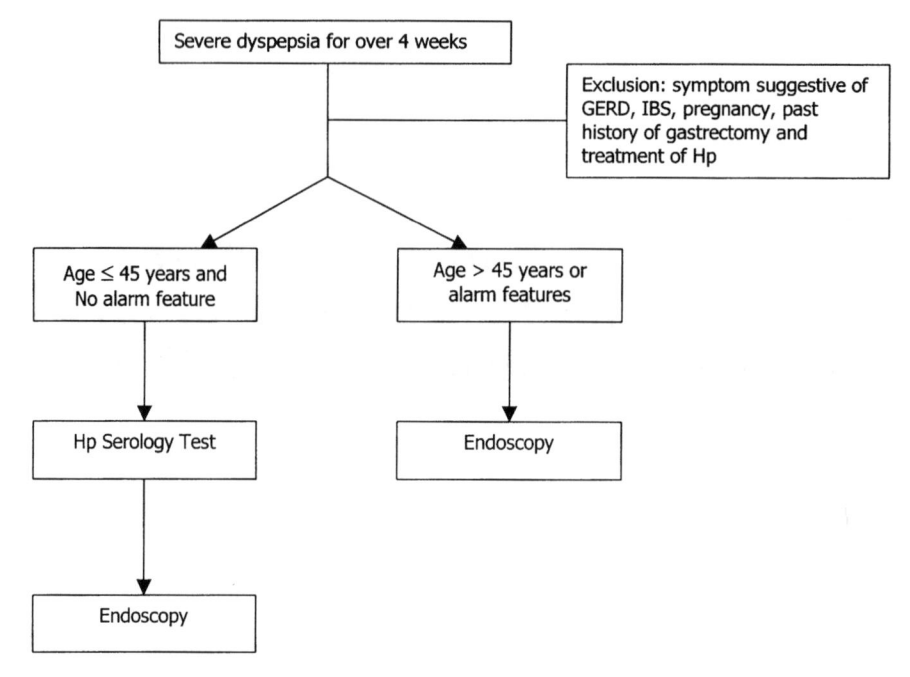

```
┌─────────────────────────────────────┐
│ Severe dyspepsia for over 4 weeks   │
└─────────────────────────────────────┘
                                    ┌──────────────────────────────┐
                                    │ Exclusion: symptom suggestive of │
                                    │ GERD, IBS, pregnancy, past   │
                                    │ history of gastrectomy and   │
                                    │ treatment of Hp              │
                                    └──────────────────────────────┘

  ┌──────────────────────┐         ┌──────────────────────┐
  │ Age ≤ 45 years and   │         │ Age > 45 years or    │
  │ No alarm feature     │         │ alarm features       │
  └──────────────────────┘         └──────────────────────┘
            │                                │
            ▼                                ▼
  ┌──────────────────────┐         ┌──────────────────────┐
  │ Hp Serology Test     │         │ Endoscopy            │
  └──────────────────────┘         └──────────────────────┘
            │
            ▼
  ┌──────────────────────┐
  │ Endoscopy            │
  └──────────────────────┘
```

Figure 1. Study design.

Patients over 45 years of age, and those with alarm symptoms (irrespective of age) were offered early endoscopy within 1 week (endoscopy group). Alarm symptoms were defined as a weight loss of 10 pounds or more over 8 weeks, recurrent vomiting, dysphagia, evidence of bleeding and anaemia. Patients who took aspirin and NSAIDs prior to the onset of symptoms were also offered early endoscopy. Patients at or below the age of 45 years without alarm symptoms were tested by *H. pylori* serology (serology group) using a whole-blood test (Flexpack, Abbott Laboratory, Chicago, IL). Endoscopic examination was also offered within 1 week of the serological test, irrespective of the result, to verify the safety of the 'test-and-treat' strategy (Figure 1).

Two thousand nine hundred and eighteen consecutive patients presented with dyspepsia in a period of 12 months, and 2627 of them were recruited into the study. The serology group consists of 1017 patients with a mean ($\pm$ SD) age of 34.1 ($\pm$ 8.2) years and 390 (38.3%) of them were male. *H. pylori* serology was positive in 522 (51.3%) cases by serology, 459 (45.1%) by biopsy urease test and 487 (47.9%) by histology. The sensitivity and specificity of serology was 88.5% and 79.2% using the biopsy urease test as the gold standard and 86.9% and 81.3% using histology as the gold standard. The endoscopy group consisted of 1610 patients with a mean ($\pm$ SD) age of 57.5 ($\pm$ 13.2) years and 666 (41.4%) of them were male. The reasons for not including them in the serology group were exceeding the age limit in 1393 patients (86.5%), use of NSAIDs in 89 (5.5%), gastrointestinal bleeding or

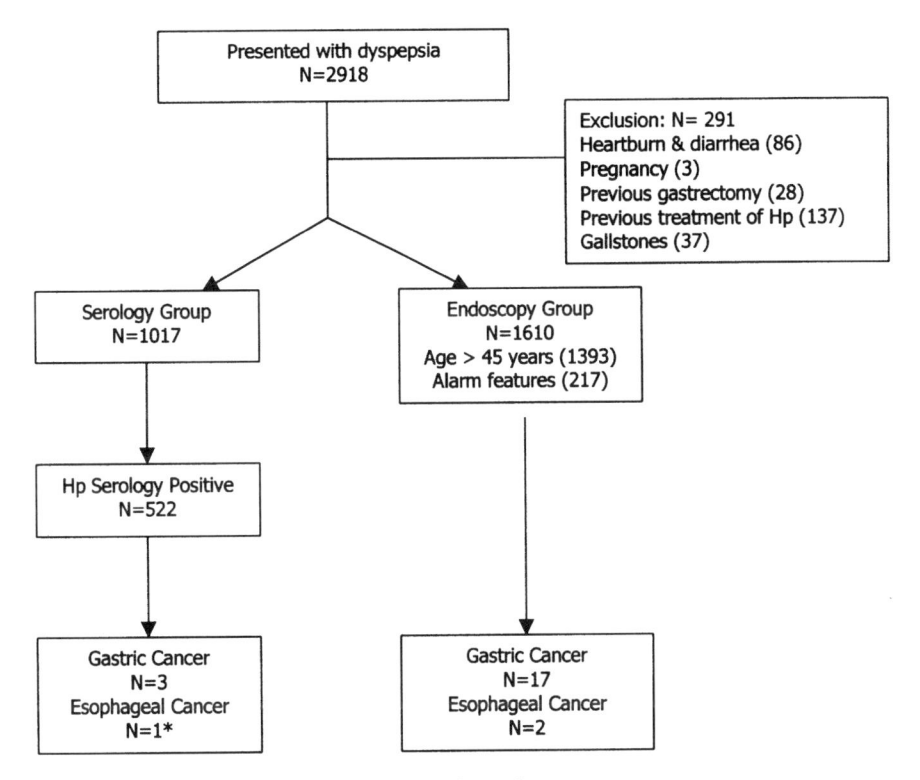

```
                    Presented with dyspepsia
                           N=2918
                              │
            ┌─────────────────┼──────────────┐
            │                 │              │
            │          Exclusion: N= 291
            │          Heartburn & diarrhea (86)
            │          Pregnancy (3)
            │          Previous gastrectomy (28)
            │          Previous treatment of Hp (137)
            │          Gallstones (37)
            ▼                                ▼
      Serology Group                   Endoscopy Group
         N=1017                            N=1610
                                   Age > 45 years (1393)
                                   Alarm features (217)
            │                                │
            ▼                                │
     Hp Serology Positive                    │
          N=522                              │
            │                                │
            ▼                                ▼
      Gastric Cancer                   Gastric Cancer
          N=3                              N=17
     Esophageal Cancer                Esophageal Cancer
          N=1*                             N=2
```

Figure 2. Outcome of patients recruited into the study.

anaemia in 80 (5%), dysphagia in 29 (1.8%) and weight loss in 19 (1.2%) (Figure 2).

No endoscopic abnormalities were found in 603 (59.3%) cases in the serology group and 795 (49.4%) in the endoscopy group. Four patients (0.4%) in the serology group were diagnosed with malignancies by endoscopy which were subsequently confirmed by histology. Three patients had gastric cancer, two in the gastric antrum and one in the lesser curve of corpus. All three patients had a positive serology test. Nineteen patients (1.2%) in the endoscopy group were diagnosed with malignancies, including 17 cases of gastric cancer and two cases of oesophageal cancer. Fourteen out of 17 cases of gastric cancer were found to have *H. pylori* infection by histology. Among these patients, five were below the age of 45 years. Three patients presented with weight loss, one with dysphagia and one had anaemia.

Our study showed that in countries with a high incidence of *H. pylori* infection and gastric cancer, endoscopy should be recommended after testing positive for the infection. We believe that young dyspeptic patients with no alarm symptoms can be offered a non-invasive test for *H. pylori* infection. Those tested positive for *H. pylori* infection should be offered prompt endoscopic examination. Empirical therapy with an H_2 receptor antagonist and/or prokinetic agent can be safely prescribed to *H. pylori*-negative young dyspeptic patients. Patients above 45 years of age and patients who present with alarm symptoms, should be offered prompt endoscopy.

References

1. Talley NJ, Weaver AL, Tesmer DL. Zinsmeister AR. Lack of discriminant value of dyspepsia subgroups in patients referred for upper endoscopy. Gastroenterology. 1993;105:1378–86.
2. Parkin DM, Muir C, Whelan SL, Ga OYT, Ferlay J, Powell J (eds). Cancer Incidence in Five Continents, vol. VI. Lyon: IARC Scientific Publication No. 120, 1992.
3. Hong Kong Cancer Registry. Cancer incidence and mortality in Hong Kong 1995–1996. Hosp Authority. 1999;40–1.
4. Leung WK, Chan FKL, Ng EKW, Chung SCS, Sung JJY. Evaluation of three commercial enzyme-linked immunosorbent assay kits for diagnosis of *Helicobacter pylori* in Chinese patients. Diagn Microbiol Infect Dis. 1999;34:13–17.
5. Leung WK, Chan FKL, Falk M, Suen R, Sung JJY. Comparison of two rapid whole-blood tests for *Helicobacter pylori* in Chinese patients. J Clin Microbiol. 1998;36:3441–2.
6. Lam SK, Talley NJ. Report of the 1997 Asia Pacific Consensus Conference on the management of *Helicobacter* infection. J Gastroenterol Hepatol. 1998;13:1–12.

Section X
Helicobacter pylori and Gastric Malignancy

53
Rodent models for *Helicobacter*-induced gastric cancer

J. G. FOX

INTRODUCTION

Helicobacter, inflammation and gastric cancer

According to data presented in 1980, gastric cancer was the most frequent neoplasm registered in the world[1] and currently it is ranked number two in frequency. On a global basis the highest rates were historically recorded in Japan, followed by northern Europe, and in Latin Americans living in the Andes mountains[2]. It is now known that the type species *Helicobacter pylori* infects ~50% of the world population. The recent decline in the so-called intestinal type of gastric adenocarcinoma may well be due to a less frequent occurrence of *H. pylori* in socioeconomically higher populations. This correlation fits well with the white populations of the United States. However, American Indians, Hispanics, Blacks, and immigrants from northern Europe, Latin America, and Asia have higher rates of gastric cancer and likewise higher rates of *H. pylori* infection, including higher acquisition rates in children of these ethnic backgrounds[3-6]. The role of chronic persistent gastritis induced by *H. pylori* in induction of gastric adenocarcinoma has received strong epidemiological support from published independent cohort studies. A recent meta-analysis of papers published on *H. pylori* and gastric cancer risk supports these findings[7]. Results first published in 1991 indicated that *H. pylori* infection, detected many years before, significantly increases the risk of gastric cancer with an odds ratio of 4.0. The odds ratio increased to 9.0 when gastric cancer cases were restricted to those with diagnosis of more than 15 years after testing *H. pylori* positive[8-14]. It is suspected that chronic infection elicits an increase in cell proliferation, constant influx of inflammatory cells, and mutagenic events that eventually lead to cancer. Indeed, it was suggested that if *H. pylori* is causally linked to intestinal-type gastric cancer, then 70% of disease incidence should be prevented through *H. pylori* eradication[15].

A WHO Working Group of the International Agency for Research on Cancer (IARC) concluded that infection increased the risk of cancer, and classified *H. pylori* infection as representing a group I carcinogen. Nevertheless, despite the recognition of *H. pylori* as a carcinogen, the strategy of widespread screening and eradication of *H. pylori* infection has not been implemented, and has remained controversial as a public health policy, because of uncertain efficacy and in part because the majority of infected individuals will remain asymptomatic. Thus, additional information is needed regarding the factors that lead to progression along a gastric cancer pathway versus a disease-free, asymptomatic pathway, and early biomarkers that may predict gastric cancer risk in an individual patient. Furthermore, until recently there has been limited insight regarding the mechanisms involved in *H. pylori*-mediated gastric cancer, and the NIH Consensus Conference in 1993 and the IARC identified as a priority the need for animal models of *Helicobacter* infection to address early mechanisms of carcinogenesis. Development of *in-vivo* models with well-defined gastric cancer directly associated with persistent *Helicobacter* infection was also recommended.

Previously, the only naturally infected *H. pylori* hosts had been several species of non-human primates[16–18]. Primates develop a chronic gastritis when naturally or experimentally infected with *H. pylori*. However, primates have not been consistently infected experimentally after oral challenges with *H. pylori*. Also, many non-human primates harbour other gastric spiral organisms, which complicates their use as models[17,19,20]. Gnotobiotic dogs and pigs developed a chronic gastritis when experimentally infected with *H. pylori*[21,22]. However, these animals are not available to most investigators, and their cost and housing requirements, and lack of reagents, impose additional constraints. Alternative models of *Helicobacter* infections were therefore developed. We documented that *H. felis* caused a persistent gastritis in germ-free mice and rats and specific pathogen-free mice[23–25]. The ferret naturally colonized and persistently infected with *H. mustelae* has also been used to study the pathogenesis and development of gastric cancer[26–28]. These models continue to be used by laboratories worldwide to study *Helicobacter* virulence factors, therapeutic modalities, vaccination strategies and facets of epidemiology. The rodent model has been particularly useful because rodents are inexpensive, easily housed, and are well defined biologically and genetically. These models, however, lacked one important feature – they were not infected with the human pathogen, *H. pylori*. Our discovery of naturally occurring chronic *H. pylori* infection in cats provided a particularly useful model of human *H. pylori* disease[29–31]. However, the mouse can now be persistently colonized with specific strains of *H. pylori*[32–35] and the discovery that gerbils infected with *H. pylori* develop gastric cancer has prompted many laboratories to begin using these latter two rodent models[36,37]. The precise significance of direct versus indirect effects of *H. pylori*, the role of immunological responses, alterations in apoptosis and proliferation, and the importance of changes in cellular differentiation, are in part being answered using animal models of *Helicobacter*-mediated gastric cancer.

ANIMAL MODELS

Mouse models of gastric *Helicobacter* infections

The rodent model of *H. felis* was first reported in 1990[24,25]. *H. felis* is a spiral organism, closely related to *H. pylori*, that shows robust and persistent colonization of the murine stomach, inducing a chronic active gastritis and Th1 immune response in C57BL/6 mice which closely resembles that observed in human patients infected with *H. pylori*[23,38,39]. It is known that C57BL/6 mice infected with *H. felis* develop a chronic active gastritis that progresses over time to a severe gastric atrophy and invasive gastric lesions[40,41]. Infection leads to an increase in apoptotic rate, leading to a rapid loss of parietal cells and chief cells within the oxyntic glands, and the onset of achlorhydria. The induction of apoptosis, which is maximal at 6–12 weeks post-infection, is followed closely by a marked increase in the proliferation (BrdU) index. The development of atrophy and the loss of parietal and chief cell populations within the oxyntic glands are associated with a marked expansion of an aberrant spasmolytic polypeptide (SP/TFF2)-expressing mucous neck cell lineage in the *H. felis*-infected C57BL/6 mice. Over time this aberrant mucous neck cell lineage progresses to intestinal metaplasia, characterized by positive staining with Alcian blue at low pH (2.5 and 1.0), indicating the presence of both acidic and sulphated sialomucins. Thus, these studies demonstrated that the *H. felis*-infected mouse was an excellent model for the early stages (e.g. gastric atrophy and intestinal metaplasia) of progression to gastric neoplasia. Older (~12 month) *H. felis*-infected mice showed both dysplasia and atypical glandular foci with invasive characteristics. Aberrant mucous neck cells with dysplastic features were found to arise in the proliferative and metaplastic corpus mucosa. These dysplastic cells, which also stained positive with Alcian Blue (pH 2.5) and SP, eventually penetrated the muscularis mucosa and invaded into the submucosa, forming nests of cystic glands lined by mucous epithelium[41].

Many of these same histological features have been reproduced in the C57BL/6 mouse using the *H. pylori* (SS1) model[32–35]. We have recently infected 8-week-old C57BL/6 mice with *H. pylori* SS1 strain and followed them for up to 52 weeks post-inoculation[32]. Mice euthanized at 32 and 52 weeks post-infection showed persistent colonization with *H. pylori* and an identical severe atrophic gastritis to that seen with *H felis*, with loss of parietal cells, replacement by an aberrant mucous neck cell lineage, and mucus cell metaplasia[32].

ROLE OF TUMOUR SUPPRESSOR GENES IN DETERMINING SUSCEPTIBILITY TO GASTRIC CANCER IN *HELICOBACTER*-INFECTED MICE

Apc knockouts

H. pylori infection and *Apc* (adenomatous polyposis coli) gene mutations have been linked to gastric cancer in humans, but a possible synergistic interaction between these risk factors has not been examined. Both C57BL/6 wild-type and *Apc*1638 hemizygous mice were inoculated with *H. felis* at 6 weeks of age and compared at various time-points with a similar number of uninfected control mice of the same genotype[42]. Both *H. felis*-infected and -uninfected *Apc*1638 mice had a limited incidence of atypical foci of proliferation in the mucosa of the antrum and pyloric junction at 4.5 and 6 months of age, whereas gastric foci of the antrum and pylorus were present in all mice, regardless of infection status, at 7.5 months[42]. In contrast, no altered gastric mucosal foci were observed in control or infected C57BL/6 mice at any time-point. Interestingly, the *Apc*1638 mice had less epithelial proliferation and inflammation in the body of the stomach, lower anti-*H. felis* serum immunoglobulin G antibody responses, and higher bacteria and urease scores compared with wild-type *H. felis*-infected C57BL/6 mice[42]. The overall gastritis score in *Apc* mutant mice suggests that a Th2-predominant gastric phenotype was present in these mice. Thus, the *Apc*1638 truncating mutation leads to gastric dysplasia and polyposis of the antrum and pyloric junction but, in the 7.5-month-old *H. felis*-infected *Apc* mutant mouse, does not predispose strongly to gastric cancer. In addition, our data suggested this *Apc* mutation may lead to decreased immune, inflammatory, and proliferative responses to *Helicobacter* infection, inferring the possibility of a novel role for this tumour-suppressor gene in the host's response to gastric bacterial infection[42].

P53 +/− mice

Alterations in the p53 tumour-suppressor gene have also shown significant interaction with *Helicobacter* infection in affecting gastritis. We examined the effects of infection with *H. felis* in mice with targeted disruption of one p53 allele[43]. *H. felis* was inoculated by gastric intubation into C57BL/6 wild-type and p53 heterozygous knockout mice that were followed for up to 1 year, and compared with uninfected controls of the same genotype. At 6 months post-infection, the infected animals demonstrated marked inflammatory and hyperplastic responses. At 1 year post-infection the infected p53 heterozygous mice were observed to have a higher proliferative index than the infected wild-type mice[43]. This study suggested that reduction in the gene dose, and consequently in the amount of p53 produced by the normal cell, does seem to confer growth advantage in the gastric epithelium in this mouse model. However, this model is complicated by the fact that p53$^{-/+}$ and p53$^{-/-}$ have a high incidence of lymphoma, which limits their longevity and usefulness for long-term carcinogenesis studies.

ROLE OF CONCURRENT PARASITIC INFECTION ON *H. PYLORI* TUMORIGENESIS

In developing countries such as Africa the prevalence rates of *H. pylori* infection can reach 100%. Fortunately, only a small percentage of the population will develop serious disease due to *H. pylori* infection. Why some individuals develop disease and others do not is unknown; host and environmental factors as well as virulence properties of particular *H. pylori* strains probably influence disease outcome in individuals infected with the organism.

Individuals living in countries with low socioeconomic conditions have high prevalence rates of *H. pylori* infection acquired at an early age[44]. Some of these countries have high rates of gastric cancer (e.g. Colombia and Peru), whereas some populations of Africa and elsewhere with equally high *H. pylori* prevalence rates have much lower gastric cancer incidence or mortality. This paradox has been referred to as the African enigma[45]. Although this enigma has sometimes been dismissed as resulting from poor cancer registration practices combined with short life expectancy, the phenomenon extends to countries other than those in Africa, and is too widespread to be disregarded. Several carefully designed correlation studies, with consistent recording of cancer information, have identified populations which have the combination of high infection and low cancer rates even if the study overall shows a significant positive association between infection prevalence and cancer incidence[4,46]. The influence of concurrent infection with other pathogens on the immune response to *H. pylori* and its possible influence on cancer risk have not been studied. $CD4^+$ T cells can be divided into two functional subsets, Th1 and Th2, which are defined by their pattern of cytokine secretion. Th1 cells produce IL-2 and IFN-γ and promote cell-mediated immune responses; Th2 cells secret IL-4, IL-5, IL-6 and IL-10 and induce B cell activation and differentiation. The cytokines secreted by each of these subsets regulate those produced by the other subset. Indeed, recent evidence has suggested that the immune response to a variety of infectious agents is accompanied by a preferential expansion of one Th subset with a concomitant down-regulation of the other[47]. Many intracellular microbes, including bacteria, protozoa and fungi, induce Th1 responses while extracellular pathogens, particularly helminthic parasites, drive polarized Th2 responses. The degree of polarization can vary along a continuum, depending upon the nature of the infection and its persistence. The immune response elicited by both *H. pylori* infection in humans and *H. felis* infection in mice has been described as Th1-like because inflammatory cells in the respective infected host produce higher amounts of IFN-γ than IL-4[38,48]. Furthermore, serum-specific *Helicobacter* spp. IgG2a levels, an indirect measure of a Th1 immune response, are higher than IgG1. Recent work in murine models has shown that this host T cell response is the key mediator of *Helicobacter*-associated gastric pathology[49,50].

Given that concurrent infections with Th2-inducing helminth parasites are also endemic in the developing countries that exhibit a high prevalence of *H. pylori* infection, we hypothesized that helminth infections might modulate a proinflammatory Th1 response to gastric *Helicobacter* infection towards a less injurious Th2 response. We therefore examined *Helicobacter*-associated gastritis in C57BL/6 mice coinfected with *Heligmosomoides polygyrus*, a natural murine parasite with a strictly enteric life cycle[51]. *Helicobacter*-infected mice with concurrent helminth infection displayed a marked reduction in *H. felis*-associated gastric corpus atrophy despite chronic inflammation and high *Helicobacter* colonization. This finding correlated with a striking reduction in mRNA for both cytokines and chemokines associated with a Th1-type inflammatory response in the stomachs of the dually infected mice (Figure 1)[52]. The results, therefore, support our hypoth-

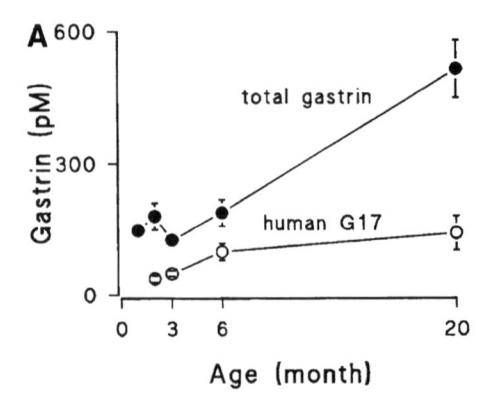

Figure 1. INS-GAS mice show loss of initial gastric acid hypersecretion and increasing serum gastrin levels over time. Serum gastrin levels in INS-GAS mice vary with the age of the mouse. Both total amidated gastrin and human amidated gastrin (human G-17, derived from the transgene) are shown[66].

esis that concurrent intestinal helminth infection can influence the progression of *H. pylori* gastritis and provide a protective effect against development of gastric atrophy and gastric adenocarcinoma. This model, as well as other well-defined parasite models, can be used to dissect the importance of this novel finding on the pathogenesis of *H. pylori* disease.

DIETARY SALT INCREASES *H. PYLORI* COLONIZATION AND SEVERITY OF GASTRITIS IN MICE

A high salt diet in humans and experimental animals is known to cause gastritis, has been associated with a high risk of atrophic gastritis and is considered a gastric tumour promoter[2,53]. In laboratory rats salt is known to cause gastritis and, when co-administered, promotes the carcinogenic effects of known gastric carcinogens[53].

Mice, in addition to rats, have been used in studies addressing gastric damage due to salt intake. Mice (strain undesignated) fed a rice diet containing highly salted food (salted codfish and yakuri sold for food consumption in Japan) developed acute gastric mucosal damage[54]. In later studies, Swiss/ICR mice fed salted (10% w/w NaCl) rice diets for 3–12 months were noted to develop hypertrophy of the forestomach but atrophy (considered a marker of premalignancy in humans) of the glandular stomach[52]. The authors emphasized that a reduction in the parietal cells accounted for the atrophy observed in the fundus of the mice[55]. Although parietal cell loss has also been noted in C57BL/6 mice infected with *H. felis*[43,56], the finding of Kodama *et al.* infers that chronic inflammation *per se* may account for parietal cell loss in the fundus of mice[55].

A recent study was undertaken to determine if excessive dietary NaCl would have an effect on colonization and gastritis in the mouse model of *H. pylori* infection. Seventy-two C57BL/6 mice were infected with *H. pylori* SS1 and 36 control mice were dosed with vehicle only. Half of the infected and control mice were fed a high-salt diet (7.5% vs 0.25%) for 2 weeks prior to dosing and throughout the entire experiment. Infected and control animals from high-salt and normal-diet groups were euthanized at 4, 8, and 16 weeks. At 8 and 16 weeks post-infection colony-forming units per gram of tissue (cfu) were significantly higher ($p < 0.05$) in the corpus and antrum of animals in the high-salt diet group compared to those on the normal diet. At 16 weeks post-infection the mice in both the normal and the high-salt diet groups developed moderate to marked atrophic gastritis of the corpus in response to *H. pylori* infection. However, the gastric pits of the corpus mucosa in mice on the high-salt diet were elongated and colonized by *H. pylori* more frequently, compared to mice on the normal diet. High-salt diets may synergize with *H. pylori* infection through expansion of cells where *H. pylori* colonizes. Indeed, the high-salt diet was associated with a significant increase in proliferation in the proximal corpus and antrum, and a multifocal reduction in parietal cell numbers in the proximal corpus, resulting in the elongation of gastric pits. Our data suggest that excessive NaCl intake enhances *H. pylori* colonization in mice, and chronic salt intake may exacerbate gastritis by increasing *H. pylori* colonization. Furthermore, elevated salt intake may potentiate *H. pylori*-associated carcinogenesis by inducing proliferation, pit cell hyperplasia, and glandular atrophy[33].

HYPERGASTRINAEMIA AND *HELICOBACTER* INFECTION

The gastric phenotype noted in hypergastrinaemic transgenic mice is distinct from that in rats with experimental hypergastrinaemia[57–59] in which ECL cell hyperplasia is common and ECL cell carcinoids develop after prolonged treatment. ECL cell hyperplasia and ECL cell carcinoids are also a feature in humans. However, in patients with mild or moderate hypergastrinaemia, particularly when *H. pylori* infection predominates in the gastric corpus, there is loss of parietal cells similar to that found in mice[60–63]. These changes are important because it is recognized from both clinical[2] and experimental[30,37,41,64] observations that gastric atrophy predisposes to carcinoma of the stomach.

Hypergastrinaemia occurs frequently in association with acid suppression and *Helicobacter* infection, but its role in the progression to gastric atrophy and gastric cancer has not been well defined. Because certain inbred strains of mice develop parietal cell loss and atrophy after *H. felis* infection[41,65], the possible role of hypergastrinaemia in accelerating the development of gastric atrophy and cancer in response to *Helicobacter* infection was evaluated. Insulin–gastrin transgenic (INS-GAS) mice and wild-type mice in the same genetic background (FVB/N) were infected with *H. felis* at 4 weeks of age and monitored for up to 7 months after inoculation. Uninfected INS-GAS and FVB/N mice were used as control animals in these studies.

INS-GAS mice initially showed mild hypergastrinaemia, increased maximal gastric acid secretion and parietal cell numbers consistent with the early elevations in serum gastrin. However, in older INS-GAS mice there was a decreasing parietal cell number and hypochlorhydria[66]. Serum amidated gastrin levels increased gradually, beginning at 6 months, with levels peaking

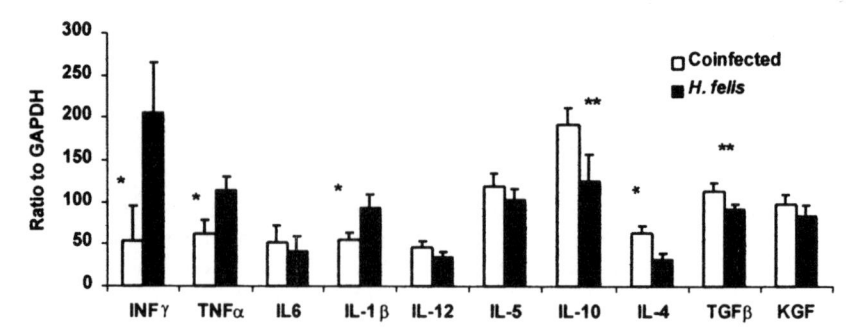

Figure 2. mRNA for cytokine gene expression was measured on gastric biopsies at 16 weeks post-infection with *H. felis* using RT-PCR. Coinfected mice had lower levels of mRNA for the Th1 cytokines TNF-α, IFN-γ and IL-1β compared to mice infected with *H. felis* alone. Furthermore, coinfected mice had significantly increased levels of mRNA for the Th2 cytokines IL-4, IL-10 and TGF-β compared to mice infected with *H. felis* alone. Error bars represent 1 standard error of the mean[42]. *$p < 0.03$; **$p < 0.04$. From ref. 52.

at 20 months to 550 pmol/L. Most of the increase in serum gastrin resulted from increased secretion of endogenous mouse amidated gastrin, with lesser changes in the level of transgene-derived human gastrin (human G-17), which increased from 49 pmol/L at 3 months to 142 pmol/L at 20 months (Figure 2).

The development of gastric atrophy was associated with increased expression of growth factors, heparin binding epidermal growth factor and transforming growth factor-α. At 20 months of age, INS-GAS mice had no evidence of increased enterochromaffin-like cell number, but instead exhibited gastric metaplasia, dysplasia, carcinoma-*in-situ*, and gastric cancer with vascular invasion. Invasive gastric carcinoma was observed in six of eight INS-GAS mice that were >20 months old[66].

H. felis infection of INS-GAS mice led to the accelerated (≤8 months) development of gastric cancer. Intramucosal carcinoma was present in 11 of 13 (85%, $p \leq 0.01$) mice, invasive submucosal carcinoma in seven of 13 (54%, $p \leq 0.01$) mice, and intravascular invasion in six of 13 (46%, $p \leq 0.05$) mice. The intramucosal carcinomas often had well-differentiated tubulacinar or microacinar architecture, resulting in irregular, cystic, or minute glandular tubules or acini formation. The epithelium ranged from hyperchromic columnar epithelium to a secretory epithelium with clear apical mucin. Intraepithelial formation of mucous acini was sometimes observed. Invasion occurred through the muscularis mucosae into the submucosa and was often associated with invasion into veins. Thrombosis was also observed in tandem with vascular invasion. Neoplastic foci, which had invaded into the submucosa and vasculature, were often enclosed by fibrous capsules. These findings support the unexpected conclusion that chronic hypergastrinaemia in mice can synergize with *Helicobacter* infection, and can contribute to eventual parietal cell loss and progression to gastric cancer[66]. Whether this model, though important to study mechanisms of gastric cancer, has a direct corollary to gastric pathophysiology in humans will require further studies.

Helicobacters as cocarcinogens

Given the generally late onset of gastric cancer in human populations, it is probable that tumour initiators as well as tumour promoters play an important role in gastric carcinogenesis. Several reviews of the pioneering work on experimental gastric carcinogenesis in rats have been published[67-69]. However, by comparison, the mouse is relatively resistant to carcinogenesis of the glandular stomach induced by nitrosoamines. For example, the administration of methyl-N-nitrosoguanidine (MNNG) to five strains of mice failed to induce gastric tumours[69]. Although mice were administered MNNG in drinking water throughout their life, adenomatous hyperplasia of the glandular stomach, but not adenocarcinoma, was noted[69]. In another study with Swiss outbred mice, administering MNNG in the drinking water with and without a salt-rich diet failed to induce glandular stomach tumours[70]. However, in one study five out of 69 Swiss albino mice developed gastric adenocarcinoma within 54–68 weeks of receiving 100 µg/ml MNNG in the drinking water[71]. Only one of the mice had a gastric tumour classified as an intestinal-type gastric adenocarcinoma.

Another widely used chemical carcinogen is N-methyl-N-nitrosourea (MNU)[72]. The action of MNU is similar to that of MNNG, resulting in the methylation of purine residues in DNA, RNA, and amino acid residues in proteins. MNU has been administered by various routes to many animal species: it is able to induce a variety of neoplasms dependent on the animal and route of administration. An interesting report described the induction of gastric cancer in the mouse treated with MNU[73]. Six-week-old male BALB/c mice were gavaged with 0.5 mg MNU per mouse (approximately 25 mg/kg) once a week for 10 weeks. Gastrointestinal tumours developed in the forestomach, glandular stomach and duodenum. Most tumours of the glandular stomach were found along the lesser curvature of the pyloric region. Adenomatous hyperplasia was present in 75% of the mice at 20 weeks and 100% of the mice at 40 weeks. Glandular stomach carcinomas also developed in a high percentage of mice and were classified into well-differentiated adenocarcinomas, poorly differentiated adenocarcinomas and signet-ring cell carcinomas.

However, a high incidence of squamous cell carcinoma in the BALB/c mice caused premature death in many animals. Subsequently, MNU was administered in the drinking water instead of oral gavage, to determine if more glandular tumours would develop. C_3H mice were given MNU in drinking water at varying concentrations for 30 weeks[74]. Mice administered 120 ppm MNU developed poorly or well-differentiated adenocarcinomas as well as signet-cell carcinomas. A disadvantage of the model was the high incidence of haemangioendothelial sarcomas of the spleen. Furthermore, no evidence of intestinal metaplasia was found in the stomachs of treated mice. Nevertheless, in many respects MNU-induced gastric carcinogenesis in the mouse appears to closely model human gastric cancer in the development of neoplasms with varying degrees of differentiation and the presence of metastases.

A short-term study was undertaken to determine whether the combination of *H. felis* infection and MNU could lead to more severe gastric pathology.

Groups of inbred BALB/c mice were either uninfected or infected with *H. felis* and dosed by gavage with 10 mg/kg MNU weekly for 5 weeks. At 18 weeks the mice receiving MNU exhibited accelerated mortality due to thymic lymphoma and forestomach carcinoma.

However, MNU dosing resulted in mucous hypertrophy and epithelial hyperplasia of the glandular stomach. Furthermore, the combination of *H. felis* infection plus MNU led to significantly greater epithelial hyperplasia compared to MNU alone ($p < 0.05$). Similar preliminary results have been found in *H. felis*-infected C57BL/6 mice receiving 5 mg/kg MNU weekly for 5 weeks[75].

In a longer-term study lasting 18 months, 6-week-old female BALB/c mice ($n = 210$) were assigned to eight groups. *H. heilmannii*-infected and -uninfected mice were treated with 150 µg/ml MNNG in the drinking water for either 20 or 38 weeks. Mice were euthanized 12 or 18 months after *Helicobacter* inoculation[70]. Neoplasia developed only in MNNG-treated mice; however, no tumours were recorded in the glandular gastric mucosa, and *Helicobacter* infection did not affect tumour incidence. The authors concluded that gastric proliferative lesions noted in *Helicobacter*-infected mice did not progress to cancer, irrespective of treatment with MNNG. Further studies using other inbred strains of mice using *H. felis*, *H. heilmannii* or *H. pylori* are required to determine whether a cocarcinogenesis model in mice is a viable hypothesis.

H. felis-induced MALT lymphoma

BALB/c mice infected with *H. felis* develop mucosal-associated lymphoid tissue (MALT) low-grade lymphoma. Lymphomas do not develop, however, until more than 20 months after infection; nearly the entire lifespan of a mouse[77]. This model may have particular importance in dissecting the association of *H. pylori* and MALT lymphoma in humans[78]. A genetic event has been postulated to initiate the transition from gastritis to low-grade MALT lymphoma[79]. Humans have an approximately balanced $\kappa:\lambda$ ratio, which facilitates distinction of lymphoma from gastritis. In humans, MALToma has been distinguished from severe gastritis by evaluating clonality using κ and λ antigen markers or immunoglobulin gene probes[78,80]. One disadvantage of studying the mouse gastric MALT lymphoma is the disparate $20:1$ $\kappa:\lambda$ ratio in mice, which has made comparisons to the human difficult. Monoclonal lesions confirmed by phenotype and genotype have regressed after antibiotic therapy for *H. pylori*, suggesting that some of these lesions may actually represent a transition to neoplasia[80].

Because low-grade B-cell MALT lymphomas of the stomach regress when *H. pylori* infection is cured by antimicrobial therapy, the authors logically decided to use the mouse model to study the effects of *H. felis* eradication and the relationship between infection and lymphoma development[81]. Antimicrobial therapy was given to one-half of the BALB/c mice infected with *H. felis*. In the study design, BALB/c mice were experimentally infected with *H. felis* as weanlings and maintained for 20 months. Groups of antibiotic-treated and untreated mice were euthanized 2, 3 and 4 months after antimicrobial therapy (i.e. 22, 23 and 24 months after *H. felis* infection). The numbers of mice with MALT decreased after *H. felis* eradication; indeed no lymphoid follicles were seen 4 months after treatment. A total of 23% (11/48) of antibiotic-treated infected mice had MALT lymphoma compared with 75% (27/36) in infected mice which were not given antibiotics. Grading the lymphomas into low-, intermediate- and high-grade lymphoma, the untreated mice had more advanced lymphoma with 36% low-grade (13/36), 39% intermediate-grade (14/36), and 6% high-grade (large B-cell) lymphoma (2/36), whereas in the treated mice the incidence was 21% (10/48), 6% (3/48), and 0% (0/48), respectively[81]. Antigenic stimulation by *H. felis* may therefore sustain growth and progression of low-grade MALT lymphoma, and primary high-grade gastric lymphomas can evolve from the transformation of these tumours. Eradication of *H. felis*, like *H. pylori* in humans, caused inhibition of low-grade MALT lymphomas or slowing down of lymphoma development towards high-grade lymphoma[81]. The *H. felis* mouse model of gastric MALT lymphoma continues to present an opportunity to address the aetiopathogenesis of MALT lymphoma before and after antimicrobial treatment of these tumours in humans.

Helicobacter-induced gastric cancer in gerbils

Recently, the gerbil has been shown to have particularly relevant features with which to address the question of the potential of *H. pylori* to induce gastric cancer. Gerbils, animals sparingly used for biomedical research, were first reported as a model for experimental *H. pylori* infection in 1991[82]. The interest in using gerbils to study gastric cancer increased when Japanese investigators noted intestinal metaplasia, atrophy, and gastric ulcer in gerbils experimentally infected with *H. pylori*[83,84]. In one study acute gastritis with erosions of the gastric mucosa occurred shortly after infection, whereas gastric ulcers, cystica profunda, and atrophy with intestinal metaplasia were observed 3–6 months post-infection[84]. Following these findings, two separate research groups have noted that gerbils infected with *H. pylori* from periods ranging from 15 to 18 months develop gastric adenocarcinoma[36,37]. In the Watanabe study the gerbils were observed for up to 62 weeks, and 37% were found to develop adenocarcinoma in the pyloric region[37]. The gastric cancers were clearly documented histologically. Vascular invasion and metastases were not observed; it is possible, however, that they may develop with longer periods of observation. It is also important to note that Honda et al., who reported *H. pylori*-associated adenocarcinoma 15 months post-inoculation, also did not record metastases or vascular invasion[36].

Interestingly, the development of cancer is preceded by invagination of atypical glands (cystica profunda) into the submucosa, considered by some to be a premalignant lesion. The histological progression in the gerbil closely resembled that observed in humans, in terms of the early appearance of intestinal metaplasia, well-differentiated histological patterns of the gastric malignancy, and antral location of the gastric cancers. The association with gastric ulcers in this model is also of interest, given recent clinical studies in human patients indicating a link between gastric ulcer disease and gastric cancer[85]. The development of metaplasia with production of predominantly acid sialomucins was associated with tumour development. Although the long-standing question as to whether the cancers arose directly from these metaplastic cells has not been answered, the tumours clearly originated deep in the gastric glands, in close proximity to these metaplastic cells. Despite the lack of labelling studies to illustrate the point, the proliferative zone in these chronically infected animals most likely extended to the base of the glands[86].

Although most of the tumours in the *H. pylori* gerbil model originated in the pyloric region of the stomach, significant changes in the oxyntic mucosa consistent with chronic atrophic gastritis were also noted. Glandular tissue in the gastric body and fundus was atrophied and replaced by hyperplastic epithelium of the pseudopyloric type. The difference between this lesion and gastric atrophy in human patients is that the gerbil corpus is not 'thinner' consequent to the pseudopyloric hyperplasia[36,37]. A similar type of gastric atrophy with loss of oxyntic glands and neck cell hyperplasia, has been reported in *H. felis*-infected C57BL/6 mice[41]. Thus, the diagnosis of atrophy has less to do with the thickness of the mucosa and more to do with the loss of oxyntic parietal and chief cell populations within the gastric glands[86]. Growing evidence suggests that the parietal cell may regulate key differentiation decisions within the gastric glands, and ablation of parietal cells using transgenic technology[87] or *H. felis* infection leads to altered glandular differentiation and neck cell proliferation, as well as changes in gastric acid and gastrin physiology[88].

The expansion of an aberrant neck cell ('regenerative hyperplasia' or 'pseudopyloric hyperplasia') in gerbils is similar to that observed in the *H. felis* mouse model. This lineage has been shown to be spasmolytic polypeptide (SP)-positive[41], and this SP-positive lineage also develops in *H. pylori*-associated gastric cancers in humans[89]. The loss of oxyntic glandular tissue in response to *H. pylori* infection suggests that the gerbil becomes achlorhydric before the development of gastric cancer. Although the precise effects of chronic *H. pylori* infection on gastric acid secretion are not known, serum gastrin levels in the *H. pylori*-infected gerbil are increased and gastric epithelial proliferation in this model appears to be gastrin-dependent[88]. The gerbil appears to be uniquely susceptible to *Helicobacter*-induced gastric neoplasia, and further characterization of the gerbil model may provide some clues to gastric cancer progression and host/bacteria interaction. The unusual susceptibility of this animal species to gastric cancer using a fairly standard laboratory-maintained *H. pylori* strain emphasizes the overriding importance of host factors in determining the progression of *Helicobacter*-induced disease[86]. However, it must be stressed that not all of the *H. pylori* gerbil studies were able to demonstrate gastric cancer in infected animals. In one study lasting 1 year, *H. pylori*-induced intestinal metaplasia but not gastric cancer[90]. In another US study the gerbils were infected with *H. pylori* for 40 weeks. Despite persistent colonization, none of the gerbils had intestinal metaplasia or dysplasia[88,91].

Another group was able to induce gastric adenocarcinoma in *H. pylori*-infected gerbils dosed with either MNU or MNNG, but was not able to detect gastric cancer in gerbils infected with *H. pylori* alone[92]. As mentioned by others, the gerbil, although a promising model to study gastric cancer,

Table 1. Rodent models of *Helicobacter*-associated gastric cancer

Attributes	Mouse	Gerbil
H. pylori colonization	++	++++
H. felis colonization	+++	NR
Known intestinal microflora	+++	+
Genetic composition	++++	+/−
Immune reagents available	++++	+/−
Gastrin-dependent	++	++
Premalignant phenotypes	++	++++
Age at tumour onset	+	++++
Antibiotic modalities	++	+/−
Nitrosamine-induced cancer	++	++++

NR = not reported.

has its limitations. The commercial sources of gerbils are few, and the animals are usually maintained as outbred stocks. Furthermore, most immune reagents needed to define immune parameters in the gerbil are not available. An unexpected finding was the observation that triple-therapy with antibiotic-impregnated wafers containing amoxycillin (3 mg/tablet), metranidazole (0.09 mg/tablet) and bismuth (0.185 mg/tablet) administered as a sole food source to gerbils for 7 days caused acute deaths. Histopathology revealed a typhlocolitis; *Clostridium difficile* was isolated using anaerobic culture and both *C. difficile* toxins A and B were confirmed using a specific ELISA (Bergin I, Fox JG. Unpublished observations). Thus, antibiotic intervention strategies designed to interrupt the carcinogenic process in gerbils may not be feasible unless *C. difficile*-free gerbils are available. Non-availability of genetically engineered gerbils, in contrast to the plethora of transgenic and knockout mice, also curtails their usefulness (Table 1).

References

1. Parkin MD, Stjhernsward J, Muir C. Estimates of the worldwide frequency of twelve major cancers. Int J Cancer. 1988;41:184–97.
2. Correa P. Human gastric carcinogenesis: a multistep and multifactorial process. First American Cancer Society Award Lecture on Cancer Epidemiology and Prevention. Cancer Res. 1992;52:6735–40.
3. Correa P, Fox JG, Fontham E et al. *Helicobacter pylori* and gastric carcinoma: serum antibody prevalence in populations with contrasting cancer risks. Cancer. 1990,66.2569–74.
4. Eurogast Study Group. An international association between *Helicobacter pylori* infection and gastric cancer. Lancet. 1993,341.1339–62.
5. Fox JG, Correa P, Taylor NS et al. *Campylobacter pylori*-associated gastritis and immune response in a population at increased risk of gastric carcinoma. Am J Gastroenterol. 1989;84:775–81.
6. Sierra R, Munoz N, Pena S et al. Antibodies to *Helicobacter pylori* and pepsinogen levels in children in Costa Rica. Cancer Epidemiol Biomarkers Prev. 1992;1:449–54.
7. Huang J-Q, Sridhar S, Chen Y, Hunt RH. Meta-analysis of the relationship between *Helicobacter pylori* seropositivity and gastric cancer. Gastroenterology. 1998;114:1169–79.
8. Forman D. *Helicobacter pylori* and gastric cancer. Scand J Gastroenterol. 1996;220:23–6.
9. Forman D, Newell DG, Fullerton F et al. Association between infection with *Helicobacter pylori* and risk of gastric cancer: evidence from a prospective investigation. Br Med J. 1991;302:1302–5.

10. Mitchell HM. The epidemiology of *Helicobacter pylori* infection and its relation to gastric cancer. In: Goodwin CS, Worsley BW, editors. *Helicobacter pylori*: Biology and Clinical Practice. Boca Raton, FL: CRC Press; 1993:95–114.
11. Nomura A, Stemmerman GN, Chyou PH, Kato I, Perez-Perez GI, Blaser MJ. *Helicobacter pylori* infection and gastric carcinoma among Japanese Americans in Hawaii. N Engl J Med. 1991;325:1132–6.
12. Parsonnet J, Friedman GD, Vandersteen DP et al. *Helicobacter pylori* infection and the risk of gastric carcinoma. N Engl J Med. 1991;325:1127–31.
13. Parsonnet J, Hanson S, Rodriguez L et al. *Helicobacter pylori* infection and gastric MALT lymphoma. N Engl J Med. 1994;330:1267–71.
14. Talley NJ, Zinsmeister AR, Weaver A et al. Gastric adenocarcinoma and *Helicobacter pylori* infection. J Natl Cancer Inst. 1991;83:1734–9.
15. Parsonnet J, Vandersteen D, Goates J, Sibey RK, Pritikin J, Chang Y. *Helicobacter pylori* infection in intestinal and diffuse-type gastric adenocarcinomas. J Natl Cancer Inst. 1991;83:640–3.
16. Dubois A, Berg DE, Incecik ET et al. Host specificity of *Helicobacter pylori* strains and host responses in experimentally challenged nonhuman primates. Gastroenterology. 1999;116:90–6.
17. Dubois A, Tarnawski A, Newell DG et al. Gastric injury and invasion of parietal cells by spiral bacteria in rhesus monkeys: are gastritis and hyperchlorhydria infectious diseases? Gastroenterology. 1991;100:884–91.
18. Shuto R, Fujioka T, Kubota I, Nasu M. Experimental gastritis induced by *Helicobacter pylori* in Japanese monkeys. Infect Immun. 1993;61:933–9.
19. Euler AR, Zurenko GE, Moe JB, Ulrich RG, Yagi Y. Evaluation of two monkey species (*Macaca mulatta* and *Macaca fascicularis*) as possible models for human *Helicobacter pylori* disease. J Clin Microbiol. 1990;28:2285–90.
20. Sato T, Takeuchi TA. Infection by spirilla in the stomach of the rhesus monkey. Vet Pathol. 1982;19(Suppl. 7):17–25.
21. Krakowka S, Morgan DR, Kraft WG, Leunk RD. Establishment of gastric *Campylobacter pylori* infection in the neonatal gnotobiotic piglet. Infect Immun. 1987;55:2789–96.
22. Radin JM, Eaton KA, Krakowka S, Lee A, Otto G. Fox JG. *Helicobacter pylori* infection in gnotobiotic beagle dogs. Infect Immun. 1990;58:2606–12.
23. Fox JG, Blanco M, Murphy JC et al. Local and systemic immune reponse in murine *Helicobacter felis* active chronic gastritis. Infect Immun. 1993;61:2309–15.
24. Fox JG, Lee A, Otto G, Taylor NS, Murphy JC. *Helicobacter felis* gastritis in gnotobiotic rats: an animal model of *Helicobacter pylori* gastritis. Infect Immun. 1991;59:785–91.
25. Lee A, Fox JG, Otto G, Murphy JC. A small animal model of human *Helicobacter pylori* active chronic gastritis. Gastroenterology. 1990;99:1315–23.
26. Fox JG, Correa P, Taylor NS et al. *Helicobacter mustelae*-associated gastritis in ferrets: an animal model of *Helicobacter pylori* gastritis in humans. Gastroenterology. 1990;99:352–61.
27. Fox JG, Dangler CA, Sager W, Borkowski R, Gliatto JM. *Helicobacter mustelae*-associated gastric adenocarcinoma in ferrets (*Mustela putorius furo*). Vet Pathol. 1997;34:225–9.
28. Fox JG, Wishnok JS, Murphy JC, Tannenbaum SR, Correa P. MNNG-induced gastric carcinoma in ferrets infected with *Helicobacter mustelae*. Carcinogenesis. 1993;14:1957–61.
29. Esteves MI, Schrenzel MD, Marini RP et al. *Helicobacter pylori* gastritis in cats with long term natural infection as a model of human disease. Am J Pathol. 2000;156:709–21.
30. Fox JG, Perkins S, Yan L, Shen Z, Attardo L, Pappo J. Local immune response in *Helicobacter pylori*-infected cats and identification of *H. pylori* in saliva, gastric fluid and feces. Immunology. 1996;88:400–6.
31. Handt LK, Fox JG, Stalis IH et al. Characterization of feline *Helicobacter pylori* strains and associated gastritis in a colony of domestic cats. J Clin Microbiol. 1995;33:2280–9.
32. Dangler CA, Taylor NS, Kobuk Z, Castriotta L, Pappo J, Fox JG. Comparison of gastric colonization and lesion development in ICR and C57BL/6 mice following long-term infection with *Helicobacter pylori* strains SS1 or H244. Gut. 1998;43:A28 (abstract).
33. Fox JG, Dangler CA, Taylor NS, King A, Koh T, Wang T. High salt diet induces gastric epithelial hyperplasia, parietal cell loss, and enhances *Helicobacter pylori* colonization in C57BL/6 mice. Cancer Res. 1999;59:4823–8.
34. Fox JG, Taylor NS, Dangler CA. Colonization and persistence of *H. pylori* in ICR mice is dependent on age of infection. Gastroenterology. 1999;116:G3117 (abstract).

35. Lee A, O'Rourke J, DeUngria MC, Robertson B, Daskslopoulos G, Dixon MF. A standardized mouse model of *Helicobacter pylori* infection: introducing the Sydney strain. Gastroenterology. 1997;112:1386–97.
36. Honda S, Fujioka T, Tokieda M, Satoh R, Nishizono A, Nasu M. Development of *Helicobacter pylori*-induced gastric carcinoma in Mongolian gerbils. Cancer Res. 1998; 58:4255–9.
37. Watanabe T, Tada M, Nagai H, Sasaki S, Nakao M. *Helicobacter pylori* infection induces gastric cancer in Mongolian gerbils. Gastroenterology. 1998;115:642–8.
38. Bamford KB, Fan X, Crow SE et al. Lymphocytes in the human gastric mucosa during *Helicobacter pylori* have a T helper cell 1 phenotype. Gastroenterology. 1998;114:482–92.
39. Mohammadi M, Nedrud J, Redline R, Lycke N, Czinn SJ. Murine CD4 T-cell response to *Helicobacter* infection: Th1 cells enhance gastritis and Th2 cells reduce bacterial load. Gastroenterology. 1997;113:1848–57.
40. Fox JG, Li X, Cahill R et al. Hypertrophic gastropathy in *Helicobacter felis* infected wildtype C57BL/6 mice and p53 hemizygous transgenic mice. Gastroenterology. 1996;110:155–66.
41. Wang TC, Goldenring JR, Ito S et al. Mice lacking secretory phospholipase A2 show altered apoptosis and differentiation with *Helicobacter felis* infection. Gastroenterology. 1998; 114:675–89.
42. Fox JG, Dangler CA, Whary MT, Edelman W, Kucherlapati R, Wang TC. Mice carrying a truncated *Apc* gene have diminished gastric epithelial proliferation, gastric inflammation and humoral immunity in respect to *Helicobacter felis* infection. Cancer Res. 1997;57:3972–8.
43. Fox JG, Li X, Cahill RJ et al. Hypertrophic gastropathy in *Helicobacter felis*-infected wildtype C57BL/6 mice and p53 hemizygous transgenic mice. Gastroenterology. 1996; 110:155–66.
44. Ally R, Mitchell HM, Segal I. cagA positive *H. pylori* aplenty in South Africa: the first systematic study of *H. pylori* infection in asymptomatic children in Soweto. Gut. 1999;45:A97–8.
45. Holcombe C. *Helicobacter pylori*: the African enigma. Gut. 1992;33:429–31.
46. Forman D, Sitas F, Newell DG, Stacey AR, Boreham J, Peto R. Geographic association of *Helicobacter pylori* antibody prevalence and gastric cancer mortality in rural China. Int J Cancer. 1990;46:608–11.
47. Abbas AK, Murphy KM, Sher A. Functional diversity of helper T lymphocytes. Nature. 1996;383:787–93.
48. Mohammadi M, Czinn S, Redline R, Nedrud J. *Helicobacter*-specific cell-mediated immune responses display a predominant Th1 phenotype and promote a delayed-type hypersensitive response in the stomachs of mice. J Immunol. 1996;156:4729–38.
49. Eaton KA, Ringler SR, Danon SJ. Murine splenocytes induce severe gastritis and delayed type hypersensitivity and suppress bacterial colonization in *Helicobacter pylori*-infected SCID mice. Infect Immun. 1999;67:4594–602.
50. Roth KA, Kapadia SB, Martin SM, Lorenz RG. Cellular immune responses are essential for the development of *Helicobacter felis*-associated gastric pathology. J Immunol. 1999; 163:1490–7.
51. Finkelman FD, Shea-Donohue T, Goldhill J et al. Cytokine regulation of host defense against parasitic gastrointesinal nematodes: lessons from studies with rodent models. Annu Rev Immunol. 1997;15:505–33.
52. Fox JG, Beck P, Dangler CA et al. Concurrent enteric helminth infection modulates inflammation, gastric immune responses, and reduces *Helicobacter* induced gastric atrophy. Nat Med. 2000;6:536–42.
53. Charnley G, Tannenbaum SR. Flow cytometric analysis of the effect of sodium chloride on gastric cancer risk in the rat. Cancer Res. 1985;45:5608–16.
54. Sato T, Fukuyama T, Urata F, Suzuki T. Studies of the causation of gastric cancer. I. Bleeding in the glandular stomach of mice by feeding with highly salted foods, and a comment on salted foods in Japan. Jpn Med J. 1959;1835:25.
55. Kodama M, Kodama T, Suzuki H, Kondo K. Effect of rice and salty rice diets on the structure of mouse stomach. Nutr Cancer. 1984;6:135–47.
56. Mohammadi M, Redline R, Nedrud J, Czinn S. Role of the host in pathogenesis of *Helicobacter*-associated gastritis: *H. felis* infection of inbred and congenic mouse strains. Infect Immun. 1996;64:238–45.

57. Hakanson R, Blom H, Carlsson E, Larsson H, Ryberg B, Sundler F. Hypergastrinaemia produces trophic effects in stomach but not in pancreas and intestines. Regul Pept. 1986;13:225–33.
58. Hakanson R, Sundler F. Trophic effects of gastrin. Scand J Gastroenterol. 1991;180:130–6.
59. Ryberg B, Axelson J, Hakanson R, Sundler F, Mattsson H. Trophic effects of continuous infusion of [Leu15]-gastrin-17 in the rat. Gastroenterology. 1990;98:33–8.
60. Eissele R, Brunner G, Simon B, Solcia E, Arnold R. Gastric mucosa during treatment with lansoprazole: *Helicobacter pylori* is a risk for argyrophil hyperplasia. Gastroenterology. 1997;112:707–17.
61. Klinkenberg-Knol E, Festen HP, Jansen JB et al. Long-term treatment with omeprazole for refractory reflux esophagitis: efficacy and safety. Ann Intern Med. 1994;121:161–7.
62. Kuipers EJ, Uyterlinde AM, Pena AS et al. Long-term sequelae of *Helicobacter pylori* gastritis. Lancet. 1995;345:1525–8.
63. Lamberts R, Creutzfeldt W, Struber HG, Brunner G, Solcia E. Long-term omeprazole therapy in peptic ulcer disease: gastrin, endocrine cell growth, and gastritis. Gastroenterology. 1993;104:1356–70.
64. Li Q, Karam SM, Coerver KA, Matzuk MM, Gordon JI. Stimulation of activin receptor II signaling pathways inhibits differentiation of multiple gastric epithelial lineages. Mol Endocrinol. 1998;12:181–92.
65. Sakagami T, Dixon M, O'Rourke J et al. Atrophic gastric changes in both *Helicobacter felis* and *Helicobacter pylori* infected mice are host dependent and separate from antral gastritis. Gut. 1996;39:639–48.
66. Wang T, Dangler CA, Chen C et al. Synergistic interaction between hypergastrinemia and *Helicobacter* infection in a mouse model of gastric carcinoma. Gastroenterology. 2000;118:36–47.
67. Bralow SP. Experimental gastric carcinogenesis. Digestion. 1972;5:290–310.
68. Klein AJ, Palmer WL. Experimental gastric carcinoma: a critical review with comments on the criteria of induced malignancy. J Natl Cancer Inst. 1941;1:559–84.
69. Sugimura T, Kawachi T. Experimental stomach cancer. Methods Cancer Res. 1973; 7:245–308.
70. Kodama M, Kodama T, Fukami H. Genetics of host response to N-methyl-N'-nitro-N-nitrosoguanidine. I: Lack of tumor production in the glandular stomach of Swiss mouse. Anticancer Res. 1992;12:441–50.
71. Sigaran MF, Con-Wong R. Production of proliferative lesions in gastric mucosa of albino mice by oral administration of N-methyl-N'-nitro-N-nitrosoguanidine. Gann. 1979; 70:343–52.
72. IARC. N-nitroso-N-methylurea. In: IARC Monographs on the Evaluation of Carcinogenic Risk of Chemicals to Man. WHO, Lyon, France. 1977:227–55.
73. Tatematsu M, Ogawa K, Hoshiva T et al. Induction of adenocarcinomas in the glandular stomach of BALB/c mice treated with N-methyl-N-nitrosourea. Jpn J Cancer Res. 1992;83:915–18.
74. Tatematsu M, Yamamoto M, Iwata H et al. Induction of the glandular stomach cancers in C3H mice treated with N-methyl-N-nitrosourea in the drinking water. Jpn J Cancer Res. 1992;84:1258–64.
75. Andrutis KA, Li X, Wang TC, Fox JG. Gastric carcinogenesis of MNU in *Helicobacter felis* infected mice. Gut. 1996;39(Suppl. 2):A79 (abstract).
76. Danon SJ, Eaton KA. The role of gastric *Helicobacter* and N-methyl-N'-nitro-N-nitrosoguanidine in carcinogenesis of mice. Helicobacter. 1998;3:260–8.
77. Enno A, O'Rourke JL, Howlett CR, Jack A, Dixon MF, Lee A. MALToma-like lesions in the murine gastric mucosa after long-term infection with *Helicobacter felis*. Am J Pathol. 1995;147:217–23.
78. Wotherspoon AC, Doglioni C, Diss TC et al. Regression of primary low-grade B-cell gastric lymphoma of mucosa-associated lymphoid tissue type after eradication of *Helicobacter pylori*. Lancet. 1993;342:575–7.
79. Calvert R, Randerson J, Evans P et al. Genetic abnormalities during transition from *Helicobacter pylori*-associated gastritis to low grade MALToma. Lancet. 1995;345:26–7.
80. Savio A, Frazin G, Wotherspoon AC et al. Diagnosis and posttreatment follow-up of *Helicobacter pylori*-positive gastric lymphoma of mucosa associated lymphoid tissue: histology, polymerase chain reaction, or both? Blood. 1996;87:1255–60.

81. Enno A, O'Rourke J, Braye S, Howlett R, Lee A. Antigen-dependent progression of mucosa associated lymphoid tissue (MALT)-type lymphoma in the stomach. Am J Pathol. 1998;152:1625–32.
82. Yokota K, Kurebayashi Y, Takayama Y et al. Colonization of *Helicobacter pylori* in the gastric mucosa of Mongolian gerbils. Microbiol Immunol. 1991;35:475–80.
83. Hirayama F, Takagi S, Kusuhara H, Iwao E, Yokoyama Y. Induction of gastric ulcer and intestinal metaplasia in Mongolian gerbils infected with *Helicobacter pylori*. J Gastroenterol. 1996;31:755–7.
84. Honda S, Fujioka T, Tokeida M, Gotoh T, Nishizono A, Nasu M. Gastric ulcer, atrophic gastritis, and intestinal metaplasia caused by *Helicobacter pylori* infection in Mongolian gerbils. Scand J Gastroenterol. 1998;33:454–60.
85. Hansson LE, Nyren O, Hsing AW et al. The risk of stomach cancer in patients with gastric or duodenal ulcer disease. N Engl J Med. 1996;335:242–9.
86. Wang TC, Fox JG. *Helicobacter pylori* and gastric cancer: Koch's postulates fulfilled (editorial). Gastroenterology. 1998;115:780–3.
87. Li Q, Karam SM, Gordon JI. Diphtheria toxin-mediated ablation of parietal cells in the stomach of transgenic mice. J Biol Chem. 1996;271:3671–6.
88. Peek R Jr, Wirth HP, Moss SF et al. *Helicobacter pylori* alters gastric epithelial cell cycle events and gastrin secretion in Mongolian gerbils. Gastroenterology. 2000;118:48–59.
89. Schmidt PH, Lee JR, Goldenring JR, Wright NA, Poulsom R. Association of an aberrant spasmolytic polypeptide-expressing cell lineage with gastric adenocarcinoma in humans. Gastroenterology. 1998;114:G2781.
90. Ikeno T, Ota H, Sugiyama A et al. *Helicobacter pylori*-induced chronic active gastritis, intestinal metaplasia, and gastric ulcer in Mongolian gerbils. Am J Pathol. 1999;154:951–60.
91. Wirth HP, Beins MH, Yang M, Tham KT, Blaser MJ. Experimental infection of Mongolian gerbils with wild-type andmutant *Helicobacter pylori* strains. Infect Immun. 1998;66:4856–66.
92. Tatematsu M, Yamamoto M, Shimizu N et al. Induction of glandular stomach cancers in *Helicobacter pylori*-sensitive Mongolian gerbils treated with N-methyl-N-nitrosourea and N-methyl-N'-nitro-N-nitrosoguanidine in drinking water. Jpn J Cancer Res. 1998;89:97–104.

54
Helicobacter pylori and gastric cancer: the risk is real

D. FORMAN

INTRODUCTION

The substance of this proposal is that the relationship between *Helicobacter pylori* infection and gastric cancer is one of major importance in terms of both public health and understanding the cancer process. The issue will be addressed from three perspectives: the worldwide burden of disease represented by *H. pylori*-associated gastric cancer; the development in understanding of carcinogenic mechanisms; and the facilitation of intervention strategies to reduce the future incidence of gastric cancer.

THE WORLDWIDE BURDEN OF GASTRIC CANCER

The latest figures from the International Agency for Research on Cancer[1,2] estimate that in 1990 there were almost 800 000 new diagnoses and 630 000 deaths from gastric cancer. It represents, after lung cancer, the second most common fatal malignancy with an increasing proportion of gastric cancer cases occurring in developing countries, notably in Asia and South America. In these continents, changes in the absolute numbers and in the age-structure of the population, towards an increased life expectancy, mean that an increasing number of gastric cancers are being diagnosed despite a general decline in age-standardized incidence. Gastric cancer is associated with an extremely poor prognosis, and 5 year survival rarely exceeds 20%[3,4] outside Japan, where surveillance programmes increase the detection rate of 'early gastric cancer'.

A group from the IARC has also estimated the proportion of gastric cancer likely to be attributable to *H. pylori* infection[5]. Even using a conservative assumption about the magnitude of the relative risk, estimating it to be 2.1, they concluded that 36% and 47% of all gastric cancers in developed and developing countries respectively resulted from the infection: a total of 337 800 cases in 1990 (Table 1). This estimate makes no allowance for the recent substantial changes in the proportion of gastric cancer that is diag-

Table 1. Estimated numbers of gastric cancer cases in developed and developing countries and numbers/fraction attributable to *H. pylori* infection

	Number of new gastric cancer cases 1990*	Estimate of new gastric cancer cases attributable to H. pylori infection**	Attributable fraction	Revised estimate of new gastric cancers attributable to H. pylori infection***	Revised attributable fraction
Developed world	315 900	112 200	36%	110 565	35%
Developing world	482 300	225 600	47%	328 000	68%

* Numbers from Parkin et al.[1].
** Numbers from Parkin et al.[5]. The attributable calculation assumes that the relative risk of cancer associated with infection is 2.1, that 50% of the population are infected in developed countries and 80% are infected in developing countries.
*** Based on Parsonnet[6]. The attributable calculation assumes that the relative risk of cancer associated with infection is 5.1, that 35% of the population are infected in developed countries and 75% are infected in developing countries. Additionally Parsonnet assumes 40% and 10% of gastric cancers arise in the proximal stomach in developed and developing countries respectively and these are not associated with infection. Parsonnet also assumes that diagnostic tests are 90% sensitive and specific in developed countries (85% in developing countries). These factors produce the attributable fractions of 35% and 68% which have then been applied to the cancer frequencies in column 1.

nosed in the cardia region of the stomach. There is no evidence that *H. pylori* infection increases the risk of such cancers, and this would reduce the total attributable burden. The IARC estimate also fails to consider the impact of serological assay misclassification. The relative risk measures used in attributable fraction calculations are derived from case–control comparisons based on serology. Reduced sensitivity and specificity in assay procedures will most likely result in an artefactual reduction in the relative risk estimate[6].

Parsonnet[7] has revised the IARC estimates by assuming that assays are 90% sensitive and specific in developed countries, 85% in developing countries. Adjustment for this would increase the relative risk estimate to a value of 5.1. She also assumed that 60% and 90% of gastric cancers are at non-cardia sites in developed and developing countries. The net effect of these revisions (Table 1) is of little consequence in developed countries, but causes a substantial increase in the estimate of *H. pylori*-attributed cancers in the developing world. The total worldwide burden for 1990 increases to over 438 000. There are in fact relatively few established causes of cancer, at any site, with an annual attributable burden of this magnitude (Table 2). Thus, on a global basis, *H. pylori* is one of a relatively short shortlist of major cancer risk factors.

MECHANISMS OF CARCINOGENESIS

From an historical perspective it is now difficult to recall how innovatory was the proposal, first made by Marshall in one of the original *H. pylori* papers[8], that a bacterial infection could be associated with gastric cancer.

Table 2. Major identified risk factors* for common cancers and crude estimates of attributable numbers of associated cancers worldwide diagnosed in 1990

Risk factor	Associated cancers	Number of cancer cases in 1990 attributable to risk factor	Basis of calculation
Tobacco smoke	Lung and many other sites	≫ 933 000 (does not include cancers apart from lung)	90% of all lung cancers[1]
Helicobacter pylori	Stomach	438 500	Table 1
Human papillomavirus	Cervix and other sites	353 400	ref. 5
Hepatitis B and C	Liver	338 600	ref. 5
Betel quid chewing	Mouth	190 300	90% of all mouth cancers[1]
Sunlight	Skin	≫ 160 000 (does not include non-melanoma)	90% of all melanoma[1]
Diet deficient in fruit and vegetables	Several sites	Uncertain	Likely to contribute to many common cancers

* This is not intended to be an exhaustive or complete listing. There would, however, appear to be few other identified cancer risk factors with an annual attributable burden of more than 100 000 cases. The author would like to hear from anyone who can suggest additions to the list.

At the time a detailed understanding of the molecular and genetic events associated with cancer was becoming appreciated, and it seemed inconceivable that bacteria, which had no direct interaction with host DNA, were involved in the process. Although *H. pylori* produces a number of toxins that may affect carcinogenesis, it would now seem that the important feature of infection is the induction of an on-going inflammatory reaction. It is likely to be the chronic stimulation of the host epithelial cells, leading to an over-expression of reactive oxygen, nitrogen oxide and similar molecules, which underlies the progressive sequence of events leading to cancer (see review in ref. 9). This model of bacterial–host interactions in cancer development has now found applicability in understanding the mechanistic basis for other types of cancer[10].

It has been known for several decades (well before the discovery of *H. pylori*) that gastric cancer primarily develops in conditions of hypoacidity. One of the major concerns about the *H. pylori*–gastric cancer relationship has always been how this infection could therefore also be associated with diseases of hyperacidity, notably peptic ulcer. Clearly a specialized feature of the stomach is to produce acid, and understanding the influence of *H. pylori* infection on this process is going to be critical in establishing the pathways which lead to pathology and disease. Two recent papers by El-Omar and colleagues have helped in teasing apart this relationship. They showed, firstly, that relatives of patients with gastric cancer were more likely than unrelated controls to be *H. pylori*-positive themselves, and that

H. *pylori*-positive relatives were more likely to have reduced gastric acid secretion than H. *pylori*-positive controls[11]. They have then gone on to show that the H. *pylori*-positive relatives are also more likely than positive controls to have specific G to T polymorphisms in the interleukin-1β gene[12]. Individuals with these polymorphisms exhibit a reduction in gastric acid secretion and are at increased risk of gastric cancer. So we now have a model whereby H. *pylori* infection may interact differentially in individuals with and without polymorphisms affecting gastric acid output. It may only be the former which respond in a manner that increases the cancer risk.

The elegance of this model is that it builds onto our previous understanding of the carcinogenic process in the human stomach, the 'Correa model'[13], a consideration of how an environmentally acquired, common risk factor may modify the host response in different directions and with different pathological consequences, dependent on the host's genetic background. The model also brings in play the role of gastric acid secretion, an essential property of the stomach likely to hold the key to disease progression[14].

PROSPECTS FOR PREVENTION

The third aspect of the H. *pylori*–gastric cancer association which underlines its importance is based on the fact that H. *pylori* infection can be simply eradicated through antibiotic therapy. This therefore raises the prospect of preventing cancer by controlling the infection. Screening at-risk populations for the presence of infection and treating those infected (or, in the future, offering therapeutic vaccination) has several advantageous features as a cancer-prevention strategy. In comparison with screening policies for other cancers, notably breast and cervical cancer, such a strategy is relatively cheap even in communities with low rates of gastric cancer[15]. This is partly because the technology required for the conduct of a serological test is relatively 'low-tech' and does not require highly skilled staff to interpret the results. From what is known about the low level of reacquisition of infection in adult life[16], it is likely that bacterial eradication would only be required as a once-only treatment in adult life, and regular repeat screening for the infection would therefore not be necessary.

A screen-and-treat strategy is also relatively non-invasive in terms of the required intervention (compared with mammography or cervical cytological sampling) and, unlike many other approaches to cancer prevention, does not require any long-term behavioural changes from the screened population (compared with modifying smoking or dietary behaviour). There are certainly several uncertainties associated with such a strategy, including substantive concerns about the induction of antibiotic resistance and increasing the risk of diseases that might be a consequence of eradication[17]. As a result, several authors have suggested that the current state of evidence on this question necessitates appropriately powered randomized intervention trials[15,18,19] as the only reliable means of assessing benefit (including cost–benefit) against harm.

In summary, and in keeping with the timing of this meeting to the new century, it is relevant to quote a recent editorial from *Gastroenterology*[20]:

As the century closes, we can view gastric cancer with much more optimism that it was viewed 100 years ago. ... We have identified a major cause of the disease – a cause that is completely curable and potentially preventable.

Julie Parsonnet was making the point here that our knowledge of *H. pylori* infection and its pathogenic consequences has not only transformed our understanding of one of the world's major cancers but also has provided an opportunity for disease prevention.

References

1. Parkin DM, Pisani P, Ferlay J. Estimates of the worldwide incidence of 25 major cancers in 1990. Int J Cancer. 1999;80:827–41.
2. Pisani P, Parkin DM, Bray F, Ferlay J. Estimates of the worldwide mortality from 25 cancers in 1990. Int J Cancer. 1999;83:18–29.
3. Berrino F, Capocaccia R, Esteve J et al. Survival of cancer patients in Europe: the EUROCARE-2 Study. IARC Scientific Publications No. 151. Lyon: International Agency for Research on Cancer; 1999.
4. Kosary CL, Ries LAG, Miller BA, Mankey BF, Harras A, Edwards BK. SEER Cancer Statistics Review 1973–92. NIH Publication No. 96-2789. Bethesda: NIH;1995.
5. Parkin DM, Pisani P, Munoz N, Ferlay J. The global health burden of infection associated cancers. Cancer Surv. 1999;33:5–33.
6. Kleinbaum DG, Kupper LL, Morgenstern H. Epidemiologic Research. New York: Van Nostrand, Reinholdt. 1982;221–41.
7. Parsonnet J. *Helicobacter pylori*: the size of the problem. Gut. 1998;43(Suppl. 1):S6–9.
8. Marshall B. Unidentified curved bacilli on gastric epithelium in active chronic gastritis. Lancet. 1983;1:1273–5.
9. Goldstone AR, Quirke P, Dixon MF. *Helicobacter pylori* infection and gastric cancer. J Pathol. 1996;179:129–37.
10. Parsonnet J. Microbes and Malignancy: Infection as a cause of human cancers. Oxford: Oxford University Press; 1999.
11. El-Omar E, Oien K, Murray LS et al. Increased prevalence of precancerous changes in relatives of gastric cancer patients: critical role of *H. pylori* Gastroenterology. 2000;118:22–30.
12. El-Omar E, Carrington, M, Chow W-H et al. Interleukin-1 polymorphisms associated with increased risk of gastric cancer. Nature. 2000;404:398–402.
13. Correa P. Human gastric carcinogenesis: a multistep and multifactorial process – First American Cancer Society Award Lecture on Cancer Epidemiology and Prevention. Cancer Res. 1992;52:6735–40.
14. Lee A, Veldhuyzen van Zanten S. The aging stomach or the stomachs of the ages [comment]. Gut. 1997;41:575–6.
15. Parsonnet J, Harris RA, Hack HM, Owens DK. Modelling cost-effectiveness of *Helicobacter pylori* screening to prevent gastric cancer: a mandate for clinical trials. Lancet. 1996; 348:150–4.
16. Parsonnet J. The incidence of *Helicobacter pylori* infection. Aliment Pharmacol Ther. 1995, 9(Suppl. 2):45–51.
17. Forman D. Should we go further and screen and treat? Eur J Gastroenterol Hepatol. 1999; 11(Suppl. 2):S69–71.
18. Forman D. Lessons from on-going intervention studies. In: Hunt RH, Tytgat GNJ, editors. Helicobacter pylori: Basic Mechanisms to Clinical Cure *1998*. Dordrecht: Kluwer; 1998:354–61.
19. Danesh J. *Helicobacter pylori* and gastric cancer: time for mega-trials? Br J Cancer. 1999;80:927–9.
20. Parsonnet J. When heredity is infectious. Gastroenterology. 2000;118:222–4.

55
Helicobacter pylori in gastric malignancy: role of oxidants, antioxidants and other co-factors*

Z. W. ZHANG and M. J. G. FARTHING

INTRODUCTION

Gastric cancer is the second most common solid tumour worldwide. Although the overall incidence of distal gastric cancer has been decreasing over the past few decades, the incidence of adenocarcinomas of the proximal stomach and oesophagogastric junction is rising[1,2]. It is one of the most common cancers in China[3]. In the United Kingdom it accounts for almost 10 000 deaths each year[4]. About 20 000–25 000 Americans each year will be diagnosed with gastric carcinoma, and around 15 000 will die of the disease[2]. In Japan gastric carcinoma remains the most frequent cancer in both sexes, and accounts for 20–30% of all incident cancers[5].

Gastric carcinogenesis is a complex, multistep and multifactorial process, in which many factors have been implicated, such as ageing, autoimmune factors, malnutrition and chronic inflammation; or repeated exposure to bile, aspirin, alcohol and sodium chloride. Over the past few years *Helicobacter pylori* infection, the main cause of gastritis, has been strongly linked to the development of gastric carcinoma[6–8]. It has recently been shown, in a Mongolian gerbil model of *H. pylori* infection, that the formation of gastric cancer is preceded by a series of mucosal premalignant changes, such as metaplasia and atrophy[9]. However, the underlying mechanisms of *H. pylori*-associated gastric carcinogenesis remain unknown[10]. Disturbances in cell turnover in the gastrointestinal tract are believed to predispose to cancer development[11], and it is clear that this organism is capable of modifying epithelial cell turnover within gastric glands and in gastric epithelial cells in culture[12–14].

---

*A version of this manuscript has been published previously in the Chinese Journal of Gastroenterology, in Chinese. Permission has been obtained from the editor to translate the paper into English and publish it again in this book.

We have studied the effect of *H. pylori* infection on gastric epithelial cell proliferation, and found that patients infected with *H. pylori* had significantly higher proliferation rates compared to uninfected controls[13,15-17]. Recently, multidisciplinary research has shown that low intake of fresh fruits and vegetables is associated with an increased risk of epithelial cancers[18]. Although many substances are contained in fruits and vegetables, a prominent group is the antioxidants, especially vitamins C and E, and β-carotene[18]. The coexistence of *H. pylori* infection and these antioxidants in the human stomach has stimulated many studies on the relationship between these antioxidants and *H. pylori*-associated gastric carcinogenesis. Vitamins C and E and β-carotene not only reduce the formation of *N*-nitroso compounds (NOCs) or scavenge reactive oxygen metabolites (ROMs) in the stomach[19-21], but can also affect gastric cell proliferation directly or through their antioxidant activities[22-26]. However, investigation of the concentrations of these vitamins in the stomachs of patients with *H. pylori* infection suggests that colonization causes a significant reduction of gastric concentrations of these antioxidants[12]. This review examines the recent literature on the role of dietary antioxidants, vitamins C and E and β-carotene in *H. pylori*-associated gastric carcinogenesis.

H. PYLORI-ASSOCIATED GASTRIC MUCOSAL OXIDATIVE STRESS AND DIETARY ANTIOXIDANTS

Carcinogens are able to cause permanent structural changes in DNA such as base-pair mutations, deletions, insertions, rearrangements, and sequence amplification. In addition they are able to activate cytoplasmic and nuclear signal transduction pathways, and to modulate the activity of stress proteins and stress genes that influence cell growth, differentiation, and cell death. ROMs possess all these properties; therefore they are one of the most important groups of human carcinogens. The gastrointestinal tract is particularly well endowed with the enzymatic machinery necessary to form large amounts of ROMs, and this would lead to a dramatic increase of ROM production during inflammation. *H. pylori* infection induces marked infiltration of inflammatory cells within the gastric mucosa; these inflammatory cells such as neutrophils and monocytes synthesize and release copious amounts of toxic ROMs[27]. It has recently been suggested that gastric pit cells possess a phagocyte nicotinamide adenine dinucleotide phosphate (NADPH) oxidase-like activity. Live *H. pylori* and its lipopolysaccharide (LPS) can significantly increase the production of superoxide anion radicals (O_2^-) from gastric pit cells by up-regulating this enzyme[28,29]. It is evident that there is excessive ROM production during *H. pylori* infection. In a previous study, for example, a positive correlation was found between mucosal ROM production and *H. pylori* status of patients[30]. There was even a positive association between mucosal ROM production and quantitative histological and microbiological *H. pylori* assessments[31]. These ROMs are highly toxic, and can cause damage to all cellular components, including structural and regulatory proteins, carbohydrates, and DNA[32,33]. Ras-family proto-oncogenes and the p53 tumour suppressor gene are the most impor-

Table 1. Antioxidant properties of dietary antioxidants[19,52,62,106]

	O_2^-	H_2O_2	HOCl	Singlet oxygen	Peroxyl radicals	NOCs
Vitamin C	✓	✓	✓	✓		✓
Vitamin E				✓	✓	✓
β-carotene				✓	✓	✓

O_2^-: superoxide anion radicals; H_2O_2: hydrogen peroxide; HOCl: hypochlorous acid; NOC: N-nitroso compound.

tant genes related to human cancer, including gastric adenocarcinoma[34,35]. G → T transversions are frequently observed in the middle position of hotspot codon 12 of Ki-ras and H-ras, which could be produced by misreplication of 8–hydroxy-deoxyguanosine lesions induced by ROMs[36,37]. Mutations at p53 hotspot codon 248 (CGG) in gastric cancer consist of C → T and G → A transitions at the CpG dinucleotide sequence[38,39]. These base-pair changes are typically produced by deamination of 5–methyl-cytosine which is enhanced by ROMs, in particular by nitric oxide (NO)[40,41]. It has been reported that intact *H. pylori*, as well as isolated cellular components, stimulate NO synthesis[42–45].

Human tissues have access to two sources of antioxidants: the endogenous and dietary antioxidants, which may terminate or reduce the toxicity of ROM reaction[46,47]. The endogenous antioxidants are those enzymes, proteins and certain by-products of metabolism, which are synthesized and controlled endogenously; these include superoxide dismutase (SOD), catalases, glutathione peroxidases and tripeptide glutathione (GSH)[48,49]. The dietary antioxidants are those provided in food, such as vitamins C and E and β-carotene. However, the human gastrointestinal mucosa, submucosa, and muscularis/serosa contain much smaller amounts of the endogenous antioxidants than does liver[50,51]. Most of the mucosal enzyme activity is associated with epithelial cells, so the lamina propria is devoid of significant enzymatic defences against ROMs. Therefore, the endogenous antioxidants can be overwhelmed during *H. pylori* infection, resulting in oxidative modification of cellular components. The imbalance between ROMs and antioxidants created by the overproduction of ROMs within the inflamed stomach suggests that dietary antioxidant supplementation may prove important.

There is convincing evidence suggesting the role of dietary antioxidants vitamins C and E and β-carotene in protecting against ROMs. Their antioxidant properties in scavenging free radicals are shown in Table 1. Ascorbic acid and α-tocopherol act as potent, and probably the most important, hydrophilic and lipophilic antioxidants, respectively. They function at their own site individually and furthermore act synergistically. β-Carotene has lower reactivity towards radicals than does α-tocopherol, and acts as a weak antioxidant in solution. It is more lipophilic than α-tocopherol and is assumed to be present at the interior of membranes or lipoproteins, which enables it to scavenge radicals within the lipophilic compartment more efficiently than does α-tocopherol, especially at low oxygen pressure[52].

GASTRIC N-NITROSO COMPOUNDS AND DIETARY ANTIOXIDANTS

Formation of NOCs in the stomach probably constitutes a major source of human exposure to this important class of environmental carcinogens[19,53,54]. Following reduction of nitrate to nitrite by oral or gastric bacteria, nitrite can react with secondary amines and N-substituted amides to form NOCs[19]. Normally this conversion occurs under the acidic conditions (pH ≤ 4) in the stomach, and the nitrosation rate is dependent on nitrite concentration. This may be particularly important in populations with a high dietary nitrate and low dietary antioxidant intake[53,55,56]. The low levels of gastric antioxidants, especially gastric juice ascorbic acid, in these populations, might allow significant increases in NOC formation and contribute to the increased gastric cancer risk. H. pylori infection may not play an important role in acid-catalysed nitrosation, as subjects with duodenal ulcers, in whom H. pylori infection can be assumed, have normal levels of NOCs[57]. Furthermore, at low pH, nitrite can inhibit H. pylori growth[58]. However, at high gastric pH (>4), the production of NOCs is significantly facilitated by bacteria, including H. pylori in the stomach[59]. Under such conditions the reduction of nitrate to nitrite becomes by far the most important source of nitrite exposure, contributing over 90% of the total gastric nitrite load of hypochlorhydric subjects[57]. Bacteria-catalysed nitrosation, associated with increased gastric juice pH, may be more important in areas where H. pylori prevalence is high, resulting in widespread gastric atrophy at an early age, which will lead to increased non-H. pylori bacterial load in the stomach. Another two pathological conditions, in which bacteria-catalysed NOC production may play an important role in the development of gastric cancer, are gastric surgery and pernicious anaemia[60,61]. As shown in Table 1, vitamins C and E and β-carotene can all block the formation of nitrosation in the stomach[20,62,63].

H. PYLORI INFECTION AND GASTRIC VITAMIN C

Vitamin C is an acidic molecule with strong reducing activity, and is an essential component of most living tissues. Due to lack of L-gulonolactone oxidase, a key enzyme for vitamin C synthesis, humans are unable to synthesize vitamin C; therefore, dietary intake is critical for maintaining normal levels of vitamin C[64]. Low intake of foods rich in vitamin C is associated with an increased risk of gastric cancer, and patients with gastric cancer, or subjects from areas with high gastric cancer rates, have significantly lower plasma or serum vitamin C concentrations compared to controls[65,66]. Although H. pylori infection is strongly associated with low socioeconomic status, a factor related to gastric cancer and malnutrition, there is no evidence so far to suggest a close relationship between H. pylori infection and vitamin C intake[67–70]. Webb et al., in a multicentre study, investigated the relationships between plasma levels of vitamin C, as an indicator of vitamin C intake, and gastric cancer in about 1400 individuals from nine centres in seven countries worldwide. They found no association between plasma vitamin C levels and H. pylori infection. However, cigarette smoking and male gender are negatively associated with plasma vitamin C levels[67].

Vitamin C has two major forms: ascorbic acid and dehydroascorbic acid (DHA). Both forms possess vitamin C activity and are interconvertible by redox chemistry[64]. Vitamin C is unevenly distributed in different tissues, with the adrenal gland having the highest ascorbate content and plasma the lowest. All tissues tested so far have significantly higher vitamin C content than plasma[71]. Therefore, it is not surprising that both gastric mucosa and gastric juice contain significantly more vitamin C than plasma[72–74]. The presence of vitamin C in the stomach may play an important role in inhibiting the formation of NOCs and neutralizing ROMs. It is suggested that ascorbic acid is actively secreted into the normal stomach; however, the secretion mechanism is impaired in gastritis, resulting in a significant reduction in gastric juice vitamin C levels[74,75]. The decreased gastric juice vitamin C concentrations return to normal after *H. pylori* eradication, indicating the recovery of vitamin C transport machinery[65].

Gastric juice vitamin C concentration is also influenced by many other factors, including gastric pH and the severity and extent of gastritis. In the presence of hypochlorhydria (pH $\geq$ 4), ascorbic acid is very unstable and oxidized to DHA, or even irreversibly converted to 2,3-diketogulonic acid, leading to the complete loss of vitamin C activity[76]. It has been shown in previous studies that in patients with diffuse antral gastritis, a condition commonly associated with duodenal ulcer, vitamin C levels in gastric juice were normal despite the presence of *H. pylori* and associated inflammation. In contrast, however, patients with pangastritis had significantly lower gastric juice ascorbic acid concentrations compared to those with diffuse antral gastritis[73,77]; this may be due to damage to parietal cells, leading to elevation of gastric pH[78,79]. These findings may shed some light on the mechanisms relating to the paradoxical outcomes of *H. pylori* infection, duodenal ulcer and gastric cancer, which are both strongly related to *H. pylori* infection, but duodenal ulcer disease has been inversely associated with gastric cancer[80]. Furthermore, our previous study also found that patients with diffuse antral gastritis had normal levels of ascorbic acid and DHA in gastric juice. By contrast, patients with precancerous lesions, such as atrophy or intestinal metaplasia, had significantly lower concentrations of both ascorbic acid and DHA[73]. It has been reported that DHA alone, or in combination with hydroxycobalamin (vitamin B_{12}), can greatly inhibit tumour mitotic activity without inhibiting the activity of normal fibroblasts[81]. Therefore, it is possible that patients with duodenal ulcer may still have the protection of both ascorbic acid and DHA, but those with atrophy or intestinal metaplasia lack such protection against gastric cancer.

H. pylori bacterial factors, such as oxidase, may also contribute to the reduction of gastric juice vitamin C concentration[82]. We observed a remarkable reduction of gastric juice vitamin C in patients infected with *cagA*$^+$ *H. pylori* strains[73]. This finding has been recently confirmed by another study[83]. The further reduction in gastric juice vitamin C concentrations may contribute to the increased gastric cancer risk associated with *cagA*$^+$ strain infections[84]. In a recent study Mowat *et al.* examined the effect of pharmacologically induced hypochlorhydria on the gastric juice ascorbate/nitrite ratio in patients with or without *H. pylori* infection. Twenty healthy volunteers (nine positive for *H. pylori* infection) were analysed for nitrite, ascorbic acid, and total vitamin C before and 2 h after ingestion of a nitrate standard salad meal. This was repeated after 4 weeks of treatment with omeprazole, 40 mg daily. They found that nitrate reduced gastric vitamin C levels and that omeprazole further enhanced this reduction in patients with *H. pylori* infection and increased the gastric nitrite levels[85]. This study suggests that treatment with omeprazole may increase gastric cancer risk by increasing gastric concentration of nitrites and decreasing gastric juice vitamin C levels. This may be particularly important in patients with *H. pylori* infection.

H. PYLORI INFECTION AND GASTRIC VITAMIN E

Vitamin E is an essential fat-soluble vitamin that includes eight naturally occurring compounds in two classes designated as tocopherols and tocotrienols which have different biological activities. α-Tocopherol has the greatest biological activity and is the most commonly available form of vitamin E in food[86]. The most widely accepted biological function of vitamin E is its antioxidant property. It is the most effective chain-breaking lipid-soluble antioxidant in biological membranes, where it contributes to membrane stability and prevents carcinogen-induced oxidative damage and protects critical cellular structures by trapping ROMs and reactive products of lipid peroxidation within the biomembranes[87,88]. It can also react with nitrite in the stomach to inhibit nitrosation[20].

Low dietary intake and low plasma or serum levels of α-tocopherol are associated with gastric cancer and premalignant lesions, such as atrophy and intestinal metaplasia[89,90]. Furthermore, supplementation with a combination of α-tocopherol, β-carotene and selenium was shown to reduce the number of deaths from gastric cancer by 21% among 15 000 people living in Linxian County in China[55]. Several studies have reported that *H. pylori* infection has no effect on vitamin E levels in serum or plasma[91–94]. There are as yet no studies to investigate the relationship between vitamin E supplementation and *H. pylori* infection. Our recent study compared serum vitamin E levels in patients infected with *H. pylori* and uninfected controls. However, patients infected with *H. pylori* had significantly lower mucosal α-tocopherol concentrations compared to uninfected patients, though no association was found between gastric juice α-tocopherol concentration and *H. pylori* infection. In addition, mucosal α-tocopherol concentrations decreased stepwise when gastric mucosal histology progressed from normal to chronic gastritis and finally to atrophy and intestinal metaplasia, indicating that, as the *H pylori*-induced gastric histological changes progressed, gastric mucosa gradually lost the protection of vitamin E against oxidative stress and NOC carcinogens[94].

H. PYLORI INFECTION AND GASTRIC β-CAROTENE

There are several hundred carotenoids distributed widely in nature. A few of them (10%) are provitamins with potential vitamin A activity[95].

β-Carotene is the most abundant and is efficiently converted to provitamin A carotenoids in vegetables and fruits[96]. It consists of two molecules of retinal joined at the aldehyde end of their carbon chains. β-Carotene itself and/or a metabolite (e.g. retinoic acid) may play a protective role in preventing both the initiation and promotion of cancer. β-Carotene neutralizes highly active ROMs, which arise from oxidant stresses such as cigarette smoking and inflammation, and from normal cell metabolism. β-Carotene is less potent as an antioxidant than α-tocopherol because β-carotene is less reactive towards peroxyl radicals than α-tocopherol. At higher oxygen pressure, β-carotene forms β-carotene peroxyl radical. Therefore, at lower oxygen pressure, β-carotene has higher antioxidant activity[97]. Some studies have raised the possibility that β-carotene may also possess immuno-enhancing effects in some vulnerable groups of people[98].

Serum levels of β-carotene rise with increased dietary intake[99,100]. Low levels of β-carotene, which reflect low β-carotene intake, have been associated with increased gastric cancer risk[101-103]. Plasma levels of β-carotene, selenium and ascorbic acid were negatively correlated with mortality rates for gastric cancer in an observational study in China[104]. No study has shown the relationship between *H. pylori* infection and β-carotene intake. Although there is no association between *H. pylori* infection and serum or plasma β-carotene levels[92,94], gastric juice β-carotene level is decreased in patients infected with *H. pylori* compared to those uninfected, and patients with gastric atrophy and intestinal metaplasia had markedly decreased mucosal β-carotene levels compared to those without the above abnormalities[94]. Therefore, the anti-carcinogenic effect of β-carotene may be particularly important in developing countries where dietary risk factors and *H. pylori* infection are both common. In these populations, plasma levels of β-carotene may be significantly affected by low intake of fruits and vegetables, which consist of about 80% of β-carotene intake, compared to that in Western populations, where only about 25% of β-carotene intake is from fruits and vegetables[100].

CONCLUSIONS

It is increasingly evident that oxidative stress plays an important role in *H. pylori*-associated carcinogenesis. Inflammation induced by *H. pylori* infection leads to enhanced production of ROMs within the gastric mucosa and gastric lumen by inflammatory cells, such as neutrophils and macrophages and gastric epithelial cells[27]. Bacterial factors may determine the degree of inflammatory responses during the infection. Some strains, such as cytotoxic ($cagA^+/vacA^+$) strains may induce higher grades of inflammation, which is associated with enhanced production of ROMs[105]. The overproduction of ROMs during the infection consumes both endogenous and dietary antioxidants in the stomach, and causes gastric mucosal oxidative stress. This is particularly important in areas where diets contain inadequate antioxidants, as ROMs may then cause DNA damage and gene mutations. Supplementation of dietary antioxidants such as vitamins C and E and β-carotene may neutralize these toxic ROMs.

Gastric pH may play an important role in determining the outcome of the infection. As shown in Figure 1, patients with duodenal ulcer with low

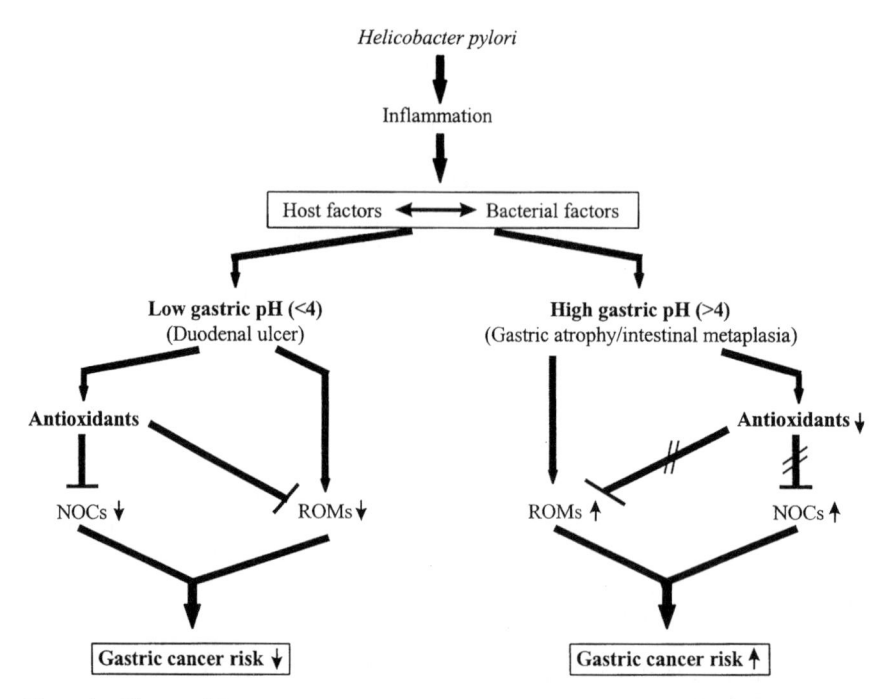

Figure 1. The possible mechanisms relating to the diverse outcomes of *H. pylori* infection, duodenal ulcer and gastric cancer. At low gastric pH (<4) and normal antioxidant levels, the production of NOCs (*N*-nitroso compounds) is inhibited and the ROMs (reactive oxygen metabolites) produced during the infection are neutralized by gastric antioxidants; therefore, the gastric cancer risk is low. However, at high gastric pH (≥4), the production of NOCs is enhanced by gastric bacteria, including *H. pylori*; unfortunately, antioxidant defence is significantly weakened by the long-standing *H. pylori* infection, high gastric pH and the formation of gastric atrophy/intestinal metaplasia. The gastric carcinogens, such as NOCs and ROMs, are both presented in gastric lumen and within gastric mucosa at high concentrations; this would lead to DNA damage and gene mutations; therefore, gastric cancer risk increased. (⊥ inhibited; ⊥̸, inhibition is blocked; ↓, decreased concentration; ↑, increased concentration).

gastric pH (<4) and normal antioxidant levels, the production of NOCs are inhibited and the ROMs produced during the infection are neutralized by gastric antioxidants; in this situation the gastric cancer risk is low. However, in patients with gastric atrophy/intestinal metaplasia with high gastric pH (≥4), the production of NOCs is enhanced by gastric bacteria, including *H. pylori*; unfortunately, antioxidant defence is significantly weakened by the long-standing *H. pylori* infection, high gastric pH and the formation of gastric atrophy/intestinal metaplasia. Therefore, NOCs and ROMs both in the gastric lumen and within gastric mucosa are at high concentrations; this would gradually lead to DNA damage and gastric carcinogenesis[10].

References

1. Whelan SL, Parkin DM, Masuyer E. Trends in cancer incidence and mortality. Lyon: IARC Scientific Publications, 1993.

2. American Cancer Society. Cancer Facts and Figures, 1995.
3. Yang GY, Zhang YC, Liu XD et al. Geographic pathology on the precursors of stomach cancer. J Environ Pathol Toxicol Oncol. 1992;11:339–44.
4. Office of Population Censuses and Surveys. Mortality Statistics by Cause. London: HMSO, 1989.
5. Tominaga S. Trends in cancer mortality, incidence and survival in Japan. Gan To Kagaku Ryoho. 1992;19:1113–20.
6. Farthing MJG. *Helicobacter pylori* infection: an overview. Br Med Bull. 1998;54:1–6.
7. Zhang ZW, Xing Y, Li SQ, Huang ZH. Seroepidemiological investigation of *Helicobacter pylori* infection in a Beijing population (Chinese). Beijing Med. 1992;23:250–2.
8. Anonymous. Schistosomes, liver flukes and *Helicobacter pylori*. IARC Working Group on the Evaluation of Carcinogenic Risks to Humans. Lyon, 7–14 June 1994. IARC Monogr Eval Carcinog Risks Hum. 1994;61:1–241.
9. Watanabe T, Tada M, Nagai H, Sasaki S, Nakao M. *Helicobacter pylori* infection induces gastric cancer in Mongolian gerbils. Gastroenterology. 1998;115:642–8.
10. Zhang ZW, Farthing MJG. Molecular mechanisms of *H. pylori*-associated gastric carcinogenesis.. World J Gastroenterol. 1999;5:369:74.
11. Fearon ER, Vogelstein B. A genetic model for colorectal tumorigenesis. Cell.1990;61:759–67.
12. Correa P, Miller MJ. Carcinogenesis, apoptosis and cell proliferation. Br Med Bull. 1998;54:151–62.
13. Patchett SE, Katelaris PH, Zhang ZW et al. Ornithine decarboxylase activity is a marker of premalignancy in long-standing *Helicobacter pylori* infection. Gut. 1996;39:807–10.
14. Zhang ZW, Patchett SE, Farthing MJG. Effect of *H. pylori* on gastric epithelial cell cycle progression. Gut. 1999;45:A39.
15. Peek RM, Jr, Moss SF, Tham KT et al. *Helicobacter pylori cagA$^+$* strains and dissociation of gastric epithelial cell proliferation from apoptosis. J Natl Cancer Inst. 1997;89:863–8.
16. Cahill RJ, Xia H, Kilgallen C, Beattie S, Hamilton H, O'Morain C. Effect of eradication of *Helicobacter pylori* infection on gastric epithelial cell proliferation. Dig Dis Sci. 1995;40:1627–31.
17. Lynch DA, Mapstone NP, Clarke AM et al. Cell proliferation in *Helicobacter pylori* associated gastritis and the effect of eradication therapy. Gut. 1995;36:346–50.
18. Block G, Patterson B, Subar A. Fruit, vegetables, and cancer prevention: a review of the epidemiological evidence. Nutr Cancer. 1992;18:1–29.
19. Kyrtopoulos SA. *N*-nitroso compound formation in human gastric juice. Cancer Surv. 1989;8:423–42.
20. Mirvish SS. Inhibition by vitamins C and E of *in vivo* nitrosation and vitamin C occurrence in the stomach. Eur J Cancer Prev. 1996;5(Suppl. 1):131–6.
21. Atanasova-Goranova VK, Dimova PI, Pevicharova GT. Effect of food products on endogenous generation of *N*-nitrosamines in rats. Br J Nutr. 1997;78:335–45.
22. Weitberg AB, Corvese D. Effect of vitamin E and beta-carotene on DNA strand breakage induced by tobacco-specific nitrosamines and stimulated human phagocytes. J Exp Clin Cancer Res. 1997;16:11–14.
23. Rock CL, Kusluski RA, Galvez MM, Ethier SP. Carotenoids induce morphological changes in human mammary epithelial cell cultures. Nutr Cancer. 1995;23:319–33.
24. Iftikhar S, Lietz H, Mobarhan S, Frommel TO. *In vitro* beta carotene toxicity for human colon cancer cells. Nutr Cancer. 1996;25:221–30.
25. Lupulescu A. The role of vitamins A, beta-carotene, E and C in cancer cell biology. Int J Vit Nutr Res. 1994;64:3–14.
26. Postaire E, Kouyate D, Rousset G et al. Plasma concentrations of beta-carotene, vitamin A and vitamin E after beta-carotene and vitamin E intake. Biomed Chromatography. 1993;7:136–8.
27. Klebanoff SJ. Oxygen metabolites from phagocytes. In: Gallin JI, Goldstein IM, Snyderman R, editors. New York: Raven Press, 1992;541–88.
28. Teshima S, Tsunawaki S, Rokutan K. *Helicobacter pylori* lipopolysaccharide enhances the expression of NADPH oxidase components in cultured guinea pig gastric mucosal cells. FEBS Lett. 1999;452:243–6.
29. Teshima S, Rokutan K, Nikawa T, Kishi K. Guinea pig gastric mucosal cells produce abundant superoxide anion through an NADPH oxidase-like system. Gastroenterology. 1998;115:1186–96.

30. Davies GR, Simmonds NJ, Stevens TR et al. Helicobacter pylori stimulates antral mucosal reactive oxygen metabolite production in vivo. Gut. 1994;35:179–85.
31. Davies GR, Banatvala N, Collins CE, Sheaff MT, Abdi Y, Clements LR, DS. Relationship between infective load of Helicobacter pylori and reactive oxygen metabolite production in antral mucosa. Scand J Gastroenterol. 1994;29:419–24.
32. Cheeseman KH, Slater TF. An introduction to free radical biochemistry. Br Med Bull. 1993;49:481–93.
33. Farinati F, Della Libera G, Cardin R et al. Gastric antioxidant, nitrites, and mucosal lipoperoxidation in chronic gastritis and Helicobacter pylori infection. J Clin Gastroenterol. 1996;22:275–81.
34. Ranzani GN. Genetic alterations in gastric cancer. Ann Ist Super Sanita. 1996;32:101–10.
35. Hirohashi S, Sugimura T. Genetic alterations in human gastric cancer. Cancer Cells. 1991;3:49–52.
36. Moriya M, Ou C, Bodepudi V, Johnson F, Takeshita M, Grollman AP. Site-specific mutagenesis using a gapped duplex vector: a study of translesion synthesis past 8-oxodeoxyguanosine in E. coli. Mutat Res. 1991;254:281–8.
37. Olinski R, Zastawny T, Budzbon J, Skokowski J, Zegarski W, Dizdaroglu M. DNA base modifications in chromatin of human cancerous tissues. FEBS Lett. 1992;309:193–8.
38. Tsuji S, Tsujii M, Sun WH et al. Helicobacter pylori and gastric carcinogenesis. J Clin Gastroenterol. 1997;25(Suppl. 1):S186–97.
39. Tsuji S, Kawano S, Tsujii M et al. Helicobacter pylori extract stimulates inflammatory nitric oxide production. Cancer Lett. 1996;108:195–200.
40. Maeda H, Akaike T. Nitric oxide and oxygen radicals in infection, inflammation, and cancer. Biochem (Mosc). 1998;63:854–65.
41. Ohshima H, Bartsch H. Chronic infections and inflammatory processes as cancer risk factors: possible role of nitric oxide in carcinogenesis. Mutat Res. 1994;305:253–64.
42. Brzozowski T, Konturek PC, Sliwowski Z et al. Lipopolysaccharide of Helicobacter pylori protects gastric mucosa via generation of nitric oxide. J Physiol Pharmacol. 1997;48:699–717.
43. Shapiro KB, Hotchkiss JH. Induction of nitric oxide synthesis in murine macrophages by Helicobacter pylori. Cancer Lett. 1996;102:49–56.
44. Ambs S, Hussain SP, Harris CC. Interactive effects of nitric oxide and the p53 tumor suppressor gene in carcinogenesis and tumor progression. FASEB J. 1997;11:443–8.
45. Forrester K, Ambs S, Lupold SE et al. Nitric oxide-induced p53 accumulation and regulation of inducible nitric oxide synthase expression by wild-type p53. Proc Natl Acad Sci USA. 1996;93:2442–7.
46. Halliwell B. Oxidation of low-density lipoproteins: questions of initiation, propagation, and the effect of antioxidants. Am J Clin Nutr. 1995;61:670–7S.
47. Dizdaroglu M. Chemistry of free radical damage to DNA nucleoproteins. In: Halliwell B, Aruoma OI, editors. DNA and Free Radicals. Chichester: Ellis Harwood; 1993;19–39.
48. Ogino K, Oka S, Okazaki Y, Takemoto T. Gastric mucosal protection and superoxide dismutase. J Clin Gastroenterol. 1988;10(Suppl. 1):S129–32.
49. Chance B, Sies H, Boveris A. Hydroperoxide metabolism in mammalian organs. Physiol Rev. 1979;59:527–605.
50. Mulder TP, Verspaget HW, Janssens AR, de Bruin PA, Pena AS, Lamers CB. Decrease in two intestinal copper/zinc containing proteins with antioxidant function in inflammatory bowel disease. Gut. 1991;32:1146–50.
51. Grisham MB, MacDermott RP, Deitch EA. Oxidant defense mechanisms in the human colon. Inflammation. 1990;14:669–80.
52. Niki E, Noguchi N, Tsuchihashi H, Gotoh N. Interaction among vitamin C, vitamin E, and beta-carotene. Am J Clin Nutr. 1995;62:1322–6S.
53. You WC, Zhang L, Yang CS et al. Nitrite, N-nitroso compounds, and other analytes in physiological fluids in relation to precancerous gastric lesions. Cancer Epidemiol Biomarkers Prev. 1996;5:47–52.
54. Joossens JV, Hill MJ, Elliott P et al. Dietary salt, nitrate and stomach cancer mortality in 24 countries. European Cancer Prevention (ECP) and the INTERSALT Cooperative Research Group. Int J Epidemiol. 1996;25:494–504.
55. Blot WJ, Li JY, Taylor PR et al. Nutrition intervention trials in Linxian, China: supplementation with specific vitamin/mineral combinations, cancer incidence, and disease-specific mortality in the general population. J Natl Cancer Inst. 1993;85:1483–92.

56. Xu GP, So PJ, Reed PI. Hypothesis on the relationship between gastric cancer and intragastric nitrosation: N-nitrosamines in gastric juice of subjects from a high-risk area for gastric cancer and the inhibition of N-nitrosamine formation by fruit juices. Eur J Cancer Prev. 1993;2:25–36.
57. Eisenbrand G, Adam B, Peter M, Malfertheiner P, Schlag P. Formation of nitrite in gastric juice of patients with various gastric disorders after ingestion of a standard dose of nitrate – a possible risk factor in gastric carcinogenesis. IARC Sci Publ. 1984;963–8.
58. Dykhuizen RS, Fraser A, McKenzie H, Golden M, Leifert C, Benjamin N. *Helicobacter pylori* is killed by nitrite under acidic conditions. Gut. 1998;42:334–7.
59. Ziebarth D, Spiegelhalder B, Bartsch H. N-nitrosation of medicinal drugs catalysed by bacteria from human saliva and gastro-intestinal tract, including *Helicobacter pylori*. Carcinogenesis. 1997;18:383–9.
60. Guadagni S, Walters CL, Smith PL, Verzaro R, Valenti M, Reed PI. N-nitroso compounds in the gastric juice of normal controls, patients with partial gastrectomies, and gastric cancer patients. J Surg Oncol. 1996;63:226–33.
61. Hall CN, Darkin D, Viney N, Cook A, Kirkham JS, Northfield TC. Evaluation of the nitrosamine hypothesis of gastric carcinogenesis in man. IARC Sci Publ. 1987;527–30.
62. Hwang H, Dwyer J, Russell RM. Diet, *Helicobacter pylori* infection, food preservation and gastric cancer risk: are there new roles for preventative factors? Nutr Rev. 1994;52:75–83.
63. Panasenko OM, Briviba K, Klotz LO, Sies H. Oxidative modification and nitration of human low-density lipoproteins by the reaction of hypochlorous acid with nitrite. Arch Biochem Biophys. 1997;343:254–9.
64. Bates CJ. Bioavailability of vitamin C. Eur J Clin Nutr. 1997;51(Suppl. 1):S28–33.
65. Correa P, Malcom G, Schmidt B et al. Review article: Antioxidant micronutrients and gastric cancer. Aliment Pharmacol Ther. 1998;12(Suppl. 1):73–82.
66. Schorah CJ. Ascorbic acid metabolism and cancer in the human stomach. Acta Gastroenterol Belg. 1997;60:217–9.
67. Webb PM, Bates CJ, Palli D, Forman D. Gastric cancer, gastritis and plasma vitamin C: results from an international correlation and cross-sectional study. Eurogast Study Group. Int J Cancer. 1997;73:684–9.
68. Vacchino MN. Poisson regression in mapping cancer mortality. Environ Res. 1999;81:1–17.
69. Stone MA, Patel H, Panja KK, Barnett DB, Mayberry JF. Results of *Helicobacter pylori* screening and eradication in a multi-ethnic community in central England. Eur J Gastroenterol Hepatol. 1998;10:957–62.
70. Boffetta P. Infection with *Helicobacter pylori* and parasites, social class and cancer. IARC Sci Publ. 1997;325–9.
71. Lewin S. Biological activity and potential. In: Lewin S, editor. Vitamin C – Its Molecular Biology and Medical Potential. London: Academic Press; 1976:75–103.
72. Waring AJ, Drake IM, Schorah CJ et al. Ascorbic acid and total vitamin C concentrations in plasma, gastric juice, and gastrointestinal mucosa: effects of gastritis and oral supplementation. Gut. 1996;38:171–6.
73. Zhang ZW, Patchett SE, Perrett D, Katelaris PH, Domizio P, Farthing, MJ. The relation between gastric vitamin C concentrations, mucosal histology, and CagA seropositivity in the human stomach. Gut. 1998;43:322–6.
74. Schorah CJ. The transport of vitamin C and effects of disease. Proc Nutr Soc. 1992;51:189–98.
75. Muto N, Ohta T, Suzuki T, Itoh N, Tanaka K. Evidence for the involvement of a muscarinic receptor in ascorbic acid secretion in the rat stomach. Biochem Pharmacol. 1997;53:553–9.
76. Schorah CJ, Sobala GM, Sanderson M, Collis N, Primrose JN. Gastric juice ascorbic acid: effects of disease and implications for gastric carcinogenesis. Am J Clin Nutr. 1991;53:287–93S.
77. Rood JC, Ruiz B, Fontham ETH et al. *Helicobacter pylori*-associated gastritis and the ascorbic acid concentration in gastric juice. Nutr Cancer. 1994;22:65–72.
78. Tani N, Watanabe Y, Suzuki T et al. Effects of inflammatory cytokines induced by *Helicobacter pylori* infection on aminopyrine accumulation in parietal cells isolated from guinea pigs. Dig Dis Sci. 1999;44:686–90.
79. Calam J. Host mechanisms: are they the key to the various clinical outcomes of *Helicobacter pylori* infection?. Ital J Gastroenterol. 1997;29:375–82.

80. Hansson LE, Nyren O, Hsing AW et al. The risk of stomach cancer in patients with gastric or duodenal ulcer disease. N Engl J Med. 1996;335:242–9.
81. Poydock ME. Effect of combined ascorbic acid and B-12 on survival of mice with implanted Ehrlich carcinoma and L1210 leukemia. Am J Clin Nutr. 1991;54:1261–5S.
82. Odum L, Andersen LP. Investigation of *Helicobacter pylori* ascorbic acid oxidating activity. FEMS Immunol Med Microbiol. 1995;10:289–94.
83. Rokkas T, Liatsos C, Petridou E et al. Relationship of *Helicobacter pylori* CagA$^+$ status to gastric juice vitamin C levels. Eur J Clin Invest. 1999;29:56–62.
84. Rugge M, Busatto G, Cassaro M et al. Patients younger than 40 years with gastric carcinoma: *Helicobacter pylori* genotype and associated gastritis phenotype. Cancer. 1999;85:2506–11.
85. Mowat C, Carswell A, Wirz A, McColl KE. Omeprazole and dietary nitrate independently affect levels of vitamin C and nitrite in gastric juice. Gastroenterology. 1999;116:813–22.
86. Murray RK. *Harper's Biochemistry*. London: Appleton & Lange, 1993.
87. Evstigneeva RP, Volkov IM, Chudinova VV. Vitamin E as a universal antioxidant and stabilizer of biological membranes. Membr Cell Biol. 1998;12:151–72.
88. Sies H, Stahl W. Vitamins E and C, beta-carotene, and other carotenoids as antioxidants. Am J Clin Nutr. 1995;62:1315–21S.
89. Choi MA, Kim BS, Yu R. Serum antioxidative vitamin levels and lipid peroxidation in gastric carcinoma patients. Cancer Lett. 1999;136:89–93.
90. Kumagai Y, Pi JB, Lee S et al. Serum antioxidant vitamins and risk of lung and stomach cancers in Shenyang, China. Cancer Lett. 1998;129:145–9.
91. Phull PS, Price AB, Thorniley MS, Green CJ, Jacyna MR. Vitamin E concentrations in the human stomach and duodenum – correlation with *Helicobacter pylori* infection. Gut. 1996;39:31–5.
92. Sanderson MJ, White KL, Drake IM, Schorah CJ. Vitamin E and carotenoids in gastric biopsies: the relation to plasma concentrations in patients with and without *Helicobacter pylori* gastritis. Am J Clin Nutr. 1997;65:101–6.
93. Varis K, Taylor PR, Sipponen P et al. Gastric cancer and premalignant lesions in atrophic gastritis: a controlled trial on the effect of supplementation with alpha-tocopherol and beta-carotene. Helsinki Gastritis Study Group. Scand J Gastroenterol. 1998;33:294–300.
94. Zhang ZW, Patchett SE, Perrett D, Domizio P, Farthing MJG. Gastric alpha-tocopherol and beta-carotene concentrations in association with *Helicobacter pylori* infection. Eur J Gastroenterol Hepatol. 2000;12:497–503.
95. Krinsky NI, Wang XD, Tang G, Russell RM. Mechanism of carotenoid cleavage to retinoids. Ann N Y Acad Sci. 1993;691:167–76.
96. Wang XD, Tang GW, Fox JG, Krinsky NI, Russell RM. Enzymatic conversion of beta-carotene into beta-apo-carotenals and retinoids by human, monkey, ferret, and rat tissues. Arch Biochem Biophys. 1991;285:8–16.
97. Tsuchihashi H, Kigoshi M, Iwatsuki M, Niki E. Action of beta-carotene as an antioxidant against lipid peroxidation. Arch Biochem Biophys. 1995;323:137–47.
98. van Poppel G, Spanhaak S, Ockhuizen T. Effect of beta-carotene on immunological indexes in healthy male smokers. Am J Clin Nutr. 1993;57:402–7.
99. Yeum KJ, Booth SL, Sadowski JA et al. Human plasma carotenoid response to the ingestion of controlled diets high in fruits and vegetables. Am J Clin Nutr. 1996;64:594–602.
100. Yeum KJ, Ahn SH, Rupp de Paiva SA, Lee-Kim YC, Krinsky NI, Russell, RM. Correlation between carotenoid concentrations in serum and normal breast adipose tissue of women with benign breast tumor or breast cancer. J Nutr. 1998;128:1920–6.
101. Zhang L, Blot WJ, You WC et al. Serum micronutrients in relation to pre-cancerous gastric lesions. Int J Cancer. 1994;56:650–4.
102. Haenszel W, Correa P, Lopez A et al. Serum micronutrient levels in relation to gastric pathology. Int J Cancer. 1985;36:43–8.
103. Stahelin HB, Gey KF, Eichholzer M, Ludin E. Beta-carotene and cancer prevention: the Basel Study. Am J Clin Nutr. 1991;53:265–9S.
104. Kneller RW, Guo WD, Hsing AW et al. Risk factors for stomach cancer in sixty-five Chinese counties. Cancer Epidemiol Biomarkers Prev. 1992;1:113–18.
105. Axon AT. Are all helicobacters equal? Mechanisms of gastroduodenal pathology and their clinical implications. Gut. 1999;45(Suppl. 1):I1–4.
106. Rice-Evans CA. Antioxidant nutrients in protection against coronary heart disease and cancer. Biochemist. 1995;8–11.

56
Gastric markers of pre-malignancy are not reversible

R. M. GENTA and F. FRANCESCHI

INTRODUCTION

In preparing this review we have maintained the title originally assigned but shall not, however, defend such a radical position, particularly in light of evidence slowly percolating into the literature that seems to suggest that not all changes believed to lead to gastric malignancy are irreversible. Therefore, we will discuss the topic from the more moderate viewpoint that, as of today, there is insufficient evidence that cure of *Helicobacter pylori* infection results in the regression or disappearance of the lesions that are commonly referred to as 'pre-malignant changes.'

WHAT ARE PRE-MALIGNANT CHANGES?

A pre-malignant change can be defined as an alteration that occurs in a tissue and has a high likelihood of becoming a malignant tumour. For practical purposes the definition must be adapted to the subjective viewpoint from which such alterations are considered. First, for an alteration to have a predictive value it must be detectable. The detection depends on the sensitivity and reproducibility of the tools available to unmask it: a defect in the cell genome that is not detectable today may become an easy target of investigation tomorrow. Similarly, with the imperfect and limited data available to us, it is impossible to quantify a predictive value that would make a lesion qualify as 'pre-malignant' while another would not. Taking these limitations into account we will consider pre-malignant changes in the stomach as detectable alterations of the gastric mucosa that are generally believed to be necessary precursors for the development of certain types of malignant neoplasms.

When referring to pre-malignant changes in the stomach we can look at lesions that may lead to epithelial tumours, i.e. adenocarcinoma, or those that create the background for the genesis of a *marginal zone lymphoma*, better known among gastroenterologists as mucosa-associated lymphoid tissue (MALT) lymphoma. Since virtually nothing is known on what may predispose to the rare malignant gastric tumours of stromal origin (sarcomas)[1-3], these tumours will not be discussed here.

LYMPHOID FOLLICLES AS PRECURSORS OF GASTRIC MALT LYMPHOMA

The normal gastric mucosa may contain scattered lymphoid aggregates, usually located at the base of the antral or oxyntic mucosa, but lymphoid follicles with germinal centres are absent or extremely rare[4]. *H. pylori* infection promotes the recruitment of plasma cells and lymphocytes, which eventually organize in lymphoid follicles with clearly defined germinal centres and mantle zones. Lymphoid follicles may become highly prominent, and their most peripheral components (B cells) may spill into the gastric epithelium, forming complexes somewhat similar in appearance to the destructive *lymphoepithelial lesions* characteristic of the MALT lymphomas. Induced and sustained by stimuli originating from *H. pylori* antigen-sensitized T cells, monoclonal populations of B cells continuously arise and fall on the mucosal inflammatory scene. In some individuals unknown factors intervene to confer a selective advantage to one of these monoclonal populations, and a lymphoma is born[5-8]. For a certain amount of time, these monoclonal populations seem to subsist and expand in a state that could be defined as *conditional immortality*: their survival depends on the presence of *H. pylori*-sensitized T cells[9]. This is probably the stage at which these lymphomas can be cured by the eradication of *H. pylori*[10-14]. Ultimately, T cell dependence fades and the lymphoid proliferations acquire the independent neoplastic nature that characterizes malignant lymphomas. Most lymphomas of this type remain slow-growing and well differentiated; rarely, some undergo a process of de-differentiation that leads to the formation of large-cell, highly malignant neoplasms, which disseminate to local and distant lymph node stations and eventually to other organs[15].

Without lymphoid follicles, MALT lymphomas do not arise: thus, although primary gastric MALT lymphomas are very rare compared to the number of subjects that are infected with *H. pylori*, lymphoid follicles can be categorized as precursors of this type of lymphoma. Within a few months of the cure of *H. pylori* infection there is a reduction in size and number of the lymphoid follicles from the gastric mucosa; after longer periods, ranging from several months to years, most lymphoid follicles are believed to disappear[4]. Thus, cure of *H. pylori* causes regression of at least one type of premalignant lesion (Figure 1), thereby reducing and possibly eliminating the risk for the development of primary gastric MALT lymphomas.

PRECURSORS OF GASTRIC CANCER AND HOW THEY CAN BE DETECTED

The endoscopic visualization of the gastric mucosa has been until recently exclusively macroscopic. Now incorporating computer-assisted magnification techniques that may revolutionize our approach to the endoscopic

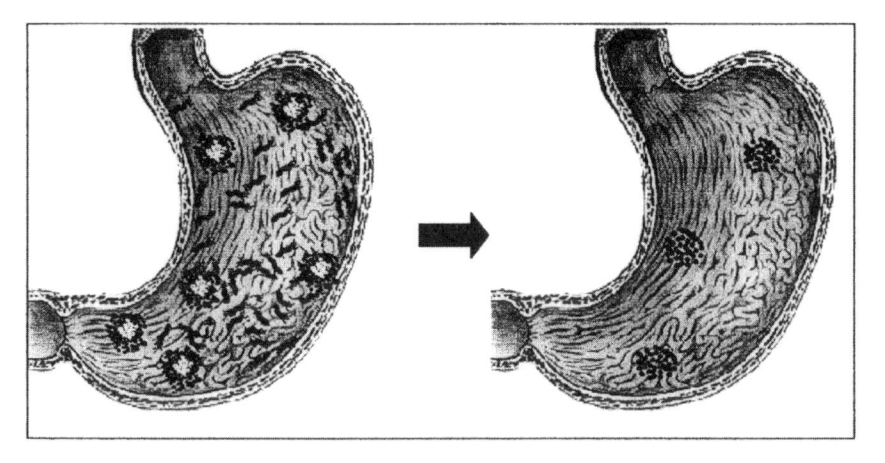

Figure 1. The genesis of primary gastric mucosa-associated lymphoid tissue (MALT) lymphomas depends on the presence of lymphoid follicles in the gastric mucosa. Lymphoid follicles are a universal part of the responses to *H. pylori* infection. The eradication of *H. pylori* results in the slow disappearance of these precursor lesions, eventually reducing or eliminating the risk for MALT lymphoma.

examination, one type of pre-malignant lesion can be detected with certainty: gastric polyps. Even so, since only adenomas are pre-malignant polyps[16], the specificity of this method is low. Furthermore, when polyps are detected there is a presumption of malignancy and they must be removed at endoscopy; thus, it would be unethical to design a study in order to determine the effects of *H. pylori* eradication on the natural course of these lesions.

Other mucosal changes such as atrophy, metaplasia, and dysplasia can be suspected by the endoscopist, but cannot be consistently recognized and assessed quantitatively[17]. Japanese endoscopists have accumulated considerable experience in the use of vital dyes used during gastroscopy to enhance the recognition of intestinal metaplasia, and several studies carried out in Japan have employed the methylene blue-enhanced endoscopic evaluation of intestinal metaplasia as a tool to measure its extension[18,19]. Although a few studies using this technique have been carried out also in North America and Europe[20], this practice has not gained wide acceptance in the West.

The histopathological evaluation of mucosal biopsy specimens has been, and continues to be, the most commonly employed method to evaluate the progression or regression of gastric disease. Histology is universally available, technically easy, and inexpensive. Until studies in various subspecialties of histopathology showed that pathologists, like radiologists and others who interpret images, have a high degree of interobserver variation[21-25], the validity of studies based on the histopathological evaluation of tissues was rarely questioned. However, after atrophy was shown to be one of the features of gastritis on which pathologists agreed the least[26-28], concerns began to arise regarding the comparability of studies performed by different pathologists. In response to the need for standardized and reproducible methods to measure atrophy, intestinal metaplasia and dysplasia in the gastric mucosa, international groups of gastric pathologists have addressed these issues and are currently attempting to validate their conclusions[29-31]. Even if these problems are resolved, and the reproducibility of pathological evaluations is brought to acceptable levels, problems of sampling, reporting (discussed below) and limited sensitivity are likely to continue to pervade histopathological studies.

The approach that may eventually provide the most reliable data on the dynamics of precursors of gastric cancer is the investigation of molecular changes that either precede or are associated with the development of neoplasia[32]. A number of such changes are now detectable by immunohistochemistry, while most changes require PCR-based methods. The advantage of evaluating such markers is that they can be detected in a more objective way (i.e. less observer-dependent) and that they may be part of a generalized field effect, thus reducing sampling-related problems. They may also be more sensitive, since molecular changes are often present before phenotypical alterations become apparent. The performance of these techniques requires more sophisticated equipment, costly reagents, and highly trained skilled personnel. Consequently, their use has so far remained largely confined to laboratories in industrialized nations. With the rapid spread of technology, however, molecular testing is becoming both easier and less expensive, and may soon become accessible to a wider and more diverse spectrum of researchers.

THE AVAILABLE EVIDENCE

A search of the indexed literature and of the abstracts presented at the Digestive Diseases Week in the United States from 1996 to 2000, identified a total of 15 peer-reviewed articles and 10 abstracts that stated either as a primary or a secondary aim the evaluation of the effects of *H. pylori* eradication on the dynamics of gastric atrophy and/or intestinal metaplasia. This is only a review of the most recent available information on this subject: it is necessarily incomplete because it does not include studies that were not presented at the United States DDW, and is not purported to be a formal meta-analysis. Therefore, we shall consider all data, irrespective of the form in which they have been published. Twelve studies were performed in Europe (10 in Western and two in Eastern Europe)[32-43]; eight studies were performed in Japan[44-50], four in the United States[51-54], and one in Australia[55]. A total of 854 patients, ranging in age from 19 to 78 years, were cumulatively evaluated at the conclusion of the studies. Although most publications indicate in the methods that the study design was 'prospective' or that 'patients were prospectively evaluated', many report clinical studies in which patients treated for *H. pylori* infection were re-evaluated at varying intervals and the respective biopsy sets were retrospectively reviewed, usually by a single pathologist in a blinded fashion. Follow-up times vary greatly, both between studies and among subjects within individual studies: they range from a minimum of 2 months[35] to a maximum of 8 years[39]. In virtually all studies the semi-quantitative assessment of atrophy and intestinal metaplasia is based on the guidelines of either the Sydney System[56] or the Updated

Sydney System[57]. Both the number of biopsy specimens evaluated and the sites from which they were obtained were stated in the majority of the studies, although only a few provided clear mapping landmarks. Biopsy protocols ranged from an unspecified number of antral biopsies to 20 mapped sites (eight antrum, eight corpus, four cardia)[53]. The most common type of biopsy protocol consisted of combinations of one or two antral and one or two corpus biopsy specimens[35,38].

Atrophy was evaluated in 20 studies: eight reported improvement, nine failed to detect any improvement or detected a progression, and three found mixed results (for example, while atrophy improved in the antrum, it worsened in the corpus). Intestinal metaplasia was assessed in 18 studies (14 of which also assessed atrophy): none reported a significant improvement of the metaplasia either in the antrum or the corpus; in two studies a possible decrease of the metaplastic areas was detected in the region of the *incisura angularis*.

PROBLEMS WITH THE STUDIES

The high level of discrepancy found between the results of these studies is not surprising, considering the variables involved. Some of the factors that could affect the individual subjects' ability to restore to normality an atrophic or metaplastic mucosa include the population (genetic make-up, diet, environmental elements), the subjects' age (one could expect a lesser ability to regenerate in older people), their condition (simple gastritis or gastric ulcer, or duodenal ulcer) and the infecting *H. pylori* strains. For example, CagA-positive strains may induce more severe inflammation, cause more tissue damage and make regeneration of glands less likely. The repercussions on the results of variables related to the design and execution of the studies may be even greater. Sampling errors, the type of biopsy protocol (or the absence of one), pathologists' inter-observer variation in the evaluation of atrophy and metaplasia, and the scales used to report histopathological changes may have a major influence on the data. A particularly important source of bias lies in the difficulties pathologists often have in separating atrophy from inflammation in the presence of active *H. pylori* infection. These issues are discussed in depth in Chapter 25 in this book. Furthermore, the biological significance of the statistical analysis of the cumulative results of multiple biopsy sites from several subjects has not been established and is far from being clear. For example, when the changes in the score of atrophy are evaluated in 10 patients, each of whom had eight biopsy specimens obtained at time-points A (before treatment) and B (after treatment), respectively, how should the results be calculated? The simplest way (used in many studies) is to average the atrophy scores of the eight biopsy sites in each patient at time-point A and at time-point B; then calculate the average of the 10 averaged scores from each patient, and perform a test (often a Student's t test or a χ^2) to determine the statistical significance of the difference between A and B. Although the final p value may show a value of less than 0.05, and lend an aura of credibility to these numerical manipulations, the biological meaning of such an exercise remains to be

Pre
3+3+0+0
IM grade: 1.5

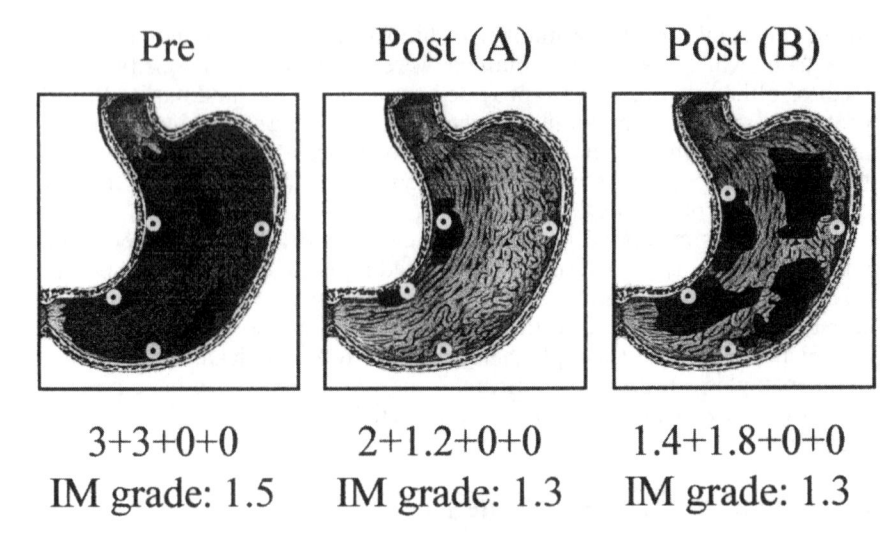

Post (A)
2+1.2+0+0
IM grade: 1.3

Post (B)
1.4+1.8+0+0
IM grade: 1.3

Figure 2. A study based on the averaging of the scores for intestinal metaplasia may yield numerical results that have little to do with what really happens in the stomach. If before treatment the 'average' gastric metaplasia score (on the Sydney System scale from 0 to 3) was 1.5, the same set of biopsy specimens may yield identical values after treatment even if the extension of metaplasia has regressed considerably (scenario A) or increased (scenario B). Today, we are not aware of any methods that could eliminate the sampling bias in this type of study.

established. Another less commonly used method is the averaging of the scores of the same biopsy site from each patient: for example, all biopsy specimens from the *angulus* are averaged, then average scores for time-points A and B are compared. This method can reveal trends that are missed if all specimens from a patient are lumped together in one value. Obviously, it can be applied only when all patients have been sampled following a standardized biopsy protocol, and this is unfortunately not the case in most studies. An example of how this type of study might yield inconsistent results is depicted in Figure 2.

CONCLUSIONS

The results of successful treatment of *H. pylori* infection in a population can be evaluated in terms of: (1) histological changes in the gastric mucosa of each infected subject; for example the effects on inflammation and the progression of lesions known to be precursors of gastric cancer, such as atrophy, intestinal metaplasia, and epithelial dysplasia, or lymphoma, such as lymphoid follicles; (2) benefits to the individual patient such as effects on dyspeptic symptoms, peptic ulcer, gastric lymphoma and gastric cancer risk; and (3) outcomes in the population, including incidence of ulcer, cancer and lymphoma. Studies that use the regression of so-called pre-neoplastic lesions as an end-point are, in our opinion, plagued by virtually insoluble problems and, although their results may point to useful directions for future research,

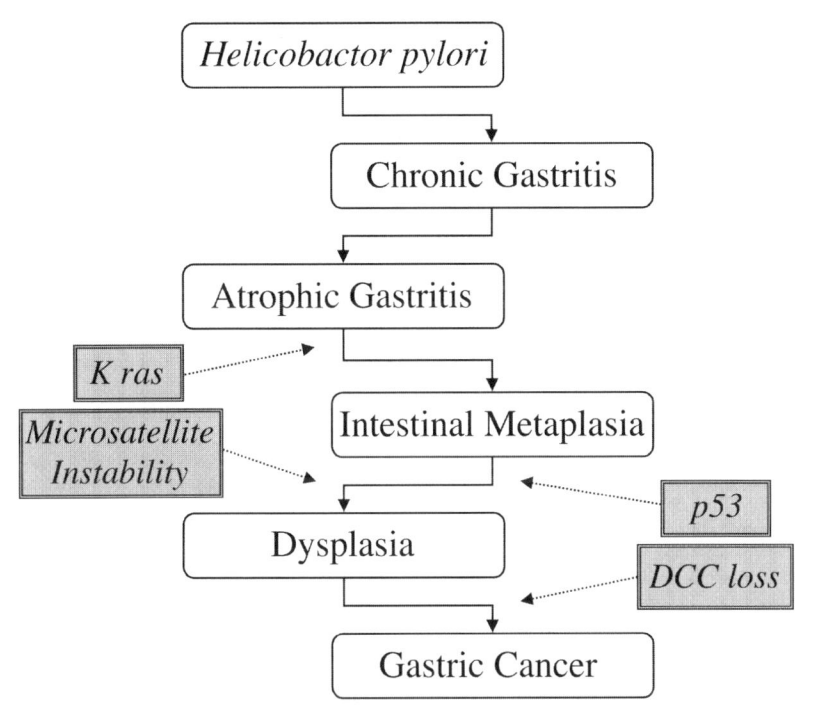

Figure 3. This modified Correa's cascade of gastric carcinogenesis shows some of the genetic changes that have been associated with the early phases of development of gastric adenocarcinoma. Although some studies have shown promising results, we are still a long way from being able to use these markers in clinical or epidemiological practice to predict an individual's or a population's cancer risk.

cannot be incorporated into the current body of indisputable evidence. Studies based on rigorously validated molecular methods to assess for genomic changes may provide useful data (Figure 3).

Very likely, however, only large randomized population-based prospective studies using the incidence of gastric adenocarcinoma as the measurable end-point will provide a body of data upon which evidence-based decisions and guidelines can be generated. Until such data are available, the decision to treat *H. pylori* infection must be based on the possible effects of eradication on other established outcomes.

References

1. Abbas JS, Massad M, Mufarrij A, Saksouk F, Kulaylat M. Gastric leiomyosarcoma: a clinicopathologic study. Int Surg. 1986;71:176–81.
2. Grant CS, Kim CH, Farrugia G, Zinsmeister A, Goellner JR. Gastric leiomyosarcoma. Prognostic factors and surgical management. Arch Surg. 1991;126:985–9.
3. Matsushita M, Hajiro K, Takakuwa H. Where does gastric leiomyosarcoma originate?. Gastrointest Endosc. 1997;46:192–3.

4. Genta RM, Hamner HW, Graham DY. Gastric lymphoid follicles in *Helicobacter pylori* infection: frequency, distribution, and response to triple therapy. Hum Pathol. 1993; 24:577–83.
5. Isaacson PG. Gastric lymphoma and *Helicobacter pylori*. N Engl J Med. 1994;330:1310–11.
6. Isaacson PG. Gastric MALT lymphoma: from concept to cure. Ann Oncol. 1999;10:637–45.
7. Isaacson PG, Spencer J. The biology of low grade MALT lymphoma. J Clin Pathol. 1995;48:395–7.
8. Wotherspoon AC, Ortiz-Hidalgo C, Falzon MR, Isaacson PG. *Helicobacter pylori*-associated gastritis and primary B-cell gastric lymphoma. Lancet. 1991;338:1175–6.
9. Hussell T, Isaacson PG, Crabtree JE, Spencer J. *Helicobacter pylori*-specific tumour-infiltrating T cells provide contact dependent help for the growth of malignant B cells in low-grade gastric lymphoma of mucosa-associated lymphoid tissue. J Pathol. 1996; 178:122–7.
10. Savio A, Franzin G, Wotherspoon AC et al. Diagnosis and posttreatment follow-up of *Helicobacter pylori*-positive gastric lymphoma of mucosa-associated lymphoid tissue: histology, polymerase chain reaction, or both? Blood. 1996;87:1255–60.
11. Wotherspoon AC, Doglioni C, De Boni M, Spencer J, Isaacson PG. Antibiotic treatment for low-grade gastric MALT lymphoma. Lancet. 1994;343:1503.
12. Wotherspoon AC, Doglioni C, Diss TC et al. Regression of primary low-grade B-cell gastric lymphoma of mucosa-associated lymphoid tissue type after eradication of *Helicobacter pylori*. Lancet. 1993;342:575–7.
13. Bayerdorffer E, Neubauer A, Rudolph B et al. Regression of primary gastric lymphoma of mucosa-associated lymphoid tissue type after cure of *Helicobacter pylori* infection. MALT Lymphoma Study Group. Lancet. 1995;345:1591–4.
14. Thiede C, Morgner A, Alpen B et al. What role does *Helicobacter pylori* eradication play in gastric MALT and gastric MALT lymphoma? Gastroenterology. 1997;113:S61–4.
15. Dogusoy G, Karayel FA, Gocener S, Goksel S. Histopathologic features and expression of Bcl-2 and p53 proteins in primary gastric lymphomas. Pathol Oncol Res. 1999;5:36–40.
16. Ho SB. Premalignant lesions of the stomach. Semin Gastrointest Dis. 1996;7:61–73.
17. Laine L, Cohen H, Sloane R, Marin-Sorensen M, Weinstein WM. Interobserver agreement and predictive value of endoscopic findings for *H. pylori* and gastritis in normal volunteers. Gastrointest Endosc. 1995;42:420–3.
18. Suzuki S, Suzuki H, Endo M, Takemoto T, Kondo T. Endoscopic diagnosis of early cancer and intestinal metaplasia of the stomach by dyeing. Int Surg. 1973;58:639–42.
19. Tatsuta M, Okuda S, Taniguchi H, Tamura H. Relation of intestinal metaplasia to the acid-secreting area. Endoscopy. 1979;11:166–71.
20. Morales TG, Bhattacharyya A, Camargo E, Johnson C, Sampliner RE. Methylene blue staining for intestinal metaplasia of the gastric cardia with follow-up for dysplasia. Gastrointest Endosc. 1998;48:26–31.
21. French METAVIR Cooperative Study Group. Intraobserver and interobserver variations in liver biopsy interpretation in patients with chronic hepatitis C. Hepatology. 1994;20:15–20.
22. Robbins P, Pinder S, de Klerk N et al. Histological grading of breast carcinomas: a study of interobserver agreement. Hum Pathol. 1995;26:873–9.
23. Page DL, Dupont WD, Jensen RA, Simpson JF. When and to what end do pathologists agree? J Natl Cancer Inst. 1998;90:88–9.
24. Cross SS. Grading and scoring in histopathology. Histopathology. 1998;33:99–106.
25. Raab SS, Geisinger KR, Silverman JF, Thomas PA, Stanley MW. Interobserver variability of a Papanicolaou smear diagnosis of atypical glandular cells of undetermined significance. Am J Clin Pathol. 1998;110:653–9.
26. Andrew A, Wyatt JI, Dixon MF. Observer variation in the assessment of chronic gastritis according to the Sydney system. Histopathology. 1994;25:317–22.
27. El Zimaity HM, Graham DY, Al Assi MT et al. Interobserver variation in the histopathological assessment of *Helicobacter pylori* gastritis. Hum Pathol. 1996;27:35–41.
28. Genta RM. Review article: Gastric atrophy and atrophic gastritis – nebulous concepts in search of a definition. Aliment Pharmacol Ther. 1998;12(Suppl. 1):17–23.
29. Genta RM. Defining atrophic gastritis and grading gastric atrophy: new challenges beyond the Sydney System. In: Hunt RH, Tytgat GN, editors. *Helicobacter pylori* – Basic Mechanisms to Clinical Cure 1998. Dordrecht: Kluwer; 1998:215–23.

30. Genta RM, Rugge M. Gastric precancerous lesions: heading for an international consensus. Gut. 1999;45(Suppl. 1):15–18.
31. Rugge M, Correa P, Dixon MF et al. Gastric dysplasia: the Padova international classification. Am J Surg Pathol. 2000;24:167–76.
32. Nardone G, Staibano S, Rocco A et al. Effect of *Helicobacter pylori* infection and its eradication on cell proliferation, DNA status, and oncogene expression in patients with chronic gastritis. Gut. 1999;44:789–99.
33. Konturek P, Pierzchalski P, Konturek SJ et al. Improvement of gastric atrophy after eradication of *Helicobacter pylori* is associated with decreased expression for interleukin-1b converting enzyme and increased gene expression for transforming growth factor α. Gastroenterology. 1999;116:G962 (abstract).
34. MacOni G, Lazzaroni M, Sangaletti O, Bargiggia S, Vago L, Porro GB. Effect of *Helicobacter pylori* eradication on gastric histology, serum gastrin and pepsinogen I levels, and gastric emptying in patients with gastric ulcer. Am J Gastroenterol. 1997;92:1844–8.
35. Oberhuber G, Wuendisch T, Rappel S, Stolte M. Significant improvement of atrophy after eradication therapy in atrophic body gastritis. Pathol Res Pract. 1998;194:609–13.
36. Ravizza M, Suriani R, Giacobbe U, Cappelletti F, Dusio P. *Helicobacter pylori* infection and intestinal metaplasia in the stomach: two years follow-up after eradication. Gastroenterology. 1998;114:G1090 (abstract).
37. Savarino V, Mela GS, Zentilin P et al. Histological and functional recovery in patients with multifocal atrophic gastritis after eradication of *Helicobacter pylori* infection. Ital J Gastroenterol Hepatol. 1999;31:4–8.
38. Stolte M, Meining A, Koop H, Seifert E. Eradication of *Helicobacter pylori* heals atrophic corpus gastritis caused by long-term treatment with omeprazole. Virchows Arch. 1999;434:91–4.
39. Tham TC, Sloan JM, Collins JS. Long-term semi-quantitative follow-up of *Helicobacter pylori* associated gastritis. Ir J Med Sci. 1997;166:132–4.
40. Tucci A, Poli L, Tosetti C et al. Reversal of fundic atrophy after eradication of *Helicobacter pylori*. Am J Gastroenterol. 1998;93:1425–31.
41. Van Der Hulst RW, van der EA, Dekker FW et al. Effect of *Helicobacter pylori* eradication on gastritis in relation to cagA: a prospective 1-year follow-up study. Gastroenterology. 1997;113:25–30.
42. Tepes B, Kavcic B, Zaletel LK et al. Two- to four-year histological follow-up of gastric mucosa after *Helicobacter pylori* eradication. J Pathol. 1999;188:24–9.
43. Kyzekova J, Mour J. The effect of eradication therapy on histological changes in the gastric mucosa in patients with non-ulcer dyspepsia and *Helicobacter pylori* infection. Prospective randomized intervention study. Hepatogastroenterology. 1999;46:2048–56.
44. Haruma K, Mihara M, Okamoto E et al. Eradication of *Helicobacter pylori* increases gastric acidity in patients with atrophic gastritis of the corpus – evaluation of 24-h pH monitoring. Aliment Pharmacol Ther. 1999;13:155–62.
45. Iijima K, Ohara S, Sekine H et al. Recovery of gastric acid secretion and mucosal atrophy after *H. pylori* eradication in severe atrophic gastritis. Gastroenterology. 1998;114:G0640 (abstract).
46. Matsukura N, Onda M, Kato S et al. Reversibility of intestinal metaplasia in the stomach after *H. pylori* eradication. Gastroenterology. 1998;114:G0901 (abstract).
47. Satoh K, Kimura K, Kihira K, Takimoto T, Tokumaru K. Change of intestinal metaplasia after *Helicobacter pylori* eradication: assessment according to the Updated Sydney System. Gastroenterology. 1998;114:G1140 (abstract).
48. Sato R, Fujioka T, Murakami K, Kodama M, Kubota T, Nasu M. Cure of *Helicobacter pylori* infection improves gastric atrophy: evaluation by five sites biopsy recommended in the Updated Sydney System. Gastroenterology. 1999;116:G1321 (abstract).
49. Satoh K, Kimura K, Takimoto T, Kihira K. A follow-up study of atrophic gastritis and intestinal metaplasia after eradication of *Helicobacter pylori*. Helicobacter. 1998;3:236–40.
50. Uedo N, Tatsuta M, Hirasawa R, Iishi H, Otani T. Eradication of *Helicobacter pylori* decreases production of interleukin 1-β and extends acid-secreting areas in gastric ulcer patients. Gastroenterology. 1999;116:G537 (abstract).
51. Genta RM, Lew GM, Graham DY. Changes in the gastric mucosa following eradication of *Helicobacter pylori*. Mod Pathol. 1993;6:281–9.

52. Morales TG, Sampliner RE, Garewal HS, Camargo E, Fennerty MB. Does eradication of *H. pylori* reverse gastric intestinal metaplasia? Long-term follow-up utilizing methylene blue staining. Gastroenterology. 1998;114:G2663 (abstract).
53. Sharma P, Topalosvki M, Sampliner RE, Mayo MS, Weston AP. *H. pylori* eradication dramatically improves inflammation in the gastric cardia (carditis). Gastroenterology. 1999;116:G1350 (abstract).
54. Weston AP, Topalosvki M, Cherian R, Dixon A. Prospective 5-year follow-up of gastric intestinal metaplasia following cure of *H. pylori* using an extensive gastric mucosal bioptic mapping protocol. Gastroenterology. 1998;114:G2907 (abstract).
55. Forbes GM, Warren JR, Glaser ME, Cullen DJ, Marshall BJ, Collins BJ. Long-term follow-up of gastric histology after *Helicobacter pylori* eradication. J Gastroenterol Hepatol. 1996;11:670–3.
56. Price AB. The Sydney System: histological division. J Gastroenterol Hepatol. 1991;6:209–22.
57. Dixon MF, Genta RM, Yardley JH, Correa P. Classification and grading of gastritis. The updated Sydney System. International Workshop on the Histopathology of Gastritis, Houston 1994. Am J Surg Pathol. 1996;20:1161–81.

57
The case for the reversibility of gastric dysplasia/neoplasia

R. H. RIDDELL

STAGES OF NEOPLASIA

'Neoplasia' refers to all stages of a process involving:

Initiation – that may or may not be recognizable morphologically.
   Sometimes *hyperplasia* that may include polyp formation in the bowel.
Dysplasia or its equivalent in other tissues.
Invasion.
Metastases.

In the stomach, initiation is complex, and there are probably multiple events, depending not only on the type of tumour (non-neoplastic polyps, adenomas, areas of epithelial dysplasia, mucosa- associated lymphoid tissue [MALT] lymphomas, stromal tumours, etc.), but variants which may occur within each of these. For example, there are not only diffuse and intestinal subtypes of gastric carcinomas, but others including pyloro-cardiac carcinomas, carcinomas of the cardia that may be reflux-associated, and also lymphoepithelial carcinoma that may be associated with Epstein–Barr virus infection.

DEFINITION AND DYNAMICS OF NEOPLASIA

While older definitions of neoplasia involve a concept that this represents 'an uncontrolled proliferation of cells', it increasingly appears that all phases of neoplasia are actually very well controlled at a molecular level. However, the fact that neoplasia occurs at all implies that the control is different from that of normal cells; that is, some clones appear to have a survival advantage over their neighbours and may grow at their expense.

Growth depends on a net excess of new cells formed over cell loss, and may be the result of numerous genetic changes involving:

1. Activation of oncogenes (e.g. myc, ras, etc.).
2. Deletion or inactivation of suppressor genes (e.g. the APC beta-catenin system, p53 and many others).

3. Defective DNA repair.
4. Up-regulation of cell growth as the result of: (a) cell growth factors and receptors that may be autostimulatory; that is, cells may both up-regulate a receptor and secretion of its ligand; (b) mutations in receptors such as c-kit may undergo mutations that enable them to be activated in the absence of ligand; (c) paracrine loops with adjacent cells that may be inflammatory or stromal, in which the loop is formed with adjacent cells in a form of cooperation that is beneficial to both. The desmoplastic reaction of many tumours may enable tumour growth in this way.
5. Gains and deletions of fragments of, or entire, chromosomes resulting in aneuploidy. As such changes progress towards invasion they tend to become closer to diploid.

Further, the whole process of neoplasia must be seen as a dynamic process involving the evolution of numerous cell clones, which compete for survival locally. If they have the opportunity they may find other parts of the body in which they are able to successfully compete with local cells (metastases), should they find that they have a survival advantage there also. These clones not only have survival advantages, but among these must be the ability to evade the host immune system, and also the ability to develop angiogenesis that allows their increased growth. The issue being addressed here is whether this whole process, in its entirety or in part, is reversible, and if so how.

REGRESSION AND FAILURE OF PROGRESSION

Anecdotal reports of either regression or failure to progress are so numerous that everyone is aware of patients who should have died of disease but did not. Some patients are either found to have no evidence of disease that was once extensive, or appear to be living with known tumour but without apparent detrimental effect. Some metastases may be intrinsically slow-growing; for example one patient was found to have a metastasis from a gastric stromal tumour 36 years after the primary was resected[1]. Other tumours, such as large-bowel carcinoid tumours, and gastric carcinoid tumours associated with pernicious anaemia, are also notorious for patients surviving a decade of more with hepatic metastases, while patients with pseudomyxoma peritonei, which is a low-grade surface adenocarcinoma, may also take well over a decade to succumb from disease. Other 'miracles' and unexpectedly long-term survivors are to be found in most cancer series. Thus, patients with stage IV colorectal carcinoma (liver metastases) rarely reach zero, and long-term (25 year) survivors in breast cancer include patients with numerous involved axillary lymph nodes[2].

There are numerous reasons why tumours do not progress. They may reflect a combination of intrinsic slow growth or, in dynamic terms, the rate of cell loss and new cell formation may be similar, but a variety of other host factors including lack of vascularity may be involved. Tumours that have stopped growing may have matured into terminally differentiated cells, although this is frequently the result of therapy, they may have undergone sclerosis or fibrosis, may be necrotic or acellular, including acellular mucin, and mucin may also undergo calcification. Indeed, in the 1960s a pathologist from Yale wrote a detailed book of patients that should have died of their tumour, including the clinical and pathology descriptions[3].

The host response is critical in tumour growth, and there are numerous reports showing an association between the intensity of the inflammatory response – usually within tumours including thymomas (which are usually locally non-aggressive despite their morphology), nasopharyngeal carcinomas, seminoma, medullary carcinoma of the breast, lymphoepithelial carcinoma of the stomach (which is frequently associated with Epstein–Barr virus in the epithelial cells), and typical and lymphoepithelial carcinoma of the large bowel. Both of these may be associated with germline or somatic mutation of mismatch repair genes, and, therefore, hereditary non-polyposis colon cancer (HNPCC) syndrome. Carcinomas from patients with this syndrome have a prominent Crohn's-like reaction, which is associated with a better prognosis stage for stage than colorectal carcinomas without these reactions[4]. Other tumours that are known to undergo spontaneous regression include melanocytic lesions such as halo naevi, malignant melanomas, and keratoacanthomas, which appear to have the same molecular abnormalities as squamous cell carcinomas, to the point that many workers now simply call them squamous cell carcinoma – keratoacanthoma type. It is also of interest that some melanomas and seminomas can undergo regression of the primary lesions, usually resulting in a scar, while metastases from those tumours are growing[5,6].

REVERSIBILITY OF GASTROINTESTINAL NEOPLASIA

In familial adenomatous polyposis there are numerous reports of polyps undergoing regression under different sets of circumstances:

1. Following ileo-rectal anastomosis in the rectal stump.
2. Following therapy with non-steroidal anti-inflammatory drugs (NSAIDs) – especially sulindac[7]. However, the mechanism by which sulindac works may not be a simple NSAID response. Nevertheless, there are considerable data showing that sporadic adenomas/carcinomas[8], and possibly HNPCC-associated tumours[9], are slowed down or prevented by NSAIDs, acting through their COX-2 pathway. It is currently unclear whether this is a delay in the early phase of adenoma formation, failure to grow, or growth at a slower rate, but the whole sequence through invasion seems retarded.
3. There are also direct observational data showing that some adenomas may spontaneously decrease in size. In one study, Hoff and colleagues followed diminutive polyps (< 5 mm) over a 2-year period before removing them. Of those followed, 35 proved to be adenomas. Of these 17 increased in size from a mean of 2.8 to 4.1 mm, but 13 remained unchanged in size and five regressed from a mean of 3.6 to 2.4 mm[10].
4. In ulcerative colitis the possibility that regression of dysplasia may occur is bedevilled by the huge sampling problem, so that dysplasia biopsied on one occasion may not be detected at a subsequent colonoscopy, simply

as a result of sampling error. However, the Seattle group have found that some patients appear to undergo at least temporary remission of both dysplasia and the associated widespread aneuploidy[11].

5. There has been a suggestion that gastric dysplasia, and possibly carcinoma, may be retarded by eradication of *Helicobacter*, and may also be accompanied by regression of the associated atrophy and intestinal metaplasia, although the latter is contentious[12–21].

REVERSIBILITY OF MALT LYMPHOMAS

Gastric MALT lymphoma

It is now well documented that lymphomas of mucosa-associated lymphoid tissue (MALT) in the stomach may undergo partial or complete regression when the stimulus that causes their proliferation is removed – i.e. gastric *Helicobacter* infection is eradicated. Although this occurs classically with low-grade MALT lymphoma, personal examples of partial regression of high-grade lesions have also been observed, and this is also documented[22].

Other interesting observations regarding this infiltrate are that there is invariably an accompanying T-cell infiltrate which may be so extensive that the possibility that the entire lesion may be driven by T-cells must be considered. In addition, these lesions may be specifically strain-dependent.

Immunoproliferative small intestinal lymphoproliferative disease (IPSID)

This lymphoma, usually associated with the production of immunoglobulin alpha heavy chains, also has a low-grade phase early in its evolution that usually responds to simple antibiotic therapy. This is a further example of probable withdrawal of the stimulus causing regression of the malignancy.

SUMMARY

Neoplasia is a very well controlled process, and not the uncontrolled process it is often made out to be. Even in tumours that appear to be highly malignant this is often dependent on feedback loops that drive cell division and that may be autocrine or paracrine. Further, well-documented regression of dysplasia is documented in the gastrointestinal tract under a variety of circumstances, in dysplastic lesions, especially large bowel adenomas. The progress of carcinomas at several sites is modified by the intensity of the inflammatory response. while even metastases may cease growing. All stages of neoplasia are, therefore, potentially reversible. Methods such as microarrays will allow direct comparison with other cells to determine which pathways are activated, and will allow understanding of the mechanisms by which these changes occur. The jump from understanding to generating therapeutic techniques such as specific monoclonal antibodies to block receptor sites is increasingly feasible and is already in practice in some areas of oncology, especially haematopoietic neoplasia. Can the gut be far behind?

References

1. Van Steenbergen W, Kojima T, Geboes K et al. Gastric leiomyoblastoma with metastases to the liver. A 36-year follow-up. Gastroenterol. 1985;89:875–81.
2. Dawson PJ, Karrison T, Ferguson DJ. Histologic features associated with long-term survival in breast cancer. Hum Pathol. 1986;17:1015–21.
3. Cole J, 1963. Yale University Press.
4. Jass JR, Ajioka Y, Allen JP et al. Assessment of invasive growth pattern and lymphocytic infiltration in colorectal cancer. Histopathology. 1996;28:543–8.
5. Elder DE, Murphy GE. Atlas of Tumor Pathology: Melanocytic Lesions of the Skin. Washington, DC: Armed Forces Institute of Pathology; 1991.
6. Mostofi FK, Price EB Jr. Burnt out testicular tumors. In: Tumors of the Male Genital System. Washington, DC: Armed Forces Institute of Pathology; 1973.
7. Stoner, GD, Budd GT, Ganapathi R et al. Sulindac sulfone induced regression of rectal polyps in patients with familial adenomatous polyposis. Adv Exp Med Biol. 1999;470:45–53.
8. Baron JA, Sadler RS. Nonsteroidal antiinflammatory drugs and cancer prevention. Annu Rev Med. 2000;51:511–23.
9. Hawk E, Lubet R, Limburg P. Chemoprevention in hereditary colorectal cancer syndromes. Cancer. 1999;86(Suppl. 1):2551–63.
10. Hoff G, Foerster A, Vatn MH, Sauar, J. Larsen S. Epidemiology of polyps in the rectum and colon. Recovery and evaluation of unresected polyps two years after detection. Scand J Gastroenterol. 1986;21:853–62.
11. Brentnall TA, Haggitt RC, Rabinovtich PS et al. Risk and natural history of colonic neoplasia in patients with primary sclerosing cholangitis and ulcerative colitis. Gastroenterology. 1996;110:331–8.
12. Kyzekova J. Mour J. The effect of eradication therapy on histological changes in the gastric mucosa in patients with non-ulcer dyspepsia and *Helicobacter pylori* infection. Prospective randomized intervention study. Hepatogastroenterology. 1999;46:2048–56.
13. Hsu PI, Lai KH, Tseng HH et al. Impact of *Helicobacter pylori* eradication on the development of MALT, gland atrophy and intestinal metaplasia of the antrum. Chung Hua I Hsueh Tsa Chih (Taipei). 2000;63:279–87.
14. Satoh, K, Kimura K, Takimoto T, Kihira K. A follow-up study of atrophic gastritis and intestinal metaplasia after eradication of *Helicobacter pylori*.
15. Ciok J, Dzieniszewski J, Lucer C. *Helicobacter pylori* eradication and antral intestinal metaplasia – two years follow-up study. J Physiol Pharmacol. 1997;48(Suppl. 4):115–22.
16. Forbes GM, Warren JR, Glaser ME, Cullen DJ, Marshall BJ, Collins BJ. J Gastroenterol Hepatol. 1996;11:670–3.
17. Tham TC, Sloan JM, Collins JS. Long-term semi-quantitative follow-up of *Helicobacter pylori*-associated gastritis. Ir J Med Sci. 1997;166:132–4.
18. Tepes B, Kavcic B, Zaletel LK et al. Two- to four-year histological follow-up of gastric mucosa after *Helicobacter pylori* eradication. J Pathol. 1999;188:24–9.
19. Annibale B, Aprile MR, D'Ambra G, Caruana P, Bordi C, Fave GD. Cure of *Helicobacter pylori* infection in atrophic body gastritis patients does not improve mucosal atrophy but reduces hypergastrinemia and its related effects on body ECL-cell hyperplasia. Aliment Pharmacol. Ther. 2000;14:625–34.
20. Tucci A, Poli L, Tosetti C et al. Reversals of fundic atrophy after eradication of *Helicobacter pylori*. Am J Gastroenterol. 1998;93:1425–31.
21. Uemura N, Mukai T, Okamoto S et al. Effect of *Helicobacter pylori* eradication on subsequent development of cancer after endoscopic resection of early gastric cancer. Cancer Epidemiol Biomarkers Prev. 1997;6:639–42.
22. Morgner A, Miehlke S, Fischbach W et al. Complete remission of gastric high-grade B-cell MALT lymphoma after cure of *Helicobacter pylori* infection. Gastroenterology. 2000;118:A761.

58
Evaluation of the long-term outcome of *Helicobacter pylori*-related gastric mucosa-associated lymphoid tissue (MALT) lymphoma

M. STOLTE, A. MORGNER, B. ALPEN, Th. WÜNDISCH, C. THIEDE, A. NEUBAUEN and E. BAYERDÖRFFER

INTRODUCTION

On taking note, in 1992, of the very surprising finding of complete regression of low-grade mucosa-associated lymphoid tissue (MALT) lymphomas in patients receiving only *Helicobacter pylori* eradication treatment, and after confirmation of this finding by Wotherspoon et al.[1], in 1993 we in Germany initiated the MALT lymphoma study, which we concluded after we had entered 120 patients, who remain under continuing surveillance.

PATIENTS AND METHODS

To this study we admitted only patients with a histologically unequivocal diagnosis of MALT lymphoma, with replacement of the glands by the lymphoma and lymphoepithelial destruction. (Immunohistochemical methods: cytokeratin antibody, CD 20-, CD 3- and Ki 67-antibodies.) We also adhered for the most part to the recommendation of Isaacson and Norton that MALT lymphoma should be diagnosed only when the endoscopic findings are compatible with MALT lymphoma[2]. Endoscopy and biopsy follow-up examinations were performed after *H. pylori* eradication, initially at intervals of 2 months and then, after achieving remission, at intervals of 6 months (for further details see refs 3–5). In patients with partial remission, and in those showing no changes to their tumours, surgical treatment, radiotherapy or chemotherapy was recommended.

Table 1. Own results of treatment of gastric MALT lymphoma with *H. pylori* eradication ($n = 120$; median follow-up: 37.5 months (2.4–73.5))

	No.	Percentage
Complete remission	97	81
Partial remission	11	9
Non-responder	12	10

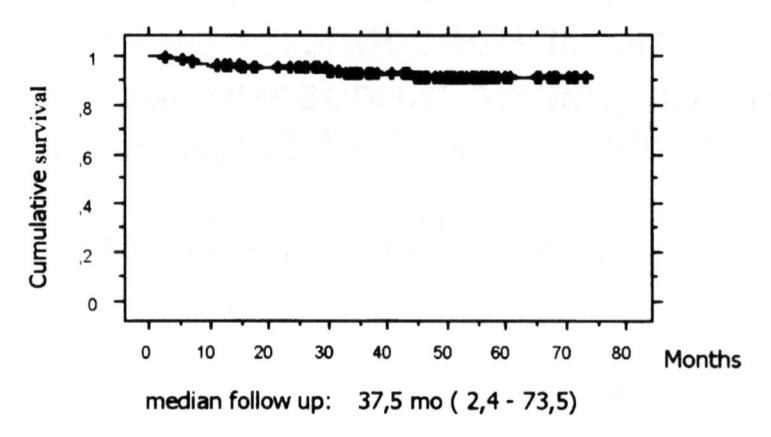

Figure 1. Kaplan–Meier analysis of the cumulative survival in 120 patients with gastric MALT lymphoma followed after eradication of *H. pylori*.

RESULTS

The median follow-up period in our 120 patients is now 37.5 months. Table 1 shows the results of eradication treatment: 81% complete remission, 9% partial remission, and 10% non-responders.

Figure 1 shows the results of the survival analysis of all our 120 patients, and Figure 2 shows the results of the event-free survival analysis of the 97 patients with continuing complete remission. Of the 12 patients with no change in the tumour, two have died of their lymphoma, and nine have been operated on. The work-up of the surgical specimens revealed a T-cell lymphoma, five secondary high-grade lymphomas and three low-grade lymphomas. Two patients received chemotherapy. Of the 11 patients with partial remission, one has died of a stroke, six have been operated, two received chemotherapy, and the remaining two have stable disease with no progression, and are still under surveillance only. The histological examination of the 15 surgical specimens shows the uncertainty of biopsy-based regression diagnosis: in cases with regression of the lymphoma in the plane of the mucosa, we found residual lymphoma in the deeper layers of the wall. Even when areas of lymphoma are found in the mucosa in the surgical specimen, the histological diagnosis of the lymphoma nevertheless remains uncertain; for in all 15 surgical specimens we have failed to detect the most important

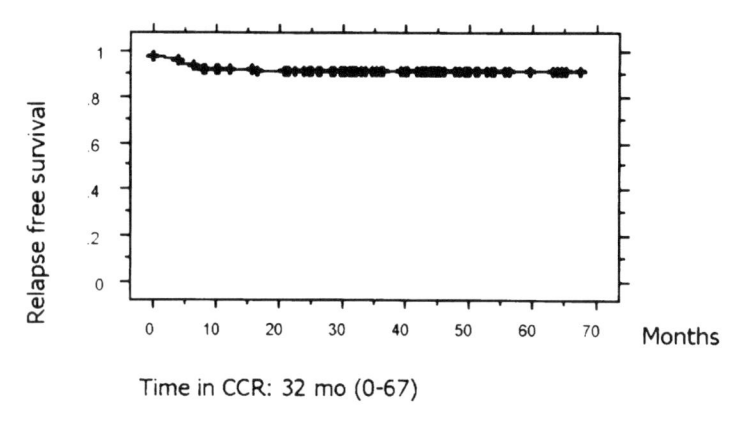

Figure 2. Kaplan–Meier analysis of the relapse-free survival in 97 patients with continuing complete remission of the gastric MALT lymphoma.

criterion for the diagnosis of MALT lymphoma, lymphoepithelial lesions, following *H. pylori* eradication.

Is it possible, on the basis of endoscopic appearance, to identify the individual patient in whom complete remission may be expected to follow *H. pylori* eradication? The answer is definitely 'No!' Only in one of our patients was the endoscopic picture normal; all the others presented with tumours, ulcers, erosions or an atypical mucosa. On the basis of endoscopic appearance it is not possible to predict whether *H. pylori* eradication will result in remission of the tumour in any given patient. Nor does the diameter of the tumour provide any clues as to its remission behaviour. The patient, a woman, with the largest tumour having a diameter of 10 cm, has now been in complete remission for 6 years after *H. pylori* eradication. This is in contrast to the depth of infiltration; only in the case of early lymphomas with infiltration of the mucosa and submucosa can complete remission be expected.

This is why endoscopic ultrasonography is of great importance in pretreatment staging, for only those lymphomas with infiltration of the mucosa and submucosa regress following *H. pylori* eradication treatment. We have never seen complete remission of lymphomas infiltrating the muscularis propria and serosa[6].

Endoscopic ultrasonography is also mandatory during follow-up examination, since our earlier studies have shown that, even in the case of early lymphomas, positive perigastric lymph nodes are present in 17.1% of cases[7]. However, in our study no perigastric lymph node recurrence has occurred to date.

We are, of course, also aware of the possible danger that, following *H. pylori* eradication, the lymphoma might be cleared only from the mucosa, while continuing to grow in the submucosa. We can thus see that assessment of the results of treatment on the basis of histological examination of a biopsy of the mucosa is unreliable.

Table 2. Results of the polymerase chain reaction (PCR) performed on the VDJ rearrangements of the immunoglobulin heavy chain prior to *H. pylori* eradication and during follow-up after complete remission of the gastric MALT lymphoma

	PCR results	
	Prior to H. pylori *eradication*	*After complete remission*
Patients	97	76
Sufficient material	90	44
Monoclonality at diagnosis	64 (71%)	20

POLYMERASE CHAIN REACTION (PCR) RESULTS

Can PCR help us out of this dilemma? So far, unfortunately, no. Already at the primary lymphoma diagnosis, prior to treatment, the PCR was positive in only 71% of cases, making it unreliable in 30% of cases. On the other hand, the PCR remains positive in 45% of cases, even in those patients with endoscopic, endosonographic and histologically diagnosed complete remission (see Table 2).

Where do the monoclonal B cells demonstrated by PCR in patients with regression of the lamina propria come from? Are the basal lymphatic aggregates, often found in addition to the signs of regression, reactive, or are they remnants of the original lymphoma? In order to answer this question we carried out PCR studies following the microdissection of superficial areas of the mucosa and basal lymphatic aggregates. It was found that the source of the monoclonal B cells is mainly located in the basal lymphatic aggregates. Further sequencing showed that the monoclonal B cells were the same as those found at the original diagnosis. Also, on dissection of superficial chronic inflammatory infiltrates we have found monoclonal bands, although only in isolated cases. The sequencing of these cells, however, was not identical with the primary clone of the lymphoma. Future examination of these patients will show whether these monoclonal cells can lead to a recurrence, and whether this can occur only after reinfection with *H. pylori*, or also in *H. pylori*-negative patients.

LONG-TERM RESULTS OF PATIENTS WITH COMPLETE REMISSION

Let us now return to the follow-up results in our 97 patients with complete remission. Sixty-four patients have exceeded the follow-up period of 3 years; 93.8% of these patients had a complete remission, and 3.1% each had partial remission or no change. The median period to complete remission was 151 days. Recurrences occurred in 10% of patients, on average 343 days after remission (see Table 3). Eleven patients have exceeded the 5-year follow-up mark; 10 of these achieved complete remission a mean of 152 days after *H. pylori* eradication. One of these patients experienced a recurrence 128 days after complete remission (see Table 4). Of the 97 patients with complete remission of the lymphoma, four have died in the meantime. The causes of death were stroke, myocardial infarction and arterial embolism.

Table 3. Long-term results of patients with a follow-up period of more than 3 years

Patients	64
Complete remission	93.8%
Partial remission	3.1%
No change	3.1%
Time until complete remission	151 days (45–777)
Recurrences	6 (10%)

Table 4. Long-term results of patients with a follow-up period of more than 5 years

Patients	11
Complete remission	90.9%
No change	9.1%
Time until complete remission	162 days (60–458)
Recurrences	1 (10%)

RECURRENCES

In our study we have so far diagnosed nine recurrences, including one high-grade lymphoma in the nose, and eight local recurrent lesions, one following reinfection with *H. pylori*, and five that occurred in the absence of *H. pylori* reinfection. In the case of the patient with *H. pylori* reinfection, *H. pylori* eradication therapy again resulted in complete remission of the lymphoma. In the other five patients the endoscopic appearance remained normal, and the subsequent histological examinations failed to reveal any lymphoma. With regard to the evaluation of remission and recurrence we are thus faced with the risk of sampling error. This can be well demonstrated in one of our patients with partial remission who underwent gastrectomy 22 months after the initial diagnosis. In the grossly unremarkable stomach the histological large-area sections showed multiple microscopically small foci of lymphoma.

The results of further follow-up examinations will have to determine whether the histological finding of a tiny focus of lymphoma and/or positive PCR following endoscopic complete remission of lymphoma has any significance at all, whether any of these cases can be classified as 'stable disease', or whether these cells may still give rise to a recurrence.

RESULTS FROM THE LITERATURE

In reviewing the literature and summarizing the results of treatment of low-grade MALT lymphoma with *H. pylori* eradication (refs 8–17 and B. Dragosics, personal communication), we find early complete remission rates of between 60% and 93% (see Table 5). On conclusion of our first study we recruited our patients to the second German MALT lymphoma study. In this study, too, after a follow-up period of 3–69 months, the preliminary results are similarly good (see Table 6). Similar results showing

Table 5. Data on complete remission inductions in low-grade gastric MALT lymphomas after *H. pylori* eradication

First author	Year	Number of patients	Complete remission (%)
Stolte	1992	16	60
Wotherspoon	1993	6	83
Bayerdörffer	1995	33	69
Savio	1995	12	92
Roggero	1995	26	60
Fischbach	1996	15	93
Montalban	1997	9	89
Pinotti*	1997	49	67
Neubauer†	1997	50	80
Nobre-Leitao†	1998	17	100
Thiede	2000	84	81
Dragosics	2000	19	84
Stolte†	2000	120	81

*Follow-up study by Roggero et al.[11].
†Follow-up studies by Bayerdörffer et al.[9].

Table 6. Preliminary results of a second German gastric MALT lymphoma study (Fischbach, personal communication)

Patients	83
Follow-up	3–69 months
Complete remission	62%
Partial remission	13%
No change	11%
In surveillance	14%

Table 7. Results of treatment of low-grade gastric MALT lymphoma with *H. pylori* eradication in Japan

First author	Year	Number of patients	Complete remission (%)
Kato	1999	19	84
Nakamura	1999	37	35
Suzuki	1999	16	88
Oda	1999	30	50
Yamashita	1999	25	64
Suekane	1999	22	68

complete remission in 35–84% of patients have also been published in Japan (see Table 7[18–23]).

It remains to be noted that, in the case of *H. heilmannii* gastritis, in comparison with *H. pylori* gastritis, more MALT lymphomas apparently occur. In our material, collected over the past 10 years. The figures were 1.47% compared with 0.66%, respectively (see Table 8), and that these lymphomas too can be cured by eradication therapy[24].

Even in individual cases of high-grade MALT lymphoma, *H. pylori* eradication can lead to complete regression of the tumour (see Table 9)[25].

Table 8. Frequency of gastric MALT lymphoma in patients with *H. pylori* gastritis and in patients with *H. heilmannii* gastritis (own material 1988–98)

	No. of patients	No. of gastric MALT lymphomas
H. pylori gastritis	163 680	1745 (0.66%)
H. heilmannii gastritis	543	8 (1.47%)

Table 9. Regression of high-grade gastric MALT lymphoma after *H. pylori* eradication

First author	Year	No. of patients
Kolve	1997	3
Tiemann*	1997	2
Ng	2000	1
Own material*	2000	9

*Not published.

CONCLUSION

In conclusion, our study confirms that *H. pylori* and *H. heilmannii* gastritis is a pre-MALT lymphoma condition, and that eradication therapy results in complete remission in 80% of cases, but that some 5% relapses per year must be expected. The question as to how often high-grade lymphomas can remit completely by *H. pylori* eradication treatments remains to be determined. The diagnosis of complete remission, however, is uncertain, as is demonstrated in particular by the findings of monoclonal PCR in 45% of these patients. These monoclonal B cells derive from the basal lymphatic aggregates.

Further follow-up investigations will need to show the significance of this B cell monoclonality. Are we dealing here with a non-proliferative, stable disease? Is further regression over the course of time to be expected, or is there a danger of relapse? We hope that, during the course of our further investigations over the next few years, we shall be able to provide answers to these questions.

References

1. Wotherspoon AC, Doglioni C, Diss TC et al. Regression of primary low-grade B-cell lymphoma of mucosa associated lymphoid tissue type after eradication of *Helicobacter pylori*. Lancet. 1993;342:575–7.
2. Isaacson PG, Norton AJ. Extranodal Lymphomas. Edinburgh: Churchill Livingstone, 1994.
3. Stolte M, Eidt S, Bayerdörffer E, Fischer R. *H. pylori*-associated gastric lymphoma. In: Hunt RH, Tytgat GNJ, editors. *Helicobacter pylori*: Basic Mechanisms to Clinical Cure. Dordrecht: Kluwer; 1995:498–503.
4. Stolte M, Morgner A, Meining A et al. Clinical presentation, diagnosis, and treatment of *Helicobacter pylori*-related gastric lymphoma. In: Hunt RH, Tytgat GNJ, editors. *Helicobacter pylori*: Basic Mechanisms to Clinical Cure. Dordrecht: Kluwer; 1996:222–31.
5. Stolte M, Morgner A, Meining A et al. Early and long-term results of *Helicobacter pylori* cure of MALT lymphoma – what are the pitfalls? In: Hunt RH, Tytgat GNJ, editors. *Helicobacter pylori*: Basic Mechanisms to Clinical Cure. Dordrecht: Kluwer; 1998:373–80.

6. Sackmann M, Morgner A, Rudolph B et al. Regression of gastric MALT lymphoma after eradication of *Helicobacter pylori* is predicted by endosonographic staging. MALT Lymphoma Study Group. Gastroenterology. 1997;113:1087–90.
7. Eidt E, Stolte M, Fischer R. Factors influencing lymph node infiltration in primary gastric malignant lymphoma of the mucosa associated tissue. Pathol Res Pract. 1994;190:1077–81.
8. Stolte M. *Helicobacter pylori* gastritis and gastric MALT-lymphoma. Lancet. 1992; 339:745–6.
9. Bayerdörffer E, Neubauer A, Rudolph B et al. Regression of primary gastric lymphoma of mucosa-associated lymphoid tissue type after cure of *Helicobacter pylori* infection. MALT Lymphoma Study Group. Lancet. 1995;345:1591–4.
10. Savio A, Franzin G, Wotherspoon AC et al. Diagnosis and posttreatment follow-up of *Helicobacter pylori*-positive gastric lymphoma of mucosa-associated lymphoid tissue; histology, polymerase chain reaction, or both? Blood. 1996;87:1255–60.
11. Roggero E, Zucca E, Pinotti G et al. Eradication of *Helicobacter pylori* infection in primary low-grade gastric lymphoma of mucosa-associated lymphoid tissue. Ann Intern Med. 1995;122:767–9.
12. Fischbach W, Kolve ME, Engemann R, Greiner A, Stolte M. Unexpected success of *Helicobacter pylori* eradication in low-grade lymphoma. Gastroenterology. 1996;110:A512.
13. Mantalban C, Manzanal A, Boixeda D et al. *Helicobacter pylori* eradication for the treatment of low-grade gastric MALT lymphoma: follow-up together with sequential molecular studies. Ann Oncol. 1997;8(Suppl. 2):37–9.
14. Pinotti G, Zucca E, Roggero E et al. Clinical features, treatment and outcome in a series of 93 patients with low-grade gastric MALT lymphoma. Leuk Lymphoma. 1997;26:527–37.
15. Neubauer A, Thiede C, Morgner A et al. Cure of *Helicobacter pylori* infection and duration of remission of low-grade gastric mucosa-associated lymphoid tissue lymphoma. J Natl Cancer Inst. 1997;89:1350–5.
16. Nobre-Leitao C, Lage P, Cravo M et al. Treatment of gastric MALT lymphoma by *Helicobacter pylori* eradication: a study controlled by endoscopic ultrasonography: Am J Gastroenterol. 1998;93:732–6.
17. Thiede C, Wündisch T, Neubauer B et al. Eradication of *Helicobacter pylori* and stability of emissions in low-grade gastric B-cell lymphomas of the mucosa-associated lymphoid tissue: results of an ongoing multicenter trial. Rec Res Cancer Res. 2000;156:125–33.
18. Kato T et al. Regression of gastric low-grade MALT lymphoma after eradication of *Helicobacter pylori*. Stomach Intest. 1999;34:1345–52.
19. Nakamura T et al. The changes of the endoscopic, roentgenographic and pathological findings of gastric MALT lymphoma after cure of *H. pylori* infection. Stomach Intest. 1999;34:1353–66.
20. Suzuki T et al. Clinicopathological features of MALT lymphoma. Stomach Intest. 1999;34:1367–79.
21. Oda I et al. Endoscopic evaluation of *Helicobacter pylori* eradication. Stomach Intest. 1999;34:1381–8.
22. Yamashita H et al. Histological features of low-grade MALT lymphoma showing complete regression after *Helicobacter pylori* eradication and prediction time of its effectiveness – the value of clinical typing based on endosonographic findings. Stomach Intest. 1999; 34:1389–96.
23. Suekane H et al. Clinical course and practical guideline after eradication of *Helicobacter pylori* – the value of clinical typing based on endosonographic findings. Stomach Intest. 1999;34:1397–409.
24. Morgner A, Lehn N, Andersen LP et al. *Helicobacter heilmannii*-associated primary gastric low-grade MALT lymphoma: complete remission after curing the infection. Gastroenterology. 2000;118:821–8.
25. Ng WW, Lam CP, Chau WK et al. Regression of high-grade gastric mucosa associated lymphoid tissue lymphoma with Helicobacter pylori after triple antibiotic therapy. Gastrointest Endosc. 2000;51:93–6.

Section XI
Treatment of *Helicobacter pylori* Infection

59
Current state-of-the-art management for *Helicobacter pylori* infection: global perspective

D. A. PEURA

INTRODUCTION

Helicobacter pylori infects more than half the population of the world. Most are unaware that they are even infected. They remain asymptomatic throughout life and survive without any harmful infection-related clinical sequelae. However, some develop duodenal or gastric ulcers, and a small proportion MALT lymphoma or gastric cancer. Yet others suffer from non-specific dyspeptic symptoms with no obvious cause found other than *H. pylori* infection and its associated gastritis.

Cure of infection cures most ulcer disease[1] and MALT lymphoma[2] (when superficial and of low grade), thereby averting the morbidity and mortality associated with disease recurrence and complications. While *H. pylori* eradication prevents some early gastric cancers in high-risk patients (those having undergone prior successful endoscopic resection of early gastric cancers)[3], the effect of screening and testing the general population to obviate future stomach cancer remains to be determined. Clinical results obtained when treating infection in those that have non-specific symptoms, especially if diagnostic studies are normal, are inconsistent and unpredictable.[4] Recent data imply that, in certain situations, *H. pylori* may modulate gastric physiology and clinical outcome in a direction favourable to the infected host[5,6]. The long-term implications of such positive interactions remain controversial at best, and their clinical significance remains unproven.

Global elimination of *H. pylori* is a noble goal that would have a major impact on present and future world health. While noble, some question if this goal is appropriate, since infection remains at a symbiotic stage in most and, as previously noted, may actually benefit some. While such controversy is interesting, it is irrelevant, since a goal of total elimination of *H. pylori* infection remains logistically as well as economically unrealistic. Primary prevention of infection may eventually be feasible when effective vaccines become available but, until then, diagnostic and treatment recommendations will target those most likely to benefit. Such specific management recommendations are based on a number of factors, many of which vary throughout the world. The prevalence and seriousness of *H. pylori*-related disease, and the likelihood of altering its clinical course, guide diagnostic and treatment decisions. Cost, accuracy and availability of the various diagnostic options, and the necessity to establish a clinical diagnosis as well as confirm *H. pylori* infection, are practical issues which determine what test is most appropriate. The likelihood of antibiotic-resistant organisms, availability and cost of medications, and possibly clinical indication or bacterial strain (eradication of infection may be more successful in those with certain clinical conditions[7] or in those infected with specific bacterial strains[8]), influence choice of treatment regimen and duration of therapy.

Given different treatment indications, and the demographic and socio-economic diversities of the patient populations being treated, state-of-the-art management of *H. pylori* varies somewhat worldwide. Nevertheless, from a global perspective, fundamentals of management are quite similar, no matter where it is provided. Testing and treatment are offered to those most likely to benefit. Diagnostic tests need to be accurate, cost-effective and provide necessary clinical information. The ideal therapy must be effective, simple, well tolerated with few side-effects. The presence of antibiotic-resistant organisms should have minimal impact on the success of the first-line treatment regimen, and when unsuccessful, treatment should minimize development of secondary antibiotic resistance that could confound subsequent therapy. Treatment duration and drug dosage should be sufficient to guarantee maximal efficacy. This is especially important since the 'true cost' of managing *H. pylori* infection is related to the consequences of failed eradication rather than the direct expense of the treatment pharmaceuticals. Working parties from the United States, Canada, Europe and the Asian Pacific region developed guidelines intended to assist physicians within the respective regions to appropriately manage *H. pylori* infection. Management guidelines were generally based on published clinical evidence and/or accepted expert opinion. Regional practices and clinical experience also guided recommendations.

UNITED STATES MANAGEMENT GUIDELINES

The National Institutes of Health Consensus Development Conference was the first to propose generalized *H. pylori* management guidelines[9]. The Panel concluded that *H. pylori* testing and treatment should be reserved for individuals with active or past history of duodenal ulcer. While data were available for gastric ulcer, complicated ulcers, dyspepsia and cancer, the consensus reached was that such data were insufficient to recommend routine testing and treatment.

The NIH Guidelines were updated in 1997, at the time of the American Digestive Health Foundation's International *H. pylori* Update Conference[10]. Consensus recommendations reinforce the treatment of patients with past

Table 1. United States guidelines for management of *H. pylori*

Active or past ulcer	Yes	Test only if Rx planned
MALT lymphoma	Yes	Treated when test positive
Gastric cancer	No	Use effective Rx
Asymptomatic persons	No	F/U testing limited
GERD/long-term PPIs		
NUD	No	
Dyspepsia	No	
NSAIDs alone	NS	

or active duodenal ulcer but expanded testing and treatment recommendations to those with gastric ulcer, complicated ulcer disease, MALT lymphoma and early gastric cancer. The Update statement further confirmed that data were lacking to advise population screening to prevent gastric cancer, but did suggest treating those who, even if asymptomatic, tested positive. Considerable controversy surrounded recommendations relating to *H. pylori* eradication in the setting of dyspepsia, especially with no obvious ulcer found. The Update Panel concluded that testing dyspeptic patients for *H. pylori* should be done only on a case-by-case basis.

The most recent US guidelines for management of *H. pylori* infection were published in 1998[11] on behalf of the Ad hoc Committee on Practice Parameters of the American College of Gastroenterology. These guidelines were approved by the respective Governing Boards of the American College of Gastroenterology, the American Society for Gastrointestinal Endoscopy and the American Gastroenterological Association. These guidelines reiterated and further reinforced those proposed by the International *H. pylori* Update Conference. Testing for infection should be done only if treatment is planned. Primary indications for such testing and subsequent treatment include patients with past or present complicated or uncomplicated duodenal and gastric ulcer, or those with gastric MALT lymphoma. Testing in the setting of dyspepsia should be done on a case-by-case basis. The guidelines also noted that there were insufficient data to warrant routine treatment of all patients on chronic proton pump inhibitor therapy (a recommendation of some European Consensus Groups)[12]. Diagnostic tests should be appropriate to the clinical situation. If endoscopy is necessary for patient care, then a biopsy urease test is the test of choice unless there is a clinical situation such as ongoing proton pump inhibitor use, which would reduce the sensitivity of urease testing. In such a case histology, although more expensive, would be appropriate. Culture of organisms from endoscopically obtained biopsy tissue was not routinely recommended. When endoscopy is not clinically indicated, office-based serology or urea breath testing is recommended. The latter test is especially useful when documenting bacterial eradication since post-treatment endoscopy is usually not indicated. Treatment regimens should include antibiotic doses and treatment of sufficient duration to ensure maximum efficacy. A proton pump inhibitor or ranitidine bismuth citrate (no longer available in the United States), clarithromycin and amoxycillin or metronidazole or proton pump inhibitor, bismuth, metronidazole and tetracycline given for 2 weeks were thought to

Table 2. European guidelines for management of *H. pylori*

Active or past ulcer	Yes	UBT noninvasive test of choice
MALT lymphoma/EGC	Yes	Early referral for EGD
Severe gastritis	Yes	Determine PUD and cancer risk
Dyspepsia (young healthy)	Yes	Use effective Rx
NUD		
FHx gastric cancer	Yes	
Long-term PPIs	Yes	
NSAIDs alone	Yes	
Other: pt request, prevent cancer, family, extra-GI	No	

achieve the highest eradication rates and were recommended therapies. Post-treatment follow-up testing was recommended only in the setting of complicated ulcer disease, MALT lymphoma or recurrent symptoms.

EUROPEAN MANAGEMENT GUIDELINES

The European *Helicobacter pylori* Study Group met in Maastricht in 1997 to develop unified consensus *H. pylori* management guidelines for the European region[12]. Formulated consensus statements and recommendations stem from presentations of evidence-based literature, expert opinion and conventions dictated by local practice opinion. Similarities between the European guidelines and those of the United States included recommending treatment for individuals with active or past ulcer disease, MALT lymphoma or early gastric cancer. Differences included recommending the testing and treatment of those with evidence of severe endoscopic gastritis and those receiving long-term proton pump inhibitors for gastro-oesophageal reflux disease. Further recommendations, although not strongly supported by the published data, included testing and treating young, healthy patients with dyspepsia, those with non-ulcer dyspepsia, those with a family history of gastric cancer and those receiving NSAIDs. The Maastricht report downplayed the role of serology, especially quick office-based tests, and suggested that the urea breath test be considered the non-invasive test of choice, both for primary infection and to document eradication. The key to patient management was determining the likelihood of underlying peptic ulcer disease or cancer risk in the population being evaluated. Primary-care physicians were urged to consider early referral for endoscopy; any patient not responding to therapy was thought to have a significant risk for underlying ulcer or cancer. Similar to United States guidelines, use of effective therapy was emphasized with the therapy of choice being a proton pump inhibitor and two antibiotics, with selection based on the likelihood of antibiotic-resistant organisms being present. Seven days treatment was thought to be adequate and, if primary therapy failed, endoscopy with culture and sensitivity testing was recommended prior to prescribing a second course of treatment.

Table 3. Canadian guielines for management of *H. pylori*

Active or past ulcer	Yes	Test only if Rx planned
MALT lymphoma	Yes	Treat all who test positive
Gastric cancer (high risk)	Yes	Use effective Rx
Severe gastritis	Yes	F/U testing limited
Asymptomatic persons	No	Early endoscopy in children
GERD/long-term PPIs	No	
NUD	No	
Dyspepsia (young healthy)	Yes	
NSAIDs alone	No	

CANADIAN MANAGEMENT GUIDELINES

The first Canadian *Helicobacter pylori* Consensus Conference took place in April of 1997, at which time it was recommended that patients with active or past ulcer disease or gastric MALT lymphoma be tested and treated for *H. pylori* infection[13]. Although, admittedly, data were equivocal, testing and treatment was recommended for young, otherwise healthy patients with chronic dyspepsia on a case-by-case basis, those at a high risk of gastric cancer (such as Japanese-Canadians or those with a family history) or those with severe histological gastritis. Testing was not recommended for patients with gastro-oesophageal reflux disease unless they were being treated with long-term proton pump inhibitor therapy, in which case testing and treatment could be offered on a case-by-case basis. Testing was thought to be inappropriate in asymptomatic individuals without previous peptic ulcer disease or in individuals when treatment was not planned. Biopsy urease testing or histology were felt to be appropriate techniques when endoscopy was planned for clinical reasons while culture was generally unnecessary. When endoscopy was not clinically indicated, urea breath testing for primary diagnosis or follow-up after treatment was the preferred diagnostic method. Emphasis was placed on using effective therapy which was proton pump inhibitors, clarithromycin, amoxycillin or metronidazole twice daily for 1 week. Seven to 14 days of bismuth, metronidazole and tetracycline with a proton pump inhibitor or an H_2-receptor antagonist was recommended as second-line therapy. Only those with complicated ulcer disease, MALT lymphoma or recurrent symptoms after treatment deserved follow-up testing to confirm bacterial eradication. These original recommendations were updated in June 1998[14], at which time recommendation for testing and treating patients was again extended to those with ulcer-like dyspepsia, and ranitidine bismuth citrate plus two antibiotics was added as a possible recommended first-line treatment option. The urea breath test was also deemed to be the non-invasive diagnostic method of choice, with serology no longer being recommended. Paediatric guidelines were also established in Canada and were very similar to those recommended for adults[15]. However, early upper endoscopy with multiple biopsies was thought to be the optimal approach to investigate paediatric patients with chronic or recurrent upper abdominal symptoms. Treatment recommendations were

Table 4. Asia–Pacific guidelines for management of H. pylori

Active or past ulcer	Yes	% HP and disease vary
MALT lymphoma/EGC	Yes	Dx methods variable
Dyspepsia	Yes	EGD for Dx and F/U
NSAIDs alone	No	Use effective Rx
NSAIDs and dyspepsia	Yes	
FHx gastric cancer	No	
Asymptomatic and family	No	

extended to include family members of treated children, although there was no proven benefit to this practice.

ASIAN PACIFIC CONSENSUS

The Asian pacific H. pylori Consensus Conference convened in August 1997 and was faced with a formidable task of developing guidelines applicable to populations diverse in the prevalence of H. pylori and clinical disease outcomes[16]. The Asian Pacific Group did recommend testing and treating those with active or past ulcer disease, MALT lymphoma, early gastric cancer and those on NSAIDs with dyspepsia. It was not recommended to test asymptomatic individuals or those on NSAIDs alone, or those solely with a family history of gastric cancer. A recommendation was made, after apparently much discussion, to test and treat individuals who are young and otherwise healthy with dyspeptic complaints. Such individuals, however, should be referred early for endoscopy, if there is lack of response because of the high prevalence of ulcer and gastric cancer in Asian countries.

As with other Consensus Guidelines, effective therapy was stressed, with a proton pump inhibitor and two antibiotics being the treatment of choice. The test to diagnose H. pylori would vary somewhat depending on the population being tested. For example, serology would be appropriate in a population in which the prevalence of cancer would be low, such as Australia or New Zealand, while endoscopic testing might be preferable in those areas where ulcer and cancer risk is high, such a China or Japan.

GLOBAL CONSENSUS AND DIFFERENCES

All guidelines agreed that effective therapy should be used, and generally this was a proton pump inhibitor and two antibiotics, with the choice depending on the likelihood of the presence of antibiotic-resistant organisms. Quadruple therapy, i.e. proton pump inhibitor, bismuth, metronidazole and tetracycline, was an acceptable alternative and a good second-line therapy in those who had failed initial treatment.

The duration and dose of therapy varied somewhat. In the United States 10–14 days of therapy is recommended, while in most other parts of the world 7-day treatment is thought to be sufficient. In the US and Canada the dose of clarithromycin recommended is 500 mg, while in other parts of the world 250 mg appears to suffice. Choice and dose of nitroimidazole and other antibiotics also vary, due primarily to drug availability and cost.

Consensus regarding treatment of active or past ulcer disease is related to the strong evidence that ulcer, especially duodenal ulcer, can be cured in most people with eradication of *H. pylori*. Similar consensus in treatment of MALT lymphoma stems from long-lasting cure of the disease with *H. pylori* eradication (albeit no controlled trials). Differences relating to recommendations concerning dyspepsia result form inconsistent symptom relief with bacterial eradication. Studies suggesting that treatment benefits patients with non-ulcer dyspepsia or undiagnosed dyspepsia come largely from centres with a high background prevalence rate of *H. pylori* infection and peptic ulcer disease[17,18]. Studies showing no benefit have generally been done in the areas with a low prevalence of *H. pylori* and ulcer disease.

There is currently no evidence that testing for and treating *H. pylori* will reverse the risk for subsequent development of cancer. Nevertheless, in high cancer areas of the world, guidelines suggest early endoscopy to exclude cancer, and limiting non-invasive testing to only very young individuals with a minimal risk of gastric cancer. Until data show reduced risk, there will be no guidelines specifically recommending population screening, although cost modelling does show that this may be cost-effective in certain situations[19].

The worldwide indications for *H. pylori* eradication and specific treatment vary. Global guidelines relate to differences in prevalence of infection, distinct clinical disease manifestations and the cost and availability of various diagnostic methods and treatments. However, from a global perspective, when dealing with *H. pylori* infection, it is important to do the right thing for the right reason in each region of the world.

References

1. Malfertheiner P, Leodolter A, Peitz U. Cure of *Helicobacter pylori*-associated ulcer disease through eradication. Bailliere's Clin Gastroenterol. 2000;14:119–32.
2. Bayerdoerffer E, Morgner A, Thiede C et al. Cure of *Helicobacter pylori* infection is associated with long-term remission in limited stages of low-grade gastric MALT lymphoma. Gastroenterology. 1999;116:A375.
3. Uemure N, Mukai T, Okamoto S et al. Effect of *Helicobacter pylori* eradication on subsequent development of cancer after endoscopic resection of early gastric cancer. Cancer Epidemiol Biomarkers Prev. 1997;6:639–42.
4. Gisbert JP, Pajares JM. *Helicobacter pylori* test-and-treat strategy for dyspeptic patients. Scand J Gastroenterol. 1999;34:644–52.
5. Blaser MJ. *Helicobacter pylori* and gastric diseases. Br Med J. 1998;316:1507–10.
6. Labenz J. Consequences of *Helicobacter pylori* cure in ulcer patients. Bailliere's Clin Gastroenterol. 2000;14:133–45.
7. Schmid CH, Whiting G, Cory D et al. Omeprazole plus antibiotics in the eradication of *Helicobacter pylori* infection: a meta-regression analysis of randomized, controlled trials. Am J Ther. 1999;6:25–36.
8. Go MF, Li L, Frantz J et al. HP cagA and vacA from U.S. duodenal ulcer (DU) patients and association with eradication. Gut. 1999;45(Suppl. III):A108.
9. NIH Consensus development panel on *Helicobcter pylori* in peptic ulcer disease. *Helicobacter pylori* in peptic ulcer disease. J Am Med Assoc. 1994;272:65–9.
10. The report of the Digestive Health Initiative SM International Update Conference on *Helicobacter pylori*. Gastroenterology. 1997;113(Suppl. 6):S4–8.
11. Howden CW, Hunt RH. Guidelines for the management of *Helicobacter pylori* infection. Ad Hoc Committee on Practice Parameters of the American College of Gastroenterology. Am J Gastroenterol. 1998;93:2330–8.

12. Current European concepts in the management of *Helicobacter pylori* infections. The Maastricht Consensus Report. The European *Helicobacter pylori* Study Group. Gut. 1997;41:8–13.
13. Hunt R, Thomson AB. Canadian *Helicobacter pylori* consensus conference. Canadian Association of Gastroenterology. Can J Gastroenterol. 1998;12:31–41.
14. Hunt RH, Fallone CA, Thomson AB. Canadian *Helicobacter pylori* Consensus Conference update: infections in adults. Canadian *Helicobacter* Study Group. Can J Gastroenterol. 1999;13:213–17.
15. Sherman P, Hassall E, Hunt RH et al. Canadian *Helicobacter* Study Group Consensus Conference on the approach to *Helicobacter pylori* infection in children and adolescents [Review]. Can J Gastroenterol. 1999;13:553–9.
16. Lam SK, Talley NJ. Report of the 1997 Asia Pacific Consensus Conference on the management of *Helicobacter pylori* infection. J. Gastroenterol Hepatol. 1998;13:1–12.
17. McColl KEL, Murray L, El-Omar E et al. Symptomatic benefit from eradicating *Helicobacter pylori* infection in patients with nonulcer dyspepsia. N Engl J Med. 1998;339:1869–74.
18. Heaney A, Collins JSA, Watson RGP et al. A prospective randomised trial of a 'test and treat' policy versus endoscopy based management in young *Helicobacter pylori*-positive patients with ulcer-like dyspepsia, referred to a hospital clinic. Gut. 1999;45:186–90.
19. Parsonnet J, Harris RA, Hack HM et al. Modeling cost effectiveness of *H. pylori* screening to prevent gastric cancer: a mandate for clinical trials. Lancet. 1996;384:150–4.

60
Guidelines for therapy of *Helicobacter pylori* infection – a world perspective

S.-K. LAM

INTRODUCTION

Since the NIH consensus meeting on *Helicobacter pylori* held in 1994[1], there have been a number of consensus meetings held in various regions of the world, notably Europe[2], Canada[3-5], Asia[6], South America[7], and South Africa[8], and similar meetings have also been held at a national level in many countries. These meetings reflect the intense interest of gastroenterologists and medical practitioners around the world on the subject, and they also represent efforts to focus on regional and national characteristics of the infection and its management. A common objective is to facilitate the transfer of scientific information and therapeutic strategies to primary-care doctors. Has the world reached a consensus? What is the world strategy? Have these meetings been successful in passing their messages to the community physicians.

In general there are, indeed, common grounds, so that a global consensus does exist, and while geographical variations will mean variations in strategy, the general principles remain similar.

TREATMENT OF *H. PYLORI* INFECTION

In broad principle the treatment should be simple, effective and safe. Acceptable eradication rates for the treatment of *H. pylori* infection are 90% or greater on a per-protocol analysis and 80% or greater on an intent-to-treat analysis[2,6,8]. Until a specific anti-infective agent becomes available, the following regimens are recommended by most workers[9-18].

1. Proton-pump inhibitor (PPI) in standard dose or ranitidine bismuth citrate (RBC) 400 mg + clarithromycin 500 mg + amoxycillin 1 g, each given twice daily for 7 days.
2. PPI in standard dose or RBC 400 mg + clarithromycin 500 mg + metronidazole 400 mg, each given twice daily for 7 days.

3. PPI in standard dose + amoxycillin 1 g + metronidazole 400 mg, each given twice daily for 7 days.
4. Colloidal bismuth subcitrate 120 mg four times daily, metronidazole 400 mg twice daily + tetracycline 500 mg four times daily for 14 days.
5. PPI in standard dose twice daily + colloidal bismuth subcitrate 120 mg four times daily + metronidazole 400 mg twice daily + tetracycline 500 mg four times daily for 7 days.

In general, the amoxycillin-containing combinations are recommended over those containing metronidazole, particularly where rates of metronidazole resistance exceed 30%. If clarithromycin is not available, regimens 3 and 4 may be considered, although it is appreciated that these regimens yield, on average, a 10% lower eradication rate than the clarithromycin-containing regimens. Following treatment failure the same or a different regimen may be used; for example, by substituting amoxycillin for metronidazole. Regimen 5 is a suitable alternative for treatment failure.

PEPTIC ULCER

All consensus meetings agreed that *H. pylori*-related duodenal ulcer and gastric ulcer, including active, inactive and bleeding ulcer, should be given eradication treatment for healing as well as for the prevention of relapse, because the evidence in support has been irrefutable[9,11,13-15,19-22].

LOW-GRADE LYMPHOMA

All would also agree that low-grade gastric mucosa-associated lymphoid tissue (MALT) lymphoma associated with *H. pylori* should be treated by eradication, although the evidence was less overwhelming. Complete remission occurred in approximately 75% of patients up to 2 years after successful treatment of *H. pylori* infection[23-25]. Patients with this condition should be managed by specialists in major centres since additional treatment modalities may be required, and all patients will need expert follow-up.

NON-ULCER OR FUNCTIONAL DYSPEPSIA

This was defined recently as persistent or recurrent pain or discomfort centred in the upper abdomen of at least 12 weeks duration, which need not be consecutive, within the preceding 12 months, with no evidence of organic disease[26]. Double-blind, randomized studies have been performed to examine the effect of *H. pylori* eradication on symptoms. These have clearly shown that there is no short-term benefit. Long-term (i.e. 1 year after eradication) benefit has been demonstrated by one study[27], but refuted by two others[28,29]. It remains possible that subgroups of patients with non-ulcer dyspepsia may be related to cytotoxin-producing strains of *H. pylori*[30], and such patients may show a better response to eradication treatment[31].

In Europe eradication is recommended because it is believed to bring substantial cost benefits[32,33]. In Asia it is recommended that eradication

GUIDELINES FOR THERAPY – WORLD PERSPECTIVE

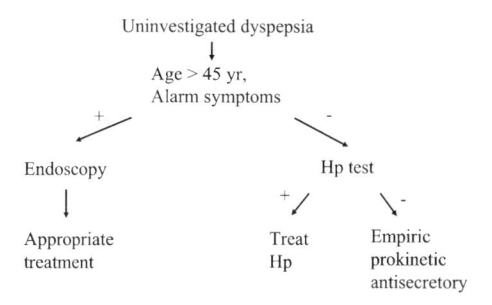

```
                    Uninvestigated dyspepsia
                              ↓
                         Age > 45 yr,
                       Alarm symptoms
              +      ↙              ↘      -
         Endoscopy                    Hp test
              ↓                    +  ↙    ↘ -
        Appropriate              Treat     Empiric
         treatment                Hp       prokinetic
                                           antisecretory
```

Figure 1. Algorithm for regions with low incidence of gastric cancer.

treatment be considered on a case-by-case basis[6,34]. As details of *H. pylori* infection and its complications become better known to the general public, more and more patients will request to have *H. pylori* testing and to be given treatment when positive. In general, treatment should be offered only after a discussion with the patient concerning the implications of treatment. Patients should be advised that treatment of the infection may not alleviate their symptoms in the short term, and they should be made aware of the possible adverse effects of therapy.

MANAGEMENT OF UNINVESTIGATED DYSPEPSIA

It is now generally recognized that the approach to uninvestigated dyspepsia depends on how common gastric cancer occurs in a given locality.

Algorithm 1 (Figure 1)

For countries with a high incidence of gastric cancer, such as China and Russia, this algorithm has been recommended. Countries with a high incidence of gastric cancer tend to have a high background prevalence of *H. pylori* infection. Therefore, a test for *H. pylori* infection might be regarded as a 'cancer test'. Endoscopy is recommended as the investigation of choice. Any non-invasive test for *H. pylori* infection should be locally validated and have a sensitivity and specificity of 90% or greater. Alarm factors include an age cut-off (range 30–50 years depending upon the national gastric cancer incidence rate, e.g. in China the onset age can be down to 30 years of age), or symptoms of weight loss, vomiting, dysphagia, anaemia, gastrointestinal bleeding, a positive family history of gastric cancer, a fear of gastric cancer, and/or a perceived need for reassurance about gastric cancer.

Algorithm 2 (Figure 2)

For countries with a low incidence of gastric cancer, such as the USA or some European countries, this algorithm, which has been modified for easy understanding, has been recommended. Countries with a low incidence of gastric cancer have an intermediate or low prevalence of *H. pylori* infection. Therefore, a test for *H. pylori* infection might be regarded as an 'ulcer test'. This approach represents the test-and-treat strategy for patients under 45

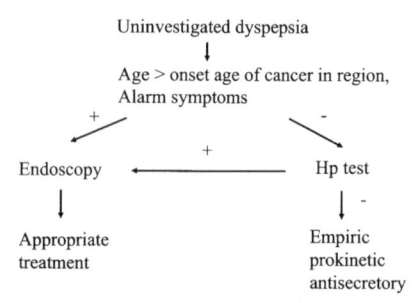

```
              Uninvestigated dyspepsia
                        ↓
           Age > onset age of cancer in region,
                   Alarm symptoms
              +                       −
                         +
        Endoscopy  ←─────────────  Hp test
           ↓                          ↓ −
       Appropriate                 Empiric
        treatment                 prokinetic
                                 antisecretory
```

Figure 2. Algorithm for regions with high incidence of gastric cancer.

years of age in Western countries where the prevalence of gastric cancer is low. A recent prospective randomized trial of the 'test-and-treat' policy versus endoscopy-based management in young patients with ulcer-like dyspepsia showed that the eradication group fared better at 12 months in both dyspepsia score and quality of life[35].

It should also be appreciated that there are countries with a high prevalence (> 70%) of *H. pylori* infection, in which endoscopy is either not affordable or not readily available. In these localities it can be envisaged that an affordable acid-reducing drug is given for the initial treatment. This, in effect, becomes an 'indirect ulcer test'. If this fails it has been recommended that *H. pylori* treatment be given without prior testing. If symptoms persist, referral should be sought. These recommendations are based on pragmatism rather than evidence.

NON-STEROIDAL ANTI-INFLAMMATORY DRUGS (NSAIDs)

H. pylori eradication for NSAID-naive subjects, i.e. before initiating NSAIDs, remains controversial. A randomized but single-blind study showed that eradication treatment reduced the risk of ulceration 10-fold from 26% to 2.5%[36]. Two small meta-analysis studies showed that use of NSAIDs in subjects infected with *H. pylori* was associated with a modest increase in the risk for ulcer of 8% to 16%[37,38]. However, in patients on chronic NSAIDs, ulcer occurrence was the same in patients treated with eradication as in those treated with placebo[39]. In patients who had been on chronic NSAIDs and who developed peptic ulcer, healing was better and relapse was less frequent in those who had *H. pylori* infection[40,41]. Furthermore, healing of gastric ulcer after eradication treatment in such patients was lower compared with omeprazole treatment alone, and ulcer/dyspepsia relapse was not different with or without eradication treatment[42]. In NSAID users presenting with bleeding gastric ulcers, *H. pylori* eradication was ineffective when compared with omeprazole in preventing further bleeding. Thus, eradication treatment is not advisable at this time before initiating NSAIDs, and is also not advisable in chronic users of NSAIDs who have a gastric ulcer, since this may retard healing and shorten subsequent remission.

The NSAID issue may become a non-issue if it can be confirmed that replacement with COX-2 specific inhibitors is associated with much fewer gastrointestinal side-effects. However, it remains necessary to evaluate the use of low-dose aspirin in coronary and stroke patients who are positive for *H. pylori* infection.

PREVENTION OF GASTRIC CANCER BY *H. PYLORI* ERADICATION

H. pylori infection has been regarded as a group 1 carcinogen[43], and one of Koch's postulates has been satisfied that *H. pylori* is a cause of gastric cancer in Mongolian gerbils[44]. Evidence remains controversial that eradication of *H. pylori* infection reverses atrophic gastritis and/or intestinal metaplasia[45], although a 5-year study reported improvement of atrophic gastritis in CagA-positive subjects[46]. Large chemoprevention studies looking at eradication of *H. pylori* infection are in progress[47], and until these data become available it is the consensus that eradication is not recommended for cancer prevention.

Even if the results of the interventional studies prove positive, it should be noted that in high gastric cancer areas such as Changle, China (80/100 000), one needs to screen and treat, using a conservative efficacy rate of 30%, 1800 subjects to prevent one cancer; whereas in low gastric cancer areas such as the USA (6.8/100 000), the number needed to prevent one cancer will increase to 23 000.

SUMMARY PERSPECTIVES

Many uncertainties and controversies with regard to therapy discussed in previous consensus meetings have now been ironed out, although many still remain. Eradication treatment is indisputable for *H. pylori* infection-related peptic ulcer. Eradication for non-ulcer dyspepsia lacks convincing evidence, which at best is marginal. Eradication remains uncertain for the group of patients who have no past or present evidence of ulcer disease, who have not taken NSAIDs previously, and who are starting these drugs for the first time. For chronic NSAID users with peptic ulcer, eradication may result in unfavourable healing and relapse, and is not advised. Eradication is not advisable for cancer prevention until the results of the interventional studies become available.

It is a general impression that, the test-and-treat approach for dyspeptic patients under the age of 45 in low cancer prevalence regions of the world is not well received by primary-care physicians. It is possible that general practitioners are confused by the uncertainties reported for non-ulcer dyspepsia, and the confusion is made worse by beneficial claims of prokinetic agents for this condition. NSAID ulcers appear to be another confusing area, since NSAID dyspepsia is poorly understood.

References

1. NIH Consensus Conference. *Helicobacter pylori* in peptic ulcer disease. J Am Med Assoc. 1994;272:65–9.

2. European *Helicobacter pylori* Study Group. Current European concepts in the management of *Helicobacter pylori* infection. Maastricht Consensus Report. Gut. 1997;41:8–13.
3. Hunt R, Thomson AB. Canadian *Helicobacter pylori* Consensus Conference. Canadian Association of Gastroenterology. Can J Gastroenterol. 1998;12:31–41.
4. Hunt RH, Fallone CA, Thomson AB. Canadian *Helicobacter pylori* Consensus Conference update: infections in adults. Canadian Helicobacter Study Group. Can J Gastroenterol. 1999;13:213–17.
5. Sherman P, Hassall E, Hunt RH et al. Canadian *Helicobacter* Study Group Consensus Conference on the approach to *Helicobacter pylori* infection in children and adolescents. Can J Gastroenterol. 1999;13:553–9.
6. Lam SK, Talley NJ. Report of the 1997 Asia Pacific Consensus Conference on the management of *Helicobacter pylori* infection. J Gastroenterol Hepatol. 1998;13:1–12.
7. De Paula las Rua L, Aleixo A. Brazilian consensus on *Helicobacter pylori* and associated diseases. Acta Gastroenterol Latinoam. 1996;26:255–60.
8. South African Medical Association, South African Gastroenterology Society Working Group. Diagnosis and management of dyspepsia – clinical guideline, 1999. S Afr Med J. 1999;89:897–907.
9. Huang JQ. Eradication of *Helicobacter pylori*: problems and recommendations. J Gastroenterol Hepatol. 1997;12:590–8.
10. Huang JQ, Chiba N, Wilkinson J, Hunt RH. Which combination therapy can eradicate >90% *Helicobacter pylori* infection? A meta-analysis of amoxicillin, metronidazole, tetracycline and clarithromycin containing regimens. Gastroenterology. 1997;112: A19.
11. Hunt RH. Eradication of *Helicobacter pylori* infection. Am J Med. 1996;100 (Suppl. 5A):425–50S.
12. Hunt RH, Lam SK. *Helicobacter pylori*: from art to a science. J Gastroenterol Hepatol. 1998;13:21–8.
13. Penston J G. Clinical aspects of *Helicobacter pylori* eradication therapy in peptic ulcer disease. Aliment Pharmacol Ther. 1996;10:469–86.
14. Unge P. Pooled analysis of anti-*Helicobacter pylori* treatment regimens. Scand J Gastroenterol. 1996;31:27–40.
15. Van der Hulst RWM, Tytgat GNJ. Treatment of *Helicobacter pylori* infection: a review of the world literature. Helicobacter. 1996;1:6–19.
16. Lind T, Veldhuyzen van Zanten S, Unge P et al. Eradication of *Helicobacter pylori* using one-week triple therapies combining omeprazole with two antimicrobials: the Mach 1 study. Helicobacter 1996;1:138–44.
17. Axon ATR, Ireland A, Smith MJL, Roopram PD. Ranitidine bismuth citrate and clarithromycin twice daily in eradication of *Helicobacter pylori*. Aliment Pharmacol Ther. 1997;11:81–7.
18. Lind T, Megraud F, Unge P et al. The MACH2 study: role of omeprazole in eradication of *Helicobacter pylori* with 1-week triple therapies. Gastroenterology. 1999;116:248–53.
19. Lam SK, Ching CK, Lai KC et al. Does treatment of *Helicobacter pylori* with antibiotics alone heal duodenal ulcer? A randomised double-blind placebo-controlled study. Gut. 1997;41:43–8.
20. Lam SK. Current strategies in ulcer management with special reference to the use of antibiotics. Yale J Biol Med. 1997;70:27–31.
21. Wong BCY, Lam SK, Lai KC et al. Triple therapy for *Helicobacter pylori* eradication is more effective than long-term maintenance anti-secretory treatment in the prevention of recurrrence of duodenal ulcer: a prospective long-term follow-up study. Aliment Pharmacol Ther. 2000 (In press).
22. Lai KC, Wong WM, Hui WM, Wong BCY, Hu WHC, Lam SK. Eradication of *Helicobacter pylori* in patients with duodenal ulcer haemorrhage – 5 years follow up. Gastroenterology. 1997;112(Suppl.):A190.
23. Wotherspoon AC, Doglioni C, Diss TC et al. Regression of primary low-grade B-cell gastric lymphoma of mucosa-associated lymphoid tissue type after eradication of *Helicobacter pylori*. Lancet. 1993;342:575–7.
24. Roggero E, Zucca E, Pinotti G et al. Eradication of *Helicobacter pylori* infection in primary low-grade gastric lymphoma of mucosa-associated lymphoid tissue. Ann Intern Med. 1995;122:767–9.

25. Bayerdorffer E, Neubauer A, Rudolph B et al. Regression of primary gastric lymphoma of mucosa-associated lymphoid tissue after cure of *Helicobacter pylori* infection. Lancet. 1995;345:1591–4.
26. Talley NJ, Stanghellini V, Heading RC, Koch KL, Malagelada JR, Tytgat GNJ. Functional gastroduodeal disorders. Rome II: a multinational consensus document on functional gastrointestinal disorders. Gut 1999;45(Suppl. II):II37–42.
27. McColl K, Murray L, El-Omar E et al. Symptomatic benefit from eradicating *Helicobacter pylori* infection in patients with nonulcer dyspepsia. N Engl J Med. 1998;339:1869–74.
28. Blum AL, Talley NJ, O'Morain C et al. Lack of effect of treating *Helicobacter pylori* infection in patients with non-ulcer dyspepsia. N Engl J Med. 1998;339:1875–81.
29. Talley NJ, Vakil N, Ballard II ED, Fennerty MB. Absence of benefit of eradicating *Helicobacter pylori* in patients with nonulcer dyspepsia. N Engl J Med. 1999;341:1106–11.
30. Ching CK, Lam SK. Nonulcer dyspepsia: association with chronic *Helicobacter pylori* infection-related gastritis? J Clin Gastroenterol. 1995;21(Suppl. 1):S140–5.
31. McColl KEL, El-Omar E, Kelman AW et al. UK MRC trial of *H. pylori* eradication therapy for non-ulcer dyspepsia. Gut 1998;42(Suppl. 1):A3.
32. Sonenberg A. Cost benefit analysis of testing for *Helicobacter pylori* in dyspeptic patients. Am J Gastroenterol. 1996;91:1773–7.
33. Briggs AH, Sulpher MJ, Logan RPH, Aldous J, Ramsay ME, Baron JH. Cost-effectiveness of screening for *Helicobacter pylori* in management of dyspeptic patients under 45 years of age. Br Med J. 1996;312:1321–5.
34. Talley NJ, Lam SK, Goh KL, Fock KM. Dyspepsia consensus: management guidelines for uninvestigated and functional dyspepsia in the Asia-Pacific region: First Asian Pacific working party on functional dyspepsia. J Gastroenterol Hepatol. 1998;13:335–53.
35. Heancy A, Collins JSA, Watson RGP, McFarland RJ, Bamford KB, Tham TCK. A prospective randomised trial of a 'test and treat' policy versus endoscopy based management in young *Helicobacter pylori* positive patients with ulcer-like dyspepsia, referred to a hospital clinic. Gut. 1999;45:186–90.
36. Chan FKL, Sung JY, Chung SCC et al. Randomised trial of eradication of *Helicobacter pylori* before non-steroidal anti-inflammatory drug therapy to prevent peptic ulcers. Lancet. 1997;350:975–9.
37. Goldstein JL, Agrawal NM, Silverstein F et al. Influence of *H. pylori* infection and/or low dose aspirin on gastroduodenal ulceration in patients treated with placebo, celecoxib or NSAIDs. Gastroenterology. 1999;116:G0759.
38. Huang JQ, Lad RJ, Sridhar S, Sumanac K, Hunt R. *H. pylori* infection increases the risk of non-steroidal anti-inflammatory drug (NSAID)-induced gastroduodeal ulceration. Gastroenterology. 1999;116:G0836.
39. Lai KC, Lam SK, Hui WM et al. Can eradication of *Helicobacter pylori* prevent future development of peptic ulcers in patients receiving long-term continuous nonsteroidal anti-inflammatory drugs. Gastroenterology. 1998;114:G0787.
40. Yeomans ND, Tulassay Z, Juhasz L et al. A comparison of omeprazole with ranitidine for ulcers associated with nonsteroidal antiinflammatory drugs. N Engl J Med. 1998; 338:719–26.
41. Hawkey CJ, Karrasch JA, Szczepanski L et al. Omepraole compared with misoprostol for ulcers associated with nonsteroidal antiinflammatory drugs. N Engl J Med. 1998; 338:727–34.
42. Hawkey CJ, Tulassay Z, Szozepanski L et al. Randomised controlled trial of *Helicobacter pylori* eradication in patients on non-steroidal anti-inflammatory drugs: HELP NSAIDs Study. Lancet. 1998;352:1016–21.
43. Schistosomes, liver flukes and *Helicobacter pylori*. In: IARC Monographs on the evaluation of carcinogenic risks to humans. Lyon: IARC; 1994;61:177–220.
44. Watanabe T, Tada M, Nagai H, Sasaki S, Nakao M. *Helicobacter pylori* infection induces gastric cancer in Mongolian gerbils. Gastroenterology. 1998;115:642–8.
45. Asaka M, Kato M, Kudo M et al. Relationship between *Helicobacter pylori* infection, atrophic gastritis and gastric carcinoma in a Japanese population. Eur J Gastroenterol Hepatol. 1995;7:S7–10.
46. van der Hulst RWM, ten Kate FJW, Rauws EAJ et al. The relation of CagA and the long-term sequelae of gastritis after successful cure of *Helicobacter pylori* infection: a long-term follow-up study. Gastroenterology. 1998;114:G1302.
47. Forman D. Lessons from ongoing intervention studies. In: Hunt RH, Tytgat GNJ, editors. *Helicobacter pylori*: Basic Mechanisms to Clinical Care, 1998. Kluwer; 1998;354–60.

61
Bismuth triple and quadruple studies for *Helicobacter pylori* eradication in Canada

C. A. FALLONE

INTRODUCTION

Since the discovery of *Helicobacter pylori* infection by Marshall and Warren[1] there have been many attempts at eliminating this infection with different antibiotic combinations. Bismuth was one of the first agents used in this regard. When used in combination with other antibiotics it continues to be one of the choices for *H. pylori* treatment recommended by several recent Consensus Conferences[2-4]. Several studies on *H. pylori* eradication have been carried out in Canada but relatively few have examined combinations which include bismuth. The purpose of this chapter is to describe the different studies which have examined bismuth triple and quadruple therapies in Canada.

In order to identify all Canadian studies either published or presented in abstract form on bismuth triple and quadruple therapies, a Medline search using the keywords *Helicobacter* and bismuth was carried out from 1976 to November 1999. Similarly, abstract databases from the following meetings were searched: Digestive Disease Week from 1995 to 1999, European *Helicobacter pylori* Study Group Meeting from 1994 to 1999 and the Canadian Digestive Week from 1998 to 1999. In addition, e-mails were sent to key investigators in Canada asking for any publications or abstracts that they may have published on the topic. The abstracts thus retrieved were subsequently reviewed for both a Canadian setting or Canadian author. The search was limited to human studies presented in English. Meta-analyses, cost-effectiveness analyses, and review articles were excluded. The trials were then segregated depending on whether they dealt with bismuth subsalicylate, colloidal bismuth subcitrate, or ranitidine bismuth citrate (RBC).

BISMUTH SUBSALICYLATE STUDIES

In the form of bismuth subsalicylate (Peptobismol), the availability of bismuth in Canada antedates the discovery of *H. pylori*. It was used commonly for symptoms of dyspepsia and diarrhoea. Israel and Hassall examined the use of bismuth subsalicylate for the eradication of *H. pylori* and published their results in 1993[5]. In 29 children with endoscopically documented duodenal ulcer disease and *H. pylori* antral gastritis, who were treated solely with bismuth with or without antibiotics, all ulcers had healed. This was without any use of acid suppression. The treatment used was 6 weeks of bismuth subsalicylate and amoxycillin initially and, if this failed, it was combined with a 4-week course of metronidazole. Patients who were compliant had clearance of *H. pylori* from antral biopsy specimens immediately after treatment in six of 12 children treated with bismuth subsalicylate alone, one of five treated with amoxycillin alone, nine of nine treated with amoxycillin and bismuth subsalicylate and three of three treated with amoxycillin, bismuth subsalicylate and metronidazole. However, at a mean of 6.5 months after treatment the numbers of biopsy specimens clear of *H. pylori* were as follows: monotherapy one of five; dual therapy four of four; and triple therapy three of three. In their non-compliant patients the rate of *H. pylori* eradication was significantly lower and duodenal ulcers recurred in all children with persistent or recurrent *H. pylori* infection. This study was important because it was one of very few studies performed in the paediatric population, not only in Canada but also elsewhere in the world. It also gave strong support for a causal relationship between *H. pylori* and duodenal ulcer disease in children.

In the adult population Veldhuyzen van Zanten and colleagues also examined this form of bismuth both retrospectively and prospectively. In 1996 they presented a retrospective analysis at the Canadian Digestive Disease Week[6]. At that time triple therapy with bismuth subsalicylate, metronidazole, and either amoxycillin or tetracycline was considered to be the best treatment for eradication of *H. pylori*. They retrospectively reviewed the charts of patients who had been treated with these combinations at their hospital from 1991 to 1995. They found 56 patients, 44 of whom had been successfully eradicated of *H. pylori* infection (78.6%). Those that were treated with the tetracycline combination had a slightly higher success rate at 81.6%, 31/38) compared to those that were treated with amoxycillin (70.6%, 12/17). Their conclusion that the tetracycline combination was superior to amoxycillin was similar to that of a previously published meta-analysis[7].

Prospectively, Veldhuyzen van Zanten *et al.*[8] conducted another study in which they randomized patients suffering from non-ulcer dyspepsia to either triple therapy (bismuth subsalicylate 302 mg q.i.d., amoxycillin 500 mg t.i.d., and metronidazole 500 mg t.i.d.) or an identical placebo. This study was aimed at assessing symptom response to *H. pylori* eradication, and they found no significant differences in outcomes between the two groups. *H. pylori* was, however, eradicated in 26 of the 27 (96%) ptients in the active treatment group compared to only one of 22 (5%) in the placebo group. Although higher than most studies, this eradication rate is consistent with other per-protocol eradication rates.

Although the bismuth triple therapies showed excellent success, the fact that patients had to take several medications four times a day for a prolonged period was the impetus for the development of simpler, less frequent or shorter treatments. Investigators and physicians thus turned to the proton pump inhibitor combinations. Dual therapy consisted of omeprazole with amoxycillin and subsequently, because of improved efficacy, triple therapy consisting of a proton pump inhibitor such as omeprazole given with two antibiotics became more popular. Attempts to simplify the bismuth-containing regimens were also made. Two groups in Canada specifically examined a less frequent bismuth therapy in the community. Chiba and Marshall[9] examined the success rate of a 7-day treatment with omeprazole 20 mg b.i.d., Pepto-Bismol 2 tab b.i.d., metronidazole 500 mg b.i.d. and tetracycline 500 mg b.i.d. Twenty-seven patients had completed this open study at the time of presentation, including patients with duodenal ulcer disease, gastric ulcer disease, non-ulcer dyspepsia and gastro-oesophageal reflux disease. The intention-to-treat eradication rate was 21/27 (78%), whereas the per-protocol rate was 21/25 (84%). In a similar study reported by Lahaie and Farley[10] the same medication combination for 7 days resulted in a lower eradication rate of 67% (12/18). The b.i.d. dosing of this quadruple therapy, hence, did not seem to be as effective as the q.i.d. dosing at least in these two Canadian communities.

COLLOIDAL BISMUTH SUBCITRATE STUDIES

Colloidal bismuth subcitrate is another form of bismuth. It is not currently commercially available in Canada, although it is available in other parts of the world. It too has been shown to have anti-*H. pylori* properties and to work in eradication of this infection. We conducted a randomized, placebo-controlled, clinical trial comparing colloidal bismuth subcitrate (120 mg per os b.i.d.) and metronidazole (500 mg per os t.i.d.) with either amoxycillin (500 mg per os t.i.d.) or placebo[11]. The study was conducted in 85 patients with endoscopically confirmed duodenal ulcer disease. The intention-to-treat eradication rate was 87% (33/38) in the triple-therapy group compared to 66% (31/47) in the dual therapy group (95% confidence interval for the difference: 4–38%). In the per-protocol analysis, eradication rates were superior at 97% (28/29) in the triple therapy group compared to 82% (27/33) in the dual therapy group. The study demonstrated that triple therapy was superior to dual therapy and that triple therapy had excellent eradication rates.

Axcan Pharma, the distributor of colloidal bismuth subcitrate in Canada, has carried out two studies on colloidal bismuth subcitrate combination therapy for *H. pylori* infection and is in the process of carrying out a third study with a combination capsule, which includes bismuth, metronidazole and tetracycline. The first study[12] was a multicentre, Canadian, double-blind, randomized, placebo-controlled trial. It included seven clinical sites but all biopsy specimens were interpreted by one central pathologist. The patients were randomized in a 2 to 1 scheme receiving either active treatment or placebo respectively. The active treatment consisted of colloidal bismuth subcitrate (Bi_2O_3) 120 mg with metronidazole 250 mg and 500 mg of tetracycline, all given q.i.d. for 14 days. Eradication was determined by histology obtained 27–35 days after the end of treatment. Of the 95 patients randomized, 92 completed therapy. Fifty-seven of these had received active therapy whereas 35 received a placebo. Fifty-one of the 57 patients (89.5%) on active treatment achieved eradication compared to only one of 35 (2.9%) on placebo (per-protocol analysis, $p < 0.001$). The individual eradication rates across the seven different sites were 83%, 89%, 91%, 100%, 100%, 100% and 100%. There was no metronidazole susceptibility testing done in this study but the consistency of results across sites and with previous studies confirms the excellent eradication rate with this combination. Interestingly, there was no statistically significant difference in the eradication rate when using this bismuth triple therapy between patients with duodenal ulcer ($n = 12$, rate = 92.3%), gastric ulcer ($n = 14$, rate = 87.5%), or non-ulcer dyspepsia ($n = 18$, rate = 85.7%). The treatment was well tolerated with only three patients having to discontinue the study because of adverse events. Two of these (3.5%) were in the bismuth triple therapy group and stopped because of moderate nausea and moderate bloating and one (2.9%) in the placebo group stopped because of severe abdominal pain. There were no clinically significant abnormalities reported in the laboratory tests. The conclusion of this study was that bismuth triple therapy given for 14 days was highly effective against H. pylori infection regardless of metronidazole resistance for first-line therapy of this infection. Its success rate in patients who had previously failed therapy, particularly if they underwent treatment with a metronidazole-containing regimen, cannot be deduced from this study as the rate of metronidazole resistance may certainly be higher in this population. The effect of metronidazole resistance on treatment outcome, however, was addressed by the second study.

The second study[13], sponsored by Axcan Pharma, examined a shorter treatment but with the addition of a proton pump inhibitor (quadruple therapy). The dose of tetracycline was also reduced with this combination compared to the first study. The aim of this study was not only to look at the eradication rate of this treatment of shorter duration but also to assess the effect of metronidazole resistance on this outcome. There were 164 patients included in this study. These were patients with H. pylori infection confirmed by histology and C13 urea breath test. The patients were treated for 7 days with bismuth subcitrate (Bi_2O_3) 120 mg, metronidazole 250 mg, and tetracycline 250 mg all given q.i.d. together with omeprazole 20 mg given b.i.d. Patients were 18–75 years of age with a history of peptic ulcer or non-ulcer dyspepsia. Eradication was defined as two negative C13 urea breath tests performed both 1 and 3 months after treatment. Metronidazole resistance was defined as strains with minimal inhibitory concentration of ≥ 8 μg/ml by E test. This was again a Canadian multicentre study with 12 clinical sites, but only one central pathologist and one central microbiology laboratory. The results were reported at the Digestive Disease Week in 1999 and consisted of a per-protocol eradication rate of 84%. The rate in metronidazole-sensitive strains was 91% whereas it was only 67% in resistant ones. A modified intention-to-treat analysis gave a 78% eradication rate with 84% in the metronidazole-sensitive strains and 66% in the resistant ones. Although the eradication rates appear to be slightly inferior to the longer triple therapy regimens with higher tetracycline dose observed with the first study, this 7-day quadruple therapy combination did still demonstrate adequate eradication rates. Again, in this study the adverse effects requiring discontinuation of treatment were few, occurring in only 1.2% of subjects. Adverse events included mild to severe abdominal pain, headaches and moderate diarrhoea.

The most recent Canadian study examining bismuth therapy is one that is currently under way. This study, led by Loren Laine and Richard Hunt and sponsored by Axcan Pharma, is a Canadian–American multicentre study. Patients with duodenal ulcer disease, who have not undergone previous *H. pylori* eradication treatment, will be tested for the presence of *H. pylori* infection and then randomized to one of two treatments. Metronidazole susceptibility will also be determined during this study. This study will be a head-to-head comparison of the two most successful anti-*H. pylori* therapies. Specifically, bismuth quadruple therapy will be compared to a proton pump inhibitor triple therapy. Omeprazole 20 mg given b.i.d. together with three BMT single capsules given q.i.d. all for 10 days will be compared to omeprazole 20 mg, amoxycillin 1000 mg and clarithromycin 500 mg all given b.i.d. for 10 days. The BMT single capsules consist of colloidal bismuth subcitrate 40 mg, metronidazole 125 mg and tetracycline 125 mg. These single capsules will simplify the treatment for patients in that they would only have to take this one type of medication together with the omeprazole rather than two types of antibiotics. The total number of capsules actually taken, however, is still quite high at 14, compared to eight with the proton pump inhibitor triple therapy. The aim of the study is to compare the eradication rates using both of these combinations of treatment, and to determine the effects of metronidazole resistance on these eradication rates. Eradication will be determined by two urea breath tests, both at 1 and 3 months, and patients who have failed eradication will undergo a repeat gastroscopy in order to test for antibiotic susceptibility of the *H. pylori* infection in that patient. The results of this study promise to be very interesting, as not only will we find out patient preference for either the proton pump inhibitor triple therapy or the bismuth quadruple therapy, but also the efficacy of these treatments overall, as well as in patients with metronidazole resistance.

RANITIDINE BISMUTH CITRATE (RBC)

Ranitidine bismuth citrate is a new molecule formed by the combination of ranitidine with bismuth. It has been shown to have anti-*H. pylori* properties not only *in vitro* but also *in vivo*. Canada has participated in international multicentre studies examining the efficacy of ranitidine bismuth citrate in the treatment of ulcer disease and *H. pylori* infection. In a study presented at the Digestive Disease Week 1995[14] 232 patients with active duodenal ulcers were treated with different combinations of ranitidine bismuth citrate (RBC). Patients received either RBC 400 mg b.i.d. for 28 days, or RBC in co-prescription with clarithromycin 250 mg q.i.d. for the initial 14 days, or RBC 800 mg b.i.d. given with the same dose of clarithromycin. *H. pylori* infection was eradicated in only 2% of the patients receiving RBC monotherapy, whereas the RBC 400 mg with clarithromycin had a 94% success rate and the RBC 800 mg with clarithromycin had an 84% success rate. The duodenal ulcers were healed in 89% and 93% of the dual therapy groups respectively. Hence, this study demonstrated that this new agent was useful in duodenal ulcer treatment and in the eradication of *H. pylori* infection when given for a 4-week period and combined with a 1-week course of clarithromycin. Paré et al.[15] published another multicentre, randomized, double-blind study involving 530 duodenal ulcer patients. Patients were randomized to receive a 14-day b.i.d. dual therapy of either RBC 400 mg or omeprazole 20 mg, both given with clarithromycin 500 mg followed by a further 14-day treatment with either RBC 400 mg b.i.d. or omeprazole 20 mg q.d. They found a 90% eradication rate in patients who received the RBC dual therapy compared to only 66% of patients who received the omeprazole dual therapy (per-protocol, $p < 0.001$). The intention-to-treat eradication rates were 77% and 60% respectively ($p < 0.001$). These are slightly inferior to the proton pump inhibitor triple therapy success rates[16,17]. Ulcer healing rates were above 95% in both groups. Again, adverse events were quite few with only 3% of the RBC group having to withdraw because of adverse events. This study, therefore, demonstrated that RBC with clarithromycin was a simple, effective, dual therapy regimen for the eradication of *H. pylori* infection. It led the way to a further study in Canada using RBC with two antibiotics. The results of this study, however, have not yet been presented.

SUMMARY

Bismuth has played, and continues to play, an important role in the treatment of *H. pylori* infection. There have been few studies performed in Canada for each of the different subtypes of bismuth. Bismuth subsalicylate studies performed in Canada have achieved a per-protocol eradication rate as high as 96% in some small studies. Ranitidine bismuth citrate has also achieved per-protocol eradication rates $>90\%$ in studies with very large numbers of subjects. The intention-to-treat rates, however, have been slightly disappointing, with only 77% reported in the study by Paré et al.[15]. Colloidal bismuth subcitrate triple and quadruple therapies have also shown eradication rates above 84% (per-protocol) with one study having as high a per-protocol eradication rate as 97% and an intention-to-treat rate of 87%[11]. It will be very interesting to see the results of the Axcan-sponsored study comparing bismuth quadruple therapy to proton pump inhibitor triple therapy in the eradication of *H. pylori* infection.

References

1. Marshall DJ, Warren JR. Unidentified curve bacilli in the stomach of patients with gastritis and peptic ulceration. Lancet. 1984;1:1311–14.
2. Current European Concepts in the Management of *Helicobacter pylori* infection. The Maastricht Consensus Report. Gut. 1997;41:8–13.
3. The Report of the Digestive Health Initiative International Update Conference on *Helicobacter pylori*. Gastroenterology. 1997;113(Suppl.):S4–8.

4. Hunt RH, Fallone CA, Thomson ABR. Canadian *Helicobacter* Study Group. Canadian *Helicobacter pylori* Consensus Conference Update: Infections in Adults. Can J Gastroenterol. 1999;13:213–17.
5. Israel BM, Hassall E. Treatment and long-term follow-up of *Helicobacter pylori* associated duodenal ulcer disease in children. J Pediatr. 1993;123:53–8.
6. Dunne D, Veldhuyzen van Zanten S. The efficacy of bismuth triple therapy for *Helicobacter pylori* infection. Can J Gastroenterol. 1996;10(Suppl. A):57A.
7. Chiba N, Rao BV, Rademaker JW, Hunt RH. Meta-analysis of the efficacy of antibiotic therapy in eradicating *Helicobacter pylori*. Am J Gastroenterol. 1992;87:1716–27.
8. Veldhuyzen van Zanten S, Malatjalian D, Tanton R et al. The effect of eradication of *Helicobacter pylori* (Hp) on symptoms of non-ulcer dyspepsia (NUD): a randomized, double-blind, placebo controlled trial. Gastroenterology. 1995;108:A250.
9. Chiba N, Marshall C. Omeprazole, bismuth, metronidazole and tetracycline (OBMT) quadruple therapy given twice daily for *H. pylori* eradication in a community gastroenterology practice. Gastroenterology. 1998;114:A91.
10. Lahaie RG, Farley A. Efficacy of OBMT in a twice daily (BID) dosage for the eradication of *H. pylori*: a preliminary study. Gastroenterology. 1998;114:A190.
11. Fallone CA, Loo VG, Jospeh L, Barkun J, Kostyk R, Barkun AN. Predictors of failure of *Helicobacter pylori* eradication and predictors of ulcer recurrence: a randomized, controlled trial. Clin Invest Med. 1999;22:185–94.
12. Veldhuyzen van Zanten S, Farley A, Marcon N et al. Efficacy of colloidal bismuth subcitrate, metronidazole and tetracycline HCl in eradication of *H. pylori*: a randomized, placebo-controlled study. Gastroenterology. 1998;114:A322.
13. Lahaie R, Farley A, Dallaire C et al. Bismuth-based quadruple therapy with colloidal bismuth substrate + tetracycline + metronidazole (M) + omeprazole in eradication of M-sensitive and M-resistant *Helicobacter pylori*. Gastroenterology. 1999;116:A227.
14. Bardhan KD, Dallaire C, Eisold H, Duggan AE. GR122311X (ranitidine bismuth citrate) with clarithromycin for the treatment of duodenal ulcer. Gastroenterology. 1995;108:A53.
15. Paré P, Farley A, Romaozinho JM, Bardhan KD, French PC, Roberts PM. Comparison of ranitidine bismuth citrate plus clarithromycin with omeprazole plus clarithromycin for the eradication of *Helicobacter pylori*. Aliment Pharmacol Ther. 1999;13:1071–8.
16. Lind T, Veldhuyzen van Zanten S, Unge P et al. Eradication of *Helicobacter pylori* using one-week triple therapies combining omeprazole with two antimicrobials: the MACH I Study. Helicobacter. 1996;1:138–44.
17. van Zanten SJ, Bradette M, Farley A et al. The DU-MACH study: eradication of *Helicobacter pylori* and ulcer healing in patients with acute duodenal ulcer using omeprazole based triple therapy. Aliment Pharmacol Ther. 1999;13:289–95.

62
Approach to *Helicobacter pylori* infection in children

E. HASSALL

INTRODUCTION

Increasingly, it has become recognized that there are widely disparate approaches to suspected or proven *Helicobacter pylori* infection in children, even within the subspeciality of paediatric gastroenterology. With this recognition has come concern that tests and treatments in the paediatric age group are being used in excess of their established benefits, and that some of the approaches might be compromising the best care of children. In addition, evidence in paediatrics has indicated that, although some of the issues regarding *H. pylori* infection are similar in children and adults, there are also some important differences. In recognition of this, initiatives have recently been undertaken by paediatric gastroenterologists, together with colleagues in other fields, to clarify the issues of importance in children, and to make rational recommendations for health-care providers to the paediatric age group. These initiatives have taken the form of groups meeting in various countries to establish consensus as to how best to approach the issues around *Helicobacter* infection in children. The consensus guidelines emanating from these groups have important practical implications for all practitioners involved in the care of children.

In this chapter the focus is on the special issues regarding children, i.e. the differences from adults. Thus, as a basis for the consensus recommendations, the sequelae of *H. pylori* infection in children are discussed, as is the relationship of symptoms to *H. pylori* infection. Also discussed are the processes by which consensus was achieved by groups in various countries. Finally, the recommendations themselves are outlined.

SEQUELAE OF *H. PYLORI* INFECTION IN CHILDREN

In children, as in adults, *H. pylori* infection causes gastritis[1]. It is associated with primary peptic ulcer diseases[2-4], and very rarely with MALT lymphoma[5]. The special aspects of these entities in children are outlined below.

However, to put this in context, it is important to point out that the great majority of children with *H. pylori* infection do not develop any of these disorders, nor do they develop symptoms attributable to the infection. This appears to be true of children even more so than of adults.

Primary peptic ulcer disease

While there is a paucity of prevalence figures in children, it is well accepted that primary peptic ulcer disease is much less common in children than adults. For example, in our own unit in a tertiary children's hospital with a referral population of some 3.5 million, we diagnose only about four to six new primary ulcers per year. Of these, duodenal ulcers are more prevalent than are gastric ulcers; in our experience over a 14-year period, with all ulcers diagnosed endoscopically, when NSAID-related ulcers are excluded, duodenal ulcers were some 25–30 times more prevalent than gastric ulcers. That some peptic ulcer disease is *H. pylori*-related in children is shown by studies in which antibiotic treatment alone resulted in the resolution and non-recurrence of duodenal ulcers[6,7].

While most primary peptic ulcers are *H. pylori*-related, a significant and apparently increasing proportion are *H. pylori*-negative or 'idiopathic'. This has implications for the approach to suspected ulcer disease, as discussed below. *H. pylori*-negative duodenal ulcer is an important entity present in about 15–20% of children with duodenal ulcers who have not taken NSAIDs and have no serological or histological evidence of *H. pylori*[1,8]; although there are few data in children, the figure may be higher, as has recently been shown in adults[9–11].

Gastritis

Although the infection is said to be acquired primarily in early childhood, in the US the prevalence of *H. pylori* gastritis in children appears to be age-dependent, with *H. pylori* accounting for few cases under the age of 5 years[12]. While the prevalence of *H. pylori* gastritis does appear to rise with age (to become, in our unit, the commonest identifiable cause of gastritis in teenagers) it is still relatively uncommon[1].

In children the commonest reported types of *H. pylori* gastritis are diffuse antral gastritis and non-ulcer pangastritis, but since paediatric reports seldom refer to corpus histology, pangastritis may be underreported[1]. In occasional children we have seen focal intestinal metaplasia in corpus and in antral biopsies, but without atrophy; therefore these findings are of questionable significance (Jevon G, Hassall E, Dimmick JE, unpublished observations). Experience from our own institution has shown the greatest severity of inflammation and highest diagnostic yields to be in the antrum, cardia and body, in that order (Jevon G, Hassall E, Dimmick JE, unpublished observations). In our own patients antral gastritis scores were higher in those with *H. pylori*-associated duodenal ulcer than in those without ulcers, and virtually absent in those with *H. pylori*-negative ulcer disease[3,8]. In a study from France the authors purported to demonstrate 'deterioration in the histologic features of the gastric mucosa' over a 2-year period in asymptomatic children infected with *H. pylori*[13]. However, there were major deficiencies in ascertainment of tissue and scoring of gastritis. These problems notwithstanding, the numbers they report indicate a degree of inflammation that appears to be minimal, even if it did increase slightly with time, in a tiny sample size of patients overall. Of most significance, there was no gastric atrophy or intestinal metaplasia seen.

Endoscopic and histological features in children

The severity and depth of *H. pylori* gastritis are variable but, in general, inflammation is most intense in the antrum, then cardia, and least in the body[14]; similarly, our own highest diagnostic yields of *H. pylori* have come from antrum, cardia, and corpus, in that order.

In *H. pylori* infection endoscopy may show normal gastric mucosa, or reveal erythema, erosions, ulcers and, especially in children, antral nodularity[1,15]. It has been our experience that, when *H. pylori* gastritis is associated with duodenal ulcer in children, a striking diffuse nodularity of the antrum is always present; when *H. pylori* causes gastritis alone ('primary gastritis'), this nodularity is seen in only some 50–60% of cases[3]. We have not seen this nodularity in cases of true non-*H. pylori* duodenal ulcer disease, nor in any of the some 5000 upper gastrointestinal endoscopies at which neither ulcer disease nor *H. pylori* was present over the past 14 years. Nodularity is sometimes not visible at first examination of the antrum but, once biopsies have been taken, oozing blood acts as a vital stain, making visible a confluent carpet of nodules; we have coined the term 'haematochromoendoscopy' for this phenomenon (Weinstein WM, Hassall E). The antral nodularity evident at endoscopy persists for months or years, even after eradication of *H. pylori* and ulcer healing.

The absence of endoscopic abnormalities in some 50% of children with *H. pylori* infection[3], and the patchy nature of the infection and of gastric MALT lymphomas, serves to emphasize the need to take biopsies from the gastric antrum, body and cardia, as an integral part of diagnostic endoscopy[14,16,17].

Whereas children with *H. pylori*-associated duodenal ulcers have a nodular antrum and impressive histological gastritis, those who are *H. pylori*-negative by histology plus serology or breath test have no nodularity, and virtual absence of histological gastritis[8]; it appears to be a different disease.

MALT lymphoma

Primary lymphoproliferative disorders of the stomach in children are low-grade and extremely rare, with some five pediatric cases reported in the past decade, and these have been responsive to eradication therapy for *H. pylori*[5].

Gastric adenocarcinoma

Fortunately, cancers of the gastrointestinal tract are rare in children, accounting for less than 5% of all malignancies in children[18,19]. Of these, only some 0.05% are primary gastric adenocarcinoma[20], the commonest primary gastric malignancies in children being lymphomas and sarcomas. Between 1960 and 1993 only 17 cases of primary gastric adenocarcinoma were reported under age 21 years; of these only one patient was under the age of 10 years, the rest being of median age 15 years[20].

CLINICAL PRESENTATIONS IN CHILDREN

Peptic ulcer disease

In the paediatric age group abdominal pain is a very common reason for seeking medical advice, and it is also the commonest presenting symptom of acid-peptic disorders in general. In children of age 10–12 years and above the symptoms may be similar to those in adults. While epigastric pain or discomfort, which is meal-related or -exacerbated, and particularly that which awakens the child from sleep often is a symptom of peptic ulcer disease[3,4,6], it is sometimes a presenting symptom of more common disorders such as non-ulcer dyspepsia, so-called 'recurrent abdominal pain', or constipation, or other peptic disorders, such as upper gastrointestinal Crohn's disease, allergic gastritis, etc. Younger children may not be able to localize the pain to the epigastrium, and may present with anorexia and irritability, especially with meals. Other presenting symptoms include anorexia, nausea, early satiety, recurrent vomiting or anaemia. Weight loss occurs less often. Gastrointestinal bleeding may occur with antecedent epigastric pain or other symptoms, but painless bleeding may be the only manifestation of ulcer disease; up to 25% of children with primary duodenal ulcers have this 'silent' presentation, while some 25% present with bleeding and antecedent pain, and the rest present with abdominal pain or recurrent vomiting[3,4]. Epigastric tenderness is an unreliable physical sign of gastritis or ulcer disease.

Symptoms and *H. pylori* primary gastritis

To date, several lines of evidence have shown that, in the absence of peptic ulcer disease, chronic *H. pylori* gastritis very seldom is the cause of abdominal pain in children. Serological studies have shown that some 30% of infected children are asymptomatic[21]. Furthermore, the prevalence of *H. pylori* antibodies is similar in children with recurrent abdominal pain to those who are asymptomatic[21,22]. In another study, of children coming to endoscopy, symptoms in those with *H. pylori* gastritis alone could not be differentiated from those without *H. pylori* infection[23].

In a study designed to determine whether eradication of *H. pylori* infection resulted in improvement or resolution of symptoms in children, Gormally et al. showed that *H. pylori* gastritis, in the absence of endoscopically proven ulcer disease, did not cause symptoms[24]. In that study, eradication of infection resulted in resolution of symptoms in all patients with ulcer diseases. In contrast, only some 30% of children with gastritis alone improved symptomatically, as did some in whom eradication failed. In a large multicentre study from Germany[25], symptom assessment could not distinguish between children with *H. pylori* gastritis, and 'functional pain'. In that study, of children with *H. pylori*-positive gastritis, symptoms improved or resolved in 87% of children with successful eradication of the organism, but also in 93% of those with failed eradication, and 80% of those with 'functional pain'.

An analysis of 45 paediatric reports showed that there was strong evidence for an association between *H. pylori* gastritis and duodenal ulcer disease in children, but weak evidence for an association with gastric ulcer, and weak or no evidence for an association with recurrent abdominal pain[26].

A major problem with all the paediatric studies is the short period of follow-up; a 4–8-week follow-up after eradication treatment does not allow for the likely presence of a placebo effect of both testing (e.g., endoscopy) and treatment. Longer follow-up studies are clearly necessary, with a randomized, double-blind, placebo-controlled design.

CONSENSUS GROUPS

The past 2 years have seen considerable activity directed towards setting up guidelines for a rational or evidence-based approach to suspected or established *H. pylori* disease in children. The first guidelines to be published pertaining specifically and solely to paediatric issues concerning *H. pylori* were those of the Canadian *Helicobacter* Study Group, in September 1999[27]. Some 10 months previously, in November 1998, a meeting was held in British Columbia, convened by the Study Group, comprising 30 participants representing the fields of paediatric and adult gastroenterology, infectious diseases, family medicine, epidemiology, government, and industry. Following a series of talks on issues relevant to *H. pylori* infection, workshop groups met to evaluate evidence, and recommend an approach to issues such as 'Whom to test', 'What diagnostic test/s to use', and 'Whom to treat'. The 'mini-consensus' of each working group was then presented to the group as a whole, and consensus achieved after debate on each issue.

In September 1998 the European Society for Pediatric Gastroenterology, Hepatology and Nutrition [ESPGHN] and the European *Helicobacter pylori* Study Group arranged a multidisciplinary meeting in Budapest, comprising 38 individuals from 19 countries. This very diverse group reached a consensus which was published in February 2000[28].

Beginning in September 1998 a group of nine individuals appointed by the North American Society for Pediatric Gastroenterology and Nutrition [NASPGN] began a process to establish clinical practice guidelines for managing *H. pylori* infection in childhood. This group, consisting of paediatric gastroenterologists, a general paediatrician, and an epidemiologist, used an evidence-based approach, ranking the quality of evidence available, and a 'nominal group technique' to achieve consensus; the latter required unanimous consensus by participants. The group 'convened' by means of several conference calls and one face-to-face meeting. Opinions and draft manuscripts were exchanged by e-mail. The group's recommendations were presented to the annual meeting of NASPGN in Denver in October 1999, and a draft manuscript will be sent out in April 2000 to some 600 members of NASPGN for comment. Submission for publication as an official position paper of the society is planned for June 2000.

In November 1998, the Japanese Society for Pediatric GI met in Kobe to address issues relevant to that country, and the process of reaching consensus is in progress.

Interestingly, the published recommendations of those groups that reached consensus, i.e. the Canadian and European paediatric groups[27,28], are virtually the same. This is somewhat remarkable, given the number and diversity of participants in the different consensus groups, and the somewhat different processes used to reach consensus.

The guidelines are summarized below.

General considerations behind the guidelines

The prevalence of gastric infection with *H. pylori* varies between countries and socioeconomic groups but, even where it is common, children are considerably less susceptible to peptic ulcers and other pathological sequelae than are adults. As a result the risk-to-benefit ratios of diagnostic studies and treatments for *H. pylori* are probably different in adult and paediatric populations; therefore, specific guidelines for approaches in children are required. Some of the rationale for these is as follows, with further comments given for each specific recommendation.

While abdominal pain and other gastrointestinal symptoms or signs are common in children, the prevalence of paediatric *H. pylori* infection in developed countries is low and, in the absence of peptic ulceration, *H. pylori* is rarely a cause of such symptoms[21-26]. Therefore *H. pylori* should be considered in the differential diagnosis of the cause of the child's symptoms only *after* other more common causes, and testing for *H. pylori* infection should not be part of the initial investigative strategy.

While certain diagnostic tests have greater up-front costs than others, the expense is often more apparent than real, as there are significant financial and social costs associated with failure to reach an accurate diagnosis. These include the costs of more tests, more doctor visits, inappropriate treatment, and missed school or work. It should not be surprising, therefore, that a more expensive test which is definitive may result in overall cost savings[29-31]. The cost–benefit of testing the large numbers of children who present with abdominal pain for a lower prevalence of peptic ulcer disease than in adults is likely to be considerably higher, on a case-by-case basis, than in adults. Simply put, there is probably higher cost of attempting to diagnose those relatively few peptic ulcers in children by using non-definitive testing, than there is in adults. When the cost of endoscopy is below certain levels[30,31], as it is in many countries or health-care systems, it becomes the most economical test to perform in children. This is in addition to the clear psychosocial benefits to children and families of prompt, accurate diagnosis.

Although eradication of infection is appropriate in the small number of children and adolescents with proven *H. pylori*-associated duodenal or gastric ulcer disease, there is no convincing evidence that cure benefits the much larger proportion of infected patients with gastritis alone.

Given these concerns, and the low prevalence of this infection in children in North America and Western Europe, a general test-and-treat approach was not considered prudent, evidence-based, or cost-effective.

Whom to test, how to test

1. Testing for *H. pylori* is appropriate only when treatment is planned if the test is positive.

2. The goal of diagnostic testing should be to determine the cause of presenting symptoms rather than the presence of *H. pylori* infection. Given the important distinction between *H. pylori* infection, and *H. pylori* disease, this is a central premise of the guidelines.
3. A test-and-treat strategy is not advised for the optimal care of children. This is discussed above.
4. Antibody tests utilizing whole blood, serum, or saliva are not recommended. The sensitivity and specificity of antibody assays in whole blood, serum and saliva are poor unless used in the populations in which they were initially developed. Furthermore, antibody levels may remain elevated for years after eradication or resolution of *H. pylori* infection, therefore a positive test does not necessarily mean that infection is present at the time of testing. In addition, the cut-off values for children are different from those in adults. These issues are discussed in detail elsewhere[32].
5. Upper gastrointestinal endoscopy with multiple biopsies is the optimal approach to investigation of the patient with chronic upper abdominal symptoms or suspected peptic ulcer disease. There is an extensive differential diagnosis of causes of upper gastrointestinal symptoms in a child. Endoscopy with biopsies is the only test that allows for rapid and definitive diagnosis of upper gastrointestinal mucosal diseases; prompt, accurate diagnosis usually enables institution of appropriate therapy, cessation of further testing, and a rapid return of the child to school and social activities. Endoscopy is the only acceptable diagnostic test in children with upper gastrointestinal bleeding, recurrent vomiting or persistent undiagnosed abdominal pain.

    Accurate diagnosis of the aetiology of peptic ulcer(s) obviously has important implications for treatment, as illustrated by the different treatments for *H. pylori*-associated and *H. pylori*-negative ulcer disease. When *Helicobacter*-negative ulcer disease is diagnosed, multiple biopsies of the stomach, duodenum, and oesophagus must be carefully examined for evidence of Crohn's disease; in addition, a fasting plasma gastrin level should be obtained to exclude one of the rare G-cell disorders or Zollinger–Ellison syndrome.

    However, the performance of endoscopy in children is a fairly specialized undertaking, the least problematic aspect of which is actual passage of an appropriate-sized endoscope, and the taking of biopsies, or intervention of endoscopic haemostasis. Many other cognitive and practical paediatric skills are important to ensure the appropriate, safe, and humane performance of endoscopy in children[33]. Drawbacks of the test are that it is invasive, more expensive than non-endoscopic tests, and availability is limited in some areas.
6. In children whose peptic ulcer was previously diagnosed by a contrast study, and who have recurrent or persistent symptoms, endoscopy with biopsies should be performed to confirm the presence of an ulcer and to determine whether *H. pylori* is present. Upper gastrointestinal contrast studies are notoriously inaccurate for the diagnosis of ulcer disease in children, with poor sensitivity, and a high rate of false-positivity. Reports

of duodenal 'spasm' or 'irritability', 'duodenitis', 'poor filling of the duodenal cap', and 'possible ulcer disease' are common in children and are not reliable predictors of the presence of ulcer disease[4,34,35]. Even when X-rays are said to show an ulcer/s definitively, their aetiology cannot be determined. Although antral nodularity associated with *H. pylori* disease may occasionally be seen on a contrast study, such nodularity often persists even when *H. pylori* infection is no longer present[3,6].

7. Urea breath tests are not an appropriate alternative to upper endoscopy for primary diagnosis of *H. pylori* infection in children. The sensitivity and specificity of labelled urea breath tests, which are non-invasive, are close to those of endoscopic biopsies for the presence of *H. pylori* infection. However, a positive breath test does not confirm or exclude the presence of disease-causing symptoms, such as an ulcer, other gastritides, gastropathies, or oesophageal disease. Similarly, in the event of a negative result, this indirect testing cannot rule out alternative diagnoses[36]. Results in adults and children are affected by current use of antibiotics, bismuth salts, and acid-suppressing medications, and by the presence of other non-urease-producing organisms, including flora resident in the oral cavity[37,38]. Breath testing is expensive, but it is less so than endoscopy. Use of the urea breath test is usually more appropriate than repeat endoscopy to confirm successful eradication of *H. pylori* infection.

8. Screening for *H. pylori* infection in asymptomatic individuals is not warranted. Screening for *H. pylori* infection is costly, and at this point in time has no established public health benefits in asymptomatic children.

9. Family members of previously infected patients who have benefited from *H. pylori* eradication can be considered for testing and treatment. It is rational, but unproven, that testing and treating family members for *H. pylori* infection may be justified by a possible reduced risk of reinfection in a child who has benefited from eradication. However, projected benefits should be weighed against the risks and costs of this strategy.

Whom to treat

In general, treatment should be given only after *H. pylori* disease has been accurately diagnosed. Eradication therapy is recommended for children who have both proven active *H. pylori* infection plus symptomatic gastrointestinal disease. Treatment is not generally recommended in the absence of either active infection or symptomatic disease. Proven active *H. pylori* infection is defined as either positive histopathology from endoscopic biopsy or a positive culture.

1. The indications for treatment are peptic ulcer disease proven to be current and associated with *H. pylori*, and MALT lymphoma. Abdominal pain which is not due to peptic ulcer disease is not an indication for treatment. However, if the presence of *H. pylori* infection is established to be current, whatever the indication for the test, treatment should be offered to the child.

2. Gastritis without peptic ulcer disease. The finding of *H. pylori* gastritis in the absence of peptic ulcer disease during diagnostic endoscopy poses a dilemma for the paediatric gastroenterologist. In adults and children there is insufficient evidence to support either initiating or withholding eradication treatment in this situation. The Canadian paediatric group recommended treatment following a positive test, no matter why the test was performed; the European group addressed only the issue of biopsy-proven *H. pylori*-positive gastritis, recommending treatment in this circumstance.

How to treat

Most paediatric treatment trials have been uncontrolled, and conducted in single centres with a small number of patients, using regimens proven to be effective in adults. Although these provide some evidence that regimens effective in adults will provide similar efficacy in children, there are important unanswered questions about the relative risk of adverse events and how, or whether, doses should be modified by chronological age, body weight or surface area. Due to a relative absence of data it is difficult to make specific recommendations that are rigorously evidence-based for treatment of *H. pylori* in children. Rather, data from some studies in children and some in adults are extrapolated with the understanding that modifications may be necessary once appropriate trials are conducted in the paediatric age group. It is important to recognize that the relative efficacy and the relative risk of adverse events may well be different in children from those in adults.

The currently recommended regimens generally include a proton pump inhibitor in combination with antibiotics. At this time, in adults, there do not appear to be major differences between the efficacy of omeprazole, lansoprazole, and pantoprazole, for healing peptic ulcers. However, at present, in children there is little published experience with lansoprazole, and even less with pantoprazole, but dosing regimens, efficacy and safety have been established for omeprazole use in children with erosive oesophagitis[39-41]. Although the regimens have not been well tested in children, one currently in favour includes omeprazole 1–2 mg/kg per day in two divided doses, plus clarithromycin with either metronidazole or amoxycillin in age-appropriate therapeutic doses, for 2 weeks[42]. Although 1-week therapy has been used[43], its efficacy in children requires further validation. The various regimens that have been used in children are summarized elsewhere[44].

References

1. Dohil R, Hassall E, Jevon G, Dimmick J. Gastritis and gastropathy of childhood. J Pediatr Gastroenterol Nutr. 1999;29:378–94.
2. Dohil R, Hassall E. Peptic ulcer disease in children. In: Tytgat GN, editor. Bailliere's Best Practice and Research in Clinical Gastroenterology. 2000;14:53–74.
3. Hassall E, Dimmick JE. Unique features of *Helicobacter pylori* disease in children. Dig Dis Sci. 1991;36:417–23.
4. Drumm B, Rhoads JM, Stringer DA, Sherman PMM, Ellis LE, Durie PR. Peptic ulcer disease in children: etiology, clinical findings, and clinical course. Pediatrics. 1988;82:410–14.
5. Blecker U, McKeithan, Hart J, Kirschner BS. Resolution of *Helicobacter pylori*-associated gastric lymphoproliferative disease in a child. Gastroenterology. 1995;109:973–7.

6. Israel DM, Hassall E. Treatment and long-term follow up of *Helicobacter pylori*-associated duodenal ulcer disease in children. J. Pediatr. 1993;123:53–8.
7. Rowland M, Imrie C, Bourke B, Drumm B. How should *Helicobacter pylori* infected children be managed? Gut. 1999;43:136–9.
8. Hassall E, Hiruki T, Dimmick JE. True *Helicobacter pylori*-negative duodenal ulcer disease in children. Gastroenterology. 1993;104:A96.
9. Peura DA. The problem of *H. pylori* negative idiopathic ulcer disease. In: Tytgat GN, editor. Baillier's Best Practice and Research in Clinical Gastroenterology. 2000;14:109–18.
10. Graham DY. Large U.S. clinical trials report a high proportion of *H. pylori* negative duodenal ulcers at study entry as well as a high recurrence rate after cure of the infection: have we all been wrong? Gastroenterology. 1998;114A:17.
11. Jyotheeswaran S, Shah AN, Jin HO, Potter GD, Ona FV, Chey WU. Prevalence of *Helicobacter pylori* in peptic ulcer patients in greater Rochester, NY: is empirical triple therapy justified? Am J Gastroenterol. 1998;93:574–8.
12. Snyder JD, Hardy SC, Thorne GM, Hirsch BZ, Antonioli DA. Primary antral gastritis in young American children. Low prevalence of *Helicobacter pylori* infections. Dig Dis Sci. 1994;39:1859–63.
13. Ganga-Zandzou PS, Michaud L, Vincent P et al. Natural outcome of *Helicobacter pylori* infection in asymptomatic children. Pediatrics. 1999;104:216–21.
14. Genta RM, Huberman RM, Graham DY. The gastric cardia in *H. pylori* infection. Hum Pathol. 1994;25:915–19.
15. Czinn SJ, Dahms BB, Jacobs GH et al. *Campylobacter*-like organisms in association with symptomatic gastritis in children. J Pediatr. 1986;109:80–3.
16. Sheu BS, Lin XZ, Yang HB, Su IJ. Cardiac biopsy of stomach may improve the detection of *H. pylori* after dual therapy. Gastroenterology. 1997;112:A288.
17. El-Zimaity HMT, Malaty HM, Graham DY. Need for biopsies targeted to the cardia, corpus and antrum in gastric MALT lymphoma. Gastroenterology, 1998;114:A591.
18. Pickett LK, Briggs HC. Cancer of the gastrointestinal tract in children. Pediatr Clin N Am. 1959;14:223–34.
19. Goldthorn JF, Canizaro PC. Gastrointestinal malignancies in infancy, childhood, and adolescence. Surg Clin N Am. 1986;66:845–61.
20. McGill TW, Downey EC, Westbrook J, Wade D, de la Garza J. Gastric carcinoma in children. J Pediatr Surg. 1993;28:1620–1.
21. van der Meer SB, Forget PP, Loffeld RJFL, Stobberingh E, Kuijten RH, Arends JW. The prevalence of *Helicobacter pylori* serum antibodies in children with recurrent abdominal pain. Eur J Pediatr. 1992;151:799–801.
22. Gormally SM, Drumm B. *Helicobacter pylori* and gastrointestinal symptoms. Arch Dis Child. 1994;70:165–6.
23. Reifen R, Rasooly I, Drumm B, Millson ME, Murphy K, Sherman PM. *Helicobacter pylori* infection in children: is there specific symptomatology? Dig Dis Sci. 1994;39:1488–92.
24. Gormally SM, Prakash N, Durnin MT et al. Association of symptoms with *Helicobacter pylori* infection in children. J Pediatr. 1995;126:753–6.
25. Koletzko S, Kindermann A, Faus-Kessler GSF et al. A prospective multi-center study on symptoms and outcome in children with abdominal pain with and without *Helicobacter pylori* [HP] infection. Gastroenterology 1999;116:A218.
26. MacArthur C, Saunders N, Feldman W. *Helicobacter pylori*, gastroduodenal disease, and recurrent abdominal pain in children. J Am Med Assoc. 1995;273:729–34.
27. Sherman P, Hassall E, Hunt RH et al. Canadian *Helicobacter* Study Group Consensus Conference on the approach to *H. pylori* infection in children and adolescents. Can J Gastroenterol. 1999;13:553–9.
28. Drumm B, Koletzko S, Oderda G, and the European Task Force on *Helicobacter pylori*. *Helicobacter pylori* infection in children. A consensus statement. J Pediatr Gastroenterol Nutr. 2000;31:207–14.
29. Sonnenberg A. Cost–benefit analysis of testing for *Helicobacter pylori* in dyspeptic subjects. Am J Gastroenterol. 1996;9:1773–7.
30. Fendrick AM, Chernew ME, Hirth RA, Bloom BS. Alternative management strategies for patients with suspected peptic ulcer disease. Ann Intern Med. 1995;123:260–8.
31. Olsen AD, Fendrick M, Deutsch D et al. Evaluation of initial noninvasive therapy in pediatric patients presenting with suspected ulcer disease. Gastrointest Endosc. 1996;44:554–61.

32. Nedrud JG, Czinn SJ. Host, heredity and *Helicobacter*. Gut. 1999;45:323–4.
33. Hassall E. NASPGN Position Paper: Requirements for training to ensure competence of endoscopists performing invasive procedures in children. J Pediatr Gastroenterol Nutr. 1997;24:345–7.
34. Gyepes MT, Smith LE, Ament ME. Fiberoptic endoscopy and upper gastrointestinal series: comparative analysis in infants and children. Am J Roentgenol. 1977;128:53–6.
35. Liebman W. Fiberoptic endoscopy of the gastrointestinal tract in infants and children. Am J Gastroenterol. 1977;68:362–6.
36. Jones NL, Bourke B, Sherman PM. Breath testing for *Helicobacter pylori* infection in children: a breath of fresh air? J Pediatr. 1997;131:791–3.
37. Bazzoli F, Zagari M, Fossi S et al. Urea breath test for the detection of *Helicobacter pylori* infection. Helicobacter. 1997;2:S34–7.
38. Kalach N, Benhamou PH, Briet F, Raymond J, Dupont C. The ^{13}carbon urea breath test for the noninvasive detection of *Helicobacter pylori* in children: comparison with culture and determination of minimum analysis requirements. J Pediatr Gastroenterol Nutr. 1998;26:291–6.
39. Gunasekaran TS, Hassall E. Efficacy and safety of omeprazole for gastroesophageal reflux in children. J Pediatr. 1993;123:148–54.
40. Hassall E, Israel DM, Shepherd R, Radke M, Dalväg A, Junghard O, Lundborg P, and the International Pediatric Omeprazole Study Group. Omeprazole for chronic erosive esophagitis in children: a multicenter study of dose requirements for healing: an interim report. Gastroenterology. 1997;112:A143.
41. Hassall E. For the International Pediatric Omeprazole Study Group. Omeprazole for maintenance therapy of erosive esophagitis in children. Gastroenterology. 2000;118:A658.
42. Dohil R, Israel DM, Hassall E. Effective two-week antibiotic therapy for *H. pylori* disease in children. Am J Gastroenterol. 1997;92:244–7.
43. Walsh D, Goggin N, Rowland M, Durnin M, Moriarty S, Drumm B. One week treatment for *Helicobacter pylori* infection. Arch Dis Child. 1997;76:352–5.
44. Gold BD. Current therapy for *H. pylori* infection in children and adolescents. Can J Gastroenterol. 1999;13:571–9.

63
What role for clarithromycin in the treatment of *Helicobacter pylori* infection?

R. CLANCY, T. BORODY and C. CLANCY

Antibiotic-induced eradication provides a platform for the management of *Helicobacter pylori* infection. The continuous evaluation of optimal eradication therapies has been driven by analysis of outcomes of sequential clinical trials, which include three antimicrobial agents. A combination of triple antimicrobial therapy (bismuth/metronidazole/tetracycline) established the gold standard with reported eradication rates in excess of 90%. Concern regarding side-effects and a complicated regimen led to alternative strategies. Dual therapy, which included a single antibiotic, gave unreliable and variable results (20–90% eradication), giving way to numerous trials of 'modified' triple therapies, especially a proton pump inhibitor (PPI) + clarithromycin, and either metronidazole or amoxycillin. Eradication rates of around 90% in some of these trials has led to the widespread use of 'modified' triple-therapy regimens, which include clarithromycin for primary eradication of *H. pylori* infection. However, data have accumulated to seriously question the widespread use of clarithromycin in therapeutic regimens for primary eradication in Western countries.

The question of the role of clarithromycin in the management of *H. pylori* infection must be considered within a broader framework of management of this and other infective diseases. An emerging problem in the Western world is that of symptomatic infection that has not been eradicated by antibiotics. For example, in Australia, about 60 000 patients are treated for *H. pylori* infection each year, with in excess of 20% per annum (say 12 000) failing to eradicate the organism. Although risk factors – in terms of the bacteria, the antibiotic regimen, and compliance – can be identified, eradication failure is neither predictable nor well understood. What is clear, however, is that there is an increasing reservoir of resistant *H. pylori* of which many are now resistant to major antibiotics used for their eradication. Clinicians are seeing more patients with persistent disease following failed eradication therapy, and cure of the infection becomes increasingly more difficult with recurrent 'eradication' therapy. Despite the increase in antibiotic resistance within the *H. pylori* 'pool' following failed eradication, failure cannot be accounted for entirely in terms of traditional clinical or microbiological factors. Host factors, as a cause of eradication failure, take on a particular interest when it is recognized that antibiotic-induced reduction in antigen load is followed by a shift in the mucosal T lymphocyte cytokine repertoire towards a Th0 pattern[1], which may reflect impaired host resistance. It follows that, for the management of *H. pylori* infection, the best antibiotic regimen should be used for primary eradication, mindful of both antibiotic sensitivities and practical considerations related to compliance. The best opportunity to eradicate the bacterium is with primary treatment, chosen with an optimal 'salvage' therapeutic regimen in mind.

Clarithromycin is a 14-membered ring macrolide antibiotic, a derivative of erythromycin, compared with which it has a similar spectrum of activity and clinical uses, but is more acid-resistant, has more consistent absorption, and has a longer half-life. Clarithromycin was trialled although never advocated as a single antibiotic for the treatment of *H. pylori* infection in the early 1990s, but monotherapy gave a poor response and was linked to the development of resistance[2]. By the mid-1990s confidence in a primal position for clarithromycin was reflected in industry statements such as 'needlessly adding a second antibiotic to the highly effective ranitidine bismuth citrate plus clarithromycin regimen is unwarranted'[3]. However, statements from the ACG Practice Parameters Committee concerning 'the impact of clarithromycin resistance on subsequent response to antibiotic combinations' voiced contemporary caution[4]. Results showing 90% *H. pylori* eradication using clarithromycin in triple-therapy regimens led to widespread use of this antibiotic, but review of data relevant to changing patterns of drug resistance, and consideration of the wider issues in the management of *H. pylori* infection, suggest review of this practice.

First, significant increases in resistance to clarithromycin throughout the Western world through the second half of the 1990s have been described. Initial levels of resistance of 0–2%[5,6] in isolates from untreated patients encouraged an optimistic future, and were supported by high eradication rates in therapeutic trials. However, by the late 1990s significantly higher levels of resistance were being described from multiple Western centres[7–9], commonly at the level of 8–15%, with higher and increasing levels reported in some countries[10]. This is consistent with recent data on triple therapy containing clarithromycin given over 1 week. Lamouliatte *et al.* reported a meta-analysis of French studies, which included 434 patients given a PPI, clarithromycin and amoxycillin, and found an eradication rate of 75%[11], while three similar studies in the USA reported intent-to-treat eradication rates of 69%, 73%, and 83%[12]. Quadruple therapy, which included ranitidine bismuth citrate, gave an eradication rate of 78%, contrasting significantly with the over 90% eradication reported several years before[13]. These latter studies are of interest in the context of the emergence of clarithromycin-resistant strains of *H. pylori*, which were described as an 'important new phenomenon in the United States'[14]. The prevalence of clarithromycin resistance in the United States increased from 4% in 1993–4, to 12.6% in 1995–6, due in part to an increase in patients with failed therapy[15]. Of particular concern in this US study was the increase in secondary resistance (to 25%) over a short period. Recently developed molecular techniques identifying defects in binding of macrolides to the 23S rRNA components of the bacterial ribosome[16] demonstrate an even higher incidence of bacterial variants compared to conventional methods.

Second, resistance to clarithromycin reduces the response rate to eradication therapy containing that antibiotic (see also above). While some consider that resistance to metronidazole can be overcome by the addition of clarithromycin, but not amoxycillin, to the therapeutic regimen, clarithromycin resistance generally predicts failure of eradication therapy, especially if associated with metronidazole resistance[17]. In a study of 102 consecutive patients in Spain[18], eradication in patients with clarithromycin-resistant *H. pylori* infection was 20% vs 83% in patients with sensitive strains ($p < 0.001$). The authors conclude that 'the 80% efficiency goal will be difficult to reach in areas with a high (>10%) primary clarithromycin resistance if currently recommended proton pump inhibitor–triple therapies are used'.

Third, there is a profound and rapid increase in clarithromycin resistance in isolates from patients with failed therapy. In most Western studies this incidence has been 25–30%[19], though levels of around 60% are reported in Europe and Asia[20]. A potential risk with clarithromycin-based therapy is the occurrence of clonal expansion of resistant mutants in multiple-strain infections[21], due to selection.

Fourth, there has been insufficient regard for the importance of resistance to metronidazole in determining the failure of clarithromycin-containing dual antibiotic eradication regimens, as a number of trials suggest little downside to subjects with primary resistance to metronidazole, provided clarithromycin is included in the triple-therapy regimen. An important study by Buckley *et al.*[22] used standard 1-week triple therapy, containing metronidazole and clarithromycin, in 87 patients with primary metronidazole and clarithromycin resistance rates of 36% and 3.5%, respectively. The overall eradication rate was 81%; for sensitive isolates it was 98%, but was significantly reduced (57%) for isolates resistant to metronidazole and 0% in cases of dual resistance ($p < 0.001$). Secondary resistance to clarithromycin, however, was 58%. The presence of metronidazole resistance can thus be a significant cause of treatment failure with triple therapy, leading to selection of strains with dual resistance that are difficult to eradicate, and may contribute to the increasing prevalence of clarithromycin resistance in the community.

Fifth, the extensive use of macrolide antibiotics in general, and clarithromycin in particular, which is anticipated to be used more extensively for 'new' infections such as *Chlamydia pneumoniae*, is expected to increase community levels of antibiotic resistance. This concern has led to a reluctance in some countries, such as Finland, to use clarithromycin for *H. pylori* eradication, because macrolides are currently the most effective antibiotic for other serious infectious diseases[23]. The rapid increase in resistance, seen in primary infections, may in part reflect this mechanism.

Sixth is the major 'new' problem of large numbers in the West who have failed eradication therapy. This is discussed in general terms above, identifying two principles: (a) the best 'rescue' treatment is effective primary eradication; (b) primary eradication must be begun, with a plan for management of eradication failure in mind. Tytgat, in his 'reflections for the next millennium'[24], highlights the falling percentage of peptic ulcer disease patients in eradication trials, with a predicted decrease in eradication rates, because *H. pylori* infection in chronic dyspepsia patients appears more resistant to eradication. It is likely that altered host–parasite relationships underlie infection in subjects with non-ulcer gastritis, emphasizing the importance of developing new strategies for the eradication, or control of infection in these patients, given the stepped-up resistance to antibiotic therapy in those who repeatedly fail therapy.

WHAT IS THE ROLE OF CLARITHROMYCIN?

We believe clarithromycin has little or no role in primary eradication therapy, except perhaps in those subjects with duodenal ulcer in communities with low levels (<2%) of clarithromycin resistance, where the convenience, effectiveness and acceptance of clarithromycin-containing triple therapy have been demonstrated. The inclusion of bismuth (as ranitidine–bismuth citrate) may be useful, given evidence that this combination does not appear to generate significant clarithromycin resistance in those who fail to eradicate *H. pylori* following therapy[25]. The importance of drug interactions with clarithromycin remains a conditioning factor[26].

The major place for clarithromycin-containing therapy is in those patients failing to eradicate *H. pylori* following primary therapy and who have *H. pylori* sensitivity to clarithromycin. In this group eradication rates of 80% can be expected. Again, combination with bismuth maybe important[25].

H. pylori-related gastritis has changed dramatically over the past 10 years, in part due to 'cure' of those with peptic ulcer disease, and in part due to subtle changes in the host–parasite relationship, possibly contributed to by the widespread and inappropriate use of antibiotics. This latter issue is perhaps less understood with *H. pylori* infection than it is for episodic infections. The 1990s has witnessed the coming, and the re-assessment, of clarithromycin as a lead antibiotic in the eradication of *H. pylori* infection. There is nothing new in this, in the saga of infectious disease. The answer is to be smart about how we use clarithromycin. In our view we need to be very smart and very quick, before the macrolides are relegated to the history of chronic gastritis. The future will be to better understand those host and parasite factors that make a difference to the outcome of infection.

References

1. Ren Z, Pang G, Lee R et al. The circulating T cell response to *Helicobacter pylori* infection in chronic gastritis. Helicobacter (Submitted).
2. Peterson W, Graham DY, Marshall B. Clarithromycin as monotherapy for eradication of *Helicobacter pylori*: a randomised double blind trial. Am J Gastroenterol. 1993;88:1860–4.
3. Webb DD. 'Letter'. J Am Med Assoc. 1996;276:1136.
4. Soll AH. 'Letter'. J Am Med Assoc. 1996;276:1136–7.
5. Van Zwet AA, Bner WA, Schneeberger P et al. Prevalence of primary *Helicobacter pylori* resistance to metronidazole and clarithromycin in the Netherlands. Eur J Clin Microbiol Infect. 1996;115:861–4.
6. Glupezynski Y, Binette A, Lang P et al. Evolution of primary resistance to antimicrobial agents in Belgium between 1995 and 1998. Gut. 1998;43:A48.

7. Iovene MR, Romano M, Pelloni AP et al. Prevalence of antimicrobial resistance in 80 clinical isolates of *H. pylori*. Chemotherapy. 1999;45:8–14.
8. Xia HY, Buckley M, Keene C et al. Clarithromycin resistance in *H. pylori* prevalence in untreated dyspeptic patients. J Antimicrobial Chemother. 1996;37:473–81.
9. Cayla R, Lamouliatte H, Brugmann D et al. Pre-treatment resistances of *H. pylori* to metronidazole and macrolides. Acta Gastroenterol Belg. 1993;56:65.
10. Fedorak R, Archombault A, Flamm R et al. Antimicrobial susceptibility of *H. pylori* in Canada. Gastroenterology. 1997;112:A115.
11. Lamouliatte H, Cayla R. *H. pylori* eradication with a one week triple therapy: meta analysis of French studies. Gastroenterology. 1998;114:A194.
12. Laine L, Suchiver L, Connors A et al. Twice daily triple therapy with omeprazole, amoxycillin and clarithromycin for *H. pylori* eradication in duodenal ulcer disease: results of 3 multicenter double blind US trials. Gastroenterology. 1998;114:A193.
13. Smoat DT, Hinds T, Ashktorab V et al. Effectiveness of a ranitidine bismuth citrate triple therapy for treating *H. pylori*. Gastroenterology. 1998;114:A290.
14. Vakil N, Cutler A. Ten-day triple therapy with ranitidine bismuth citrate, amoxycillin, and clarithromycin in eradicating *H. pylori*. Am J Gastroenterol. 1999;94:1197–9.
15. Vakil N, Hahn B, McSorley D. Clarithromycin-resistant *H. pylori* in patients with duodenal ulcer in the United States. Am J Gastroenter. 1998;93:1432–5.
16. von Doorn L, Debets-Ossenkopp Y, Morais A et al. Rapid detection by PCR and reverse hydridization of mutations in the *Helicobacter pylori* 23S rRNA gene, associated with macrolide resistance. Antimicrob Agents Chemother. 1999;43:1779–82.
17. Adamek R, Suerbaum S, Pfaffenbach B et al. Primary and acquired *H. pylori* resistance to clarithromycin, metronidazole and amoxycillin – influence on treatment outcome. Am J Gastroenterol. 1998;93:380–9.
18. Ducons J, Santolaria S, Guiro R et al. Impact of clarithromycin resistance on the effectiveness of a regimen for *H. pylori*: a prospective study of 1-week lansoprazole, ampicillin, and clarithromycin in active peptic ulcer. Aliment Pharmacol Ther. 1999;13:775–80.
19. Boyanova L, Spassova Z, Krastev Z et al. Characteristics of trends in macrolide resistance among *H. pylori* strains isolated in Bulgaria over four years. Diag Microbiol Infect Dis. 1999;34:309–13.
20. Megraud F, Doermann HP. Clinical relevance of resistant strains of *H. pylori*: a review of current data. Gut. 1998;43:S61–5.
21. Matsuoka M, Yoshida Y, Hayakawa R et al. Simultaneous colonisation of *H. pylori* with and without mutations in the 23S rRNA gene in patients with no history of clarithromycin exposure. Gut. 1999;45:503–7.
22. Buckley MJ, Xia HX, Hyde D et al. Metronidazole resistance reduces efficiency of triple therapy and leads to secondary clarithromycin resistance. Dig Dis Sci. 1997;42:2111–15.
23. Bayerdorffer E, Kind T, Dite P et al. Omeprazole, amoxycillin, and metronidazole for the cure of *H. pylori* infection. Eur J Gastroenterol Hepatol. 1999;11:S19–22.
24. Tytgat G. *Helicobacter pylori* – reflections for the next millennium. Gut. 1999;45:145–7.
25. Midolo PD, Lambert JR, Kerr TG. Ranitidine bismuth citrate can overcome *in-vitro* antibiotic resistance to *H. pylori*. Gut. 1997;41:A12.
26. Choosing a macrolide. Prescrire Int. 1999;8:183–7.

64
What is the role of bismuth in *Helicobacter pylori* antimicrobial resistance?

S. VELDHUYZEN VAN ZANTEN and N. CHIBA

INTRODUCTION

Bismuth compounds have been used as therapeutic agents for more than two centuries. Use of bismuth compounds is well established in the treatment of *Helicobacter pylori*-associated gastritis and *H. pylori*-associated duodenal and gastric ulcers.[1-4] There is also convincing evidence that bismuth compounds are efficacious in the treatment of traveller's diarrhoea[3,5], acute diarrhoea in children[3,5], dyspepsia[6], microscopic colitis[7] and ulcerative colitis[8,9], although bismuth-containing compounds are not the current standard of care. In microbiology there are opportunities for bismuth regimens in the future. Apart from activity against *H. pylori* infection there is also evidence for antibacterial activity of bismuth compounds against *Salmonella*, *Treponema*, *Neisseria* and more recently *Clostridium difficile*[5,10].

FUNDAMENTAL CHEMISTRY OF BISMUTH COMPOUNDS

The fundamental chemistry of bismuth compounds is poorly understood[5]. Marked differences in the pharmacological behaviour of different bismuth preparations exist, but it is not appropriate to assume that all bismuth compounds will have similar activity in the gastrointestinal tract[5,11-13]. This is also true for the use of bismuth compounds in the treatment of *H. pylori* infection[14,15].

Surprisingly, the exact chemical structure of bismuth subsalicylate (BSS, PeptoBismol®) and colloidal bismuth subcitrate (CBS, Denol®) is not known[5]. It is clear that the chemical structure of these compounds is very complex. The proposed structures for BSS and CBS are shown in Figure 1[5]. Several structures have been proposed for colloidal bismuth subcitrate (CBS) but none of them can be considered definitive to date. Figure 1 shows one of the proposed structures for CBS[5]. It consists of a citrate anion ($C_6H_4O_7^{4-}$)

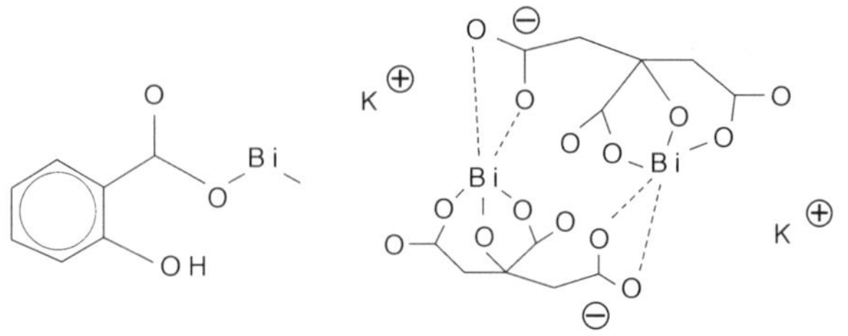

Figure 1. Proposed structures of BSS and CBS (adapted from ref. 5); exact structures are unknown.

intimately bound to elemental bismuth molecules, which are located in the centre, surrounded by an appropriate number of potassium or ammonium (NH_4) cations to balance the charge and finally coordinated with numerous water molecules[5]. One of the proposed formulations[5] for CBS is tripotassium dicitrato bismuthate $K_3(NH_4)_2Bi_6O_3(OH)_5(C_6H_5O_7)_4$. This is the chemical formula for CBS listed in the Merck Index, and obviously a very complex structure. In contrast to BSS and CBS, much more is known about the exact structure of the newly developed bismuth compound ranitidine bismuth citrate (RBC, Pylorid®)[16,17]. This compound is highly soluble in water.

Apart from a poor understanding of the fundamental chemistry it is also largely unknown what happens to bismuth compounds in the acidic environment of the stomach. The low pH and the aqueous environment of the stomach will alter bismuth compounds. There is speculation that the preferred bismuth compounds in the stomach may be bismuthyl ion (BiO+) which is not very water-soluble, followed by bismuth oxychloride (BiOCl), which is highly water-soluble[5].

RESISTANCE TO ANTIBIOTICS

The mechanisms by which bismuth acts against *H. pylori* organisms are largely unknown[5]. Like other heavy metals such as zinc and nickel, bismuth compounds do interfere with the activity of the urease enzyme[18], the high activity of which is a characteristic feature of the organism. There is evidence that bismuth is directly bactericidal, although the minimal inhibitory concentration (MIC) and bactericidal concentrations are relatively high for *H. pylori*[5,14,15]. Other proposed mechanisms include interference with the mucosal attachment of *H. pylori* organisms to surface epithelial cells and changes in the mucous microenvironment and mucosal surface[2,5,16,19].

BISMUTH AND ANTIMICROBIAL RESISTANCE

Primary resistance is defined as resistance to antibiotics that was present prior to treatment. Secondary resistance is resistance which develops following treatment in strains which were originally sensitive. The study by Goodwin *et al.* reported in 1988 was the first to suggest that the use of bismuth compounds could prevent the development of secondary resistance[20]. The study showed that 70% of *H. pylori* strains recovered from patients treated with the dual combination cimetidine and tinidazole became resistant following failed attempted eradication, as compared to only 9% of strains from patients treated with a combination of CBS and tinidazole[20].

Williamson and Pipkin wrote an excellent review on the question of whether the use of bismuth compounds can prevent or overcome resistance to antibiotics, in a previous edition of this book[21]. They addressed the same questions that will be addressed in this review. Three aspects will be discussed on the topic of bismuth and resistance, and these are:

1. the addition *in vitro* of bismuth to antibiotics leads to synergy in bacterial effect
2. addition of a bismuth compound may help overcome primary resistance
3. addition of bismuth may help prevent the development of secondary resistance.

IDENTIFICATION OF RELEVANT STUDIES

The literature on this topic is difficult to review, as few studies are available which compare the different treatment regimens head to head. Several studies to date have been published only in abstract form. Many studies did not test the *H. pylori* strains for resistance to antibiotics. A problem in reviewing this topic is that antibiotic resistance of *H. pylori* organisms is poorly defined in the literature. This is especially true for metronidazole resistance. For metronidazole resistance most studies use either an E-test or the agar dilution method. Usually strains with MICs greater than 8 µg/ml or 16 µg/ml are considered resistant. There is much more uniformity in the way that clarithromycin resistance is defined. Usually *H. pylori* strains with MICs >2 µg/ml are classified as resistant to clarithromycin.

THE IMPACT OF TREATMENT SUCCESS ON RESISTANCE

What is clear from the literature is that *the most important predictor for overcoming primary resistance and prevention of secondary resistance is the use of a treatment regimen which has a high cure rate of the infection.* This is more important than any other aspect of the treatments used. Currently, the highest cure rates are achieved with the combination of a proton pump inhibitor or the RBC bismuth compound together with clarithromycin and either amoxycillin or metronidazole[22–26]. Both regimens achieve cure of the infection in 80–85% of cases. A good alternative, but more complicated regimen, is quadruple therapy consisting of a proton pump inhibitor together with 'classic' bismuth triple therapy consisting of a bismuth compound, metronidazole and tetracycline[27–29]. The success rate of this therapy is similar to the proton pump inhibitor or RBC-based triple therapies, or perhaps slightly higher.

IN-VITRO EVIDENCE FOR SYNERGY OF BISMUTH COMPOUNDS WITH ANTIBIOTICS IN KILLING CAPACITY AND PREVENTION OF RESISTANCE

This topic was carefully reviewed by Williamson and Pipkin[2]. *In vitro* there are convincing data that there is a synergistic rather than an additive effect when RBC is combined with clarithromycin or metronidazole[21,30]. This synergy was also found in *H. pylori* strains that were resistant to clarithromycin[21,30–32]. However, generally speaking *in-vitro* evidence for anti-*Helicobacter* activity is not a good predictor for clinical efficacy. Therefore, it is unclear what the clinical significance of this observation is. Studies confirming this synergy *in vivo* have not been reported. There are also *in-vitro* data demonstrating that in the presence of RBC fewer strains became resistant to metronidazole or clarithromycin when those drugs were added to the culture plates[21,33,34].

DUAL THERAPY DATA AND PRIMARY RESISTANCE

There is some evidence that ranitidine bismuth citrate (RBC) when given with clarithromycin for 14 days is able to overcome primary resistance better as compared to the combination of omeprazole and clarithromycin for 14 days. This was shown in the study by Megraud *et al.* in which 11/12 (92%) strains which were resistant prior to treatment were eradicated compared to 3/8 (38%) treated with the omeprazole combination[35]. In clarithromycin-susceptible and intermediate resistant strains the success rate of therapy was 82% (208 of 254). The study of Megraud *et al.* was carried out in Europe. The results, however, could not be confirmed in a US study reported by Perschy *et al.*[36]. In this study the combination of RBC and clarithromycin given for 14 days was successful in only 3/38 (8%) strains that were resistant prior to treatment.

DUAL THERAPY DATA AND SECONDARY RESISTANCE

There is also evidence that the combination of RBC and clarithromycin may prevent secondary resistance. In the same study by Megraud *et al.* as reported above, RBC and clarithromycin given for 14 days led to development of secondary clarithromycin resistance in only one of 39 patients (3%)[35]. This was significantly lower than seen in the 14-day combination of omeprazole and clarithromycin, in which eight of 44 patients (18%) acquired secondary resistance to clarithromycin. The difference between the two groups was just below the conventional significance level, $p = 0.046$.

Osato *et al.*, in another study of 446 patients, found that acquired clarithromycin resistance occurred in 19/29 (66%) of patients who failed the RBC and clarithromycin combination[37]. This is in contrast to the omeprazole–clarithromycin combination in which 41/49 (84%) strains in patients in whom eradication was not successful turned out to be resistant to clarithromycin. The difference in resistance frequency was statistically significant ($p < 0.05$). These data suggest that the addition of RBC may reduce the development of secondary resistance. It should be noted that the rate of acquired resistance was markedly different between these two studies, but the reasons for this difference are unknown.

Although the dual therapy data with RBC and clarithromycin are interesting, the clinical relevance of the findings is minimal as dual therapy is not recommended, since better results can be obtained with triple therapy consisting of RBC and clarithromycin together with either metronidazole or amoxycillin.

TRIPLE THERAPY DATA

There are interesting data concerning the combination of bismuth compounds given together with metronidazole (M) and tetracycline (T)[38,39]. In the study reported by Kung *et al.* the cure rate overall of *H. pylori* infection was 46/50 (92%) for RBC given together with metronidazole and tetracycline as compared to 41/50 (84%) for the combination of CBS and metronidazole and tetracycline[38]. The RBC–MT combination was also better able to overcome metronidazole resistance, as 25/25 (100%) of resistant strains were eradicated compared to 12/16 (75%) for CBS–MT[38]. This study supports the contention that there may be differences among bismuth compounds in their anti-*Helicobacter* activity. As with the studies mentioned above, this result was repeated in another study from the United States in which RBC–MT given for 7 or 10 days led to cure of the infection in only 60% of strains[39]. Currently, triple therapy consisting of bismuth with metronidazole and tetracycline is uncommonly used as first-line therapy.

Finally, there are interesting data concerning RBC triple therapy with clarithromycin and metronidazole being able to overcome metronidazole resistance. In a recent study, published only in abstract form, the results of nine clinical trials were pooled[40]. It was shown that the relative risk of overcoming metronidazole resistance was 1.18 (95% confidence interval 1.03–1.46) when compared to the combination of a proton pump inhibitor given together with clarithromycin and metronidazole. This result was not explained by an overall higher eradication rate with the combination of RBC and clarithromycin and metronidazole, which was estimated to be around 87%. These data do suggest that, when clarithromycin is used with metronidazole and RBC, there may be a slight advantage over the use of similar proton pump inhibitor combinations.

CONCLUSION

Much of the fundamental chemistry of bismuth compounds is poorly understood. It is unknown how bismuth compounds help kill *H. pylori*. Data are suggestive, but not conclusive, that bismuth compounds may help to overcome primary resistance and prevent the development of secondary resistance. The evidence is strongest for the dual combination of ranitidine bismuth citrate and clarithromycin. There is some evidence that the triple combination of RBC together with clarithromycin and metronidazole is better able to overcome metronidazole than the combination of a proton pump inhibitor with the same two antibiotics but further studies are required to confirm this observation.

Acknowledgement

Dr Veldhuyzen van Zanten is the recipient of a Nova Scotia Clinical Scholar Award.

References

1. Lambert JR. Clinical indications and efficacy of colloidal bismuth subcitrate. Scand J Gastroenterol. 1991;26(Suppl. 185):13–21.
2. Marhall BJ, Armstrong JA, Francis GJ, Nokes NT, Wee SH. Antibacterial action of bismuth in relation to *Campylobacter pyloridis* colonization and gastritis. Digestion. 1987; 37(Suppl. 2):16–30.
3. Gorbach SL. Bismuth therapy in gastrointestinal diseases. Gastroenterology. 1990; 99:863–75.
4. Tillman LA, Drake FM, Dixon JS, Wood JR. Review article: Safety of bismuth in the treatment of gastrointestinal diseases. Aliment Pharmacol Ther. 1996;10:459–67.
5. Bryant GG, Burford N. Bismuth compounds in preparations with biological or medicinal relevance. Chem Rev. 1999;99:2601–57.
6. Hailey FJ, Newsom JH. Evaluation of bismuth subsalicylate in relieving symptoms of indigestion. Arch Intern Med. 1984;144:269–72.
7. Fine KD, Lee EL. Efficacy of open-label bismuth subsalicylate for the treatment of microscopic colitis. Gastroenterology. 1998;114:29–36.
8. Gionchetti P, Rizzello F, Venturi A *et al.* Long-term efficacy of bismuth carbomer enemas in patients with treatment-resistant chronic pouchitis. Aliment Pharmacol Ther. 1997; 11:673–8.
9. Pobbioli G, Miglioli M, Campieri M. Long-term efficacy of bismuth carbomer enemas in patients with treatment-resistant chronic pouchitis. Aliment Pharmacol Ther. 1997; 11:673–8.
10. Mahony DE, Lim-Morrison S, Bryden L *et al.* Antimicrobial activities of synthetic bismuth compounds against *Clostridium difficile*. Antimicrob Agents Chemother. 1999;43:582–8.
11. Sandha GS, LeBlanc R, Veldhuyzen van Zanten SJO *et al.* Chemical structure of bismuth compounds determines their gastric ucler healing efficacy and anti-*Helicobacter pylori* activity. Dig Dis Sci. 1998;43:2727–32.
12. Koo J, Ho J, Lam SK, Wong J Ong GB. Selective coating of gastric ulcer by tripotassium dicitrato bismuthate in the rat. Gastroenterology. 1982;82:864–70.
13. Nwokolo CU, Lewin JF, Hudson M, Pounder RE. Transmucosal penetration of bismuth particles in the human stomach. Gastroenterology. 1992;102:163–7.
14. Burford N, Veldhuyzen van Zanten SJO, Agocs L *et al.* Anti-*Helicobacter pylori* properties of new bismuth compounds. Gastroenterology. 1994;106:A59.
15. Midolo PD, Norton A, von Itzstein M, Lambert JR. Novel bismuth compounds have *in vitro* activity against *Helicobacter pylori*. FEMS Microbiol Lett. 1997;15:229–32.
16. Stables R, Campbell CJ, Clayton NM *et al.* Gastric anti-secretory, mucosal protective, antipepsin and anti-*Helicobacter* properties of ranitidine bismuth citrate. Aliment Pharmacol Ther. 1993;7:237–46.
17. Sadler PJ, Sun H. Ranitidine bismuth (III) citrate. J Chem Soc Dalton Trans. 1995; 1395–401.
18. Kodak Ektachem Clinical Products Division. Ammonia Test Methodology. Publication MP2-33, 1985.
19. Elder JB. Recent experimental and clinical studies on the pharmacology of colloidal bismuth subcitrate. Pharmacology of CBS. Scand J Gastroenterol. 1986;21(Suppl.122):14–16.
20. Goodwin CS, Marshall BJ, Blincow ED, Wilson DH, Blackburn S, Phillips M. Prevention of nitroimidazole resistance in *Campylobacter pylori* by co-administration of colloidal bismuth subcitrate: clinical and *in vitro* studies. J Clin Pathol. 1998;41:207–10.

21. Williamson R, Pipkin GA. Does bismuth prevent antimicrobial resistance of *Helicobacter pylori*? In: Hunt RH, Tytgat GN, editors. Bismuth and eradication of *H. pylori*. Basic Mechanisms to Clinical Cure 1998. Lancaster: Kluwer; 1998:416–25.
22. Lind T, Veldhuyzen van Zanten SJO, Unge P et al. Eradication of *Helicobacter pylori* using one week therapies combining omeprazole with two antimicrobials – The MACH 1 Study. Helicobacter. 1996;1:138–44.
23. Lind T, Megraud F, Unge P et al. The MACH 2 Study: Role of omeprazole in eradication of *Helicobacter pylori* with one-week triple therapies. Gastroenterology. 1999;116:248–53.
24. Veldhuyzen van Zanten SJO, Bradette M, Farley A et al. The DU-MACH Study: Eradication of *Helicobacter pylori* and ulcer healing in patients with acute duodenal ulcers using omeprazole-based triple therapy. Aliment Pharmacol Ther. 1999;13:289–95.
25. Sung JJY, Chan FKL, Wu JCY et al. One-week ranitidine bismuth citrate in combinations with metronidazole, amoxicillin and clarithromycin in the treatment of *Helicobacter pylori* infection: the RBC-MACH study. Aliment Pharmacol Ther. 1999;13:1079–84.
26. Van der Wouden EJ, Thijs JC, van Zwet AA, Kooy A, Kleibeuker JH. The influence of metronidazole resistance on the efficacy of ranitidine bismuth citrate triple therapy regimens for *Helicobacter pylori* infection. Aliment Pharmacol Ther. 1999;13:297–302.
27. De Boer Wink, Driessen W, Jansz A, Tytgat G. Effect of acid suppression on efficacy of treatment for *Helicobacter pylori* infection. Lancet. 1995;345:817–20.
28. De Boer W, van Etten RJXM, Schade RWB, Ouwehand ME, Schneeberger PM, Tytgat GNJ. 4-Day lansoprazole quadruple therapy: a highly effective cure for *Helicobacter* infection. Am J Gastroenterol. 1996;91:1778–82.
29. van der Hulst RWM, van der Ende A, Homan A, Roorda P, Dankert J, Tytgat GNJ. Influence of metronidazole resistance on efficacy of quadruple therapy for *Helicobacter pylori* eradication. Gut. 1998;42:166–9.
30. Coudron P, Stratton C. Utilization of time-kill kinetic methodologies for assessing the bactericidal activities of ampicillin and bismuth, alone and in combination, against *Helicobacter pylori* in stationary and logarithmic growth phases. Antimicrob Agents Chemother. 1995:66–9.
31. Osato MS, Graham DY. Ranitidine bismuth citrate enhances clarithromycin activity against clinical isolates of *H. pylori*. Gastroenterology. 1997;112:A1057.
32. Osato MS, Graham DY. Overcoming clarithromycin resistance with the combination of clarithromycin and ranitidine bismuth citrate. Gut. 1997;41(Suppl. 1):A104 and A105(09/386).
33. McLaren A, Donnelly C, McDowell S, Williamson R. The role of ranitidine bismuth citrate in significantly reducing the emergency of *Helicobacter pylori* strains resistant to antibiotics. Helicobacter. 1997;1:21–6.
34. López-Brea M, Domingo D, Sánchez I, Alarcón T. Synergism study of ranitidine bismuth citrate and metronidazole against metronidazole resistant *H. pylori* clinical isolates. Gastroenterology. 1997;112:A201.
35. Mégraud F, Pichavant R, Palegry D, French PC, Roberts PM, Williamson R. Ranitidine bismuth citrate (RBC) co-prescribed with clarithromycin is more effective in the eradication of *Helicobacter pylori* than omeprazole with clarithromycin. Gut. 1997;41(Suppl. 1):A92(09/337).
36. Perschy TB, McSorley DJ, Sorrells SC, Webb DD. Ranitidine bismuth citrate in combination with clarithromycin is effective against *H. pylori* strains with susceptible or intermediate clarithromycin sensitivity. Gastroenterology. 1997;112:A257.
37. Osato M, Graham DY, Vakil N et al. Development of clarithromycin resistance is 2.7 times less likely with ranitidine bismuth citrate than with omeprazole. Gastroenterology. 1998;114:A249(G1022).
38. Kung N, Sung J, Yuen N et al. One-week ranitidine bismuth citrate versus colloidal bismuth subcitrate-based anti-*Helicobacter* triple therapy; a prospective randomized controlled trial. Am J Gastroenterol. 1999;94:721–4.
39. Knigge K, Kelly C, Peterson WL, Fennerty MB. Eradication of *Helicobacter pylori* infection after ranitidine bismuth citrate, metronidazole and tetracycline for 7 to 10 days. Aliment Pharmacol Ther. 1999;13:323–6.
40. Gisbert JP, Gonzalez L, Calvet X, Gabriel R, Pajares JM. Proton pump inhibitor versus ranitidine bismuth citrate plus two antibiotics for one week. A meta-analysis of its efficacy on *Helicobacter pylori* eradication. Gastroenterology. 2000;118(Suppl 2):abstract 2666.

65
Risk factors for failure of *Helicobacter pylori* eradication therapy

N. BROUTET, S. TCHAMGOUÉ, E. PEREIRA and
F. MÉGRAUD

INTRODUCTION

During the past decade effective therapies have been developed to cure *Helicobacter pylori* infection, following the work of Bazzoli et al.[1] and Lamouliatte et al.[2]. Current treatments are based on combinations of a proton-pump inhibitor (PPI) and clarithromycin, with a second antibiotic being either amoxycillin or metronidazole.

Large multicentre trials, especially the MACH 1[3] and MACH 2[4] studies, have confirmed the excellent results of pilot studies leading to eradication rates higher than 90%. Unfortunately, in subsequent years such good results have not been reproduced everywhere, especially in southern Europe, where resistance to antibiotics is known to be higher[5]. Compliance, usually considered as an important cause of failure, has rarely been proven to be responsible. Other factors could also be involved.

In this chapter we will review resistance to antibiotics as a cause of failure of PPI-based triple therapies and we will present preliminary results of a study carried out in France on risk factors for failure of *H. pylori* treatment in a cohort of patients.

RESISTANCE TO ANTIBIOTICS AS A CAUSE OF FAILURE

Among the antibiotics commonly used to treat *H. pylori* infections, clarithromycin and metronidazole are essentially the most effective. However, the situation is quite different for these two antibiotics in a number of ways.

Mechanism

Although the genetic background concerning macrolide resistance is now well known and monomorphic, it is complex and not yet fully understood for metronidazole.

For macrolide resistance, a point mutation on the 23S rRNA can occur in position 2142 or 2143, as a transition or transversion[6]. The consequence is a conformational modification of the ribosomal structure, which does not allow macrolide binding[7]. To be active, the nitro function of a nitroimidazole must be reduced to hydroxylamine, a compound which has a deleterious effect on DNA. An oxygen-intensive nitroreductase, coded by the gene *rdxA*, seems to play a major role in this reduction. Goodwin *et al.* have shown an association between null mutations on the *rdxA* gene and metronidazole resistance[8]. Other mutations on *rdxA*, leading to stop codons and truncated proteins, have been found[9,10]. Other enzymes, such as the flavin oxidoreductase, could also be involved, and render the mechanism of resistance much more complex than that of clarithromycin. Furthermore, in contrast to clarithromycin, which selects only resistant mutants appearing randomly, nitroimidazole induces such mutations.

Detection methods

A first consequence of these different mechanisms of resistance is the ability to detect it. Macrolide resistance can be accurately detected by any phenotypic method, including the most simple, the disc diffusion method[11], and a reference method has been proposed by the NCCLS and European researchers[12]. Furthermore, because of the restricted number of mutations, it has been feasible to design methods to detect this resistance at the molecular level[13–15].

In contrast, at this time, only the dilution agar method can be considered to be relatively accurate for the detection of metronidazole resistance, even if its reproducibility is not perfect. The other phenotypic methods, including the Etest, led to a large number of discrepancies. Furthermore, because of the complexity of the mechanism at the genomic level, it is not yet possible to develop a molecular test.

Epidemiology

Macrolide resistance is still at a low level, and virtually absent in some countries; it may reach 20% in certain groups of patients elsewhere. As for other resistances with this genetic background, i.e. chromosomal mutation, they are irreversible and the prevalence increases steadily under selective pressure. Such pressure is probably not due only to *H. pylori* eradication treatments, but also to the treatment of respiratory tract infections.

In contrast, metronidazole resistance is reported to be high in most countries (33% in Europe[5]) and virtually 100% in developing countries. However, this resistance is sometimes reversible, probably due to the fact that metronidazole can be reduced by different metabolic pathways, which can be activated or not, according to the environmental conditions.

Clinical relevance

Macrolide resistance has an important impact on the outcome of treatment with PPI-based triple therapies. Meta-analyses or analyses of pooled data have shown that the cure rate is between 0% and 50%, when the *H. pylori* strain is resistant, while it is approximately 90% when the strain is susceptible. Such a dramatic impact is not found with metronidazole resistance[16,17]. In the MACH 2 trial, which was designed for the purpose of evaluating resistance, the rate of eradication decreased by 20% when the *H. pylori* strain was resistant[4]. A similar result was also found in a meta-analysis[18]. However, increasing the duration of treatment appears to improve the eradication rate in the case of metronidazole resistance.

RISK FACTORS FOR FAILURE OF *H. PYLORI* ERADICATION THERAPY IN A COHORT OF PATIENTS IN FRANCE

A population with low rates of eradication is the best suited group in which to try to identify risk factors for failure of *H. pylori* therapy. Such is the case in France, where resistance to antimicrobial agents, especially clarithromycin, could be a cause of failure[19], but does not fully explain the results obtained. A study of treatment failures was therefore undertaken in France.

Material and methods

All multicentre, randomized, double-blind, comparative studies carried out in France for *H. pylori* eradication using triple therapies, completed before December 1999, and for which the diagnostic tests were centralized, were included.

These studies had the same design, i.e. inclusion of patients after an endoscopy, where the CLO test and another invasive test were positive, a follow-up visit at the end of the treatment to evaluate tolerance and compliance, and another follow-up visit 1 month later, during which a urea breath test (UBT) was carried out to evaluate *H. pylori* eradication. In cases in which the UBT was not performed, the results of endoscopy-based tests were considered.

The data files received from the different sponsors of these trials (six pharmaceutical companies) were homogenized and fused into a final database. A per-protocol population of each of these studies constituted the study population of the present analysis. The variables selected were related: (1) to the patient: sociodemographic and behavioural data, and endoscopic diagnosis; and (2) to the treatment received.

The different treatment arms were classified into four categories: (1) those which included a double dose of PPI + amoxycillin (1 g b.i.d.) and clarithromycin (b.i.d.) for 7 days, which is the most widely used regimen amongst those approved in clinical practice in France; (2) those with the same regimen but with a single dose of PPI for 7 days; (3) those including metronidazole, regardless of the other antibiotic and antisecretory drug; (4) those which did not fit into the three previous groups, especially treatments including other macrolides (roxithromycin, azithromycin) than clarithromycin, and other doses of antibiotics.

Results

Fifteen trials were identified but three were not completed in 1999 and, for one, the tests were not performed centrally so 11 trials with 27 treatment arms were included, representing 3270 randomized patients.

Table 1. Risk factors for failure of *H. pylori* eradication therapy in a cohort of 2751 patients in France (1990–98)

	Total no.	Treatment failure		p-Value
		No.	Percentage	
Gender				
Female	761	193	25.4	0.62
Male	1726	422	24.4	
Tobacco				
Non-smoker	1459	372	25.5	0.13
Smoker	854	242	28.3	
Geographical origin				
Born in France	1803	458	25.4	0.3
Others	338	99	29.3	
Region of inclusion				
North	1012	261	25.8	0.17
Centre	836	199	23.8	
South	891	247	27.7	
Endoscopic diagnosis				
DU	1838	403	21.9	$<10^{-6}$
NUD	913	308	33.7	
Other macroscopic lesions:				
Gastritis				
Absent	655	171	26.1	0.39
Present	953	267	28	
Duodenitis				
Absent	1062	292	27.5	0.74
Present	546	146	26.7	
Oesophagitis				
Absent	424	146	34.4	0.84
Present	25	9	36	
Treatment group				
PPI × 2, amox 1 g bd, clari 500 mg bd	1029	194	18.9	$<10^{-6}$
PPI × 1, amox 1 g bd, clari 500 mg bd	856	229	26.8	
PPI, imidazole, 2nd antibiotic	391	121	30.9	
Others	475	167	35.2	
Observance				
Poor (<85%)	116	39	33.6	0.22
Good (>85%)	1811	513	28.3	
Side-effects				
Absent	1433	333	23.2	0.54
Present	625	153	24.5	

DU, duodenal ulcer; NUD, non-ulcer dyspepsia; Amox, amoxycillin; Clari, clarithromycin.

We considered for analysis the records of patients with complete data at entry, who had taken the drugs and for whom the outcome was known. The final database concerned 2751 patients. The mean age of these patients was 47.5 years, 66% were male, 85% were born in France, and 37% were smokers. The global rate of eradication failure was 25.8% (95% CI: 24–27).

The description of the sample, including a comparison of eradication rates between the different patient characteristics, is presented in Table 1.

There was a large proportion of males, which is usual in clinical trials concerning this type of disease. This can be explained by the high proportion

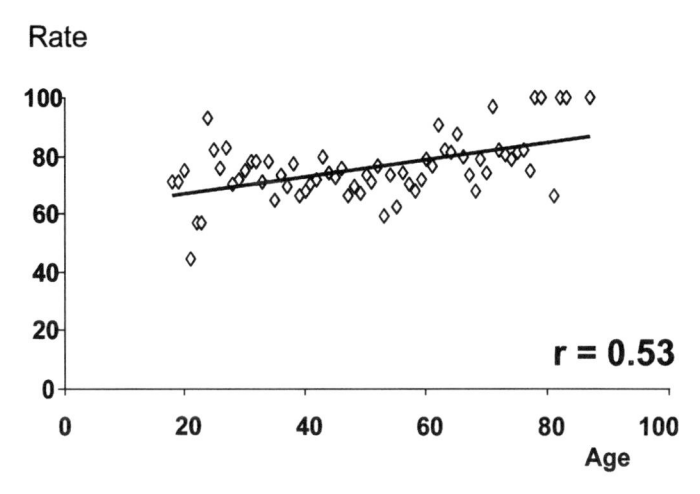

Figure 1. Eradication rate of *Helicobacter pylori* according of age (global).

of duodenal ulcer (DU) patients, who are more likely to be male, and by the more frequent exclusion of females due to child-bearing age. However, the failure rate was not significantly different between males and females (24.4% vs 25.4%, respectively).

The mean age of the patients who experienced failure was slightly lower than that of those who were cured (46.8 years vs 48.5 years) and, because of this large sample, this difference was statistically significant ($p = 0.007$). The eradication rate according to age is presented in Figure 1. A weak correlation was found ($r^2 = 0.53$) between a higher rate of failure and young age.

Thirty-seven per cent were smokers, i.e. slightly more than the rate of smokers in the general population in France (30%). However, the failure rate of smokers was not significantly different from non-smokers (28.3% vs 25.5%, respectively). The same was seen for alcohol consumption.

The geographical origin of the patients included in trials can also be associated with failure. Approximately 10% of the French population are immigrants, and in this study 15.7% of the patients were born outside Europe. The failure rate was higher in immigrants in this study (29.3%) vs 25.4% for the others but was not statistically significant.

France is a country lying midway between northern Europe and the Mediterranean countries, which have different eradication rates with triple therapies. For this reason we looked at the failure rate in the northern, central, and southern parts of the country, but did not find a statistically significant difference.

Among the 2751 patients, 66.8% were DU patients and 33.2% were non-ulcer dyspepsia (NUD) patients. There was a highly statistically significant difference between these two groups. The failure rate was 21.9% in DU patients vs 33.7% in the NUD group ($p < 10^{-6}$). In contrast, there was no association with other macroscopic lesions of the gastrointestinal tract assessed by fibreoptic endoscopy, i.e. with oesophagitis, gastritis and duodenitis, etc. There was also a statistically significant difference in the failure rate according to the treatment group. In group 1, which received the most popular regimen in France, i.e. OAC with a double dose of PPI, the failure rate was 18.9%. It increased to 26.8%, when only a single dose of PPI was used. The arms including nitroimidazoles were less successful (30.9% failure) as well as the groups containing various treatment regimens (35.2%). Globally, there were few patients with a bad compliance (6%) and there was no impact on the failure rate.

Thirty per cent of the patients reported side-effects of the treatment used, but this finding did not appear to lead to an increased risk of failure.

Discussion

The construction of such a cohort with individual data to analyse risk factors for eradication failure has its drawbacks. The first is that the risk factors were not the primary goal of these clinical trials, and the study designs were not properly adapted. The second drawback was to deal with data collection performed with differently constructed questionnaires, necessitating considerable efforts to homogenize the data when possible, and leading to an important loss of information. Thirdly, the missing data constitute a problem which jeopardizes the value of the results. For example, in this study, data on the important risk factor of antibiotic resistance, were not available in most of the trials and could not be considered. However, this is counterbalanced by the important power of such a study, because of the large number of patients included and the exhaustive nature of the trials considered.

The essential result is the major difference (12%) in failure rates between DU and NUD patients. Such a result was already reported in a meta-analysis by Huang and Hunt[20], while in most of the individual studies performed there was a trend for this result, although the power was not sufficient to reach significance. The reasons for this difference are not yet clearly understood. It could be due to patient differences, especially differences in the status of the gastric mucosa; to environmental differences such as smoking habits; or to differences due to the infecting strain of *H. pylori*, such as antibiotic resistance or cag status.

With regard to treatment regimens, the most commonly used treatment in France (PPI-A-C) with a double dose of PPI turned out to be more effective than a similar treatment with a single dose of PPI. Because of the diversity of the other treatment regimens used, we had to group them artificially, and again this is a limitation of this study.

These results are preliminary, but point out the importance of considering DU and NUD independently. A multivariate analysis will be performed in order to define in each group of patients what the independent risk factors are.

References

1. Bazzoli F, Zagari RM, Fossi S et al. Efficacy and tolerability of a short term, low dose triple therapy for eradication of *Helicobacter pylori*. Gastroenterology. 1993;104:A40.

2. Lamouliatte H, Cayla R, Mégraud F et al. Amoxicillin–clarithromycin–omeprazole: the best therapy for *Helicobacter pylori* infection? Acta Gastroenterol Belg. 1993;56:140.
3. Lind T, van Zanten SV, Unge P, Spiller R et al. Eradication of *Helicobacter pylori* using one-week triple therapies combining omeprazole with two antimicrobials: the MACH1 study. Helicobacter. 1996;3:138–44.
4. Lind T, Mégraud F, Unge P et al. The MACH2 study: role of omeprazole in eradication of *Helicobacter pylori* with 1-week triple therapies. Gastroenterology. 1999;116:248–53.
5. Glupczynski Y, Mégraud F, Andersen LP, Lopez-Brea M. Antibiotic susceptibility of *H. pylori* in Europe in 1998: results of the third multicentre study. Gut. 1999;45(Suppl. 3):A3.
6. Versalovic J, Shortridge D, Kliber K et al. Mutations in 23S rRNA are associated with clarithromycin resistance in *Helicobacter pylori*. Antimicrob Agents Chemother. 1996;40:477–80.
7. Occhialini A, Urdaci M, Doucet-Populaire F, Bébéar CM, Lamouliatte H, Mégraud F. Macrolide resistance in *Helicobacter pylori*: rapid detection of point mutations and assays of macrolide binding to ribosomes. Antimicrob Agents Chemother. 1997;41:2724–8.
8. Goodwin CS, Marshall BJ, Blincow ED, Wilson DH, Blackbourn S, Philipps M. Prevention of nitroimidazole resistance in *Campylobacter pylori* by coadministration of colloidal bismuth subcitrate: clinical and *in vitro* studies. J Clin Pathol. 1988; 41:207–10.
9. Jenks PJ, Ferrero RL, Labigne A. The role of the *rdxA* gene in the evolution of metronidazole resistance in *Helicobacter pylori*. J Antimicrob Chemother. 1999;43:753–8.
10. Jenks PJ, Labigne A, Ferrero RL. Exposure to metronidazole *in vivo* readily induces resistance in *Helicobacter pylori* and reduces the efficacy of eradication therapy in mice. Antimicrob Agents Chemother. 1999; 43:777–81.
11. Fauchère JL. Validation of a disk diffusion method for macrolide susceptibility testing of *Helicobacter pylori*. Gut. 1999;45(Suppl. 3):A9.
12. Glupczynski Y, Andersen LP, Lopez-Brea M, Mégraud F. Toward standardisation of antimicrobial susceptibility testing of *H. pylori*: preliminary results by a European multicentre study group. Gut. 1998;43(Suppl. 2):A47.
13. Marais A, Monteiro L, Occhialini A, Pina M, Lamouliatte H, Mégraud F. Direct detection of *Helicobacter pylori* resistance to macrolides by a polymerase chain reaction/DNA enzyme immunoassay in gastric biopsy specimens. Gut. 1999;44:463–7.
14. Van Doorn LJ, Debets-Ossenkopp YJ, Marais A et al. Rapid detection, by PCR and reverse hybridization, of mutations in the *Helicobacter pylori* 23S rRNA gene, associated with macrolide resistance. Antimicrob Agents Chemother. 1999;43:1779–82.
15. Gibson JR, Saunders NA, Burke B, Owen RJ. Novel method for rapid determination of clarithromycin sensitivity in *Helicobacter pylori*. J Clin Microbiol. 1999;37:3746–8.
16. Dore MP et al. Effect of pretreatment antibiotic resistance to metronidazole and clarithromycin on outcome of *Helicobacter pylori* therapy: a meta-analytical approach. Dig Dis Sci. 2000;45:68–76.
17. Houben MHMG, van de Beek D, Hensen EF et al. A systematic review of *Helicobacter pylori* eradication therapy – the impact of antimicrobial resistance on eradication rates. Aliment Pharmacol Ther. 1999;13:1047–56.
18. Van der Wouden EJ, Thijs JC, van Zwet AA, Sluiter WJ, Kleibeuker JH. The influence of *in vitro* nitroimidazole resistance on the efficacy of nitroimidazole-containing anti-*Helicobacter pylori* regimens: a meta-analysis. Am J Gastroenterol. 1999;94.1751–9.
19. Broutet N, Guillon F, Sauty E et al. Survey of the *in vitro* susceptibility of *Helicobacter pylori* to antibiotics in France. Preliminary results. Gut. 1998;43(Suppl. 2):A11.
20. Huang JQ, Hunt RH. Are one-week anti-*H. pylori* treatments more effective in patients with peptic ulcer disease (PUD) than in those with non-ulcer dyspepsia (NUD)? A meta-analysis. Am J Gastroenterol. 1998;93:1639.

66
Strategies for therapy failures: Choice of 'back-up' regimen determined by primary treatment for *Helicobacter pylori* infection

W. A. DE BOER

AN OVERALL APPROACH TO THERAPY – INTRODUCTION

Much is known about *H. pylori* therapy in new patients. We have studies on hundreds of different therapies. Many regimens look alike, but often the daily dose of the antibiotic, the choice of the acid suppressant or the number of doses per day differ. Review articles in which the data of all these studies are pooled and summarized give us a good overview of the cure rates we can expect[1,2]. Although recrudescence of the infection occurs occasionally, true reinfection is extremely rare[3,4]. We also know a lot about the impact of bacterial resistance on the outcome of primary therapy; both metronidazole and clarithromycin resistance have a negative impact on the outcome of the treatment[2,5–7]. Amoxicillin and tetracycline resistance are non-existent or extremely rare.

There are many therapies that can achieve the required efficacy level of an 80% intention to treat (ITT) and a 90% per protocol (PP) cure rate. We cannot conclude that any of these adequate therapies is either superior or inferior to the others[8,9]. The choice of primary treatment depends heavily on the local prevalence of resistance, and the personal preference of the physician.

We believe that another issue should also be considered in this selection: the further therapeutic options that remain if therapy fails[9]. Even the best therapies fail in 5–20% of cases and, as in any other infection, the development of future resistance should be a major concern[10–12]. Our aim is to cure the infection in 100% of our patients[13]. Only after the infection is cured do ulcers or ulcer bleeding not recur[14]. No ulcer patient should leave our care until we have documented proof by endoscopy, breath test or 6-month follow-up serology that *H. pylori* is eliminated[15]. This means that in case of treatment failure a second therapy must be prescribed, and if necessary even a third or fourth therapy. Ideally, follow-up therapy is guided by susceptibility data, but this information is often unavailable. Therefore, empiric 'back-up' therapies are usually prescribed.

In designing a treatment strategy we should not focus on the results of primary therapy alone. An adequate strategy for treating this infection should use two therapies which, if used consecutively, come as close to the 100% cure rate as possible. These two therapies should preferably not contain the same antibiotics, and they must supplement each other. We need to look for studies in which a fixed combination of two therapies was prescribed consecutively in a given group of patients. We look for combinations of therapies: one primary regimen and one 'back-up' regimen. Future trials must study combinations of therapies. Authors must also focus on reporting antimicrobial susceptibility before and after therapy[5,7,12,16] and on finding the optimal complementary 'back-up' regimen to their initial therapy.

SECOND-LINE THERAPY

The literature on second-line therapy is very difficult to analyse; hundreds of different first-line therapies are combined with the same number of different second-line therapies. The number of possible combinations is endless. Many studies have used primary treatments that are no longer in use today, especially dual therapy with a proton-pump inhibitor (PPI) with amoxycillin. Furthermore, the number of failures after most modern therapies is usually small, which leads to wide 95% confidence intervals for the published results of re-treatment. Some patients do not receive the second-line treatment, for reasons that are often unknown, and a selection bias is often present in re-treatment studies.

The most important problem, however, is that in many studies cure is determined by urea breath test, and susceptibility data are not given. This makes such data useless as they cannot be adequately analysed or compared[5,7,16]. We can only determine whether the reported results also apply to other populations if the data on antimicrobial resistance are provided. In order to analyse the literature on 'back-up' therapies it is therefore imperative to know the number of patients with secondary resistance, and studies should focus more on this issue[7,9,12,16]. In general, it is more difficult to succeed with second-line therapy[17–20], and repeated regimens might need to be prolonged. There are bacteria that can be killed easily (steep kill-curve) and bacteria that are more difficult to kill. During treatment the substrains with the steepest kill-curve will disappear first. The bacteria that are the least susceptible remain if therapy fails[21]. Bacteria of this 'difficult-to-kill' substrain then increase their numbers and repopulate the stomach. Moreover, such remaining strains are likely to have become resistant to one or both key antibiotics. For obvious reasons, non-compliers are over-represented in the group of failures. These factors may all explain the reported lower cure rates of retreatment.

A few authors have observed that in some patients, due to as-yet-unknown factors, the infection cannot be made to disappear[17,22], but this is not a general feeling[23,24]. In our experience this happens only rarely. Several authors, however, have warned against a rising number of failures and the problems with retreatment[11,12]. There is increasing support for the notion that only the best primary treatment should be used; the primary therapy may be the best opportunity to treat the infection[11–13,17,25]. Afterwards it becomes harder and harder to cure the patient.

QUADRUPLE THERAPY AS SECOND-LINE THERAPY

Quadruple therapy (PPI, bismuth, tetracycline, metronidazole) for 1 week duration was recommended as the optimal second-line therapy in several guidelines[8,26]. If this therapy would perform optimally, independent of which primary regimen was prescribed, retreatment would be very simple. Unfortunately this is not the case. In clinical studies 7-day quadruple therapy proved to be extremely effective after dual therapy with amoxycillin[27] and after a regimen with amoxycillin and clarithromycin[28–31]. Results, however, were less good after a regimen that contains metronidazole[32–35], although this has not been a universal finding[21,23,36–40]. It is clear from several studies that secondary metronidazole resistance is a major problem, which is harder to overcome than primary metronidazole resistance. Apparently, the large number of 'difficult-to-kill' *H. pylori* which have also become resistant to metronidazole are problematic even when using quadruple therapy. Quadruple therapy, therefore, is not the sole solution for treatment failures. It is the choice of the primary therapy, and the secondary resistance that must be assumed to have occurred, that dictates the choice of the second-line therapy. Some data, however, suggest that by increasing the length of therapy beyond 7 days quadruple therapy will achieve excellent results as a 'back-up' regimen, even in the case of secondary metronidazole resistance[23,36,37,40,41]. In this circumstance it is also important to use at least 1200 mg (3 × 400 mg), but preferably 1500 mg (3 × 500 mg) or 1600 mg (4 × 400 mg) of metronidazole[42].

A LOGICAL AND RATIONAL FRAMEWORK FOR THERAPY

We have previously proposed using either a regimen based on clarithromycin or a regimen based on metronidazole as primary treatment[9]. The choice of the second-line treatment depends solely on which therapy has been used initially, and different antibiotics need to be selected for the 'back-up' regimen. If a clarithromycin-based regimen was used first, a metronidazole-based regimen should be used afterwards and vice-versa, as shown in Figure 1.

As previously stated, we do not favour an initial regimen with both clarithromycin and metronidazole[9]. Such therapies are effective, but they are not superior to other therapies and other arguments must, therefore, be considered in the selection process. Use of this regimen poses a problem for those who fail. We must realize that such regimens lead at least to single, but more often to double resistance[11,32,33,40,43,44] against both key antibiotics. This is of particular importance in areas with a high prevalence of primary metronidazole resistance, where more failures and thus more double resistance will be a consequence of its use[44]. There is no logical empiric

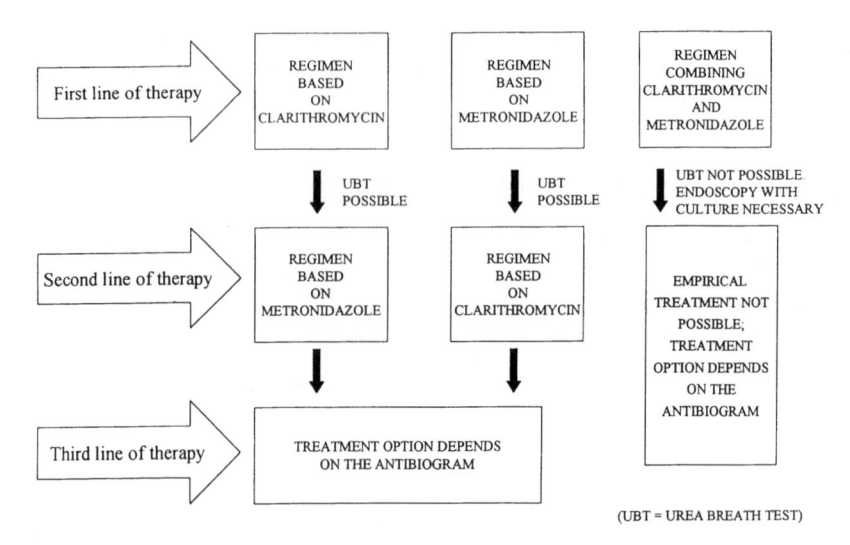

Figure 1. General principles of empirical treatment.

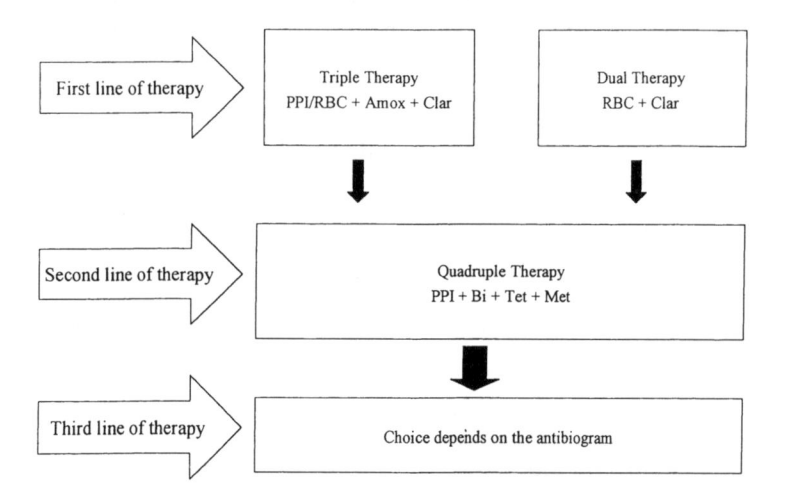

Figure 2. Treatment strategy in area with low primary prevalence of clarithromycin resistance.

second-line treatment available afterwards and endoscopic biopsies for culture and susceptibility testing seem to be mandatory to select a further therapy. Some groups have reported major problems with re-treating patients who received this treatment[34]. Especially when such a regimen is used in primary care, a lower cure rate than that achieved in randomized trials might actually make double resistance a true clinical problem. We, therefore, prefer the use of either a regimen based on clarithromycin (with or without amoxycillin) (Figure 2) or a regimen based on metronidazole (with tetracycline) (Figure 3). The background of this choice has been dis-

STRATEGIES FOR THERAPY FAILURES

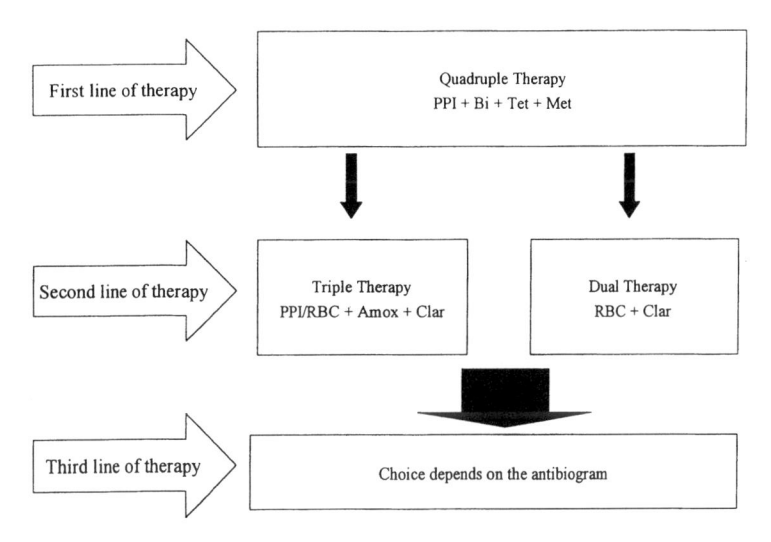

```
First line of therapy  →  Quadruple Therapy
                          PPI + Bi + Tet + Met
                                    ↓
Second line of therapy →  Triple Therapy              Dual Therapy
                          PPI/RBC + Amox + Clar       RBC + Clar
                                    ↓
Third line of therapy  →  Choice depends on the antibiogram
```

Figure 3. Treatment strategy in area with high primary prevalence of clarithromycin resistance.

cussed elsewhere[9]. If the regimen fails, the patient should receive the supplementary therapy. The choice of the second-line therapy is clear from the beginning, and does not depend on culture results. An easier and cheaper follow-up schedule can, therefore, be used[15]. This means that each therapy chosen as initial therapy has a fixed second-line treatment that belongs to it. Preferably, this should be an evidence-based selection of two connected therapies, supported by clinical studies. The general practitioner can re-treat without the need for consulting a specialist. Because all regimens are less efficacious for re-treatment as compared to their efficacy when used as primary treatment, we advise that the course of the secondary therapy should be extended to at least a 10-day treatment period.

In the rare case that a second-line therapy also fails, the choice of the third therapy should always be guided by culture and susceptibility testing (Figures 1–3)[12]. Some patients fail therapy due to non-compliance and we prefer admission and treatment with the antibiotic regimen in the hospital for patients who have been non-compliant with the previous two attempts[45]. This holds true especially for patients with ulcer complications, who have a high recurrence rate. Elective admission for a third-line therapy might be cost effective in such non compliant patients.

CLARITHROMYCIN-BASED REGIMENS AS BACK-UP AFTER METRONIDAZOLE-BASED REGIMENS

Two early studies demonstrated that PPI–amoxycillin–clarithromycin triple therapy achieved high cure rates after a metronidazole-based therapy[46,47]. This has subsequently been confirmed in more recent studies[38,39,41,48–50]. The results of these studies are shown in Table 1, and they support the use of a triple therapy with a PPI, amoxycillin and clarithromycin after failure

Table 1. Clarithromycin-based second-line therapy after failed metronidazole-based regimens

Primary treatment	Ref.	Secondary therapy	Cure of re-treatment	
Metro-based	46	(O20 × 2/A500 × 3/C250 × 3) × 7 days	18/21	(86%)
Metro-based	47	(O20 × 2/A750 × 2/C250 × 2) × 10 days	18/18	(100%)
Bis–amo–metro	48	(PPI × 2/A1000 × 2/C500 × 2) × 14 days	92/114	(81%)
Ome–amo–metro	41	(O20 × 2/A1000 × 2/C500 × 2) × 7 days	17/20	(85%)
Metro-based	49	(L/A/C) × 7 days	10/11	(90%)
Metro-based	38	(PPI × 2/A1000 × 2/C500 × 2) × ? days	26/35	(74%)
Metro-based	39	(RBC × 2/A1000 × 2/C250 × 2) × 7 days	28/33	(85%)
Bis–amo–metro	50	(L/A/C) × 10 days	8/8	(100%)

O = omeprazole, L = lansoprazole, PPI = proton-pump inhibitor, A (amo) = amoxycillin, C = clarithromycin, metro = metronidazole, bis = bismuth.

of a regimen with metronidazole, but without clarithromycin. The preferred treatment duration for re-treatment is 10 days. The available data do not allow us to calculate an overall cure rate for the two regimens together but, judging from the result depicted in Figure 1, a high overall cure can be expected.

METRONIDAZOLE-BASED REGIMENS AS BACK-UP AFTER CLARITHROMYCIN-BASED REGIMENS

The most widely investigated metronidazole-based therapy is quadruple therapy with a PPI, bismuth, metronidazole and either tetracycline or amoxycillin. The combination with tetracycline is superior to the combination with amoxycillin and should probably be preferred[42]. Some have, however, reported adequate re-treatment results with a quadruple therapy that uses amoxycillin[23,51–54]. One study suggests that quadruple therapy is superior to a triple therapy with a PPI, amoxycillin and metronidazole in this clinical setting[41]. A 7-day treatment duration is sufficient when quadruple therapy is used after a failed regimen with clarithromycin, as shown in Table 2. However, as discussed, if the primary regimen contained metronidazole, quadruple therapy retreatment should probably be prescribed for 14 days.

Replacing the PPI and the bismuth compound by 'RBC' in quadruple therapy has been shown to achieve adequate results in two re-treatment studies[41,55], but more data are needed and presently we still prefer to use the acid suppressant and the bismuth compound as separate drugs. Replacing the PPI by high-dose H_2-receptor antagonists is possible, but gives a slightly lower rate of eradication[56,57].

Several studies, which used first a triple therapy with a PPI, amoxycillin and clarithromycin and standard quadruple therapy as second-line treatment allow us to calculate the per-protocol (PP) and intention-to-treat (ITT) overall cure rates, after two consecutive treatments[28,30,31,58,59]. These results are shown in Table 3. Based on these data, one can conclude that this combination of therapies cures ≥ 95% of patients, and very few will subsequently need endoscopy with culture and susceptibility testing to select the third-line therapy (Figure 1). This combination of therapies, which uses

Table 2. Metronidazole-based second-line therapy after failed clarithromycin-based regimens

Primary treatment	Ref.	Secondary therapy	Cure of re-treatment
L/A/C	58, 78	(L30 × 2/B120 × 4/M500 × 3/T500 × 4) × 7 days	20/21 (95%)
O/A/C	60	(O20 × 2/B120 × 4/M250 × 4/T500 × 4) × 7 days	17/30 (57%)
O/A/C	60	(RBC × 2/M250 × 4/T500 × 4) × 7 days	25/30 (83%)
PPI/A/C	55	(RBC × 2/Ti500 × 2/T500 × 3) × 14 days	31/36 (86%)
C-based	38	(PPI × 2/B120 × 4/M400 × 3/T500 × 4) × ? days	13/14 (93%)
0/A/C	31	(PPI × 2/B120 × 4/M500 × 3/T500 × 3) × 7 days	27/31 (87%)
O/A/C	30	(PPI × 2/B120 × 4/M500 × 3/T500 × 4) × 7 days	33/39 (85%)
O/A/C	28	(O20 × 2/B120 × 4/M500 × 3/T500 × 4) × 7 days	3/3 (100%)
O/A/C	59	(O20 × 2/B240 × 2/M500 × 3/A750 × 3) × 7 days	14/20 (70%)
O/A/C	41	(O20 × 2/B120 × 4/M250 × 4/T500 × 4) × 7 days	7/9 (78%)
O/A/C	41	(O20 × 2/A1000 × 2/M500 × 2) × 7 days	10/21 (48%)
O/A/C	41	(O20 × 2/A1000 × 3/M500 × 3) × 7 days	14/24 (58%)
O/C	41	(O20 × 2/A1000 × 2/M500 × 2) × 7 days	8/8 (80%)

O = omeprazole, L = lansoprazole, PPI = proton-pump inhibitor, A = amoxycillin, C = clarithromycin, M = metronidazole, T = tetracycline, Ti = tinidazole, B = bismuth, RBC = ranitidine bismuth citrate.

Table 3. Overall cure rates after two consecutive treatments

Ref.	First treatment	Cure rate	Second treatment	Overall cure PP	Overall cure ITT
58	O/A/C	79/102 (77%)	O/B/M/T	99/100 (99%)	99/102 (97%)
30	O/A/C	294/337 (87%)	O/B/M/T	327/332 (98%)	327/337 (97%)
31	O/A/C	205/245 (84%)	O/B/M/T	232/236 (99%)	232/245 (95%)
28	O/A/C	60/71 (85%)	O/B/M/T	63/66 (95%)	63/71 (89%)
59	O/A/C	73/99 (74%)	O/B/M/A	87/93 (94%)	87/99 (88%)
			Total:	808/827 (98%)	808/854 (95%)

different antibiotics in the two consecutive attempts, can be regarded as evidence-based.

RANDOMIZED TRIALS BETWEEN TWO SECOND-LINE THERAPIES

Only a few studies have directly compared two or more second-line therapies. Some are truly randomized, others just give the results of re-treatment with different regimens in a single centre[22,35,39,41,49,51,54,56,60-67]. Only recently did some head-to-head comparison trials appear in the literature on patients treated with modern triple regimens. These studies are usually small, and most used quadruple therapy as reference therapy, together with a comparator. Quadruple therapy achieved either superior or equivalent results in all of the trials except one. In this particular study, 60 patients who were treated with a PPI, amoxycillin and clarithromycin were randomized to standard quadruple therapy or RBC with tetracycline and metronidazole, both for 1 week[60]. Exchanging the 'PPI plus colloidal bismuth citrate' for 'RBC' proved to be significantly better with an odds ratio of 3.9 (95% CI 1.02–15).

The disappointing results of quadruple therapy in this particular study are surprising, not in line with the literature and cannot be easily explained. The results of the RBC regimen, however, are as expected. A similar regimen with RBC, tetracycline and tinidazole for 2 weeks also achieved 86% (31/36) eradication after failure of a clarithromycin-based therapy[55]. RBC with another tetracycline (minocycline) and amoxycillin for 2 weeks also cured 17/19 (89%), who had failed PPI, clarithromycin and tinidazole in a small study[68]. The results of RBC–TET–MET are also in line with previous reports on this regimen when used as primary treatment[69].

The study by Lee et al. was not randomized, but the outcome suggested that if a PPI-triple therapy is used as a 'back-up' regimen it should always be given for 14 days. Quadruple therapy for 7 days achieved equivalent results to the 14-day PPI-triple therapy[61], but was significantly better then the 1-week PPI-triple therapy.

The randomized study on re-treatment by Houben et al. demonstrated a significant difference in favour of quadruple therapy as compared to 1-week PPI-triple[62]. Furthermore, they showed good results (5/7 (71%)) for 1-week quadruple therapy, when used as third-line therapy[62]. These data are in line with the results of Katelaris et al., who reported a cure rate of 13/17 (77%) for quadruple therapy when used as third, fourth or fifth treatment[38]. The data from Gisbert lend further support for the superiority of quadruple therapy over a 1-week PPI-triple therapy with a PPI, amoxycillin and metronidazole[41].

NEW ALTERNATIVES

In the somewhat older literature dual therapy with a PPI and amoxycillin was ineffective as second-line therapy in several studies[18,19]. Recently this regimen with an increased dose of the PPI and the amoxycillin was again proposed as a regimen for patients in whom secondary resistance was encountered. Peitz et al. treated 33 patients, of whom 14 had been treated once with a regimen of clarithromycin plus metronidazole, and 17 had been treated by multiple regimens. Their patients received omeprazole 40 mg t.i.d. and amoxycillin 1000 mg t.i.d. for 2 weeks. Overall 27/33 (82%) were cured[70].

Jaup treated 45 patients, who had failed one or two previous attempts with a PPI-triple therapy, with omeprazole 40 mg t.i.d. and amoxycillin 750 mg t.i.d. and reported a cure rate of 36/45 (80%)[71].

In contrast van der Hulst et al. used the same high-dose re-treatment after a previous dual therapy and cured only 7/25 (28%)[72]. Kayser used 14-day re-treatment with lansoprazole 60 mg b.i.d. and amoxycillin 1000mg b.i.d. and also cured only 5/22 (23%)[27]. Chen used a lower dose for re-treatment but, nevertheless, reported a cure rate of 23/36 (63.8%)[66]. Neville used 14-day dual therapy after triple therapy with a PPI, clarithromycin and metronidazole, and cured 23/47 (48.9%) in a study in which the dose schedule was not mentioned[34], but was 22/30 (73%) in another study[65].

It is clear that the data are somewhat contradictory and more data are needed before high-dose dual therapy can be advised outside clinical trials.

At present the regimen can best be used in patients with dual resistance, who have already failed several previous attempts to cure the infection.

A combination of a PPI, amoxycillin and rifabutin was also proposed as 'back-up' regimen[73]. Data from Italy[74] and Germany[75] support its use. Cure rates were >80% with a dose of 300 mg rifabutin/day either prescribed as 300 mg u.i.d.[74] or 150 mg b.i.d.[75] for 7–10 days. More data are clearly needed, especially regarding the impact of secondary resistance on the performance of this rescue therapy. The cost of rifabutin, however, is not reimbursed in many countries, and the availability of the drug may be a problem.

Ciprofloxacin is another antibiotic that has been tried for re-treatment but the combination of a PPI with amoxycillin and ciprofloxacin was found to be ineffective in patients with dual resistance[76].

Furazolidone was tried for resistant *H. pylori* in a small group of 12 patients, and has been proposed as salvage therapy[77]. More data on this drug, used in a second-line regimen, are needed.

RECOMMENDATIONS FOR THERAPY

Local (geographical) prevalence of antimicrobial resistance determines whether it is better to start with a regimen based on clarithromycin or one based on metronidazole[1,2,5–9]. Presently, clarithromycin resistance is below 10% in most populations, except southern Europe[79]. Therefore, one can usually start with a regimen based on clarithromycin (14 days of ranitidine bismuth citrate–clarithromycin dual therapy or 7-day proton pump inhibitor–amoxycillin–clarithromycin triple therapy or 7-day ranitidine bismuth citrate–amoxycillin–clarithromycin triple therapy) and use 7-day quadruple therapy (proton pump inhibitor–bismuth–tetracycline–metronidazole) as second-line treatment (Figure 2). Different antibiotics are used in the subsequent attempts and prospective studies show a 98% overall PP cure and 95% ITT cure rate with this approach (Table 3). Ranitidine bismuth citrate–clarithromycin dual therapy is used in case of penicillin allergy.

The order can, of course, be reversed, and treatment can also start with a regimen based om metronidazole; this is the preferred approach if the prevalence of clarithromycin resistance has increased to levels >15%. Bismuth triple therapy and 7-day proton pump inhibitor triple therapy with metronidazole and amoxycillin are less effective in primary metronidazole resistant strains[2,3,9], whereas quadruple therapy seems to perform well in metronidazole-resistant strains[2,3,6]. It can, therefore, be employed in almost all populations and we choose quadruple as first-line therapy in this scenario (Figure 3). The main problem with quadruple therapy used to be its rather complex dosing schedule. The recent introduction of an all-in-one single–triple monocapsule, which combines bismuth, metronidazole and tetracycline in a single capsule, greatly improves the convenience of the regimen for both the patient and the physician[80,81].

Since there are equally effective regimens, there is no logical reason to prefer a regimen containing both clarithromycin and metronidazole. Clearly studies have demonstrated difficulties in re-treating patients who failed to be cured with this therapy, and culture and susceptibility testing is mandatory to select an adequate salvage therapy. The aforementioned problems cannot be ignored, and we suggest refraining from or restricting the use of these therapies until a valid empiric 'back-up' therapy is available.

In general, one can increase the likelihood of cure by increasing the length of therapy. Although 7-day treatment is standard for proton-pump inhibitor or ranitidine bismuth citrate triple therapies in Europe, an individual physician can improve his/her success rate by always prescribing a 10–14-day treatment course in patients in whom a previous therapy failed, or in whom the consequence of failure can be life-threathening, as is the case in patients presenting with ulcer complications such as bleeding.

References

1. Lahey RJF, van Rossum LGM, Jansen JBMJ et al. Evaluation of treatment regimens to cure *Helicobacter pylori* infection – a meta-analysis. Aliment Pharmacol Ther. 1999;13:857–64.
2. van der Wouden EJ, Thys JC, van Zwet AA et al. The influence of *in vitro* nitroimidazole resistance on the efficacy of nitroimidazole containing anti-*Helicobacter pylori* regimens: a meta-analysis. Am J Gastroenterol. 1999;94:1751–9.
3. van der Hulst RWM, Rauws EAJ, Koycu B et al. *Helicobacter pylori* reinfection is virtually absent after successful eradication. J Infect Dis. 1997;176:196–200.
4. Gisbert JP, Pajares JM, Garcia-Valriberas R et al. Recurrence of *Helicobacter pylori* infection after eradication: incidence and variables influencing it. Scand J Gastroenterol. 1998;33:1144–51.
5. de Boer WA, Tytgat GNJ. How to treat *H. pylori* infection. Should treatment strategies be based on testing bacterial susceptibility? A personal viewpoint. Eur J Gastroenterol Hepatol. 1996;8:709–16.
6. Houben MHMG, van de Beek D, Hensen EF et al. A systematic review of *Helicobacter pylori* eradication therapy: the impact of antimicrobial resistance on eradication rates. Aliment Pharmacol Ther. 1999;13:1047–55.
7. Graham DY. Antibiotic resistance in *Helicobacter pylori*: implications for therapy. Gastroenterology. 1998;115:1272–7.
8. Anonymous. Current European concepts in the management of *Helicobacter pylori* infection. The Maastricht Consensus Report. Gut. 1997;41:8–13.
9. de Boer WA, Tytgat GNJ. Treatment of *Helicobacter pylori* infection. BMJ. 2000;320:31–4.
10. Leibovici L, Shraga I, Andreassen S. How do you choose antibiotic treatment? BMJ. 1999;318:1614–8.
11. Miyaji H, Azuma T, Ito S et al. Susceptibility of *Helicobacter pylori* isolates to metronidazole, clarithromycin and amoxicillin *in vitro* and in clinical treatment in Japan. Aliment Pharmacol Ther. 1997;11:1131–6.
12. Hazell SL. Will *Helicobacter pylori* be the next organism for which we will have exhausted our treatment options? Eur J Clin Microbiol Infect Dis. 1999;18:83–6.
13. de Boer WA, Tytgat GNJ. The best therapy for *Helicobacter pylori* infection. Should efficacy or side effect profile determine our choice? Scand J Gastroenterol. 1995;30:401–7.
14. Hopkins RJ, Girardi LS, Turney EA. Relationship between *H. pylori* eradication and reduced duodenal and gastric ulcer recurrence: a review. Gastroenterology. 1996;110:1244–52.
15. Katelaris PH, Jones DB. Testing for *Helicobacter pylori* infection after antibiotic treatment. Am J Gastroenterol. 1997;92:1245–7.
16. Graham DY, de Boer WA, Tytgat GNJ. Choosing the best anti-*Helicobacter* therapy: effect of antimicrobial resistance. Am J Gastroenterol. 1996;91:1072–6.
17. Borody TJ, Shortis NP. Treatment of patients with failed eradication – a personal view. In: Hunt RH, Tytgat GNJ editors. *Helicobacter pylori*; Basic Mechanisms to Clinical Cure 1996. Dordrecht: Kluwer; 1996:357–65.
18. van der Hulst RWM, van 't Hoff BWM. Treatment of *Helicobacter pylori* eradication failure. Gastroenterol Int. 1997;10:153–60.

19. Atherton JC, Hawkey CJ, Spiller RC. Retreatment of *Helicobacter pylori* infection with amoxicillin and omeprazole in patients failing this regimen is less successful than initial treatment. Gastroenterology. 1994;106:A42.
20. Moshkowitz M, Konikoff FM, Peled Y et al. One week triple therapy with omeprazole, clarithromycin and tinidazole for *Helicobacter pylori*: differing efficacy in previously treated and untreated patients. Aliment Pharmacol Ther. 1996;10:1015-9.
21. van Doorn LJ, Schneeberger PM, Nouhan N et al. Importance of *Helicobacter pylori* cagA and vacA status for the efficacy of antibiotic treatment. Gut. 2000;46:321-6.
22. Borody TJ, Shortis NP, Chongnan J et al. Eradication failure after *H. pylori* treatment – further therapies. Gastroenterology. 1996;110:A67.
23. Seppala K, Sipponen P, Nuutinen H et al. Intent to treat metronidazole resistant *H. pylori* infection to 100% of cure. Therapy with quadruple therapy and its modifications. Gastroenterology. 1995;108:A216.
24. Tucci A, Poli L, Caletti G. Treatment of the ineradicable *H. pylori* infection. Am J Gastroenterol. 199;94:1713-15.
25. Borody TJ, Shortis NP, Reyes E. Eradication therapies for *Helicobacter pylori*. J Gastroenterol. 1998;33(Suppl. X):53-6.
26. Lam SK, Talley NJ. Report of the 1997 Asia Pacific Consensus Conference on the management of *Helicobacter pylori* infection. J Gastroenterol Hepatol. 1998;13:1-12.
27. Kayser S, Flury R, Zbinden R et al. Comparative effect of lansoprazole/amoxicillin and omeprazole/amoxicillin for eradication of *Helicobacter pylori* in duodenal ulcer patients. Schweiz Med Wochenschr. 1997;127:722-7.
28. De Koster E, De Reuck, Jonas C et al. French triple works fine in Brussels. Gastroenterology. 1997;112:A99.
29. Lee JM, Fallon C, Breslin NP, Hyde DK. *H. pylori* eradication: quadruple therapy is effective in triple therapy failures. Gastroenterology. 1997;112:A195.
30. Huelin Benitez J, Jimenez Perez M, Duran Campos A et al. Quadruple therapy with omeprazole, tetracycline, metronidazole and bismuth as a second option after failure of a first eradication therapy. Gut. 1998;43(Suppl. 2):A86.
31. Borda F, Martinez A, Echarri A et al. Clinical practice results of quadruple treatment in *Helicobacter pylori* eradication failure with OCA-7. Gut. 1998;43(Suppl. 2):A81.
32. Goddard AF, Logan RPH, Atherton JC, Hawkey CJ, Spiller RC. Maastricht consensus report regimen for second-line treatment of *H. pylori* infection: how does it perform in practice? Gut. 1997;41(Suppl. 1):A96.
33. Peitz U, Nusch A, Sulliga M, Becker T, Stolte M, Borsch G. Second-line treatment of *Helicobacter pylori* infection. Gut. 1997;41(Suppl. 1):A104.
34. Neville P, Barrowclough S, Moayyedi P. Second-line eradication for *H. pylori* after failure of therapy with proton pump inhibitor (PPI), clarithromycin and metronidazole: results of a case series. Gastroenterology. 1999;116:A266.
35. Peitz U, Sulliga M, Nusch A et al. Randomised study on two second line treatments after failed metronidazole–clarithromycin therapy. Gut. 1999;45(Suppl. III):A114.
36. Canena JM, Pinto AS, Reis JA et al. Safe profile of quadruple therapy using combination of omeprazole and bismuth. Gastroenterology. 1999;116:A131.
37. Pieramico O, Zanetti MV. Treatment with quadruple therapy after triple therapy failure in patients infected with *H. pylori* resistant strains. Gastroenterology. 1999;116:A282.
38. Katelaris P, Nguyen TV, Robertson G. Efficacy of repeat treatments after initial failure of *Helicobacter pylori* eradication therapy. Gastroenterology. 1999,116.A205.
39. Yakovenko A, Grigoriev P, Yakovenko E et al. Ranitidine bismuth citrate (RBC)-based triple therapies for recurring *Helicobacter pylori* eradication. Gut. 1999;45 (Suppl. III):A117-18.
40. Graham DY, Osato MS, Hoffman J et al. Metronidazole quadruple therapy for infection with metronidazole resistant *Helicobacter pylori*: a prospective study. Gut. 1999;45(Suppl. 2):A120.
41. Gisbert JP, Boixeda D, Barmejo F et al. Re-treatment after *Helicobacter pylori* eradication failure. Eur J Gastroenterol Hepatol. 1999;11:1049-54.
42. de Boer WA. Bismuth triple therapy: still a very important drug regimen for curing *Helicobacter pylori* infection. Eur J Gastroenterol Hepatol. 1999;11:697-700.
43. Kist M, Strobel S, Folsch UR et al. Prospective assessment of the impact of primary antimicrobial resistance on cure rates of *Helicobacter pylori* infections. Gut. 1997;41(Suppl. 1):A90.

44. Buckley MJM, Xia HX, Hyde DM et al. Metronidazole resistance reduces efficacy of triple therapy and leads to secondary clarithromycin resistance. Dig Dis Sci. 1997;42:2111–5.
45. Marusic M, Katicic M, Presecki et al. Eradication of *H. pylori* infection in hospitalized and non-hospitalized patients. Gut. 1997;41(Suppl. 3):A166.
46. Reilly TG, Ayres RCS, Poxon V, Walt RP. *Helicobacter pylori* eradication in a clinical setting: success rates and the effect on the quality of life in peptic ulcer. Aliment Pharmacol Ther. 1995;9:483–90.
47. Lerang F, Moum B, Haug JB et al. Highly effective second-line anti-*Helicobacter pylori* therapy in patients with previously failed metronidazole based therapy. Scand J Gastroenterol. 1997;32:1209–14.
48. Mera R, Realpe JL, Bravo LE et al. Eradication of *Helicobacter pylori* infection with proton pump based triple therapy in patients in whom bismuth based triple therapy failed. J Clin Gastroenterol 1999;29:51–5.
49. Fennerty MB, Nathan M, Kelly C et al. A randomized trial of lansoprazole, amoxicillin, clarithromycin (LAC) vs lansoprazole, bismuth, metronidazole, tetracycline (LBMT) in the retreatment of patients failing *H. pylori* therapy. Gastroenterology. 199;116:A161.
50. Avidan B, Melzer E, Bar-Meir S. Second-line treatment for the eradication of *Helicobacter pylori* following failure of primary therapy. Eur J Gastroenterol Hepatol. 1999;11:A8.
51. Di Mario F, Salandin S, Dal Bo N et al. Retreatment after failure of *Helicobacter pylori* eradication: quadruple therapy vs ranitidine bismuth citrate two week therapy. Gut. 1999;45(Suppl. III):A115.
52. Della Libera M, Bramati S, Bovo G et al. Re-treatment of patients with persistent *Helicobacter pylori* infection. Gastroenterology 1999;116:A144.
53. DiMario F, Dal bo N, Salandin S et al. The 'very bad' *H. pylori*: experience on 69 consecutive patients after the failure of the second eradication treatment. Gastroenterology. 199;116:A148.
54. Borody TJ, Brandl S, Andrews P et al. *H. pylori* eradication failure – further treatment possibilities. Gastroenterology. 1992;102:A43.
55. Rinaldi V, Zullo A, De Francesco V. *Helicobacter pylori* eradication with proton pump inhibitor based triple therapies and re-treatment with ranitidine bismuth citrate-based triple therapy. Aliment Pharmacol Ther. 1999;13:163–8.
56. Michopoulos S, Tsibouros P, Sotiropoulos M et al. Randomized comparison of omeprazole and ranitidine when used for *H. pylori* eradication in 'quad' treatment (second line) of patients with erosive duodenitis or duodenal ulcer disease. Gut. 1999;45(Suppl. 2):A118.
57. Chiba N, Hunt RH. Bismuth, metronidazole and tetracycline and acid suppression in *H. pylori* eradication: a meta-analysis. Gut. 1996;39(Suppl. 2):A36–7.
58. Gomollon F, Ducons JA, Ferrero M et al. Quadruple therapy is effective for eradicating *Helicobacter pylori* after failure of triple proton pump inhibitor-based therapy: a detailed, prospective analysis of 21 consecutive cases. Helicobacter. 1999;4:222–5.
59. Garcia-Romero E, Del Val E, Cuquerella J et al. Erradicacion de *Helicobacter pylori* con terapia triple de 6 dias en pacientes con ulcera duodenal (UD). Eficacia de una cuadruple terapiua de 7 dias en los francos. Gastroenterol Hepatol. 1997;20:525.
60. Gisbert JP, Gisbert JL, Marcos S et al. Seven day 'rescue' therapy after *Helicobacter pylori* treatment failure: omeprazole, bismuth, tetracycline and metronidazole versus ranitidine bismuth citrate, tetracycline and metronidazole. Aliment Pharmacol Ther. 1999;13:1311–6.
61. Lee JM, Breslin NP, Hyde DK et al. Treatment options for *Helicobacter pylori* infection when proton pump inhibitor-based triple therapy fails in clinical practice. Aliment Pharmacol Ther. 1999;13:489–96.
62. Houben MHMG, Tuinman PR, van de Beek D et al. PPI-triple therapy failure in *Helicobacter pylori* infection: re-treatment with PPI-triple therapy or quadruple therapy? Thesis, University of Amsterdam, 2000.
63. Choi IJ, Park MJ, Kim YS et al. Comparison of the efficacy of two quadruple therapies for *Helicobacter pylori* eradication in patients with primary treatment failure. Gastroenterology. 1999;116:A137.
64. DiMario F, Salandin S, Dal Bo N et al. Retreatment after failure of *Helicobacter pylori* eradication: quadruple vs ranitidine bismuth citrate 2 weeks therapy. Gastroenterology. 1999;116:A149.
65. Neville P, Axon A, Moayyedi P. Addition of metronidazole to omeprazole and amoxicillin for second line *H. pylori* eradication does not influence eradication rates: results of a single blinded randomised trial. Gastroenterology. 1999;116:A266.

66. Chen CY, Chen CY, Chang TT et al. What is the best rescue therapy for omeprazole plus amoxicillin? Gut. 1996;39(Suppl. 3):A144.
67. Sheu BS, Wu JJ, Yang HB, Huang AH, Lin XZ. One week proton pump inhibitor based triple therapy eradicates residual *Helicobacter pylori* after failed dual therapy. J Formos Med Assoc. 1998;97:266–70.
68. Cudia B, Romano M, Gioe FP et al. Rescue therapy including ranitidine bismuth citrate (RBC) + minocicline (MIN) + amoxicillin (AMOX) for eradication of *Helicobacter pylori* in previous HP treatment failure. Gut. 1997;41(Suppl. 1):A103.
69. de Boer WA, Haeck PWE, Otten MH et al. Optimal treatment of *Helicobacter pylori* with ranitidine bismuth citrate (RBC): a randomized comparison between two 7-day triple therapies and a 14-day dual therapy. Am J Gastroenterol. 1998;93:1101–7.
70. Peitz U, Glasbrenner B, Ellenrieder V et al. Re-treatment of *H. pylori* infection with high dose omeprazole–amoxicillin after failure with metronidazole–clarithromycin combination. Gut. 1999;45(Suppl. III):A111.
71. Jaup BH. Dual rescue therapy for eradication of *H. pylori* in previous triple therapy failure. Gut. 1999;45(Suppl. III):A118.
72. van der Hulst RWM, Weel JFL, Verheul SB et al. Treatment of *Helicobacter pylori* infection with low or high dose omeprazole combined with amoxicillin and the effect of early retreatment. Aliment Pharmacol Ther. 1996;10:165–71.
73. Perri F, Festa V, Andriulli A. Treatment of antibiotic resistant *Helicobacter pylori* infection. N Engl J Med. 1999;339:53.
74. Perri F, Festa V, Quitadamo M et al. 'RAP'-treatment for *Helicobacter pylori* infected patients after failure of standard triple therapies: a dose response study. Gut. 1999;45(Suppl. III):A107.
75. Bock H, Heep M, Lehn N. Rifabutin, Amoxicillin and lansoprazole eradication of *H. pylori* after multiple therapy failures. Gut. 1999;45(Suppl. III):A109.
76. Lamarque D, Tankovic J, Berrhouma A et al. Triple therapy using ciprofloxacin for eradication of clarithromycin and metronidazole-resistant *Helicobacter pylori*. Gut. 1997;41 (Suppl. 1):A104.
77. Graham DY, Hoffman J, Osato MS et al. New therapy for metronidazole or clarithromycin resistant *Helicobacter pylori*: FOC or FOM. Gastroenterology. 1998;114:A138–9.
78. Santolaria S, Guirao R, Ducons JA et al. Effectividad de la pauta 'cuadruple' en los francasos de erradicacion: analisis detallado segun las resistencias a claritromicina y metronidazol. Gastroentreol Hepatol. 1998;21:519.
79. Megraud F. Epidemiology and mechanism of antibiotic resistance in *Helicobacter pylori*. Gastroenterology. 1998;115:1278–82.
80. de Boer WA, van Etten RJXM, van de Wouw BAM et al. Bismuth based quadruple therapy for *Helicobacter pylori* – a single triple capsule plus lansoprazole. Aliment Pharmacol Ther. 2000;14:85–89.
81. de Boer WA, van Etten RJXM, Schneeberger PM, Tytgat GNJ. A single drug for *Helicobacter pylori* infection: first results with a new bismuth triple monocapsule. Am J Gastroenterol. 2000;95:641–5.

67
Quadruple should be first-line therapy for *Helicobacter pylori* infection

T. J. BORODY

INTRODUCTION

Classic quadruple therapy is the combination of a proton pump inhibitor (PPI) and the classic triple therapy, which consists of bismuth, tetracycline hydrochloride and metronidazole. Quadruple therapy has been conventionally relegated to the position of 'last resort' therapy or 'salvage therapy' following eradication failure[1]. It initially emerged as an improvement of classic triple therapy in that it reduced the patient's symptoms during the treatment through the use of a PPI and at the same time significantly improved the eradication rate. Going back in history to the development of *Helicobacter pylori* eradication therapies, those who remember will note that monotherapy with bismuth was soon followed by dual therapy using bismuth and amoxycillin, and later by triple therapy of bismuth + amoxycillin + metronidazole – changing the amoxycillin for tetracycline to avoid penicillin allergies. As the credibility of *H. pylori* as a cause of ulcer disease and stomach cancer grew, there evolved a 'race' for the development of a monotherapy or 'magic bullet' to eradicate all helicobacters. To simplify triple therapy downsizing from triple to double therapy was attempted, and passed through a phase of multiple trials of a combination of omeprazole and amoxycillin; that experiment unfortunately failed[2]. Soon there came a return to triple therapy but with a shift away from bismuth towards a combination of PPIs and two antibiotics such as clarithromycin and metronidazole or clarithromycin and amoxycillin – as reviewed by Misiewicz[3]. The race for the 'single magic bullet' died when it was realized that chronic infections appear to require multiple antibiotics for efficient eradication. Classic triple therapy was maligned for its complexity and side-effects[4]. Meanwhile, PPI-clarithromycin + amoxycillin or nitroimidazole combinations began progressively falling from favour as clarithromycin resistance increased[5,6] and clarithromycin-based therapies began to lose efficacy[7,8].

Hence, history has come full circle and the quadruple therapy which was relegated to the position of an 'agent of last resort' is starting to look good again.

Quadruple therapy has indeed come a long way, and it owes a great debt to Dr Wink de Boer who, during and after publication of his PhD thesis[9], continued trials with quadruple therapy and maintained interest in the subject through his ongoing publications[10].

In this debate the virtues of quadruple therapy will be presented. These virtues will be reviewed, compared and contrasted with what is otherwise available for patients with *H. pylori* infection. Quadruple therapy should be first-line therapy for *H. pylori* infection for the following reasons:

Highest efficacy therapy

Of all the widely tested therapies quadruple therapy heads the list as the most efficacious first-line therapy. These results come from Europe and also Asia and Australia[15,17,18] and report an eradication rate of over 90%, which is generally greater than that obtained with proton pump based triple therapies. Indeed it is clear that quadruple therapy is a powerful treatment as it can achieve 90% eradication even when given for only 4 days[29,30]. With an eradication rate of over 90% the eradication failure rate is less than 10%. For a patient who has for years suffered with chronic dyspepsia the physician needs to make a serious decision before giving his patient therapy with an eradication rate of say 80% and an eradication failure rate of 20% – knowing that one out of five will need to be re-treated to obtain a 90% eradication. Using quadruple therapy the treating physician will not need to face >20 out of 100 patients failing PPI triple therapy to tell them that they will require biopsy, culture and re-treatment dependent on sensitivity to clarithromycin. Perhaps we should warn our patients who are being given a PPI triple therapy of the increased risks that attend its use in the event of eradication failure, and the need for further antibiotic therapy. Perhaps one of the reasons for the unsurpassed eradication rate of quadruple therapy is its ability to manage not only metronidazole-sensitive but also the majority of metronidazole-resistant strains, and it can therefore be used in all populations. Even in populations where metronidazole resistance is over 50%[12,14], quadruple therapy has reached over 95% eradication rate in the large trials. Furthermore, in the event of quadruple therapy failure as a first-line treatment, the number of patients that require re-treatment is significantly lower. With the availability of clarithromycin for second-line therapy this gives the patient a highly effective combination, without exposing large segments of the population to clarithromycin, potentially leading to irreversible resistance. Metronidazole remains an important component of quadruple therapy and, with the need to combine at least three drugs in any *H. pylori* therapeutic protocol, metronidazole will continue to be a key candidate. One of the important observations on metronidazole resistance is that, in spite of high resistance rates (e.g. >50%), when included in quadruple therapy the cure rate of metronidazole-resistant and -sensitive bacteria remains high as the therapy approaches 7 days of treatment (Table 1). Since quadruple therapy does not contain clarithromycin it is not affected by its rising resistance. On

Table 1. Results achieved with quadruple therapy for 1 week when given as primary treatment (PPI + bismuth salt + metronidazole + tetracycline)[a]

Reference	PPI used	Cure rate overall		MTZ sensitive	MTZ resistant
		No.	Percentage		
12	Omeprazole	70/74	95	NA[b]	NA[b]
13	Omeprazole	66/67	98	NA[b]	NA[b]
14	Omeprazole	53/54	98	27/28	3/3
15	Omeprazole	37/40	93	26/28	5/5
16	Omeprazole	31/35	89	20/22	3/3
	Lansoprazole	30/32	94	12/14	0/0
17	Omeprazole	140/147	95	93/96	35/37
18	Omeprazole	49/53	92	NA[b]	NA[b]
19	Omeprazole	50/50	100	NA[b]	NA[b]
20	Omeprazole	74/82	90	42/43	32/39+
21[c]	Omeprazole	48/52	92	NA	NA
22	Lansoprazole	114/130	89	NA	NA
23	Omeprazole	24/40	60	NA	NA
24	Omeprazole	107/107	100	51/51	56/56

NA = not available; + = significant difference between cure rate in sensitive and resistance strains.
[a] Prevalence of metronidazole resistance in Hong Kong 53%.
[b] After ref. 11.
[c] Metronidazole was given for only 3 days.

the other hand, clarithromycin-containing therapies face increasing failure rates and decreasing recommendations as 'primary treatment' as community clarithromycin resistance rises above just 10%[25]. In a sense quadruple therapy largely overcomes metronidazole resistance, and bismuth and tetracycline resistance is rare. With metronidazole resistance overcome by quadruple therapy this treatment suffers little from microbial resistance, thought to be the main determinant of success in eradication therapy[4,26].

Rising clarithromycin resistance

With a documented rise in *H. pylori* resistance to clarithromycin[5], and without expensive and time-consuming pre-treatment sensitivity testing, clarithromycin-based therapies are progressively falling below the target of 80% eradication by intention to treat analysis. Eradication rates in some regions are falling to levels of around 60-70%[7,8] and eradication failure rates rising to over 30%. Sensitivity-blind therapy in such circumstances is equivalent to 'Russian roulette' with a 1:3 failure rate. This is clearly clinically unacceptable. The greater the use of clarithromycin in therapies the greater the development of community-wide resistance and this is a powerful reason why clarithromycin-based therapy use should be limited as soon as possible and quadruple therapy introduced as first-line therapy for *H. pylori* to save the loss of a valuable clarithromycin-based second-line therapy.

The penicillin allergy question

Quadruple therapy does not contain amoxycillin. The most commonly used PPI triple therapy contains amoxycillin. Around 9% of patients claim that they are 'sensitive' or 'allergic' to penicillin, and from a legal point of view these patients must be excluded from the use of an amoxycillin-containing PPI-based triple therapy. With trials analysed on an ITT basis the clarithromycin:amoxycilin:PPI-based triple therapy efficacy should be discounted by a figure of around 9% to be compared realistically with other ITTs. Patients who have been selected for trials using PPI-AC have had 9% of their number removed because of an exclusion criterion of 'penicillin allergy'. This disadvantages quadruple therapy and seems an inaccurate evaluation of efficacy. ITT should include all patients, and 'failure' should appear if a patient was excluded due to penicillin allergy. Otherwise, this therapy only addresses the non-penicillin allergic subgroup of the population, and the very definition of ITT is transgressed. In other words, a PPI-based triple therapy with clarithromycin and amoxycillin is actually 9% less efficacious than the ITT figure ascribed to it.

Quadruple therapy as a rescue therapy

Two International Consensus Conferences have recommended quadruple therapy as a rescue treatment after eradication failure. This recommendation is not because quadruple therapy is inefficacious or impotent, but because it has power to be a 'rescue therapy' in a situation where primary therapy has not done the job. This very recommendation indicates that quadruple therapy can cure even those patients who fail the current recommended first-line PPI triple therapy. This recommendation makes the statement that quadruple therapy is indeed potent. If it is so potent quadruple therapy should be the first to be used – to prevent eradication failure and minimize the need for second-line therapy[10].

Quadruple therapy does not expose patients to clarithromycin

Exposure of bacteria to antibiotics which fail to eradicate the infection as monotherapy can stimulate the selection of resistant strains. It is a bold statement, indeed, that exposure of patients to clarithromycin could harm them in the long term. However, such a statement can be backed up by evidence. A short exposure to clarithromycin could jeopardize future antibiotic treatment for a variety of important conditions. Importance of macrolides in community-acquired atypical pneumonia is an example of the need to preserve the efficacy of antimicrobials[27]. *Mycobacterium paratuberculosis* is emerging as a strong causal contender of Crohn's disease[28]. A short course of clarithromycin for *H. pylori* in a young person who is developing Crohn's disease may confound potential treatment, which requires macrolide-containing therapy used to treat *Mycobacterium paratuberculosis* in the intestine[31]. Quadruple therapy does not expose patients to clarithromycin with these shortcomings.

No 'big pharma' for quadruple therapy

It is probably true to say that had quadruple therapy been championed by a large pharmaceutical company it might have become the leading treatment and the PPI-based triple therapy would not have eventuated. We can never underestimate the developmental and marketing impetus that can be given to a therapy when finance and high levels of expertise are behind the project. Furthermore, we might have exposed less of the world to the macrolides required for more serious diseases.

Potential clarithromycin bowel effects

Although clearly not a widespread phenomenon, pseudomembranous colitis (PMC) from clarithromycin-based therapy has been recorded[32] and two deaths documented[33]. Particularly when combined with amoxycillin, PMC is more likely. Quadruple therapy has an in-built safety against PMC as demonstrated by its widespread use – probably due to bismuth, tetracycline and metronidazole having anti-Clostridial activity. This does not mean that quadruple therapy is excluded as a cause for PMC, but the likelihood is reduced.

Side-effects and compliance

All therapies display adverse effects. PPI triple therapy as well as quadruple therapy have side-effects. However, numerically quadruple therapy and PPI triple therapy are not far apart in complications, as reflected by comparable dropout rates of around 3% for both types of therapy[16,35-37]. Compliance is a factor of patients and of therapy. Compliance is generally not a problem, with good results reported with the use of quadruple therapy in primary care[36]. Even if the 'missed dose' rate was higher in quadruple therapy, there is a certain reserve of efficacy in quadruple therapy which PPI triple therapy does not have. Moreover, quadruple therapy is taken four times daily, whereas PPI triple therapy is twice daily. Thus, if a single dose of PPI triple therapy is missed, 50% of that day's doses have been missed, while the figure is only 25% for quadruple therapy. This gives quadruple therapy greater reserve and probably helps buffer quadruple therapy from some compliance problems.

CONCLUSION

Although quadruple therapy appears to be more complicated it is the most effective therapy which reduces 'resistant' scars on our patients. Use of quadruple therapy initially allows for a more effective second-line therapy if required – a less common phenomenon. If we are to give patients the highest efficacy, lowest eradication failure, and avoid creating resistance in non-*Helicobacter* infections quadruple therapy should be given as first-line treatment for *H. pylori* infection.

References

1. Malfertheiner P, Megraud F, O'Morain C et al. Current European concepts in management of *Helicobacter pylori* infection – the Maastricht Consensus Report. The European *Helicobacter pylori* Study Group (EHPSG). Eur J Gastroenterol Hepatol. 1997;9:1–2.

2. Tytgat G, Noach L. *H. pylori* Eradication. *Helicobacter pylori* – Basic Mechanisms to Clinical Cure. Proceedings of International Symposium, Florida. 3–6 November 1993; P550–69.
3. Misiewicz J. Management of *Helicobacter pylori* related disorders. Eur J Gastroenterol Hepatol 1997;9(Suppl. 1):S17–20.
4. de Boer W, Tytgat G. The best therapy for *Helicobacter pylori* infection. Scand J Gastroenterol. 1995;30:401–7.
5. Vakil N, Hahn B, McSorley D. Clarithromycin resistant *Helicobacter pylori* in the United States. Am J Gastroenterol. 1998,93:1432–5.
6. De Koster E, Cozzoli A, Vandenborre C et al. *Helicobacter pylori* resistance to macrolides increases, to imidazoles remains stable. AGA Digestive Diseases Week, 10–16 May 1997:A1619.
7. Realdi G, Dore MP, Carta M et al. Failure of Bazzoli's regimen (omeprazole–metronidazole–clarithromycin) therapy for *H. pylori* infection in Sardinia. Gastroenterology. 1998;114:A226.
8. Bigard MA, Delcher JC, Riachi G, Thibault P, Barthelemy P. One week triple therapy using omeprazole, amoxycillin and clarithromycin for the eradication of *Helicobacter pylori* in patients with non-ulcer dyspepsia: influence of dosage of omeprazole and clarithromycin. Aliment Pharmacol Ther. 1998;12:383–8.
9. de Boer W. *Helicobacter pylori* – studies on epidemiology diagnosis and therapy. Thesis, Universiteit van Amsterdam.
10. de Boer W. Quadruple therapy: first- or second-line anti-*Helicobacter pylori* therapy? Res Clin For. 1998;20:43–7.
11. de Boer W. Quadruple therapy – second- or first-line eradication regimen? Clinical pharmacology and therapy for *Helicobacter pylori* infection. Prog Basic Clin Pharmacol Basel: Krager 1999;11:212–26.
12. Hosking SW, Ling TKW, Yung MY et al. Randomised controlled trial of short term treatment to eradicate *H. pylori* in patients with duodenal ulcer. Br Med J. 1992;305:502–4.
13. Hosking SW, Ling TW, Chung SCS et al. Duodenal ulcer healing by eradication of *H. pylori* without anti-acid treatment. Randomised controlled trial. Lancet. 1994;343:508–10.
14. de Boer WA, Driessen WMM, Jansz AR. Tytgat GNJ. Effect of acid suppression on efficacy of treatment for *Helicobacter pylori*. Lancet. 1995;335:817–20.
15. de Boer, Driessen WMM, Jansz AR, Tytgat GNJ. Quadruple therapy compared with dual therapy for eradication of *Helicobacter pylori* in ulcer patients. Eur J Gastroenterol Hepatol. 1995;7:1189–94.
16. de Boer WA, van Etten RJXM, Lai JYL, Schneeberger PM, van de Wouw BAM, Driessen WMM. Effectiveness of quadruple therapy using lansoprazole instead of omeprazole in curing *Helicobacter pylori* infection. Helicobacter. 1996;1:145–50.
17. Borody TJ, Andrews P, Shortis NP, Hyland I. Seven-day therapy for *Helicobacter pylori*. Gastroenterology. 1995;106:A62.
18. Sung JJY, Leung VKS, Chung SCS et al. Triple therapy with sucralfate, tetracycline and metronidazole for *Helicobacter*-associated duodenal ulcers. Am J Gastroenterol. 1995; 90:1424–7.
19. Kung NNS, Sung JJY, Yuen NWI et al. Anti-*Helicobacter* treatment in bleeding ulcers. Randomized controlled trial comparing 2-day vs 7-day bismuth quadruple therapy. Am J Gastroenterol. 1997;92:438–41.
20. van der Hulst RWM, van der Ende A, Homan A, Roorda P, Dankert J, Tytgat GNJ. Influence of metronidazole resistance on efficacy of quadruple therapy for *Helicobacter pylori* eradication. Gut. 1998;42:166–9.
21. Vautier G, Scott BB. A one week quadruple eradication regimen for *Helicobacter pylori* in routine clinical practice. Aliment Pharmacol Ther. 1997:11:107–8.
22. Bolin TD, Korman MG, Engelman JL, Nicholson FB. Lansoprazole and bismuth triple therapy in the eradication of *Helicobacter pylori*. Gastroenterology. 1997;112:A76.
23. Phull PS, Griffiths AE, Halliday D, Jacyna MR. One week treatment for *Helicobacter pylori* infection: a randomised study of quadruple therapy versus triple therapy. J Antimicrob Chemother. 1995;36:1085–8.
24. Chan FKL, Yung MY, Lint TKW, Leung WK, Chung SCS. What is the true impact of metronidazole resistance on the efficacy of bismuth triple therapy? Gut. 1998; 43(Suppl. 2):A85.

25. de Boer W, Tytgat G. Treatment of *Helicobacter pylori* infection. Br Med J. 2000;320:31–4.
26. de Boer W, Tytgat G. How to treat *Helicobacter pylori* – should treatment strategies be based on testing bacterial susceptibility? A personal viewpoint. Eur J Gastroenterol Hepatol. 1996;8:709–16.
27. Bayerdorffer E *et al.* Omeprazole, amoxycillin and metronidazole for the cure of *Helicobacter pylori* infection. Eur J Gastroenterol Hepatol. 1999;11(Suppl. 2):S19–22.
28. Hermon-Taylor J. The causation of Crohn's disease and treatment with antimicrobial drugs. Commentary. Ital J Gastroenterol Hepatol. 1998;30:607–10.
29. de Boer WA, Driessen WMM, Tytgat GNJ. Only four days of quadruple therapy can effectively cure *Helicobacter pylori* infection. Aliment Pharmacol Ther. 1995;9:633–8.
30. de Boer WA *et al.* Four day lansoprazole-quadruple therapy is very effective in curing *Helicobacter pylori* infection. Am J Gastroenterol. 1996;91:1778–82.
31. Borody T, Pearce L, Bampton P, Leis S. Treatment of severe Crohn's disease using rifabutin–macrolide–clofazimine combination: interim report. Gastroenterology. 1998;114:A938.
32. Borody TJ, Shortis NP, Chongnan J. Reyes E, O'Shea J. Eradication failure (EF) after *H. pylori* treatment – further therapies. Gastroenterology. 1996;110:A67.
33. Teare JP, Booth JC, Brown JL, Martin J, Thomas HC. Pseudomembranous colitis following clarithromycin therapy. Eur J Gastroenterol Hepatol. 1995;3:275–7.
34. Lerang G *et al.* Simplified 10-day bismuth triple therapy for cure of *Helicobacter pylori* infection: experience from clinical practice in a population with a high frequency of metronidazole resistance. Am J Gastroenterol. 1998;93:212–16.
35. Chiba N, Hunt RH. Bismuth, metronidazole and tetracycline (BMT) $\pm$ acid suppression in *H. pylori* eradication. A meta-analysis. Gut. 1996;39 (Suppl. 2):A36–7.
36. de Boer WA *et al.* One-day intensified lansoprazole-quadruple therapy for cure of *Helicobacter pylori* infection. Aliment Pharmacol Ther. 1997;11:109–12.

68
Quadruple therapy should be second-line treatment for *Helicobacter pylori* infection

A. AXON

INTRODUCTION

Triple therapy comprising a combination of bismuth (B), metronidazole (M) and tetracycline (T) was the first effective anti-*Helicobacter* combination to be used in clinical practice. From the beginning, however, it was unpopular because it was a complicated regimen. Although some centres reported excellent results, with over 90% success, others obtained disappointing 60% cure rates. It took some years to realize that the variations in results were partly a reflection of whether or not acid-suppressive drugs were used in addition to the triple therapy. Some centres routinely added an H_2-receptor antagonist to heal the peptic ulcer; others did not do this but relied upon the healing properties of the bismuth. The importance of acid suppression in *H. pylori* eradication regimens was recognized only when it was noted that the combination of omeprazole with amoxycillin (A) was effective, whereas amoxycillin on its own was not. It is still unclear why acid suppression benefits *H. pylori* eradication regimens. It appears that bismuth triple therapy is less effective in patients infected with metronidazole-resistant organisms, whereas if acid suppression is added to the regimen the combination is successful even with these otherwise resistant organisms. A similar situation obtains with a combination of clarithromycin (C) and metronidazole. In the absence of acid suppression, metronidazole-resistant organisms survive, whilst acid suppression seems to render them more susceptible.

Bismuth triple therapy (BTT) lost its popularity before this important fact was realized, because of the variability of published results, the complexity of the combinations, the 2 weeks therapy recommended and the fact that side-effects were a frequent problem. Today the situation is different. The addition of a proton pump inhibitor to bismuth, tetracycline and metronidazole provides a 1-week therapy which is effective, active against metronidazole-resistant organisms and has fewer side-effects. It is still rather

Table 1. Percentage eradication rates for *H. pylori* regimens according to two recently published meta-analyses

	Per-protocol		Intention-to-treat	
	Houben et al.[1]	Laheij et al.[2]	Houben et al.[1]	Leheij et al.[2]
Rbc–CM	92	91	87	78
PPI–BTM	92	91	87	82
PPI–AC	84	86	81	80
PPI–CM	90	87	86	83
Rbc–AC		88		81

Rbc = ranitidine bismuth citrate; C = clarithromycin (or other macrolide); M = metronidazole (or other nitroimidazole); PPI = proton pump inhibitor; A = amoxycillin.

cumbersome for general use. It is, in short, an effective tool that should be added to the armamentarium deployed against *H. pylori* infection; the question is at what point should it be prescribed.

FIRST-LINE THERAPY

So many different combinations of antibiotics and acid suppressants have been used in different geographical locations, for patients with different ages, genders, diseases and ethnic backgrounds that it is difficult to provide all-embracing advice for clinicians. Recently, two excellent meta-analyses have been published that have independently analysed the data and have provided results that are similar[1,2]. Table 1 shows the results obtained from the best combinations. On a per-protocol basis eradication rates for the best treatments range from 84% to 92%. On intention-to-treat analysis, however, figures range from 78% to 87%. The variation between the effectiveness in the two meta-analyses makes it difficult to come down strongly for any one of the four regimens on the basis of successful treatment, and the decision as to which combination should be chosen as a first-line treatment has to be based on other factors.

In reality, if success rates of 80–85% confirmed eradication are to be expected in a clinical trial it is likely that treatment in the community will be less successful, probably ranging from 75% to 80%. The problem with this is that up to 25% of patients treated will be failures, and it is this substantial minority who represent the greatest challenge in management. It is clear, therefore, that when considering the choice of a first-line treatment we should not consider this in isolation, but should ensure that the medication does not compromise a second line of attack if the first combination fails.

WHAT ARE THE REASONS FOR ERADICATION FAILURE?

Previous work has shown that the main reason for treatment failure is poor patient compliance. No matter how good the treatment is, if the patient does not take it then it will not work. Most patients with poor compliance probably take some drug but discontinue it either from boredom, fear, forgetfulness, laziness or side-effects. It is this group which represents the biggest problem because they are patients who do want treatment, but having taken an inadequate course, now harbour resistant organisms. The second cause for failure of treatment is antibiotic resistance. Increasing numbers of *H. pylori* infections are developing resistance; many to nitroimidazoles, some to macrolides, but others to tetracycline and a few to amoxycillin. It is important to recognize that, if a patient is infected with an organism that is resistant, treatment with a combination that contains that antibiotic may still work; but if it does not, there is a real risk that the patient will then be resistant to both antibiotics. The third cause of failure of treatment is what could be described as 'constitutional'. Occasionally one meets a patient in whom all attempts to eradicate the infection have met with failure. Not all of these patients have resistant organisms, and many of them are fully compliant. Whether failure in these cases is due to an organism that is resistant *in vivo*, as opposed to *in vitro*, or whether the patient has some genetic or environmental influence that prevents the antibiotics from working is unclear. These cases are uncommon but, as the cause of failure is not understood, a logical approach to their management is not possible.

CHOOSING A STRATEGY

It follows from the above that in choosing the strategy that will cure as many individuals as possible it is necessary to focus on the problems of compliance and antibiotic resistance. It is expensive and impractical to obtain antibiotic sensitivity on all patients who require eradication therapy. Furthermore, controversy still surrounds the importance of metronidazole resistance because, as indicated earlier, the use of acid suppression in addition to metronidazole and another antibiotic will often lead to a successful outcome in spite of apparent metrnonidazole resistance. A logical approach would be to use a first-line treatment containing one group of drugs, followed if necessary by a second regimen comprising completely different drugs. In this way, if the first therapy fails or induces resistance to the other antibiotic of the combination the second therapy, by using completely different antibiotics, should give the best chance of success.

A consideration of Table 1 suggests that the use of a PPI plus CM, although perhaps the most effective primary treatment, is maybe not the best one to use initially. This is because all of the best combinations use either clarithromycin or metronidazole, therefore, it would be impossible to use a completely different combination if one starts with these two antibiotics. The alternatives are to use PPI–AC followed by PPI–BTM (or ranitidine bismuth citrate (Rbc)). By doing this the whole range of effective treatment will have been provided independently over the protocol. At present, quadruple therapy (PPI–BMT) is preferred to Rbc–TM because quadruple therapy has been used in a larger number of studies and considerable experience has been gained with it, whereas to date the RBC combination with metronidazole and tetracycline has not been evaluated fully. If then PPI–AC and PPI–BMT are the two combinations to be used in the treatment protocol the next question is in which order should they be used?

Table 2. Success rates for the secondary eradication of *H. pylori* from some recent studies

Pieramico et al.[3]	20/21
Choi et al.[4]	16/22
Lee et al.[5]	15/20
Peitz et al.[6]	17/29
Neville[7]	16/32
Gisbert et al.[8]	17/29
Chan et al.[9]	5/7
Total	106/160 = 60%

PPI–AC involves taking three drugs twice a day for a week. The dose of amoxycillin is high, two capsules have to be taken for this, so a daily dose of four tablets twice a day is used for that regimen. The dose schedule of quadruple therapy is more complicated. Most advocates have recommended colloidal bismuth subcitrate (Denol) 120 mg four times a day, tetracycline hydrocholoride 500 mg four times a day, metronidazole 400 mg three times a day and a PPI twice daily. This represents 17 tablets in a rather complicated dose schedule. The efficacy of this combination cannot be impugned on the basis of the effectiveness studies. However, from a practical perspective it would seem to be more sensible to start with the simpler posology, as this is more likely to be accepted by patients as a first treatment. It is more likely that the physician would be able to convince the patient of the importance of taking the more complicated regimen if the patient fails with the first, as patients would probably understand that, after failure with one regimen, they will have to concentrate harder with the second.

Secondary eradication treatment after failure is often referred to as 'rescue; or 'salvage' treatment. Papers published in this area are difficult to analyse. Patients who fail with their first treatment include a higher percentage of individuals who are unreliable tablet takers, others who have resistant organisms and also the 'constitutional' group, where failure will be inevitable. Analysis of results of rescue treatment are bedevilled by inconsistency in patients returning for follow-up or reflecting incomplete compliance. Furthermore, some patients submitted for rescue therapy have already had more than one previous treatment for *H. pylori* and the original primary treatments vary. All of these factors mean that secondary treatment is likely to be less satisfactory than primary treatment. Numbers are relatively small and comparison between studies is difficult. Nevertheless, quadruple therapy has found a niche as a secondary therapy and a number of studies published, mainly in abstract form, have been published and are shown in Table 2. The figures shown are, where possible, per-protocol, and a success rate of 66% is achieved, roughly 20% less than with primary treatment. Although this figure is not as satisfactory as one would hope it is probably the best that can be achieved when considering the difficulties set out earlier in this paragraph. Under the circumstances, therefore, the approach of PPI–AC followed by PPI-BMT would appear to be the most favoured treatment strategy to date. What are now needed are prospective multicentre studies comparing this approach with others. What we have learnt of the treatment of *H. pylori* infection is that, in spite of careful microbiological studies, the best therapies for *H. pylori* eradication have been achieved by empiricism rather than logic.

References

1. Houben MHMG, Van de Beek D, Hensen EF, De Craen AJM, Rauws EAJ, Tytgat GNJ. A systematic review of *Helicobacter pylori* eradication therapy – the impact of antimicrobial resistance on eradication rates. Aliment Pharmacol Ther. 1993;13:1047–55.
2. Laheij RJF, Van Rossum LGM, Jansen JBMJ, Straatman H, Verbeek ALM. Evaluation of treatment regimens to cure *Helicobacter pylori* infection – a meta-analysis. Aliment Pharmacol Ther. 1999;13:857–61.
3. Pieramico O. Treatment with quadruple therapy after triple therapy failure in patients infected with *H. pylori* resistant strains. Gastroenterology. 1999;116:A282.
4. Choi IJ, Park MJ, Kim YS *et al.* Comparison of the efficacy of two quadruple therapies for *Helicobacter pylori* eradication in patients with primary treatment failure. Gastroenterology. 1999;166:A137.
5. Lee JM, Breslin NP, Hyde DK, Buckley MJ, O'Morain CA. Treatment options for *Helicobacter pylori* infection when proton pump inhibitor-based triple therapy fails in clinical practice. Aliment Pharmacol Ther. 1999;13:489–96.
6. Peitz U, Sulliga M, Nusch A *et al.* Randomised study on the impact of resistance on second-line treatment after failed metronidazole–clarithromycin containing triple therapy. Gut. 1998;43:A82.
7. Neville P. Second-line eradication for *H. pylori* after failure of therapy with proton pump inhibitor (PPI), clarithromycin and metronidazole: results of a case series. Gastroenterology. 1999;116:A266.
8. Gisbert JP, Gisbert JL, Marcos S, Garcia Gravalos R, Carpio D, Pajares JM. Seven-day 'rescue' therapy after *Helicobacter pylori* treatment: omeprazole, bismuth, tetracycline and metronidazole vs. ranitidine bismuth citrate, tetracycline and metronidazole. Aliment Pharmacol Ther. 1999;13:1311–16.
9. Chan FKL, Sung JJY, Suen R, Wu JCY, Ling TKW, Chung SCS. Salvage therapies after failure of *Helicobacter pylori* eradication with ranitidine bismuth citrate-based therapies. Aliment Pharmacol Ther. 2000;14:91–5.

69
Helicobacter pylori infection: expectations for future therapy

C. J. HAWKEY

INTRODUCTION

Within 12 years of the discovery of *Helicobacter pylori* and recognition of its importance in ulcer disease, highly effective 1-week regimes for its eradication had become widely used[1-3]. This rapid progress was achieved with results from a relatively small number of trials that were very pragmatic and often under-powered[4], an interesting illustration of the fact that progress can, and usually does, occur in the absence of orthodox research design. As a result, management of *H. pylori*-associated peptic ulcer has been revolutionized by becoming substantially better and substantially cheaper.

There are, however, a number of trade-offs for these rapid pragmatic advances that may hinder progress in the future. First, with a few exceptions[5], trials to date have not had an explanatory design with, for example, an investigation of the extent to which individual components of a regime may synergize or provide additive effects. Often, trials have compared regimes in which more than one of the antibiotics has been different. Consequently, there is little strategic understanding of the principles of drug interaction or synergy even at a clinical level.

This lack of understanding is also seen in studies that have tried to investigate mechanistic aspects of drug regimes directly. It seems likely that antibiotics are delivered to the site of infection from the circulation rather than the gastric lumen, involving, at least for metronidazole, a process linked to acid fluxes[6]. The most cryptic component of current triple-therapy regimens is the proton pump inhibitor (PPI). Omeprazole has been shown to enhance levels of amoxycillin in gastric juice, probably simply by a process of increased concentration[7], but reduce transfer of metronidazole, probably by inhibiting acid-linked transfer mechanisms[6].

One consequence of the limitations on understanding is the lack of a set of principles to identify good treatment regimes for the future, ahead of pragmatic testing. A better understanding of the principles of *H. pylori* therapeutics may be critical, if resistance to existing antibiotics rises substantially. Thus, for example, bismuth appears able to overcome metronidazole resistance[8]. It is less clear if this is also true for clarithromycin, and the possible mechanisms involved remain obscure.

The period since 1995 has been one of 'marking time' with, for example, newer PPIs establishing that their efficacy is comparable to those originally tested. Another reason why progress has slowed is that, as the success of existing treatment has increased, the size of studies required to have sufficient power to show equivalence or improvement with a new regime has grown substantially[4]. Approximately 400 patients would be required to prove a treatment equivalent to within 5% of the best results with bismuth-based triple therapy, and more than 1000 patients would be required to show improvment[9]. Although there has been a big increase in the number of trials conducted since 1995, hardly any of them even approaches such power.

Finally, cost will become an increasing issue and disease targets of treatment widen. A net cost of £25.00 per successful eradication is outstandingly cost-effective in a patient with peptic ulcer, where the subsequent costs of peptic ulcer disease are avoided in nearly every patient treated, whatever assumptions are made about the cost of these[10]. If eradication treatment were proven to prevent some instances of a rare but important condition such as gastric cancer, and it was used in a population for this purpose, cost would become a dominant issue, particularly in countries where health-care resources are limited.

FUTURE THERAPEUTIC NEEDS

The ideal future treatment for *H. pylori* would be cheap, simple to administer, have higher rates of compliance, cause little or no bacterial resistance, hit interesting novel targets and underpin highly effective clinical management strategies. The ideal treatment for *H. pylori* is unlikely to emerge, although at least some of these principles can be expected.

Cost

There is some conflict between the requirements of pharmaceutical companies to recoup research investment and the ability of developing countries to pay for such treatment. Moreover, improvements in sanitation and some economic factors, whilst they may take a generation longer to have impact, may ultimately be more effective than drug treatments. Thus, new treatments that impact upon the less developed world may have to be natural and/or non-patentable products, or possibly a therapeutic vaccination. In this context, the observation that mastic gum chewed by the population of some Mediterranean countries with a low incidence of peptic ulcer inhibits growth of *H. pylori in vitro*[9] deserves testing therapeutically[11].

Simplicity

Current treatment regimes are relatively complex, involving several antibiotics, in part because understanding of how they work together to achieve eradication is so limited. Development of simplified regimes, even involving new antibiotics, may provide better understanding of therapeutic interaction

Compliance

Two main factors influence the success of current therapies: compliance and bacterial resistance. Systematic enhanced patient compliance packs can increase the proportion of pills in an eradication regime that patients actually take[12], but it is uncertain whether this actually influences eradication rate[13].

Resistance

It seems likely that *H. pylori* eradication treatment is currently enjoying a honeymoon period. Resistance to clarithromycin and metronidazole is widespread, and probably increasing as a result of the use of these drugs both for *H. pylori* eradication and other indications[14]. It seems likely that a time will come in the not-too-distant future when therapy will fail more often because of increasing resistance, and then eradication rates will fall, perhaps substantially. How can this be avoided? First, greater understanding of the extent to which bismuth overcomes metronidazole resistance, and a clearer understanding of whether this also extends to clarithromycin resistance, would in the short term be important. It may be that other divalent cations, taken up by *H. pylori*'s avaricious and promiscuous nickel uptake system[15,16] may mimic the effects of bismuth.

In the longer term, development of resistance to future antibiotics might be reduced if their use was dedicated solely to treatment of *H. pylori*. This, in turn, implies development of an antibiotic targeted at a unique colonization, persistence, survival or virulence factor in *H. pylori*, since it is unlikely that commercial pressures would allow an antibiotic to have activity against other bacteria and be restricted to *H. pylori*. Thus, it may be that the 40% of the genome of *H. pylori* whose function is unknown[17,18] could be more fertile soil than the 60% with functions attributed by homology with other bacteria.

TARGETS FOR FUTURE ANTIBIOTICS

Elucidation of the *H. pylori* genome has been important in identifying potential new targets for treatment[16]. Whilst progress since the genome was first published[17] appears to have been slow, with no new antibiotics so far appearing, this is not surprising given commercial secrecy and a long lead time for new drug development. Amongst targets that may be attractive are outer membrane proteins (for vaccination), adherence mechanisms[19–21], *H. pylori*'s unique and potent urease mechanisms by which *H. pylori* maintains a neutral intercellular pH[22], the uptake and extrusion of divalent cations[16], chemo-sensing[23] or motility mechanisms[24] and key metabolic pathways including fumarate reductase[15], as well as the type-4 secretory system that has recently been described[25]. Use of oligosaccharides to 'mop-up' lipoprotein surface adhesions on *H. pylori* and prevent adherence to host oligosaccharide receptors has recently been shown to achieve eradication in infected monkeys[26]. Perhaps loosening adherence might move *H. pylori* to sites where other antibiotics in combination could be more effective?

Whilst vaccination against urease has not been very successful, urease may remain an important drug target, particularly intracellular urease that appears important in maintaining intrabacterial homeostasis[22].

THERAPEUTIC STRATEGIES

Critical therapeutic targets are likely to be defined, particularly for drug development, but may also be targets for vaccine developments. Given the evidence that *H. pylori* infection can sometimes be beneficial to patients, an attractive approach would be just to target, via virulence mechanisms, those bacteria associated with disease. Unfortunately our knowledge of bacterial characteristics that distinguish pathogens from possible commencals[27] is too rudimentary for this to be realistic at present. The question that is increasingly emerging is the extent to which treatment should be aimed in a blunderbuss fashion at large patient populations. One example of this is the 'test-and-treat' strategy. This is, in some ways, unappealing as it undervalues the importance of precise disease diagnosis. Nevertheless, it may be a valid strategy if established by empirical assessments. This will need to include the effect on patient behaviour compared to current more conventional strategies such as endoscopic diagnosis. Results from Nottingham suggest that, whilst the latter is more costly initially, it is better than a test-and-treat strategy in reducing future consultation and drug use, and achieving patient satisfaction with treatment[28].

More difficult to evaluate will be the impact of a population approach to the prevention of gastric cancer in countries where this is common. If eradication in childhood is the critical time to prevent later gastric cancer, it may be impossible to prove the value of this approach and decisions on such strategies may have to be taken on the basis of the balance of probabilities.

TRIAL PRINCIPLES FOR FUTURE THERAPIES

When genuinely new treatments emerge, larger trials than currently conducted are likely to be needed to establish whether there are genuine therapeutic improvements. Ironically, if eradication rates fall because of widespread resistance to current antibiotics, trials will not need to be so large to show an improvement on the reduced efficacy of these regimes! An alternative or complementary strategy would be initially to evaluate regimes over a shorter time-course and/or to use a more sensitive surrogate endpoint (e.g. clearance of faecal antigen) before embarking on definitive large-scale trials. An argument can be made that the *Helicobacter* investigators community is well placed for a collaborative initiative to identify and then answer key therapeutic questions, particularly if they involve the kind of cheap therapies that might not appeal to industry, but nevertheless, have particular potential in the developing world.

References

1. Bazzoli F, Gullini S, Zagari RM et al. Effect of omeprazole and clarithromycin plus tinidazole on the eradication of *Helicobacter pylori* and the recurrence of duodenal ulcer. Gut. 1995;37(Suppl. 1):5.
2. Bazzoli F. Italian omeprazole triple therapy – a 1-week regimen. Scand J Gastroenterol. – Suppl. 1996;215:118.
3. Labenz J., Stolte M, Ruhl GH et al. One-week low-dose triple therapy for the eradication of *Helicobacter pylori* infection. Eur J Gastroenterol Hepatol. 1995;7:9–11.
4. Sherwood 2000 in preparation
5. Peterson WL, Ciociola AA, Sykes DL, McSorley DJ, Webb DD and the RBC *H. pylori* Study Group. Ranitidine bismuth citrate plus clarithromycin is effective for healing duodenal ulcers, eradicating *H. pylori* and reducing ulcer recurrence. Aliment Pharmacol Ther. 1996;10:251–61.
6. Goddard AF, Jessa MJ, Barrett DA et al. Effect of omeprazole on the distribution of metronidazole, amoxicillin, and clarithromycin in human gastric juice. Gastroenterology. 1996;111:358–67.
7. Sherwood PV, Wibaud JI, Goddard AF, Barrett DA, Shaw PN, Spiller RC. Acid secretion determines gastric metronidazole transfer. Gastroenterology. 1999;116:A309.
8. Houben MHMG, van de Beek D, Hensen EF, De Craen AJM, Rauws EAJ, Tytgat GNJ. A systematic review of *Helicobacter pylori* eradication therapy – the impact of antimicrobial resistance on eradication rates. Aliment Pharmacol Ther. 1999;13:1047–55.
9. Borody TJ, Brandl S, Andews P, Ferch N, Jankiewicz E, Hyland L. Use of high efficacy, lower dose triple therapy to reduce side effects of eradicating *Helicobacter pylori*. Am J Gastroenterol. 1994;89:33–8.
10. Duggan AE, Tolley K, Hawkey CJ, Logan RFA. *H. pylori* eradication in duodenal ulcer disease: what determines cost effectiveness? Br Med J. 1998;316:1648–54.
11. Huwez FU, Thurlwell D, Cockayne A, Ala-Aldeen DA. Mastic gum kills *Helicobacter pylori*. N Engl J Med. 1998;339:1946.
12. Lee M, Kem JA, Canning A, Egan C, Tataronis G, Francis F. A randomized controlled trial of an enhanced patient compliance programme for *Helicobacter pylori* therapy. Arch Intern Med. 1999;159:2312–16.
13. Henry A, Batey RG. Enhancing compliance not a prerequisite for effective eradication of *Helicobacter pylori*: the HelP Study. Am J Gastroenterol. 1999;94:811–15.
14. Megraud F. Risk factors for failures. In: Hunt RH, Tytgat GJ, editors. *Helicobacter pylori*: Basic Mechanisms to Clinical Cure 2000; this volume.
15. Hazell S. What are the biochemical and physiological implications of the new genetic information? In: Hunt RH, Tytgat GJ, editors. *Helicobacter pylori*: Basic Mechanisms to Clinical Cure 2000; this volume.
16. Marais A, Mendz GL, Hazell SL, Megraud F. Metabolism and genetics of *Helicobacter pylori*: the genome era. Microbiol Mol Biol Rev. 1999;63:642–74.
17. Tomb J-F, White O, Kerlavage AR et al. The complete genome sequence of the gastric pathogen *Helicobacter pylori*. Nature. 1997;388:539–47.
18. Alm RA, Ling L-SL, Moir DT et al. Genomic-sequence comparison of two unrelated isolates of the human gastric pathogen *Helicobacter pylori*. Nature. 1999;397:176–80.
19. O'Toole PW, Janzon L, Doig P, Huang J, Kostrzynska M, Trust TJ. The putative neuraminyllactose-binding hemagglutinin HpaA of *Helicobacter pylori* CCUG 17874 is a lipoprotein. J Bacteriol. 1995;177:6049–57.
20. Boren T, Roth KA, Larson G, Normark S. Attachment of *Helicobacter pylori* to human gastric epithelium mediated by blood group antigens. Science. 1993;262:1892–5.
21. Zopf D, Roth S. Oligosaccharide anti-infective agents. Lancet. 1996;347:1017–21.
22. Sachs G. Urease regulations. In: Hunt RH, Tytgat GJ editors. *Helicobacter pylori*: Basic Mechanisms to Clinical Cure 2000; this volume.
23. Jackson CJ, Kelly DJ, Clayton CL. The cloning and characterization of chemotaxis genes in *Helicobacter pylori*. Gut. 1995;37:A71.
24. O'Toole PW, Kostrazynska M, Trust TJ. Non-mobile mutants of *Helicobacter pylori* and *Helicobacter mustelae* defective in flagellar hood production. Mol Microbiol. 1994;14:691–703.

25. Sega ED, Cha J, Falkow S, Tompkins LS. Altered states: involvement of phosphorylated CagA in the induction of host cellular growth changes by *Helicobacter pylori* Proc Natl Acad Sci USA. 1999;96:14559–64.
26. Mysore JC, Wiggington T, Simon PM, Zopf D, Heman-Ackah LM, Dubois A. Treatment of *Helicobacter pylori* infection in rhesus monkeys using a novel antiadhesion compound. Gastroenterology. 1999;117:1316–25.
27. Graham DY. vacA, cagA, iceA and babA are not useful for assessing *H. pylori* virulence. In: Hunt RH, Tytgat GJ, editors. *Helicobacter pylori*: Basic Mechanisms to Clinical Cure. 2000; this volume.
28. Duggan AE, Elliott C, Hawkey CJ, Logan RFA. Randomised controlled trial of four dyspepsia management strategies in primary care with 12 months follow-up. Gastroenterology. 2000 (In press).

70
A *Helicobacter pylori* vaccine is essential

S. BANERJEE and P. MICHETTI

HELICOBACTER PYLORI-RELATED DISEASE: THE MAGNITUDE OF THE HEALTH PROBLEM

Helicobacter pylori is one of the most successful of bacterial pathogens. By some estimates over one half of the world's human population is infected with this organism[1]. The prevalence of this infection varies widely between population groups. Whereas in developed countries such as the United States around 30–40% of the population is infected with *H. pylori*[2], the prevalence of the infection in developing countries may be as high as 80–90%[3,4]. *H. pylori* is the most frequent cause of chronic gastritis[5] and is a major aetiological agent in the development of gastric and duodenal ulcers. It is also associated with the development of gastric mucosa-associated lymphoid tissue (MALT) lymphomas and non-cardia gastric adenocarcinomas.

An estimated 5–15% of *H. pylori*-infected subjects will develop peptic ulceration[1]. Worldwide, an estimated 6 000 000 people develop duodenal ulcer each year. Although early studies suggested that *H. pylori* infection was associated with 95% of duodenal ulcers, this may not hold true in areas of low *H. pylori* prevalence, where association rates of 50–60% have been reported for duodenal and gastric ulcers, with lower association rates in whites[6,7]. Regardless, on a global scale the burden of peptic ulcer disease due to *H. pylori* infection is enormous.

Up to 1% of subjects infected with *H. pylori* for > 20 years develop gastric cancer. Gastric cancer ranks 14th as a cause of death worldwide, and is the second commonest cause of cancer-related death[8], with an estimated 750 000 people dying from the disease each year[8,9]. *H. pylori* is estimated to cause 55% of non-cardia gastric cancers[10], and was declared a human Group 1 carcinogen by a working party of the IARC-WHO in 1994[11]. Although the incidence of gastric cancer has been falling over recent decades in the developed world[12], the absolute number of deaths from gastric cancer worldwide will continue to increase over coming decades due to evolving demographics. Improved health care in developing countries, with resultant increases in population and life expectancy, will lead to larger numbers of infected subjects living long enough to develop gastric cancer. These changing demographics are expected to increase gastric cancer deaths to 900 000 per year over the course of the next decade, elevating its ranking to the 8th commonest cause of death worldwide[13]. As survival following the diagnosis of gastric cancer is appallingly short, prevention of the disease by elimination of known carcinogenic factors such as *H. pylori* infection is a desirable and logical intervention.

In summary, it is estimated that *H. pylori* infection results in 5 000 000 new cases per year worldwide of significant gastroduodenal disease, including peptic ulceration and gastric cancer[1]. It is, therefore, a global health problem of considerable magnitude, which mandates an effective and wide-reaching solution.

ARGUMENTS AGAINST ERADICATING *H. PYLORI*

Proponents of *H. pylori* argue that the organism, which has cohabited with humans since the earliest of times, may be a commensal with potentially beneficial effects on upper gastrointestinal physiology, possibly resulting in protection from gastro-oesophageal reflux and consequently from distal oesophageal adenocarcinoma[14]. It has been noted that the incidence of reflux oesophagitis[15] and adenocarcinoma of the lower oesophagus and cardia[16,17] has been increasing over the same time period that prevalence rates of *H. pylori* infection have been falling, raising the possibility of a negative correlation. Prevalence studies have been contradictory and unhelpful, with some studies showing no difference in the prevalence of *H. pylori* infection in patients with reflux oesophagitis and in controls[18,19], while others suggest a decreased prevalence of infection[20,21]. Labenz et al. reported that 26% of patients with duodenal ulcers who underwent eradication of *H. pylori* developed reflux oesophagitis over the subsequent 3 years, compared with only 13% of patients with continuing infection[22]. However, this observation does not confirm direct causality, as the development of reflux was correlated with weight gain. Withdrawal of antisecretory therapy following *H. pylori* eradication may also result in symptomatic unmasking of previously present gastro-oesophageal reflux. Indeed, several subsequent studies have failed to find increased gastro-oesophageal reflux following *H. pylori* eradication[23–27]. Thus, overall, evidence that *H. pylori* infection offers any protection against reflux oesophagitis and oesophageal cancer is scanty, indirect and far from convincing.

It has also been argued that a further beneficial aspect of *H. pylori* infection is that the presence of associated gastritis may improve immune responses against other ingested gastrointestinal pathogens[14]. Mattsson et al. found that only *H. pylori*-positive volunteers developed vaccine-specific antibody-secreting cells (ASCs) in the gastric antrum following ingestion of oral B subunit whole-cell cholera vaccine[28], although duodenal ASCs and serum antibody levels were similar in both *H. pylori*-positive and *H. pylori*-negative volunteers. The authors suggest that *H. pylori*-induced gastritis may facilitate local antigen uptake due to impaired mucosal integrity, and may up-regulate the local immune response. However, the relevance of this observation is debatable, as gastric inflammation may impair generation of secretory IgA and as *H. pylori* infection has recently been associated with an increased risk of bacterial enteric infection. A recent study has indicated that *H. pylori*-specific IgA in the gastric juice of infected humans is predominantly of the non-secretory type[29], which has poor stability due to susceptibility to acid hydrolysis and proteolytic cleavage[30]. Moreover, gastric acid is an important non-immunological defence mechanism against ingested micro-organisms[31–33] and hypochlorhydria due to acute *H. pylori* infection, long-standing disease with atrophic gastritis, or antisecretory therapy may in fact increase susceptibility to other ingested gastrointestinal pathogens. In a recent study during an outbreak of cholera, *H. pylori* infection was associated with increased risk of *Vibrio cholera* infection and more severe dehydration in patients developing choleric diarrhoea[31].

A final question is whether some *H. pylori* strains may be beneficial to humans and so should be preferentially spared, or whether eradication efforts should encompass all strains. $CagA^+$ *H. pylori* strains are associated with a higher risk of peptic ulceration[34], atrophic gastritis[35], and non-cardia gastric adenocarcinoma[36], and arguments have been made that only $cagA^+$ strains should be targeted for eradication. Serological testing for *cagA* status would add considerably to the expense of vaccination, which may not be feasible in developing countries. An alternative approach using CagA as the vaccine antigen might allow serological testing to be dispensed with. However, although CagA has been shown to be a protective vaccine antigen in animal studies[37], it is likely that successful human vaccines will need to be multivalent with more than one antigen[38], making selective targeting of $cagA^+$ strains difficult. Moreover, this association between $cagA^+$ positive strains and gastro-duodenal disease appears restricted to Western populations, and is not seen in Asia[39,40]. $CagA^+$ and $cagA^-$ strains may also coexist in patients[41,42]. Therefore, targeting selected *H. pylori* strains for eradication is unlikely to prove practical.

WHAT IS THE BEST METHOD OF ACHIEVING GLOBAL CONTROL OF *H. PYLORI* INFECTIONS?

Having decided that eradication of *H. pylori* is a responsible and necessary public health measure, the question then arises as to the best means of tackling this problem on a global scale. The relative merits of antibiotic therapy, public health measures and vaccination are discussed.

Antibiotic therapy

With some reservations, antibiotic therapy may offer an acceptable albeit expensive means of control in wealthy societies with low prevalence and reinfection rates of *H. pylori*. Mathematical models suggest that, in areas of low prevalence, serological screening for *H. pylori* followed by antibiotic treatment may be cost-effective, comparing favourably with other cancer screening programmes. Parsonnet *et al.* estimated the cost per year of life saved using this approach would be <$25 000 in the United States, using the conservative assumption that *H. pylori* eradication would prevent 30% of gastric cancers[43]. However, antibiotic therapy, which typically yields success rates of 85–90%, is not an effective strategy for eradication on a global scale. Eradication rates can be expected to fall with time, due to acquisition of antibiotic resistance by *H. pylori*. Moreover, widespread antibiotic use can also be expected to select for resistant strains in other pathogenic bacteria. The high cost of antibiotics is also out of the reach of many developing countries, where high re-infection rates may further impair the efficacy of antibiotic-based therapies[44]. Alternative strategies are, therefore, needed to combat the infection on a global scale.

Interruption of transmission

The primary mode of transmission of *H. pylori* infection remains unclear, and it is possible that multiple modes of transmission may coexist. Epidemiological evidence indicates that person-to-person transmission occurs early in life, particularly in conditions of overcrowding. This is predominantly parent to child[45], although transmission between siblings[46] and from adults to children outside the family probably also occurs. Decreased crowding is probably responsible for the declining rates of *H. pylori* infection in the industrialized world, but similar improvements in living conditions cannot be expected to occur in developing countries for several decades. In developing countries, contaminated drinking water[47,48] and agricultural water[49] may provide additional means of transmission of infection. *H. pylori* has also recently been detected by PCR from drinking water and surface water in developed countries, although the specificity and the significance of these findings are unclear[50,51]. Public health measures such as improved sewage disposal and sanitary water supplies may therefore be helpful in selected areas, but are likely to make only a minimal impact on transmission of infection on a global scale.

Vaccines

Rupnow *et al.*, in a study using methodology developed by the American Institute of Medicine, suggested that development and use of a *H. pylori* vaccine in the USA would provide public health benefits far superior to those provided by several other vaccines, including those directed against hepatitis B, respiratory syncytial virus, influenza, varicella, rotavirus and herpes simplex virus[52]. The Institute of Medicine has also recently carried out a cost–effectiveness analysis of the benefits of investing in the development of potential new vaccines[53]. A *H. pylori* vaccine was grouped in level II on a scale of I to IV, where level I has the most favourable cost–benefit ratio. Thus, there appears to be a clear benefit in pursuing vaccine development in the industrialized world. However, in developing countries with the highest prevalence of *H. pylori* and scarce public resources, *H. pylori* vaccination compares unfavourably with vaccination against other infective diseases which cause higher morbidity and mortality in these areas[52]. Development of cheap multivalent vaccines active against several pathogens may allow circumvention of these economic obstacles.

Feasibility of vaccines

The fact that the natural host immune response is ineffective in clearing *H. pylori* infection raised the possibility that a vaccine approach might be ineffectual. However, numerous studies in animal models of infection have demonstrated the feasibility of both prophylactic and therapeutic vaccination against *Helicobacter* infections, achieving protection rates averaging 60–80%[54–59]. These studies suggest that an efficacious immune response against *H. pylori* can occur in the gastric lumen.

Human vaccine studies

Four clinical trials have thus far studied *H. pylori* vaccination in humans. An initial study from our group in asymptomatic volunteers with *H. pylori* infection confirmed the safety of orally administered recombinant *H. pylori* urease[60]. In a subsequent human study we confirmed the immunogenicity of recombinant urease administered with *E. coli* heat-labile enterotoxin (LT) as a mucosal adjuvant[61]. Administration of the vaccine to *H. pylori*-infected asymptomatic volunteers led to urease-specific humoral and cellular immune responses, and although eradication of infection was not seen, an encouraging decrease in bacterial densities on quantitative cultures of gastric biopsy specimens was noted. The main adverse event noted was diarrhoea due to the use of LT. A more recent study from our group has defined a safe and effective dose of LT (unpublished observations). DiPetrillo *et al.* recently reported development of a vaccine strain of *Salmonella typhi* modified to express *H. pylori* urease subunits A and B[62]. However, administration of the vaccine to human volunteers failed to induce immune responses against *H. pylori*, for reasons that are unclear.

Improvements necessary in human vaccines

Clarifying the basic mechanisms of protection in animal models is essential for the development of an effective human vaccine. Further human studies are required to define ideal vaccine antigens, adjuvants, and delivery systems. Immunization of mice with dual antigen preparations confers increased protection rates compared with single antigens[63,64], and it is possible that multivalent vaccines may be required for successful protection against *H. pylori* in humans. Genetically altered adjuvants, modified to diminish toxicity while retaining adjuvancy, also require further study. Alternative routes of vaccine administration need to be explored in humans, as oral vaccination may not be the optimal route for inducing gastric protection[65]. Finally, alternative antigen delivery systems need to be explored. An interesting approach is using attenuated live bacteria such as modified *Salmonella typhimurium* strains, to express and deliver *H. pylori* antigens[66,67]. With this approach more than one vaccine antigen can be delivered, purification of the antigens is not necessary and the problem of antigen denaturation and degradation in the stomach does not exist. *Salmonella* can persist in infected intestinal tissues for several weeks post-immunization, and prolonged antigenic stimulation should be possible. Potentially toxic adjuvants may not be required, but if deemed necessary to modulate the immune response, recombinant adjuvants could be included in the system. Furthermore, using this approach, only one or two immunizations will be needed. All the above advantages should result in lower costs.

The ideal vaccine

The ideal *H. pylori* vaccine must have several characteristics to be successfully used on a global scale. Successful large-scale vaccination is more likely with an oral vaccine that requires only a single administration, particularly in the developing world. Production costs should be low and the vaccine should not require cold storage. Recombinant bacterial vaccines have the best potential to satisfy these conditions. Finally, the ideal vaccine should function in prophylactic as well as therapeutic indications, to circumvent the need for screening prior to large-scale vaccination, and to provide an alternative to antibiotics for the management of individual patients.

References

1. Parsonnet J. *Helicobacter pylori*: the size of the problem. Gut. 1998;43(Suppl. 1):S6–9.
2. Malaty HM, Graham DY, Wattigney WA, Srinivasan SR, Osato M, Berenson GS. Natural history of *Helicobacter pylori* infection in childhood: 12-year follow-up cohort study in a biracial community. Clin Infect Dis. 1999;28:279–82.
3. Forman D, Sitas F, Newell DG et al. Geographic association of *Helicobacter pylori* antibody prevalence and gastric cancer mortality in rural China. Int J Cancer. 1990;46:608–11.
4. Matysiak-Budnik T, Megraud F. Epidemiology of *Helicobacter pylori* infection with special reference to professional risk. J Physiol Pharmacol. 1997;48(Suppl. 4):3–17.
5. Sipponen P. *Helicobacter pylori* gastritis – epidemiology. J Gastroenterol. 1997;32:273–7.
6. Jyotheeswaran S, Shah AN, Jin HO, Potter GD, Ona FV, Chey WY. Prevalence of *Helicobacter pylori* in peptic ulcer patients in greater Rochester, NY: is empirical triple therapy justified? Am J Gastroenterol. 1998;93:574–8.
7. Gislason GT, Emu B, Okolo P et al. Where have all the *Helicobacter* gone: etiological factors in patients with duodenal ulcers (DU) presenting to a university hospital. Gastrointest Endosc. 1997;45:AB90 (abstract).
8. Murray CJ, Lopez AD. Mortality by cause for eight regions of the world: Global Burden of Disease Study. Lancet. 1997;349:1269–76.
9. Parkin DM, Pisani P, Ferlay J. Estimates of the worldwide incidence of eighteen major cancers in 1985. Int J Cancer. 1993;54:594–606.
10. Pisani P, Parkin DM, Munoz N, Ferlay J. Cancer and infection: estimates of the attributable fraction in. 1900. Cancer Epidem Biomarkers Prev 1997;6:389–400.
11. Anonymous. Schistosomes, liver flukes and *Helicobacter pylori*. IARC Working Group on the Evaluation of Carcinogenic Risks to Humans. Lyon, 7–14 June. 1994. IARC Monogr Eval Carcinog Risks Hum. 1994;61:1–241.
12. Coleman MP, Esteve J, Damiecki P, Arslan A, Renard H. Trends in cancer incidence and mortality. IARC Sci Publ. 1993;121:193–224.
13. Williams MP, Pounder RE. *Helicobacter pylori*: from the benign to the malignant. Am J Gastroenterol. 1999;94:S11–16.
14. Blaser MJ. Hypothesis: the changing relationships of *Helicobacter pylori* and humans: implications for health and disease. J Infect Dis. 1999;179:1523–30.
15. el-Serag HB, Sonnenberg A. Opposing time trends of peptic ulcer and reflux disease. Gut. 1998;43:327–33.
16. Blot WJ, Devesa SS, Kneller RW, Fraumeni JF, Jr. Rising incidence of adenocarcinoma of the esophagus and gastric cardia. J Am Med Assoc. 1991;265:1287–9.
17. Pera M, Cameron AJ, Trastek VF, Carpenter HA, Zinsmeister AR. Increasing incidence of adenocarcinoma of the esophagus and esophagogastric junction. Gastroenterology. 1993;104:510–13.

18. Newton M, Bryan R, Burnham WR, Kamm MA. Evaluation of *Helicobacter pylori* in reflux oesophagitis and Barrett's oesophagus. Gut. 1997;40:9–13.
19. Liston R, Pitt MA, Banerjee AK. Reflux oesophagitis and *Helicobacter pylori* infection in elderly patients. Postgrad Med J. 1996;72:221–3.
20. Werdmuller BF, Loffeld RJ. *Helicobacter pylori* infection has no role in the pathogenesis of reflux esophagitis. Dig Dis Sci. 1997;42:103–5.
21. Haruma K, Hamada H, Mihara M et al. Negative association between *Helicobacter pylori* infection and reflux esophagitis in older patients: case–control study in Japan. Helicobacter. 2000;5:24–9.
22. Labenz J, Blum AL, Bayerdorffer E, Meining A, Stolte M, Borsch G. Curing *Helicobacter pylori* infection in patients with duodenal ulcer may provoke reflux esophagitis. Gastroenterology. 1997;112:1442–7.
23. Vakil N, Hahn B, McSorley D. Recurrent symptoms and gastro-oesophageal reflux disease in patients with duodenal ulcer treated for *Helicobacter pylori* infection. Aliment Pharmacol Ther. 2000;14:45–51.
24. McColl KE, Dickson A, El-Nujumi A, El-Omar E, Kelman A. Symptomatic benefit 1–3 years after *H. pylori* eradication in ulcer patients: impact of gastroesophageal reflux disease. Am J Gastroenterol. 2000;95:101–5.
25. Tefera S, Hatlebakk JG, Berstad A. The effect of *Helicobacter pylori* eradication on gastro-oesophageal reflux. Aliment Pharmacol Ther. 1999;13:915–20.
26. Odman B, Lindberg G, Befrits R et al. Symptoms of gastro-oesophageal reflux in duodenal ulcer patients after treatment for *Helicobacter pylori* during a two year follow up. Gastroenterology. 1998;A1005 (abstract).
27. Mantzaris GJ, Archavlis EM, Kourtessas D et al. Oesophagitis does not develop frequently after eradication of *Helicobacter pylori* infection. Gut. 1998;43(Suppl. 2):A96 (abstract).
28. Mattsson A, Lönroth H, Quiding-Järbrink M, Svennerholm AM. Induction of B cell responses in the stomach of *Helicobacter pylori*-infected subjects after oral cholera vaccination. J Clin Invest. 1998;102:51–6.
29. Birkholz S, Schneider T, Knipp U, Stallmach A, Zeitz M. Decreased *Helicobacter pylori*-specific gastric secretory IgA antibodies in infected patients. Digestion. 1998;59:638–45.
30. Berdoz J, Blanc CT, Reinhardt M, Kraehenbuhl JP, Corthesy B. In vitro comparison of the antigen-binding and stability properties of the various molecular forms of IgA antibodies assembled and produced in CHO cells. Proc Natl Acad Sci USA. 1999;96:3029–34.
31. Shahinian ML, Passaro DJ, Swerdlow DL, Mintz ED, Rodriguez M, Parsonnel J. *Helicobacter pylori* and epidemic *Vibrio cholerae* O1 infection in Peru. Lancet. 2000; 355:377–8.
32. Belitsos PC, Greenson JK, Yardley JH, Sisler JR, Bartlett JG. Association of gastric hypo-acidity with opportunistic enteric infections in patients with AIDS. J Infect Dis. 1992; 166:277–84.
33. Cook GC. Infective gastroenteritis and its relationship to reduced gastric acidity. Scand J Gastroenterol Suppl. 1985;111:17–23.
34. Tee W, Lambert JR, Dwyer B. Cytotoxin production by *Helicobacter pylori* from patients with upper gastrointestinal tract diseases. J Clin Microbiol. 1995;33:1203–5.
35. Fox JG, Correa P, Taylor NS et al. High prevalence and persistence of cytotoxin-positive *Helicobacter pylori* strains in a population with high prevalence of atrophic gastritis. Am J Gastroenterol. 1992;87.1554–60.
36. Blaser MJ, Perez-Perez GI, Kleanthous H et al. Infection with *Helicobacter pylori* strains possessing cagA is associated with an increased risk of developing adenocarcinoma of the stomach. Cancer Res. 1995;55.2111–15.
37. Marchetti M, Rossi M, Giannelli V et al. Protection against *Helicobacter pylori* infection in mice by intragastric vaccination with *H. pylori* antigens is achieved using a non-toxic mutant of *E. coli* heat-labile enterotoxin (LT) as adjuvant. Vaccine. 1998;16:33–7.
38. Banerjee S, Michetti P. Strategies for developing a *Helicobacter pylori* vaccine. Curr Opin Gastroenterol. 1999;15:557–61.
39. Pan ZJ, van der Hulst RW, Feller M et al. Equally high prevalences of infection with cagA-positive *Helicobacter pylori* in Chinese patients with peptic ulcer disease and those with chronic gastritis-associated dyspepsia. J Clin Microbiol. 1997;35:1344–7.
40. Kumar S, Dhar A, Srinivasan S, Jain S, Rattan A, Sharma MP. Antibodies to Cag A protein are not predictive of serious gastroduodenal disease in Indian patients. Indian J Gastroenterol. 1998;17:126–8.

41. van der Ende A, Rauws EA, Feller M, Mulder CJ, Tytgat GN, Dankert J. Heterogeneous *Helicobacter pylori* isolates from members of a family with a history of peptic ulcer disease. Gastroenterology. 1996;111:638–47.
42. Figura N, Vindigni C, Covacci A et al. cagA positive and negative *Helicobacter pylori* strains are simultaneously present in the stomach of most patients with non-ulcer dyspepsia: relevance to histological damage. Gut. 1998;42:772–8.
43. Parsonnet J, Harris RA, Hack HM, Owens DK. Modelling cost-effectiveness of *Helicobacter pylori* screening to prevent gastric cancer: a mandate for clinical trials. Lancet. 1996; 348:150–4.
44. Ramirez-Ramos A, Gilman RH, Leon-Barua R et al. Rapid recurrence of *Helicobacter pylori* infection in Peruvian patients after successful eradication. Clin Infect Dis. 1997;25:1027–31.
45. Malaty HM, Graham DY, Klein PD, Evans DG, Adam E, Evans DJ. Transmission of *Helicobacter pylori* infection. Studies in families of healthy individuals. Scand J Gastroenterol. 1991;26:927–32.
46. Goodman KJ, Correa P. Transmission of *Helicobacter pylori* among siblings. Lancet. 2000;355:358–62.
47. Klein PD, Graham DY, Gaillour A, Opekun AR, Smith EO. Water source as risk factor for *Helicobacter pylori* infection in Peruvian children. Gastrointestinal Physiology Working Group. Lancet. 1991;337:1503–6.
48. Hulten K, Han SW, Enroth H et al. *Helicobacter pylori* in the drinking water in Peru. Gastroenterology. 1996;110:1031–5.
49. Hopkins RJ, Vial PA, Ferreccio C et al. Seroprevalence of *Helicobacter pylori* in Chile: vegetables may serve as one route of transmission. J Infect Dis. 1993;168:222–6.
50. Hulten K, Enroth H, Nystrom T, Engstrand L. Presence of *Helicobacter species* DNA in Swedish water. J Appl Microbiol. 1998;85:282–6.
51. Hegarty JP, Dowd MT, Baker KH. Occurrence of *Helicobacter pylori* in surface water in the united states. J Appl Microbiol. 1999;87:697–701.
52. Rupnow MF, Owens DK, Shachter R, Parsonnet J. *Helicobacter pylori* vaccine development and use: a cost-effectiveness analysis using the Institute of Medicine Methodology. Helicobacter. 1999;4:272–80.
53. Stratton KR, Durch JS, Lawrence RS. Vaccines for the 21st century: a tool for decision making. Washington, DC: National Academy Press; 2000 (Prepublication copy can be viewed on the Internet at: http://bob.nap.edu/readingroom/books/vacc21).
54. Chen M, Lee A, Hazell S, Hu P, Li Y. Immunization against gastric infection with *Helicobacter* species: first step in the prophylaxis of gastric cancer? Zentrabl Bakteriol. 1993;280:155–65.
55. Czinn SJ, Cai A, Nedrud JG. Protection of germ free mice from infection by *Helicobacter felis* after active oral or passive IgA immunization. Vaccine. 1993;139:637–42.
56. Doidge C, Gust I, Lee A, Buck F, Hazell S, Manne U. Therapeutic immunization against *Helicobacter* infection. Lancet. 1994;343:913–14.
57. Michetti P, Corthésy-Theulaz I, Davin C et al. Immunization of BALB/c mice against *Helicobacter felis* infection with *H. pylori* urease. Gastroenterology. 1994;107:1002–11.
58. Corthésy-Theulaz I, Porta N, Glauser M et al. Oral immunization with *Helicobacter pylori* urease B subunit as a treatment against *Helicobacter* infection in mice. Gastroenterology. 1995;109:115–21.
59. Cuenca R, Blancha TG, Czinn SJ et al. Therapeutic immunization against *Helicobacter mustelae* in naturally infected ferrets. Gastroenterology. 1996;110:1770–5.
60. Kreiss C, Buclin T, Cosma M, Corthésy-Theulaz I, Michetti P. Safety of oral immunization with recombinant urease in patients with *Helicobacter pylori* infection. Lancet. 1996; 347:1630–1.
61. Michetti P, Kreiss C, Kotloff KL et al. Oral immunization with urease and *Escherichia coli* heat-labile enterotoxin is safe and immunogenic in *Helicobacter pylori*-infected adults. Gastroenterology. 1999;116:804–12.
62. DiPetrillo MD, Tibbetts T, Kleanthous H, Killeen KP, Hohmann EL. Safety and immunogenicity of phoP/phoQ-deleted *Salmonella typhi* expressing *Helicobacter pylori* urease in adult volunteers. Vaccine. 1999;18:449–59.
63. Ferrero RL, Thiberge JM, Kansau I, Wuscher N, Huerre M, Labigne A. The GroES homolog of *Helicobacter pylori* confers protective immunity against mucosal infection in mice. Proc Natl Acad Sci USA. 1995;92:6499–505.

64. Ghiara P, Rossi M, Marchetti M et al. Therapeutic intragastric vaccination against *Helicobacter pylori* in mice eradicates an otherwise chronic infection and confers protection against reinfection. Infect Immun. 1997;65:4996–5002.
65. Kleanthous H, Myers GA, Georgakopoulos KM et al. Rectal and intranasal immunization with recombinant urease induce distinct local and serum immune responses in mice and protect against *Helicobacter pylori* infection. Infect Immun. 1998;66:2879–86.
66. Corthésy-Theulaz IE, Hopkins S, Bachmann D et al. Mice are protected from *Helicobacter pylori* infection by nasal immunization with attenuated *Salmonella typhimurium* phoPc expressing urease A and B subunits. Infect Immun. 1998;66:581–6.
67. Gomez-Duarte OG, Lucas B, Yan ZX, Panthel K, Haas R, Meyer TF. Urease subunits A and B delivered by attenuated *Salmonella typhimurium* vaccine strain protects mice against gastric colonization by *Helicobacter pylori*. Vaccine. 1998;16:460–71.

Section XII
Helicobacter Infections and the Future

71
The agenda for the microbiologist

A. LEE

INTRODUCTION

There have been many 'golden ages' of microbiology. The era of Koch and Pasteur, where the aetiology of numerous infectious diseases was defined, and of Fleming, Flory and the discovery of antibiotics. Yet here, at the beginning of a new millennium, we are entering perhaps the most exciting age of microbiology, the era of genomics. This will impact greatly on the research agenda for microbiologists interested in *Helicobacter pylori* over the next few years.

A PACKET OF CHIPS

Over the past decade has come the realization that many of our early studies into the pathogenesis of *H. pylori* were flawed. They were based on *in-vitro* experimentation in situations which bore very little relevance to the gastric environment where this pathogen caused disease. We now know that bacteria have sophisticated control mechanisms that switch on and off transcription of different genes when they are needed. Increasing ability to be able to manipulate the genome, to produce isogenic mutants with one gene deleted, has allowed for increased opportunity to study the importance of the genes *in vivo* using animal models. However, these methods have not allowed identification of which genes are switched on in different environments. Microarray technology and advances in computer power now provide the tools. The *H. pylori* chip is here.

In brief, the Hp Chip or microarray is a glass or plastic slide on which has been spotted, by an automated robot or arrayer, small drops containing different short oligonucleotides representing part of the whole sequence of every gene of *H. pylori*. As the complete sequence of two strains of *H. pylori* is now known, the vast majority of the genes, i.e. nearly 1600, can be 'printed' onto the chip. With this chip, genes that are 'turned on' can be assessed. The basic principle is that, if a gene is 'turned on', messenger RNA is being transcribed which will form the template for synthesis of the protein gene product.

The best way to show the power of the microarray technology is to describe the type of experiment that will soon be done to contrast genes switched on *in vitro* with those *in vivo*.

A GENE CHIP EXPERIMENT

Goal: to compare the *H. pylori* genes transcribed by the Sydney strain SS1 in the gastric mucosa of a mouse compared to the same isolate grown in a liquid culture, i.e. *in-vivo* growth compared to *in-vitro* growth.

Step 1: After infection or growth in liquid culture, mouse stomach infected with *H. pylori* or a broth culture is homogenized and RNA is extracted.

Step 2: As messenger RNA is unstable, the molecules are reverse-transcribed by an enzyme to produce a complementary strand of more stable DNA (copy or cDNA). The cDNA from the mouse stomach (i.e. *in vivo*) is labelled with a green fluorescent marker. The cDNA from the culture (i.e. *in vitro*) is labelled with a red fluorescent marker.

Step 3: After adjusting DNA concentrations, both labelled cDNA solutions are layered on top of the Hp Chip. If a gene has been transcribed then that labelled DNA would bind to the complementary oligonucleotide sequence on the microarray. The chip is then washed well, so that only bound DNA remains.

Step 4: The chip is then placed in a special dual-colour laser scanner which automatically scans a laser beam on each spot and captures images of the fluorescent colour and intensity. Spots would be green for genes switched on only *in vivo* or red for those solely express *in vivo*. If both are expressed then a mixed colour results. The scan determines the relative activity of these genes.

Step 5: This image is captured as a digital file and analysed via complex computer analysis. A read-out is obtained identifying the *in-vivo* expressed genes.

As with all new technologies, the practice is not as simple as it appears above. Extraction of the mRNA from the mouse stomach will pose methodological challenges. However, the major problem will be the bioinformatic aspects of these studies, in particular how to analyse the mass of data in order to determine what is and what is not significant. No doubt the ever-increasing power of the computer, and growing sophistication of the bioinformation scientist will overcome this problem. So far, in the particular experiment described above, we will have identified genes that are only switched on *in vivo*. What next? It is well and good to say that gene x is only expressed *in vivo*. Next we need to know what the gene product actually does. Comparisons with homologous proteins in other bacteria can be misleading. For example, some lower bowel *Helicobacters* and *H. pylori* have the gene for urease but the function of this protein will be different *in vivo* for the different bacteria. The urease activity in the lower bowel is most likely to be nutritional as is found in ruminants. Urease-positive bacteria close to the mucosal surface can assimilate urea nitrogen via the action of the enzyme. In contrast, in the very different environment of the gastric mucosa, the enzyme is an essential component of the bacterium's acid survival mechanism. Functional genomics, i.e. what the proteins actually do as shown by the three-dimensional structure modelled as a putative protein based on the genomic sequence and compared with the protein database, is the next growth area of microbiology.

The next few years will see the publication of large numbers of experiments based on microarray technology. While trying to interpret this data, the reader should keep in mind the problems mentioned above.

THE ORIGIN OF THE SPECIES

There is remarkably extensive literature on gastric variation amongst different isolates of *H. pylori*. Much of this effort has centred on sequence variations in two genes, the cytotoxin-associated gene (*cag*A), a marker for the *cag* pathogenicity island, and the *vac*A gene that codes for a cytotoxin and is present in all *H. pylori* strains. The goal of these studies has been to determine subtypes with a particular association with disease. All these studies have failed in that objective, and it is unlikely, based on logic, that there are associations between a subtype and pattern of disease, as these are most likely determined by host factors[1]. Rather the subtypes are a consequence of a unique feature of *H. pylori* epidemiology; that is that, past childhood, the organism is difficult to acquire. This makes it more likely that non-functional genetic changes occur by chance and tend to be restricted to narrow population groups. As populations have evolved separately so have their *H. pylori*. Covacci *et al.* have observed this, and commented on *H. pylori* and genetic geography[2]. Subtypes of the *vac*A genotype have also been shown to separate along geographic lines[3]. These studies provide a wonderful opportunity for the microbiologist to learn much about bacterial evolution; an agenda of little interest to the gastroenterologist.

THE MAGIC BULLET

Myself and others, when speculating on the future of microbiological research into *H. pylori*, consistently emphasize the need for more effective therapies. The vaccine remains the major goal. However, a 'magic bullet' or monotherapy that is unique to *H. pylori*, would be a valuable addition to management options, particularly if drug resistance, for example to clarithromycin, decreases the effectiveness of current therapies. This will remain an agenda item. The chances of success have increased recently with the demonstration that there are feasible bacteria-specific targets. The exciting studies of the Sachs group described in a previous chapter (Chapter 2) have identified a protein, the product of the gene *ure*I, that inserts into the membrane of *H. pylori* and controls the influx of urea, thus controlling urease activity. Below a certain pH, protonation of a few critical histidine residues exposed on the bacterial membrane causes a conformational change allowing urea to enter the cell and provide a substrate for the acid-protective urease enzyme[4-7]. This gene product is found only in the gastric *Helicobacters*, as these are the only ones which would benefit from such a urea channel. This small area of a species-specific molecule represents the ultimate selective target. The challenge is to find the ureI inhibitor that can be delivered to the gastric mucosa.

COMPARATIVE AND STRUCTURAL GENOMICS

H. pylori was one of the first bacteria for which two complete genomes were available[8]. Comparison of these sequences provided some interesting insights[9]. Sequence variation between the strains was significantly greater at the nucleotide level than at the amino acid level. Thus, the heterogeneity of the protein did not mirror the heterogeneity of the gene sequence. Indeed, the bacterium does not have great genetic diversity at a functional level. Strain differences are restricted to a remarkably small part of the genome.

Possession of these two genomes provides the opportunity for much more revealing comparisons with the genomes of other bacteria. The number of available sequences of different bacterial species is going to increase exponentially over the next few years. Comparative and structural genomic studies between the two H. pylori sequences and this ever-growing genomic database will become increasingly productive as the truly unique genes and sequences are identified. Correlation of results of these comparisons with the known behaviour of other pathogens and likely different environments inhabited by the different bacterial species will be very productive. The very recently reported complete genome of Campylobacter jejuni, published 1 month before this Bermuda H. pylori conference, provides a good example[10].

C. jejuni is the major bacterial cause of diarrhoea worldwide. The bacterium shares many properties with H. pylori: both have a spiral morphology, both live in mucus and both are microaerophilic. The bacteria were considered close relatives. Indeed, H. pylori was initially called a Campylobacter-like organism, or CLO, by Warren and Marshall, and later called Campylobacter pyloridis[11,12]. Thus, the comparison of these two bacterial species has been awaited with interest. The expectation was that they might be very similar. This is not the case. Strong similarities were mainly restricted to housekeeping genes, the genes that code for the shared fundamental processes of all bacteria. Only 55% of C. jejuni have recognizable equivalent genes to H. pylori. In most functions the bacteria have remarkably little in common. The authors comment that 'this indicates that selective pressures have driven profound evolutionary changes to create two very different and specific pathogens appropriate to their niches from a relatively close common ancestor'[10].

One particularly interesting insight into pathogenesis was revealed in this relatively brief comparison of these genomes. There are three distinct areas where there is almost no similarity between C. jejuni and H. pylori. These regions correspond with the hypervariable areas of the C. jejuni genome and also the three areas that code for surface polysaccharide, flagellar modification and lipopolysaccharide. Hypervariability is also seen with these regions in H. pylori. The most unique sequences are thus those which code for the structures most important in the interaction of the pathogens with their host, the outer surface structures. These are the structures which one would think are similar in function, and yet are the ones that have varied most. The comparison of these areas is likely to be a feature of the many further genomic comparisons between these bacteria that will be published over the next 2 years.

THE YEAR OF THE GERBIL

The many recent publications on the consequence of infection with *H. pylori* of the small rodent, the Mongolian gerbil, reveal that at last we have available an animal model of infection that truly mimics the varying patterns of the human diseases with active chronic gastritis, gastric ulcer, and gastric adenocarcinoma. In the future this model offers much promise to the microbiologist. The impact on disease of genes identified as important by the microarray and genomic studies can be effectively assessed in this model via the use of isogenic mutants in which the genes have been deleted or disrupted. However, there are two questions that need to be answered in parallel, if the gerbil studies are to be correctly interpreted. The first is: 'Why the gerbil?' What is so special about this animal that results in such comparable outcomes of infection to the human, while in others such as mice, ferrets, cats, etc., only a subset of human disease follow *Helicobacter* infection? There is something very different about the physiology of the gerbil.

Secondly, close reading of the current literature reveals that it is only in Japan that the severe human-type pathologies are observed in the gerbil[13-19]. For example in an American study only one ulcer was seen following infection of many animals, while in the Japanese studies nearly 100% show ulceration[20].

What is different between the US and Japanese Mongolian gerbils? Inspection of the homepage of a major US gerbil website (http://comhlan.erin.krakow.pl/mirrors/g-color-palette/colors.htm) reveals the diversity of even the US gerbils. The Japanese pedigree needs further investigation. How does the lower bowel *Helicobacter* flora of these animals vary? Could this impact on the severity of *H. pylori* infection and subsequent disease expression?

BRING ON THE TWINS

Apart from the overwhelming plagues of history, the consequence of many microbial infections is that only a small proportion of those infected progress to severe symptomatic disease. This is true for malaria, helminth infection, tuberculosis, hepatitis B, and many others. *H. pylori* infection is the same. It is now becoming clear that to some extent this is a consequence of a long period of evolution of host and parasite, such that not only have parasites acquired mutations that influence the outcome of the host/parasite relationship, but also genetic changes and variations in the host genome can impact on susceptibility to disease. What has been the situation with *H. pylori* infection?

Certainly, there are some studies which show that there is likely to be a genetic basis for infection. Twin studies have suggested a 57% genetic influence on *H. pylori* acquisition with a shared rearing environment accounting for 20% and non-shared environmental factors 23%[21].

The first clearly linked genes to infectious disease were the major histocompatibility class (MHC) genes, which are involved with antigen presentation; for example, the regions that code for the MHC class molecule, the DHQ part of the gene. This is logical because this is the part of the complex that forms between the antigen-presenting cell and the T cell. The interactions involve a complex of molecules where the MHC gene products are critical for the quality of the immune response. Changes or polymorphisms in the genes coding for these molecules may enhance the immune response, thus putting those gene polymorphisms at an advantage to the host. Alternatively, the response may not be as effective. Changes in MHC I and II in the critical antigen-presentation region can result in selection of particular epitopes that result in a more effective immune response. There is a huge variation in the MHC regions and it is possible that it is the constant exposure of the host to many epitopes by many pathogens and the selective pressure for more effective binding that has contributed to MHC diversity. The selective pressure of the ever-changing pathogen results in a selection out of various polymorphisms.

An example is hepatitis C virus infection; 14% of those infected contract a very severe form of the disease called mixed cryoglobulinaemia, due to the behaviour of the gammaglobulin. This appears to be an autoimmunity, an area affected by MHC. Rashes, purpura, arthralgia, etc. result. If the hepatitis C-infected person has the two alleles HLA-B8 and DR3 there is a nearly nine-fold increased risk of contracting the severe form of the disease. In the Gambia, if a person has the MHC allele HLA-DRB1*1302 then that person has a greatly reduced risk of proceeding to persistent infection. Thus, this allele codes for an immune response that the virus cannot easily escape.

The *H. pylori* MHC associations are only just starting to appear, and have been mostly studied in Japanese populations. Thus DQA1*0102 was significantly higher in *H. pylori*-negative controls and DQA1*0301 was significantly lower in *H. pylori*-negative controls than in *H. pylori*-positive duodenal ulcer patients. The DQA1*0102 allele may contribute to resistance against *H. pylori*-associated gastric atrophy and its association with intestinal-type gastric adenocarcinoma. Absence of DQA1*0102 may be a host genetic risk factor for *H. pylori*-associated atrophic gastritis and intestinal-type gastric adenocarcinoma[22,23].

Studies with other diseases have identified a wide range of other candidate genes all involved in the interaction between host and parasite in which polymorphisms also result in different disease outcomes. These include: MBP, ICAM-1, inducible NO synthetase, Nramp 1, IL 12, TNF, IL-1 receptor, FcγR11, IgE-Rii, vitamin D receptor, T cell receptor variants, interferon γ receptor, IL-4, IL-10, etc.

A good example of polymorphisms in a candidate gene is variations in the critical promoter region for TNF-α. Two types of polymorphisms have been found in position 308; in this promoter region either a guanine or adenosine may be present. In a study in the Gambia there was found to be an increased prevalence of the TNF2 polymorphism in children with a particularly severe form of malaria. This is thought to be due to increased amounts of TNF-α transcription. TNF-α in excess can have devastating effects. With this information workers looked for the impact of this polymorphism on other diseases, and many were found. Thus, in the severe form of scarring trachoma increased TNF-α was seen in tears. Lepromatous leprosy and mucocutaneous leishmaniasis[24-26] also showed a greater proportion of TNF-α polymorphisms.

The underlying pathology of *H. pylori* is gastritis, to an extent that the likelihood of symptomatic disease is greater the more severe the gastritis. Given that this host/parasite relationship is ancient, as with any other long-standing diseases, one would predict that there will be candidate genes in which one would predict polymorphisms would impact on the presentation of the disease. This was to be the key message of this talk: that a major agenda for the microbiologist was to search for polymorphisms such as IL-5, TNF-α308A, IFN-γ receptor, etc. as correlations with disease severity are likely to be found. By coincidence this prediction actually came true in the week of the Bermuda meeting, when an article was published in *Nature* from McColl's group reporting that interleukin-1 gene cluster polymorphisms that enhance the production of interleukin-1-beta were associated with increased risk of gastric cancer[27]. This was correlated with hypochlorhydria. This timely and very important paper highlights that host genetics and *H. pylori* are likely to be a feature of research into this bacterium in the next few years.

CONCLUSION

The agenda for the microbiologist as we move from Bermuda towards the twentieth anniversary of *H. pylori* remains the same:

>Understand the pathogenesis.
>Discover the monotherapy.
>Produce the vaccine.

Now we have amazing tools at our disposal. Ask the right questions and we will get some answers!

References

1. Lee A. Peptic ulceration – *H. pylori*-initiated ulcerogenesis – look to the host. Lancet. 1993;341:280–81.
2. Covacci A, Telford JL, Del Giudice G, Parsonnet J, Rappuoli R. *Helicobacter pylori* virulence and genetic geography. Science. 1999;284:1328–33.
3. Atherton JC, Sharp PM, Cover TL et al. Vacuolating cytotoxin (vacA) alleles of *Helicobacter pylori* comprise two geographically widespread types, m1 and m2, and have evolved through limited recombination. Curr Microbiol. 1999;39:211–18.
4. Scott DR, Weeks D, Hong C, Postius S, Melchers K, Sachs G. The role of internal urease in acid resistance of *Helicobacter pylori*. Gastroenterology. 1998;114:58–70.
5. Scott D, Weeks D, Melchers K, Sachs G. The life and death of *Helicobacter pylori*. Gut. 1998;43:S56–60.
6. Scott DR, Marcus EA, Weeks DL, Lee A, Melchers K, Sachs G. Expression of the *Helicobacter pylori* ureI gene is required for acidic pH activation of cytoplasmic urease. Infect Immun. 2000;68:470–7.

7. Weeks DL, Eskandari S, Scott DR, Sachs G. A H^+-gated urea channel: the link between *Helicobacter pylori* urease and gastric colonization. Science. 2000;287:482–5.
8. Alm RA, Ling LSL, Moir DT *et al*. Genomic-sequence comparison of two unrelated isolates of the human gastric pathogen *Helicobacter pylori*. Nature. 1999;397:176–80.
9. Alm RA, Trust TJ. Analysis of the genetic diversity of *Helicobacter pylori*: the tale of two genomes. J Mol Med. 1999;77:834–46.
10. Parkhill J, Wren BW, Mungall K *et al*. The genome sequence of the food-borne pathogen *Campylobacter jejuni* reveals hypervariable sequences. Nature. 2000;403:665–8.
11. Marshall BJ. Unidentified curved bacillus on gastric epithelium in active chronic gastritis. Lancet. 1983;1:1273–5.
12. Marshall BJ, Royce H, Annear DI *et al*. Original isolation of *Campylobacter pyloridis* from human gastric mucosa. Microbiol Lett. 1984;25:83–8.
13. Hirayama F, Takagi S, Iwao E, Yokoyama Y, Haga K, Hanada S. Development of poorly differentiated adenocarcinoma and carcinoid due to long-term *Helicobacter pylori* colonization in Mongolian gerbils. J Gastroenterol. 1999;34:450–4.
14. Hirayama F, Takagi S, Kusuhara H, Iwao E, Yokoyama Y, Ikeda Y. Induction of gastric ulcer and intestinal metaplasia in Mongolian gerbils infected with *Helicobacter pylori*. J Gastroenterol. 1996;31:755–7.
15. Honda S, Fujioka T, Tokieda M, Satoh R, Nishizono A, Nasu M. Development of *Helicobacter pylori*-induced gastric carcinoma in mongolian gerbils. Cancer Res. 1998; 58:4255–9.
16. Ikeno T, Ota H, Sugiyama A *et al*. *Helicobacter pylori*-induced chronic active gastritis, intestinal metaplasia, and gastric ulcer in Mongolian gerbils. Am J Pathol. 1999;154:951–60.
17. Matsumoto S, Washizuka Y, Matsumoto Y *et al*. Induction of ulceration and severe gastritis in Mongolian gerbil by *Helicobacter pylori* infection. J Med Microbiol. 1997;46:391–7.
18. Sawada Y, Yamamoto N, Sakagami T *et al*. Comparison of pathologic changes in *Helicobacter pylori*-infected Mongolian gerbils and humans. J Gastroenterol. 1999;34:55–60.
19. Watanabe T, Tada M, Nagai H, Sasaki S, Nakao M. *Helicobacter pylori* infection induces gastric cancer in Mongolian gerbils. Gastroenterology. 1998;115:642–8.
20. Wirth HP, Beins MH, Yang MQ, Tham KT, Blaser MJ. Experimental infection of Mongolian gerbils with wild-type and mutant *Helicobacter pylori* strains. Infect Immun. 1998;66:4856–66.
21. Malaty HM, Graham DY, Isaksson I, Engstrand L, Pedersen NL. Co-twin study of the effect of environment and dietary elements on acquisition of *Helicobacter pylori* infection. Am J Epidemiol. 1998;148:793–7.
22. Azuma T, Konishi J, Tanaka Y *et al*. Contribution of HLA-dqa gene to hosts response against *Helicobacter pylori*. Lancet. 1994;343:542–3.
23. Azuma T, Ito S, Sato F *et al*. The role of the HLA-DQA1 gene in resistance to atrophic gastritis and gastric adenocarcinoma induced by *Helicobacter pylori* infection. Cancer. 1998;82:1013–18.
24. Roy S, McGuire W, Mascie-Taylor GC *et al*. Tumor necrosis factor promoter polymorphism and susceptibility to lepromatous leprosy. J Infect Dis. 1997;176:530–2.
25. Conway DJ, Holland MJ, Bailey RL *et al*. Scarring trachoma is associated with polymorphism in the tumor necrosis factor alpha (TNF-alpha) gene promoter and with elevated TNF-alpha levels in tear fluid. Infect Immun. 1997;65:1003–6.
26. Cabrera M, Shaw MA, Sharples C *et al*. Polymorphisms in tumor necrosis factor genes associated with mucocutaneous leishmaniasis. J Exp Med. 1995;182:1259–64.
27. El-Omar E, Carrington M, Chow W *et al*. Interleukin-1 polymorphisms associated with increased risk of gastric cancer. Nature. 2000;404:398–402.

72
The agenda for the immunologist

P. B. ERNST

GAPS IN OUR KNOWLEDGE

Many tools have been used to minimize the impact of an infection on a population. For example, ever since John Snow studied the pattern of diarrhoeal disease during a cholera outbreak, and prevented further spread by removing the handle from the Broad Street pump, epidemiology has been a powerful approach to understand the transmission and expression of infectious disease. The use of epidemiological approaches to identify risk factors for disease transmission or pathogenesis facilitates the design of mechanistic studies *in vitro*, as well as the implementation of targeted interventions to prevent infection, or at least the more severe manifestations of the infection. However, to date, our understanding of the transmission of *Helicobacter pylori* is such that no easily implemented change in behaviour can adequately prevent its transmission, or prevent the development of the more severe complications associated with this infection.

Even as our understanding of the epidemiology of *H. pylori* infection and its associated diseases improves, history has proven that society is generally unwilling to rely simply on education and improvements in infrastructure to prevent infectious diseases. For example, we have the technology in hand to improve water management in order to prevent several diarrhoeal diseases that plague many countries. However, the political will to redirect financial resources towards funding these measures is lacking. Venereal diseases are another example. Clearly, education and simple preventive measures could greatly reduce the impact of these infections. Despite the availability of these tools for disease prevention, research resources are usually directed towards complementary measures such as new antimicrobials and vaccine development. The application of antimicrobials as an effective measure to control the global impact of *H. pylori* infection is limited due to drug resistance, costs and complications. Thus, vaccine development remains a desirable and achievable goal.

Many advances have contributed to the current optimism about vaccine development. Our understanding of the immunopathogenesis of gastroduodenal disease associated with *H. pylori* infection has improved, thereby identifying the elements of the host response that are not effective at conferring immunity. What is lacking is a clear understanding of the effector mechanisms that would be desirable and how they can be stimulated. Using animal models it has been shown that, like humans, animals can be chronically infected, and the persistence of the bacterium is associated with a potentially deleterious pro-inflammatory immune response driven by Th1-like T cells. Thus, the fact that many different vaccine preparations either prevent or treat an infection is a source of much optimism[1-4]. However, our understanding of the host response that permits a persistent infection is incomplete and our knowledge of the mechanisms of protection is even worse.

IMMUNOLOGICAL GOALS

There are two main goals for developing a vaccine. First, it is important to understand the elements of the host response to natural infection that are not protective. Secondly, correlates of immunity – presumably some markers that are absent during natural infection – have to be identified so that vaccines can be designed strategically and their effectiveness monitored easily.

Elsewhere[5-9], as well as in this volume, the host response to natural *H. pylori* infection, and its role in the pathogenesis of disease, have been discussed. This field continues to emerge as several immune/inflammatory pathways are activated by natural infection. It is essential to completely define this host response and its impact on gastroduodenal disease so that protective mechanisms can be correctly targeted. For example, many vaccines are judged by their ability to induce antibodies but antibody responses to *H. pylori* infection may be sufficient to cause autoimmune gastritis[10]. Thus, immunopathogenesis studies suggest a better correlate of immunity is needed. Other attempts to identify correlates of immunity have used animals that lack genes encoding antibodies, various cytokines, MHC molecules or other molecules of the immune system[11-13]. For example, recent studies using mice deficient in antibody protection have shown that these animals still developed protective immunity[12]. Using IFN-γ-deficient mice, investigators have found that protection can still be induced, but it is decreased[11].

Other studies have shown that class I MHC molecules are not necessary while class II MHC molecules are[12,13]. These observations point to the important role of helper T cells in developing protective immunity.

Using this type of approach, one hopes to identify the 'magic bullet' that is necessary for protective immunity, and then to design a vaccine that can exploit these protective mechanisms. However, the process is very time-consuming as only one or two gene products can be studied at a time. This limitation not only delays the advancement but fails to detect the different complementary layers of the host response that provide redundant levels of protection. Clearly, other strategies are required to decrease the element of chance and to improve the design with which such experiments are planned.

In addition to identifying which immune responses may be protective, other key immunological issues that emerge include: how can protective

Table 1. Areas of research in immunology for the next millennium

Application of genomics
Definition of immunopathogenesis
Application of pathogenesis to other gastrointestinal disease research
Understanding oxidative stress and gastrointestinal cancer
Identification of candidate vaccine antigens
Development of effective adjuvants
Identification of inductive sites for gastric immunity
Identification of protective mechanisms
Application of surrogates of immunity to other infections

responses be selected; are they relevant for other gastrointestinal or mucosal infections; where do immune cells come from and to which sites should vaccines be targeted for ideal sensitization? All of these areas (described in Table 1) will unfold over the next 10 years and the application of genomics will expedite all of these advances.

STRATEGIES FOR ADVANCING OUR UNDERSTANDING OF IMMUNOBIOLOGY

While the use of animal models has been extremely valuable, the pace of advancement is limited for the reasons described above. One of the new techniques that will expedite the development of a vaccine is the application of high-throughput genetic profiling. These techniques allow an investigator to rapidly screen various tissues for the expression of numerous genes simultaneously. Currently, some 7000 known genes and another 35 000 expressed sequence tags (ESTs = genetic sequences of unknown function) can be probed. With the completion of the human genome project in the summer of 2000, another 60 000 or more ESTs will be identified and the process of mining the wealth of information generated by these technologies will begin.

The principles behind these techniques are elegant and intuitively simple (Figure 1). Basically, specific sequences can be bonded to a microarray 'chip' at a density of more than 800 genes/mm^2. Computer analysis is used to select for probes that have a minimum amount of homology to other known genes or ESTs, thereby decreasing the chance of any cross-reactivity. With a microarray chip containing these probes in hand, one simply isolates the RNA from a cell or tissue of interest, labels it with a fluorescent probe and hybridizes it to the microarray chip. Subsequently, the chip is scanned and the data analysed. An important component of this process is the data analysis, which includes techniques that are developing rapidly. These techniques perform a systematic interrogation of the data with the appropriate internal controls in order to decide if the expression of a gene is increased or decreased. Subsequently, various algorithms can be applied to examine the patterns of gene expression using multidimensional analysis. These complex analyses can in turn be reduced to simplified graphics presentations with which specific associations can be examined.

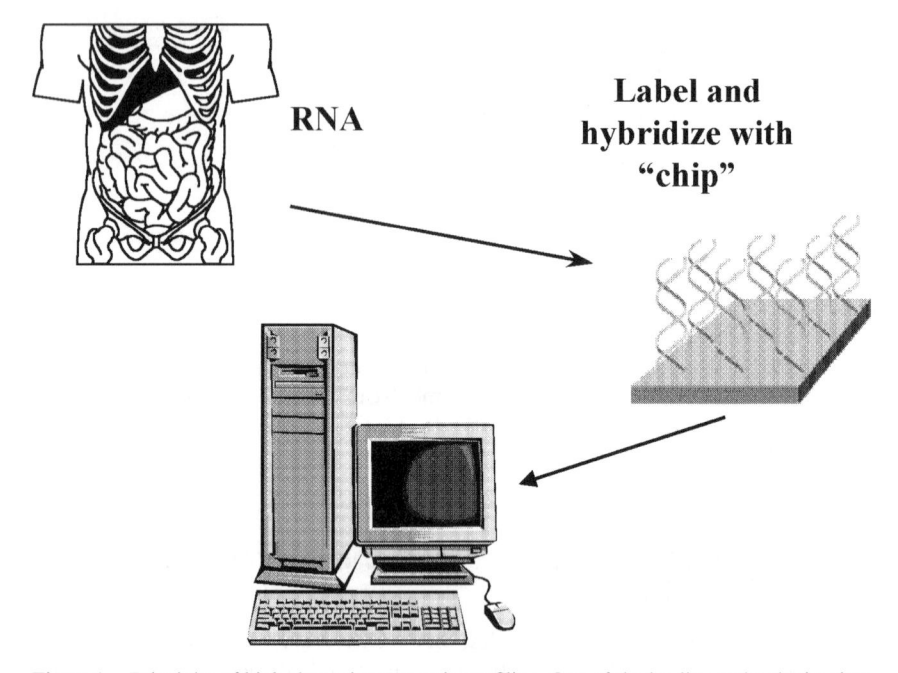

Figure 1. Principles of high-throughput genetic profiling. One of the leading technologies that is available has been produced by Affymetrix™. Using this technology, cells or tissue are used as a source of RNA, which is labelled with a fluorescent probe and hybridized to a microarray chip. Subsequently, the chip is scanned and the data analysed. Arrays are designed to include 16–20 pairs of specific, unique 25mer oligonucleotide probes representing different regions of a gene or an EST. Each region on the chip includes a match test cell paired to a mismatch control cell containing the oligonucleotide with a single mutation. The 16–20 match and mismatch control cells enable one to evaluate expression at multiple points within a gene or EST with defined controls for each point. This in turn is analysed by software that permits the relative intensity of each point to be considered simultaneously. While 20 positives out of 20 probe sites and 20 negatives in the controls would be ideal, the software will provide estimates of probability for a change in gene expression based on any variation of the response in all 16–20 cells. The techniques in data analysis perform a systematic interrogation of the data with the appropriate internal controls in order to decide if the expression of a gene is increased or decreased. Subsequently, various algorithms can be applied to examine the patterns of gene expression using multidimensional analysis. These complex analyses can in turn be reduced to simplified graphics presentations with which specific associations can be examined.

High-throughout gene profiling does not complete the task, but generates a short list of genes, perhaps 300 out of approximately 120 000 that deserve additional investigation. Changes in expression have to be confirmed with an independent assay and the function established, but a few examples will illustrate the potential power of these applications. For example, we know that mice can be persistently infected with *H. pylori* and this infection is associated with a 'non-protective' immune response. In contrast, an animal can be fully protected after immunization. Therefore, a complete expression analysis of the infected mouse versus the immunized mouse could identify genes that are only expressed in immunity. These candidates may encode proteins that are responsible for the induction or actual effector mechanisms. Should this be confirmed, then one would have a terrific target with which to direct vaccines in humans. At the least, some of the genes may encode proteins that will serve as surrogates of immunity, some of which could provide a relatively non-invasive approach to test the efficacy of vaccines under development.

Genomics will have many more applications, including the study of the bacteria themselves, the pathogenesis of gastric cancer as well as the vaccine development. In all cases the goal will be to generate a list of candidate genes that provide a set of markers that distinguishes the relative susceptibility of a subject to health or disease.

RELEVANCE OF RESEARCH IN *H. PYLORI* INFECTION

To evaluate the impact of research in *H. pylori* infection, one only has to look at the effort to date and the impact it has had. In the 100 years prior to the observation by Marshall and Warren, that gastritis and peptic ulceration were associated with an infection of spiral bacteria[14], only a few reports had speculated about the role of spiral bacteria in gastroduodenal diseases[15]. Based on a search of the National Library of Medicine using the key word '*pylori*', on 21 March 2000, more than 11 450 papers have now been published since the report by Marshall and Warren in 1984. The result of this effort has been the recognition of the role for *H. pylori* in the pathogenesis of gastroduodenal disease, and the improvement in our ability to prevent or treat these disorders.

Is the job done? Clearly not. The global impact of infection greatly exceeds the positive impact that has been achieved in Europe and North America due to the decreasing infection rate and antibiotic therapy. Other advances in the prevention or treatment of infection, including the use of vaccines, will extend the positive contributions that have been achieved to date.

A relatively ignored aspect of *H. pylori* research is the potential use of *H. pylori* infection as a model of other chronic inflammatory diseases in the digestive tract. Like *H. pylori*-related diseases, coeliac disease and inflammatory bowel diseases share the features of inappropriate immune regulatory responses to luminal antigens that damage tissue and increase the chance of developing cancer. Coeliac disease is sufficiently uncommon that research is difficult to do, while IBD research is hampered by the absence of a defined aetiology. *H. pylori* infection is still prevalent enough to provide a readily accessible model to understand the regulation of antigen-specific immune responses in the human digestive tract and their role in chronic inflammatory disease. Similarly, identification of novel protective mechanisms for *H. pylori* might well find use in the design of vaccines for other enteric infections. Hopefully, the broad relevance of *H. pylori* research will be appreciated as an important tool for studies of gastrointestinal immunology in general.

References

1. Rappuoli R. Rational design of vaccines. Nature Med. 1997;3:374–6.
2. Ghiara P, Michetti P. Development of a vaccine. Curr Opin Gastroenterol. 1995;11:52–6.

3. Doidge C, Gust I, Lee A, Buck F, Hazell S, Manne U. Therapeutic immunization against *Helicobacter pylori* infection. Lancet. 1994;343:913–14.
4. Michetti P. Oral immunization against *Helicobacter pylori* – a future concept. J Gastroenterol. 1998;33(Suppl. 10):66–8.
5. Ernst PB. The role of inflammation in the pathogenesis of gastric cancer. Aliment Pharmacol Ther. 1999;13:13–18.
6. Ernst PB, Gold BD. *Helicobacter pylori* in childhood: new insights into the immunopathogenesis of gastric disease and implications for managing infection in children. J Pediatr Gastroenterol Nutr. 1999;28:462–73.
7. Correa P, Miller MJS. Carcinogenesis, apoptosis and cell proliferation. Br Med Bull. 1998;54:151–62.
8. Crabtree JE. Role of cytokines in pathogenesis of *Helicobacter pylori*-induced mucosal damage. Dig Dis Sci. 1998;43:46–55S.
9. Ernst PB, Michetti P, Smith PD. The Immunobiology of *Helicobacter pylori*. From Pathogenesis to Prevention. Philadelphia: Lippincott-Raven; 1997.
10. Appelmelk BJ, Faller G, Claeys D, Kirchner T, Vandenbroucke-Grauls CMJE. Bugs on trial: The case of *Helicobacter pylori* and autoimmunity. Immunol Today. 1998;19:296–9.
11. Sawai N, Kita M, Kodama T et al. Role of gamma interferon in *Helicobacter pylori*-induced gastric inflammatory responses in a mouse model. Infect Immun. 1999;67:279–85.
12. Ermak TH, Giannasca PJ, Nichols R et al. Immunization of mice with urease vaccine affords protection against *Helicobacter pylori* infection in the absence of antibodies and is mediated by MHC class II-restricted responses. J Exp Med. 1998;188:2277–88.
13. Pappo, J, Torrey D, Castriotta L, Savinainen A, Kabok Z, Ibraghimov A. *Helicobacter pylori* infection in immunized mice lacking major histocompatibility complex class I and class II functions. Infect Immun. 1999;67:337–41.
14. Marshall, BJ, Warren JR. Unidentified curved bacilli in the stomach of patients with gastritis and peptic ulceration. Lancet. 1984;8390:1311–15.
15. Blum AL. An historical overview of *Helicobacter*-associated disorders. In: The Immunobiology of *Helicobacter pylori*: From Pathogenesis to Prevention. Ernst PB, Michetti P, Smith PD, editors. Philadelphia: Lippincott-Raven; 1997;xiii–xix.

73
The agenda for the histopathologist

R. H. RIDDELL

In the next few years research will be dominated by advances in research on a variety of technological fronts combining informatics and technology, and limited only by finances, and the ingenuity of combining them. These technologies will be used to help resolve, or cast new light on, the pathophysiology of *Helicobacter* infection, the diseases associated with it and their sequelae. However, histopathologists will be a fundamental part of the teams required in which each will team member will use their own areas of expertise.

The continued generation of computer and computerized hardware and software will be at the centre of this revolution. Animal research will continue both to explore new diseases in the animal kingdom that are *Helicobacter*-associated, and to create new animal models that can be used to explore the extent to which they resemble their human counterparts and also their pathophysiology. The same techniques will be used to cast new light on the pathophysiology of the spectrum of *Helicobacter*-associated diseases in humans.

At the heart of the explosion of new data that will be forthcoming will be the use of gene microarray technology (GMT) which will dominate research. Genome-wide expression monitoring of DNA, RNA and proteins, either with chip technology or using other variants of the same technique, will spearhead this approach. Increasing efficiency and complexity of these machines currently allow simultaneous examination of the actions of thousands of genes or their products, and this will increase logarithmically. Substrates/primers will become more readily available in clusters to analyse specific pathways in increasing detail. The number of pathways that can be examined simultaneously will also grow logarithmically, allowing examination of the workings of much of the genome. The combination of GMT with laser capture microscopy (LCM) may provide the keenest insights into the disease process. LCM allows removal of microscopic pieces of tissue down to virtually single cells, and even organelles, allowing the examination of specific cell types – epithelium, lamina propria cells, nerves, endothelial and stromal cells. This will allow determination not only of how each functions independently, but also the manner in which they may cooperate, as they clearly do in life and in disease. The automated combination of LCM and GMT (e.g. Taqman), is already available and will rapidly become more sophisticated; such methods will be applied to:

1. Exploration of the full range of diseases with which *Helicobacters* are associated in experimental animals and animal models, and in humans.
2. Correlation of genetically distinct subtypes of *H. pylori* with the variability of diseases seen in patients with *Helicobacter* infection, and in specific cell types within a biopsy from that patient; e.g. is the mechanism of generation of duodenal ulcers identical from patient to patient irrespective of the genetic make up of the *H. pylori* strain(s) causing it, and what is the role of heredity in increasing the probability that any specific strain of *H. pylori* may be ulcerogenic? What are the differences in mRNA in gastric and intestinal epithelia in the proximal duodenum between inflamed and non-inflamed tissue, and also in the different types of lamina propria cells in these locations? LCM will allow microdissection of all elements of biopsies of inflamed and control duodenal mucosa in humans, or of animal models to help resolve these issues.
3. What are the molecular and genetic mechanisms involved in:
   (a) The intensity of the inflammatory reactions associated with *H. pylori*?
   (b) The more unusual types of gastric pathology possibly associated with *H. pylori*? (which may also be able to confirm that these associations exist). These include lymphocytic gastritis and Menetrier's disease.
   (c) The development of atrophy in oxyntic mucosa and the antrum?
   (d) The development of mucous neck hyperplasia (pseudopyloric metaplasia)?
   (e) The development of the different subtypes of intestinal metaplasia in the antral, transitional, oxyntic, cardiac and Barrett's epithelium: are there common molecular mechanisms or do these differ depending on their aetiology and the genetic make-up of the patient (soil and seed)?
   (f) The development of dysplasia, early invasion and metastasis in both intestinal and non-metaplastic mucosa giving rise to the diffuse and other subtypes of gastric cancer, and whether these are similar irrespective of whether *H. pylori* is present or not?
4. Data capture and management. The use of these technologies will result in the generation of huge amounts of data. How such data are stored, their level of general availability, and how they are analysed will present major problems. Ideally, following its initial use by the primary investigating team, it should be possible to download such data onto web sites created specifically for that purpose, so that others doing similar work can use the data to compare with, validate or act as controls for their own work. There is huge potential for patenting issues to limit the accessibility of such data. Ideally programs for comparing results automatically on line with other microarray displays would be hugely beneficial.
5. Clinical correlation. Informatics will allow the generation of large databases of information that can be used to mine data on patients while

maintaining their anonymity, and combine this with electronic records of the results of tests, including radiology, endoscopy and pathology. These can readily be combined with experimental data generated by GMT and LCM.

It is clear that the role of the histopathologist will be essential in ensuring that these technologies are used correctly, and to be part of the teams that will be required to maintain the quality of the results that these studies will generate.

74
Helicobacter infections in the new millennium: the challenge for the clinician

A. AXON

INTRODUCTION

In looking to the future we must reflect on the past. The challenges that will confront us in the twenty-first century, although different from those encountered previously, will be similar. Human behaviour follows well-established precedents. There is no better example than the discovery of *Helicobacter pylori*. During the nineteenth century it seemed inconceivable to some that tuberculosis and puerperal sepsis might be transmissible; however, the suggestion that peptic ulcer might be caused by *H. pylori* was also met with incredulity in the late twentieth century. The idea that smoking might cause lung cancer was rejected by many in the 1960s in spite of powerful epidemiological data. In the early twenty-first century there are still some who believe that *H. pylori* does not cause gastric cancer, even though the epidemiological evidence is solid, and Koch's postulates have been satisfied in the experimental animal. These two cancers, worldwide numbers one and two as causes of death, could be eliminated within a generation if there were sufficient medical and political consensus and enthusiasm. The major *Helicobacter* challenges in the twenty-first century will be to produce the data, provide the education, and apply the political pressure to carry through policies that will lead to the elimination of gastric cancer.

THE SEED, THE SOIL AND THE WEATHER

New technologies in molecular medicine have highlighted the importance of host genetics in the outcome of infectious disease. However, it has been known for years that genetic variation is essential for the preservation of a species when attacked by an epidemic. This understanding is underlined by the analogy of 'the seed and the soil' the seed representing the infective organism, the soil the host. This is incomplete, however. No matter how healthy the seed or fertile the soil, in times of drought the harvest will fail, so the weather (or environment) also plays a fundamental role. The same principle applies in human disease.

Great epidemics of the past would not have occurred had it not been for changes in human behaviour, social activity and other environmental influences. It was the opening up of the trade routes from the East that brought the Black Death to Europe in the thirteenth and fourteenth centuries, when roughly 25% of the population died. Even earlier than this, it was the change from nomadic hunter–gatherer to farming and more settled social order that assisted the transmission of infectious organisms between individuals. Warfare has spread diarrhoeal disease and typhus. Imperialism took measles and syphilis to virgin populations. Industrialization compromised the water supply and induced epidemics of cholera. Poverty and overcrowding led to scarlet fever and tuberculosis. Social changes have had a greater influence upon infectious disease than either seed or soil. The changes that have occurred with *Helicobacter* infection are unlikely to be dissimilar.

Modern medicine has not diminished the importance of environmental factors on infectious disease. Whilst the latter half of the twentieth century witnessed a vast increase in economic prosperity in the West and the decline of tuberculosis and rheumatic fever. Sexual liberation and inexpensive travel led to the epidemic of HIV infection. Drug abuse spread hepatitis C, and medical 'advances' led to methicillin-resistant *Stapylococcus aureus* (MRSA) and resistant malaria. The use of human material for therapy caused transmission of hepatitis B and Creutzfeldt Jakob disease (CJD). Eating out and the mass production of food caused food poisoning with *Campylobacter*. Short-sighted animal husbandry led to bovine spongiform encephalopathy (BSE) and variant CJD, and has encouraged more virulent strains of *Salmonella enteriditis* to appear.

H. PYLORI IN THE NINETEENTH AND TWENTIETH CENTURIES

H. pylori may have infected mankind over the millennia; however, the clinical diseases attributed to the organism have reached prominence only within the past 200 years. Duodenal ulcer, the condition most closely associated with the infection, was excessively rare until the middle of the nineteenth century but reached epidemic proportions in the Western world during the first half of the twentieth century. Gastric ulcer, although recognized earlier, seems to have been a different disease in the nineteenth century when it particularly affected young women. The typical gastric ulcer associated with *Helicobacter* followed a similar time trend to duodenal ulcer. Gastric cancer preceded duodenal and gastric ulcer, but has declined since the middle of the twentieth century in the developed world. Whether the fall in incidence of gastric cancer can be attributed to social change, to an absolute decline in infection, or a combination of the two, is uncertain. Widely different international gastric cancer rates imply that whilst *H. pylori* is the seed, both the soil and the environment play important roles in its development. When all factors are considered, one truth remains: if the seed is not sown the plant will not grow, whatever the nature of the soil or the environment. It follows that if *H. pylori* can be eradicated from the human race *Helicobacter*-associated disease will disappear.

MEDICAL CARE IN THE DEVELOPED WORLD

Our approach to medicine in the developed world has changed in the second half of the twentieth century. Before that time most people did not seek medical advice unless they were ill. Although children were brought for immunization, healthy individuals rarely attended their doctor. Today, people are encouraged to attend well-women's clinics and well-men's clinics. Companies provide routine medical examinations or pay for personnel to undergo 'check-ups'. Women are encouraged to have regular cervical smear tests and mammography. Men are screened for testicular and prostatic cancer, hypertension and elevated cholesterol. Interest is expressed in the prevention of colonic cancer by occult blood screening, flexible sigmoidoscopy, or colonoscopy. Screening *per se* is of little value unless carried through to preventative treatment. Cone biopsy, lumpectomy, prostatectomy, polypectomy, treatment of hypertension, prescription of 'statins and aspirin are the natural follow-through. With increased longevity the screening of elderly people and medical interventions will expand.

The principles underlying medical treatment have also changed. Whereas diagnosis and cure of disease was the fundamental role of physicians and surgeons 40 years ago, today it is preservation of quality of life and tommorow it will be longevity. Patients present with conditions that are not life-threatening but are inconvenient, or cause discomfort or concern. Thus, hip and knee replacements are common; the prescription of sedatives and antidepressants, of contraceptives, and hormone replacement therapies are part of everyday life. The increase in demand for comfort and happiness in the population means that this aspect of medicine will continue to grow. Political correctness, the availability of socialized medicine provided directly by the State or through insurance linked to increasing prosperity means that in the new century demand for preventative and convenience medicines will continue to expand.

H. PYLORI IN THE TWENTY-FIRST CENTURY IN THE DEVELOPED WORLD

In the developed world the prevalence of *H. pylori* will continue to decline. Nevertheless, the infection is still responsible for many deaths. In England and Wales around 7500 people a year die from gastric cancer and over 3000 from peptic ulcer disease. *H. pylori* infection is responsible for more deaths than any other infectious disease in much of the developed world. Although the overall risk of death is falling with the decline in the rate of infection, the risk for individuals already infected will rise as people live longer and reach an age at which cancer exacts a higher toll.

The challenge for clinicians in the developed world is to undertake the clinical trials that are necessary to show that the eradication of *H. pylori* infection will protect against the development of non-cardia gastric cancer.

Although a number of studies have already been initiated, it will be some years before they have been completed. Without well-designed trials, and convincing data, governments and health providers are unlikely to provide eradication programmes.

A second challenge is to identify the risks that may accrue from the eradication of *H. pylori* infection. and the possibility that *Helicobacter* infection may offer protection against certain diseases. A specific suggestion is that the organism, by inducing hypochlorhydria, may protect against gastro-oesophageal reflux disease and possibly even cancer of the cardia and adenocarcinoma of the distal oesophagus[1]. Although the experimental evidence in support of this hypothesis is equivocal, the fact that well-respected researchers have raised this possibility places an onus upon those advocating *H. pylori* eradication to explore the potential problems that may arise from *Helicobacter* eradication, as well as the benefits.

Apart from the theoretical protective effects that *H. pylori* infection may have for humans, other concerns have been expressed concerning a programme of *H. pylori* eradication. These include the risk that antibiotic therapy may induce resistance in non-*Helicobacter* opportunists and pathogens. In reality, less than 30% of the developed world are now infected with *H. pylori*, however, the current use of antibiotics is equivalent to more than one course for every person in the community per year. It follows that the amount of antibiotic that would be required to treat all *H. pylori*-infected people is less than that used in a full year for all other infections. Its impact on the ecology, therefore, is likely to be small, relative to the antibiotics already in use. Nevertheless, the new century will see a greater concern for the environment, and before eradication policies are introduced, governments will demand a clear understanding of the risks involved in their use. This area should be addressed sooner rather than later.

These problems raise the question as to whether it would be possible to develop a specific new monotherapy for the treatment of *H. pylori* infection. The acquisition of the genome of *H. pylori* provides the potential for a designer antibiotic specific for *H. pylori*. A drug of this nature would be ineffective against other organisms and would not affect other flora. Treatment of *H. pylori* infection is less than ideal. Although PPI-based triple therapies provide a 90% cure in clinical trials, when used outside clinical trials they are less effective, and are probably even less so when used in primary care or in population treatment. There is a need for a more effective and simpler form of treatment.

Methods of testing for *H. pylori* appear at first glance to be reasonably effective. The urea breath test is extremely sensitive and specific but serology still lags behind and, although most commercial tests are marketed with an accuracy of over 90%, they still have to be evaluated in the specific community in which they are to be used. In a situation in which the incidence of infection is falling this causes problems. If a test has a 90% specificity it means that there will be 10% of false-positives in every 100 subjects tested. If the incidence of the disease in the population is only 10%, roughly half of those receiving treatment on the basis of the test will be false-positives.

It follows that if we are to pursue a policy of *Helicobacter* eradication in the normal population more accurate tests are required.

In the new century, a greater emphasis will be placed upon cost-effectiveness. The rising cost of medical care has already impelled governments to restrict the services that have been routinely offered. In the United Kingdom the National Institute for Clinical Excellence is responsible for ensuring that treatments are not introduced unless they have been shown to be effective and, to some extent, affordable. Fortunately, so far as *H. pylori* is concerned, recent data suggest that eradication of the infection from the population would be cost-effective[2]. That being the case, if eradication of *Helicobacter* did prevent cancer the intervention would be one of the few policies to pay for itself.

CHALLENGES FOR THE CLINICIAN IN THE DEVELOPING WORLD

The challenge to the clinician in the developing world is different. If the history of the twentieth century in the developed world is replayed over the next 50 years in developing countries we will expect a considerable improvement in standards of living, hygiene and general health. This will lead to a decline in infant mortality and to greater longevity. People will live to an age at which they will develop gastric cancer. In the interim it is probable that the incidence of duodenal ulcer will rise, as it did in the West in the 1940s and 1950s, 80 or so years following industrialization.

At present the economies of the developing countries are insufficient to pay for widespread eradication of *H. pylori* infection. These countries will develop at varying rates depending upon political, social and geographical differences. With improving socioeconomic status the infection rate will eventually fall, but in the foreseeable future it will remain high. An important challenge to the clinician, therefore, is to identify the manner in which the infection is spread. To date we do not know how *H. pylori* infection is transmitted. The high levels of transmission that continued in the developed world after the beginning of the twentieth century, when clean water was generally available, make it unlikely that infection will be reduced simply by improvement of the water supply. If we were able to identify the means of transmission of *H. pylori* infection it is possible that simple measures could be introduced that would drastically reduce the infection rate.

As indicated earlier, the identification of the *H. pylori* genome provides the opportunity for the development of new drugs; it also may lead to the production of a vaccine. A vaccine would be of incalculable value in the developing world, where straightforward drug treatment of the infection is likely to be followed by re-infection and could lead to the widespread emergence of resistant *H. pylori* infection.

For the practising physician in the developing world, the challenge must be to identify those patients who are at risk of the complications of *H. pylori* infection, peptic ulcer and cancer. It may be that development of serological tests predicting gastric atrophy, or genetic screening, may enable those that are more likely to develop cancer to be selected for treatment.

Infection is mainly acquired in childhood and it might be possible, using a less expensive means of testing and treating, to provide eradication therapy in early adulthood. It would be a tragedy if governments and clinicians in the developing world did not take account of what has happened in the developed countries. It would be an even greater tragedy if the world community is not prepared to provide the support that will be needed to prevent these diseases, which have been so costly in terms of health and financial expenditure over the past 100 years.

References

1. Richter JE, Falk GW, Vaezi MF. *Helicobacter pylori* and gastroesophageal reflux disease: the bug may not be all bad. Am J Gastroenterol. 1998;93:1800–2.
2. Moayyedi P, Mason J, Mason S, Duffett S, Feltbower R, Axon ATR. Population *H. pylori* screening and treatment reduces dyspepsia costs. Gastroenterology. 1999;116:A466.

Index

acetate 4
acetylcholine (Ach) 417
acetyl-CoA 4–5
achlorhydria 289
acid secretion, gastritis 386–9
acid tolerance 330–1
acid-suppressive therapy 439, 469
   rebound acid hypersecretion 391–4
acidity, environment 15–16
acquired immunodeficiency syndrome (AIDS) 25
activator protein-1 (AP-1) 38, 163
adhesins 197–8
adolescents, mucosal inflammation, severity and reversibility 175–83
Airs, Waters and Places 348
alanine 4
alkyl hydroperoxide reductase 7, 8–9
Alp protein 198
α-haemolytic streptococcus 26
α-ketoglutarate 5
α-tocopherol 515, 518
amidase gene cluster 22
amidoporin(s) 22–3
amino acids 4
ammonia 15, 240, 330
   gastric urease 367–8
   neutralisation, intrabacterial urease 16
amoxycillin 78–9, 134, 611, 623
amphibiosis 26
   relationship and humans 25–9
anaerobics, facultative 5
animal models, *Helicobacter* infections 491
antibiotics 25, 27, 78
   future, targeting 639–40
   infected hosts, decrease 46–7
   resistance, primary/secondary 594–5
   urea breath test, effect on 134–5
antibody responses, children 170–1

antigen transport 152–3
antioxidants, dietary 515(table), 520(fig.)
antireflux surgery 273
antisecretory drugs 78, 133
antral glandular atrophy 276
apoptosis 159–60
   gastric epithelial cells, infection 159–60
   NH_2Cl 160
   redox-sensitive signalling mechanisms 164(fig.)
aquaporin(s) 22–3
Archaeal genes 5
ascorbic acid 515–16
aspirin 53, 439, 461
   H.pylori-negative ulcer disease, role of 341
ASTRONAUT study 455
atrophic gastritis 229–36
   onset, long-term proton pump inhibitor therapy 255–64
   acid suppression, progression to and onset 257–63
   atrophy, progression to 256–7
Atrophy 2000 meeting 234
Atrophy Club 229
atrophy, definition (Atrophy 2000 meeting) 234
autoimmune gastritis
   antigenic mimicking 289–92
   evidence in favour/against of *H. pylori* as a cause 290–2
   pathways 291(fig.)
   via mimicking 281–6
   H. pylori-eradication, healing 282–3
   H. pylori-induced 281–2
   non-atrophic, incidence 281
   study, retrospective 283
autoimmune thrombocytopenic purpura 318–19

autonomic imbalance, effect on
    dyspepsia 414–15

BabA protein 39–40, 198
bacillus 352
Bacillus coli 363
Bacillus hoffmani 366
bacterial factors, mucosal inflammatory
    responses in children/
    adolescents 180–3
bacteriology, early 357–8
Balard, Antoine (1802–1876) 355
Barrett's oesophagus 234, 270, 277, 295–6
basal acid output 393
Bassi, Agostino (1773–1856) 347, 353
BCECF 18, 19(fig.)
Beitrage zur Biologie der Pflanzen 357
Berstad study 275
Berzelius, J. (1779–1848) 354
β-carotene 515(table)
    gastric, *H. pylori* infection 518–19
bile reflux 240
biopsy sampling 115
    gastric *vs.* stomach 230–1
    Houston modification 213
    Sydney classification system 213
    tests, based 124
biotin 9
bismuth 78, 124
    H. pylori antimicrobial resistance, role
        of 593–8
        antibiotics, resistance to 594–5
        compounds, chemistry 593–4
        dual therapy data, secondary
            resistance 596–7
        treatment success on resistance,
            impact 595
        triple therapy data 597
    triple and quadruple studies
        (Canada) 567–72
        colloidal subcitrate, studies 569–71
        ranitidine bismuth citrate,
            studies 571–2
        sub-salicylate studies 567–9
    triple therapy 631
    urea breath test, effect on 134–5
bismuth subsalicylate (BSS) 593, 594(fig.)
Bizzozero, G. (1846–1901) 361–2
Black Death 349, 674
Blasser atests 33
Book of Leviticus 348
Bordet, Jules (1870–1939) 348

bovine spongiform encephalopathy
    (BSE) 674
bovine viral diarrhoea virus 163
breast feeding 170
Brunner's glands 300, 308, 310
    neo G zone 310
Budd, William (1811–1880) 350
Bulloch, William (1868–1941) 358

C-UBT 120
c-x-c 143
cadmium 10
cag+ strains 27–8, 151
cagA+ 39–40
cagA 37–8, 127, 171–2, 199, 289
cag-associated pathogenicity island
    (cag-PAI) 199–200, 205
    virulence factor 206(fig.)
Campylobacter jejuni 9, 96
Campylobacter spp. 48–9, 97
Canadian Dyspepsia Working
    Group 439(table)
capronophilic property 5
CAR-5 249
carbon dioxide 15
    H.pylori growth, role of 4–5, 9
carbonic anhydrase 9
carcinogenesis 159
carcinogens 514
cardia 328–9(figs)
    adenocarcinoma 295
    anatomical definition 299–300
    cancer 33–4
    carditis 302–5
    histological abnormalities 301–3
    histological definition 300
    squamo-columnar junction 328
carditis 302–5
    cardia, intestinal metaplasia, *H. pylori*
        relationship 299–305
    cardia, intestinal metaplasia and reflux
        relationship 295–9
    IM, with 303–5
cathepsin E 152–3
cell death 159–60
    induction, TNF-α 158(fig.)
cell responses, digestive tract
    inflammation 207(fig.)
cellular immune response, children 172–3
ceramide 161–2
Chadwick, Edwin (1800–1890) 350
children
    antibody responses 170–1

cellular immune response 172–3
diarrhoeal disease 27
H. pylori infection, sequelae 575–8
  clinical presentations 578–9
  consensus groups 579–83
  gastric adenocarcinoma 577–8
  gastritis 576–7
  MALT lymphoma 577
  primary peptic ulcer disease 576
  immuno-inflammatory response 169–73
  mucosal inflammation, severity and reversibility 175–84
  pathogenesis (bacterial) 171–2
  transmission, infection and acquisition 169–70
  urea breath test 170
chili, protective effect 67–8
cholera 48
  hygiene 349–52
  toxin 141, 144
chronic atrophic gastritis 230, 242(fig.)
cigarette smoking 260
citric acid 133
clarithromycin 47, 587–90
  back-up, after metronidazole-based regimens 613–14
  bowel effects, potential 627
  resistance, treatment strategy 612–13(figs)
CLO test 120
Clostridium difficile 203, 593
cobalt 10
cocarcinogens 497–8
CODA 371
coeliac disease 222–3
Cohn, Ferdinand Julius (1828–1898) 357
Cohnheim, J. (1839–1884) 363
collagenous gastritis 221–3, 224(fig.)
colloidal bismuth subcitrate 569–71, 593, 594(fig.)
colonization, benefits to humans 27–8
compliance, gastric 412
cop A 10
cop P 10
coronary heart disease 115, 316–18
COX-2 pathway 143, 537
Creutzfeldt-Jakob disease 674
CRL-1739 16
Crohn's disease 221, 225, 241–2, 342, 626
cytokines 142
  apoptosis 163
  immunity, protective 145

  induction 38
  oxidative stress 163
cytolethal distending toxin 97
cytoplasmic vacuoles 152
czc A 10

Davaine, Casimir (1812–1882) 358
Denol 593
developed *vs.* developing countries, *H. pylori*, infection incidence 57
diabetes mellitus 115
diagnosis 115–20
  pitfalls 123–35
    biopsy-based tests 124
    clinical application 128
    general aspects 123–4
    results interpretation 129–30
    serology 125–8
    stool assays 117–20
diet 40, 67–8
  antioxidants 514–15, 520(fig.)
  high-salt 240
dihydrolipoamide dehydrogenase 7
discovery, *H. pylori* 368–70
diseases of civilization 32
Doenges, J.L. 366
Domagk, Gerard (1895–1964) 348
Dragstedt, L.R. (1893–1975) 365
DT-diaphorase 8
Dumas, Jean (1800–1884) 355
duodenal ulcers 32–3, 334–5, 674
  low gastric pH 520(fig.)
duodenum, children/adolescent, inflammation and gastric metaplasia 179–80
dysentery, spirochetal 363
dyspepsia
  definition 435–6, 469
  functional
    improvement in symptoms, after cure 436–7
    studies, results 436(table)
  functional, pathophysiology 411–18
    autonomic imbalance 414–15
    gastric and duodenal motor function, altered 411–12
    mechano-and chemo-sensitivity, abnormal 412–13
    psychological factors 414–15
    stress, effects 414–15
    visceral hypersensitivity, mechanisms 413–14

functional/non-ulcer, therapy guidelines,
    worldwide perspectives 560–1
H. pylori
  infection 428–9
  treatment 429–30
investigated 435
management
  arguments against 437–9
  strategy options 476(table)
no indication for H. pylori
    eradication 435–40
studies, outcome differences,
    explanation 421–5
  discordant results, explanation 423–4
  H. pylori therapy, trials 421–2
  non-ulcer dyspepsia, trials 422–3
uninvestigated 435
  therapy guidelines, algorithm
    1/2 561–2
  treatment 435, 439(table)
vs. heart disease 439
dysphagia 439
dysplasia/neoplasia, reversibility 535–8

Edkins, J.S. (1863–1940) 365–6
Ehrenberg, Christian Gottfild
  (1795–1876) 352
Ehrlich, Paul (1854–1915) 348
Eissele study 275
electron acceptors 5
elimination
  Th 2 cytokine response
    dependent 187–90
    animal evidence and
      elimination 188–9
    human evidence 189–90
  Th 2 cytokine response non-
    dependent 193–5
ELISA test 126–8
  cut-off point 130
  validity 131–2(tables)
Embden–Mayerhof–Parnas pathway 4
endoscopy 115–16
  gastric cancer 475
endosomal vesicles 152
Entamoeba histolytica 7
enteric nervous system 411
Entner–Doudoroff pathway 4
environmental factors 4, 66
eosinophilic gastritis 224(fig.), 225–6
epidermal growth factor 156
epithelial barrier, oxidative injury, role
    of 155–65

eradication, H. pylori
  arguments against 644–5
  dyspepsia, clinically useful 427–31
  hypersecretion 406–7
  PPI therapy
    atrophic gastritis during,
      prevention 263–4
    gastric consequences (debate) 397–407
ethanol 4, 156
extracellular matrix 241
extragastric manifestations 315–25

faecal antigen determination, infection
    diagnosis 115–20
Fas–Fas ligand 161–2
fatty acids 4
Fenton reaction 161
fibrosis 231–2
flavodoxin oxidoreductase 5
flavoproteins 7
Fleming, Sir Alexander (1881–1955) 348
flesh-eating bacteria 25
Flexispira rappini 95
Florey, Sir Howard (1898–1968) 348
Food and Drug Administration study 273
formate 4
Fracastoro, Girolamo (1478–1553) 347,
    350(fig.)
free radicals, generation 6
Freund's adjuvant 146
fucosyl-transferase (fuc T2) 200
fumarate 5
fumarate reductase 5, 639
fundoplication 258, 260
  Lundell study 261
fur (ferric uptake regulator) 10

gallstone disease 115
γ-glutamylcysteinyl glycine 6
gastric acid/acidity 17, 46
  central vs. peripheral
    stimulation 399–400
  pH 4, 385
  secretion 232
    regulation 399(fig.)
gastric adenocarcinoma, non-cardia 26
gastric atrophy
  mechanisms, involved 239–45
    gland loss 239–40
    metaplasia 243–5
    mucosal response 241–3
  vs. atrophic gastritis 229–30
gastric bacteriology 359–63

INDEX

gastric cancer 475, 674
  carcinogenesis, mechanisms 508–10
  Helicobacter-induced
    gerbils 499–501
    rodent models 489–501
  incidence, Southeast Asia 63–5, 67–8
  intestinal metaplasia (type III) 275
  malignant precursor, detection 526–8
  oxidants/antioxidants and co-factors, role of 513–20
  prevention, prospects 510–11
  risk is real 507–11, 520(fig.)
    worldwide burden 507–8
  vacA 198
gastric cardia *see* cardia
gastric emptying 417
  delayed 412
gastric epithelium
  infected, schematic representation 232(fig.)
  interaction 151–3
gastric *Helicobacter* spp., habitat 15–16
gastric hypersensitivity 412–13
gastric inflammation, unusual forms 221–6
gastric juice, vitamin C concentration 517
gastric MALT lymphoma 223
  H. pylori related, long-term outcome evaluation (study) 541–547
  lymphoid follicles 526, 527(fig.)
  reversibility 538
gastric metaplasia
  origins 307–11
  phenotype 307
gastric mucosal barrier 4, 155–7
  function, factors affecting 159(table)
gastric mucosal oxidative stress 514–15
gastric *N*-nitroso compounds 515–16
gastric physiology, urea breath test, impact 133–4
gastric syphilis 361
gastric ulcer
  endoscopy 116
  proximal 332–4
gastrin 392
  parietal cells, effects on 401–3
gastritis 15
  cellular response, mucosa 28(fig.)
  giant fold 221
  global view study 213–19
  H. pylori-induced (mouse model), neural dysfunction, evidence of 417–18
  Helicobacter heilmannii 75

patterns, Southeast Asia 65
gastritis mucosal atrophy 230
gastro-oesophageal junction 299–300
gastro-oesophageal reflux disease (GERD) 27, 54, 257, 259–60, 269–70
  acid suppression therapy 385
  H. pylori-positive patients, harm in eradication 276–8
gastroenteritis 49(fig.)
gastrointestinal barrier function, evaluation 156
Gastrointestinal Symptom Rating Scale 423–4
Gastrospirillum hominis infection 73–9
  diagnosis 78
  epidemiology 77
  histology 73–4
  microbiology 74
  pathology 75–7
  therapy 78–9
  transmission and reservoir 78
gene expression, environment-dependent 200
gene microarray technology 669
gene regulation, mechanisms 199–200
"generational cohort" phenomenon 57
genetic information, biochemical/physiological implications 3–11
genomics 3–4
Glasgow Dyspepsia Severity Scale 423–4
gluconeogenesis 4
glucose, metabolism 4
glucose-6-phosphate 4
glutathione 6–7
glycolysis 4
Goeppert, Heinrich Robert (1800–1884) 357
Golgi, Camillio (1844–1926) 362
Gorgas, William (1854–1920) 348
Gorham, Frank D. 366–7
graft-versus-host disease 159
Gram, Heinz Christian Joachim (1853–1938) 357
granulomatous gastritis 223–5
GRO-α 143
growth requirements 4–5
Guardia duodenalis 7
Guardia intestinalis 7
Guillain-Barré syndrome 324
gut permeability, measurement 156

H2-receptor antagonists 78, 385, 469
  rebound 401

secretory pathways, effects on 398-9
  tolerance 400
Haber-Weiss reaction 161
heartburn 439
Helicobacter acinonyx 74
Helicobacter bilis 94, 107(table)
Helicobacter bizzozeronii 74
Helicobacter canadensis 96
Helicobacter canis 95-6, 107(table)
Helicobacter cholecystis 94, 107(table)
Helicobacter cinaedi 95, 107(table), 108
Helicobacter colifelis 107(table)
Helicobacter felis 74
  induced MALT lymphoma 498-9
Helicobacter fennelliae 95, 107(table), 108
Helicobacter heilmannii see also
    Gastrospirullum hominis
Helicobacter hepaticus
  hepatitis and liver cancer
    association 83-5
  hepatobiliary disease, humans 97-8
  induced hepatitis, host
    susceptibility 87-93
  apoptosis/proliferation induction, liver
    cancer 90-1
  non-genotoxic carcinogen 92
  oxidative stress and cytotoxicity,
    biomarkers 91-2
  SCID mice 92-3
  tumour induction, mechanisms 89-90
  Koch's postulates 86
  mouse carcinogenesis studies 86-7
  Th-1 immune response, induction 85-6
  virulence determinants 96-7
Helicobacter muridarum 105, 330
Helicobacter nemestrinae 74
Helicobacter pametensis 107(table)
Helicobacter pullorum 96, 98, 107(table)
Helicobacter rappini 95, 98, 107(table), 108
Helicobacter rodencium 98, 105
Helicobacter salmonis 74
Helicobacter trogontum 107(table)
Helicobacter typhylonicus 107(table)
Helicobacter westmeadii 108
Helicobacter-cotton top 107(table)
Henley, F.G. Jacob (1809-1885) 347, 353
hepatitis 33
  Helicobacter hepaticus induced 87-93
  toxic 85
hepatitis B infection 674
  transmission 67

hepatitis C infection, drug abuse 674
hepatobiliary *Helicobacters* see *Helicobacter hepaticus*
hereditary non-polyposis colon cancer
  (HNPCC) syndrome 537
high acid output states 329(fig.)
histidines, mutation 22
histopathologist, agenda 669-71
Hop proteins 198
horseradish peroxidase 156
host factors 40
host response
  inflammation, control of 207-8
  microbial pathogenesis 203(table)
Hp Chip 655-7
HP-0824 7
HP-0825 7
HP-1103 4
HP-1164 7
HP-1458 7
HpSA (*H. pylori* stool antigen) test 117, 120
human immunodeficiency virus (HIV) 33, 163, 674
HUMARA (human androgen receptor
  gene) 242
hydrocobalamin *see* vitamin B12
hydrogen peroxide 160
hydroxyl radicals 160-1
hypercalcaemia 341-3
hyperchlorhydria, *H. pylori* induced 374
hypergastrinaemia 240
  Helicobacter infection (animal
    models) 495-7
hyperparathyroidism 341
hypochlorhydria 46, 49(fig.), 98, 517
  development, mechanisms
    involved 373-81

iceA 38-9, 199
idiopathic urticaria 320-1
immune-mediated vasculitis syndrome 223
immune/inflammatory changes 141-6
  humans 143
  mouse 143-4
immunomodulation 145-6
immunity, protective, against infection 46
immunization 144-5
immunoblot assays 126-7
immunoglobulin A 170-1
immunologist, agenda (new
  Millennium) 663-7

INDEX

immunoproliferative small intestinal lymphoproliferative disease (IPSID) 538
infected hosts, decrease 46–7
infection, *H. pylori* caused by
  acid secretion, effect on 386–9
  age/prevalence 128–9
  childhood
    consequences 176
    eradication therapy 678
    infants/toddlers 46
    natural history 180
    reversibility 183
    transmission and acquisition 169–70
  chronic, effect on dyspepsia 415–17
  diagnosis *see* diagnosis
  disappearance
    Far East, factors associated 53–5
    West, factors associated 45–50
  endoscopy-related 46
  ethnicity 57
  extrinsic barriers 47–9
  false-negative tests 341–2
  gastric cancer, sequence of events leading to 380–1
  global control, best method 645–8
  IL-4 absence, effect of 194
  inflammatory activity
    host related 203–8
    immune response, shaping 205–7
    organism related, predominantly 197–201
  mucosal barrier function 157–8
    altered, mechanisms 158–9
  NSAID-associated gastropathy 443–9
  oxidative stress 162–4
  protective role, against NSAID damage 455–6
  recurrence, Asia 55
  therapy
    guidelines, world perspective 559–60
    true cost 552
inflammatory bowel disease, rodent 108
iNOS 143
interferon γ
  apoptosis 160
  elimination, viral-induced 194
  gastric epithelial barrier during infection 158(fig.)
interleukin-12, elimination, viral induced 194
interleukin-1 32

interleukin-6 143
interleukin-8 38, 143
  secretion 197–8
intestinal *Helicobacters*, pathogens in animals 107–8
intestinal metaplasia 243–5
  gastric cancer 249–53, 275
    cancer histogenesis, role 250–1
    origin, mechanisms of 249–50
    results 251–3
    types 249
  high gastric pH 520(fig.)
intestinal mucus, ecological niche 105–6
iron
  availability 4
  transport 9–10
iron-deficiency anaemia 33, 319
irritable bowel syndrome 413

Jaworsky, Walery 360, 361(fig.)
Jenner, Sir Edward (1749–1823) 348
JHP-1029 4
JHP-1091 7
JHP-1351 7
JHP-764 7
JHP-991 7

kappas 229
Kniper's hypothesis/study 269–70, 276
Koch, Robert (1843–1910) 347–8
Kussmaul, A. (1822–1902) 363

lactate 4
Lactobacillus 361
lansoprazole 260, 385, 387
laser capture microscopy 669
Lavoisier, A. (1743–1794) 354
Leeuwenhock, Antonj van (1632–1723) 347
Letulle, M. (1853–1929) 359
Liebig, J. von (1803–1873) 354
lipids, intraduodenal 413
lipopolysaccharide 198
lower bowel *Helicobacters* 108
Lundell study 261, 270–3
lymphocytic gastritis 221–3, 224(fig.)
lymphoid follicles 176–8

M cells 142, 156–7
malnutrition 46
management *see* therapy
manganase superoxide dismutase 160
marginal zone lymphoma 525
markers (pre-malignancy) 525–31

evidence, available 528–9
studies, problems 529–30
Marshall, B.J. 370(fig.)
matrix metalloproteinase 241
maximal acid output 392–4
melanosis coli 159
menaquinone 5
Ménétrier's disease 221
mercuric reductase 7
metabolic pathways 4–6
metaplasia 232–3
Metchnikoff, Elie (1845–1916) 348
methicillin-resistant *Staphylococcus aureus* (MRSA) 674
metronidazole 6, 47, 611
   back-up after clarithromycin-based regimens 614–15
   nitroreductase, activation by 8
   quadruple therapy 623–7
Mettler, Cecilia (1909–1943) 353
microbiologist, agenda 655–61
migraine 115, 322–3
migrating motor complex 412
minimal inhibitory concentration 594
MIP-1 α 143
misoprostol 456(fig.)
mitochondria 160
MKN-28 cells 152
mono-amine oxidase 160
motility disorders 411
mucosa associated lymphoid tissue (MALT) 142
mucosa associated lymphoid tissue (MALT) lymphoma 427, 526
   Helicobacter heilmannii 76, 78
   low grade 32–3
   therapy guidelines 560
   vacA 198
mucosal eosinophilic gastroenteritis 226
mucosal immune response 142
Muhlens, P. (1874–1943) 363
Mulder study 275
Muller, Otto Friedrich (1730–1784) 352
multiple endocrine neoplasia, type I 341
Mycobacterium avium 626
Mycobacterium avium-intracellulare complex 163
Mycobacterium paratuberculosis 626
Mycobacterium tuberculosis 25, 33
myofibroblast 241

N-methyl-*N*-nitrosourea 497–8
natura abhorret vacuum 231

NDH-I dehydrogenase 5
necrosis 159
   bacterial 363
negative non-NSAID-related ulcers 339–44
Neisseria 593
neoplasia
   definition 535
   dynamics 535–6
   progression, regression and failure 536–7
   reversibility 537–8
   stages 535
nickel transport protein (Nix A) 10
nitric oxide 156
   apoptosis 160
nitro compounds 6
5-nitroimidazole 6
nodular gastritis 176–8
non-steroidal anti-inflammatory drugs (NSAIDs) 53, 116, 128, 156, 240, 398, 439
   enteropathy, induced 159
   H. pylori 461–5
   H. pylori-negative ulcer disease
      causes, possible 341–3
      role of 341
   therapy guidelines, worldwide perspectives 562–3
   ulcers, recurrence of ulcer complications, eradication effect 456–7
non-steroidal anti-inflammatory drugs (NSAIDs)-associated gastropathy 443–9
   epidemiological studies 444–7
   gastroduodenal mucosal damage, mechanisms leading 444
   H. pylori, beneficial effect, infection? 453–8
non-ulcer dyspepsia 421
   endoscopy 427
   H. pylori therapy, trials 422–3
normal flora 31
nuclear factor κB (NFκB) 38, 161
nutrition, improvement 46

Obermeyer, Otto (1843–1873) 357
OCAY study 436(table)
oesophagus, adenocarcinoma 27–8
Ogston, Alexander (1844–1929) 360
omeprazole 78, 133–4, 257–60, 385, 456(fig.), 637
   corpus glandular atrophy, intestinal metaplasia 274(tables)
   Lundell study 270–3

INDEX

OMNIUM study 455
open-reading frames (ORFs) 3
   functions 3
Oppler-Boas lactobacillus 360–1
orange juice 133
ORCHID study 436(table)
outer membrane vesicles 151–2
oxaloacetate 5
oxidative injury 160–4
oxidoreductase 8
oxygen 6–9
   electron acceptor 6
   environmental concentration, change 8
   growth, concentration necessary 4–5
   redox potential 6–9
   toxic oxygen species 6–9

p53 161–2
pancreatic metaplasia (heterotopia) 300
pantoprazole 385, 388(fig.)
parasite infection 32
parietal cells, gastrin effects on 401–3
Pasteur, Louis (1822–1895) 348, 353–7
pathogen, definition 26–7
pathogenic flora 31–4
pathogenicity, determination, host response 203–4
Pavlov, I. (1849–1936) 363
penicillin 46, 386
   allergy question, quadruple therapy 625–6
pepsin 444
   discovery 358
peptic ulcer disease 15, 26, 33
   acid tolerance 330–1
   incidence, Southeast Asia 67
   races, distribution among 63
   therapy guidelines, world perspectives 560
   transitional zones 327–32
      acid-gradient 331–2
      lability 328–30
   vacA 198
Pepto-Bismol 567, 593
periplasm buffering, intrabacterial urease 16–19
pernicious anaemia 289
phospholipase A2 444
pituitary adenylate cyclase-activating peptide (PACAP) 399–400, 402(fig.)
Pneumococcus 361
polio virus 33
polymorphonuclear leukocytes (PMNL) 6

postprandial fullness 412
Pouchett, Felix-Archmedi (1800–1872) 353
pre-malignant changes 525–6
premastication 66
prevalence, race/environmental factors in Southeast Asia, studies 57–68
primary biliary cirrhosis 98
primary sclerosing cholangitis 98
primordial *Helicobacters* 31–2
prokinetic drugs 469
promoters 200
prostaglandins 156
   NSAIDs, inhibition by 444
protein kinase C 157
Proteus vulgaris 330
proton motive force 330
proton pump inhibitors (PPI) 119, 124, 469, 637
   acid rebound 403–6
      hypersecretion 391–4
   atrophic gastritis onset, acceleration? 255–64
   bioavailability, oral 386
   effects 401
   failure, reasons 386
   gastric atrophy, development, acceleration? 269–78
   gastritis, acid control, effect of *H. pylori* infection 385–9
   H. pylori eradication, gastric consequences (debate) 397–407
   quadruple therapy 623–7
   urea breath test, effect on 134–5
pseudomembranous colitis 627
Pseudomonas aeruginosa 368
pseudopyloric metaplasia 243–5
psychological factors, effect on dyspepsia 414–15
"pump to the helix" 347–71
Pylorid 594
pyruvate 4–5

quinones 6

rabeprazole 385
racial cohort theory 66–7
ranitidine 78, 273, 387, 398
ranitidine bismuth citrate 571, 594
RANTES 143
Rayer, Pierre (1793–1867) 358
reactive oxygen species 6, 155, 160–2
rebound acid hypersecretion, acid-suppressive therapy after 391–4

rectal distension 413
Reed, Walter (1851–1902) 348
reflux oesophagitis 33–4
respiratory pathways 5
restriction fragment length polymorphism (RFLP) 97
Reynaud's phenomenon 115, 320
rosacea 321–2
Rosenow, E.C. 364–5
Ross, Sir Ronald (1857–1932) 348
rpoB-rpoC structure 4

Salmon, Daniel Elmer (1850–1914) 359
Salmonella 48, 49(fig.), 593
salt, intake 68
sarcoidosis 225
sarcomas 526
scarlet fever 674
Schwann, Theodor (1810–1882) 348, 354(fig.), 358
  zuckerpilz 353
scintigraphy 133
scleroderma 320
screening 675
Sedillot, C.E. (1804–1883) 358
Seminaria contagiosum 349
sepsis, micro-organisms, relationship 358–9
serology 125–28
  eradication, assessment following 129
  ethnicity/geographical differences 129
Shigella 47–8
Shigella dysenteriae 363
Smith, Theobald (1859–1934) 359
Snow, John (1813–1858) 347, 351(fig.)
socioeconomic standards 55
spasmolytic peptide-expressing metaplasia (SPEM) 243–5
Spirochaeta pallidum 363, 367
Spirochaeta regandi 365
spirillum 352
squamous cell carcinoma-keratoacanthoma type 537
Staphylococcus pyrogenes aureus 360
Stolte's study 292
stomach
  adenocarcinoma 27–8
  B-cell lymphoma, non-Hodgkin's 26
  pathological responses, children/adolescents 178–9
  pH 4
stool, assays 117–20
stress, effect on dyspepsia 414–15
succinate 4, 5

sucrose absorption 156
sulindac 537
superoxide 160
superoxide dismutase 515
susceptibility 45–6
syphilis 349

T cells 142
tachyphylaxis 385
terramycin 368
test meal 133
test-and-treat strategy
  arguments against it 480–1
  dyspepsia
    European perspective 475–81
    United States perspective 469–72
  evidence for it 480
  H. pylori infection, Asian perspective 483–6
  Maastricht guidelines 476–7
  European studies, considerations/evaluation since 477–80
tetracycline 611, 623–7
therapy
  cost benefits 34
  current state-of-the-art, global perspective 551–7
    Asian-Pacific consensus 555–6
    Canadian management guidelines 554–5
    European management guidelines 554
    global consensus and differences 556–7
    United States guidelines 552–4
  failures, risk factors 601–6
    antibiotics, resistance to 601–3
    France, cohort study 603–6
  failures, strategies for *H. pylori* eradication 609–18
    framework, logical and rational 611–13
    new alternatives 616–17
    second-line therapies, randomized trials between 610–11, 615–16
    therapy, recommendations 617–18
  future, expectations 637–40
  guidelines, world perspective 559–63
  quadruple, should be
    first-line therapy 623–7
    second-line therapy 631–5
thioredoxin reductase 7
thyroiditis 323–4
tinidazole 595

INDEX

tocopherol 161
tolerance 385
  oral 144
transcription regulatory sigma factor 4
transforming growth factor α (TGF-α) 156
transitional zones, normal 328(fig.)
transmission 47–8, 54
  children, infection and
      acquisition 169–70
  hypothetical cycle 49(fig.)
  micro-organisms 347
  zoonotic 95–6
trefoil peptides 156
Treponema 593
tricarboxylic acid 4
Trichomonas foetus 7
Trichomonas vaginalis 7
tripotassium-dicitrato-bismuthate
    (DeNol) 134–5
tuberculosis 674
tumour necrosis factor α (TNF-α), cell death
    induction 158(fig.)
tumour necrosis factor γ (TNF-γ),
    apoptosis 160
turmeric, protective effect 68

UK-MRC study 436(table)
ulcer colitis 234–5
Untersuchungen uber Bakteria 358
Untersuchungen uber dier Aetiologie der
    Wundinfektions Krankheiten 358
updated Sydney system 230–1
urea breath test 116, 124–5, 130–5, 428,
    439
  antibiotics, bismuth salts and PPI, use
      of 134–5, 342
  children 170
  gastric physiology, impact on 133–4
  pitfalls 133(table)
  test procedure, role of 130–3
urease 15
  activity 133
  intrabacterial
    acid activation 16
    activation, kinetic mechanism 19–20
    periplasm buffering 16–19
  system 15–23
  virulence factors 204

UreI 20–3, 330
  properties 23(table)
USA study 436(table)

vaccination 34, 46, 145–6, 643–8
  H. pylori infection, global world 645–8
  H. pylori-related disease, health problem
      magnitude 643–4
vaccines 646
  feasibility 647
  human
    improvements 647–8
    studies 647
  ideal 648
vacuolating cytotoxin A (vacA) 39, 127,
    157, 171–2, 198–9
  release, outer membrane vesicles 151–2
  s-1 39–40
vagal tone 412
vagotomy 258, 261, 365, 412
Vibrio fischeri 25
Vibrio regula 360–1
virulence factors
  disease-specific 37–40
  model, problems 204–5
visceral hypersensitivity 411, 413
vitamin B12 262, 289, 517
vitamin C 515(table)
  gastric, *H. pylori* infection 516–18
vitamin E 161, 515(table)
  gastric, *H. pylori* infection 518
vomiting 47, 412, 439

Warren, J.R. 370(fig.)
Wegener's disease 223
Wöhler, F. (1800–1882) 354
Wolinella succinogenes 5
woodchuck hepatitis virus (WHV)
    infection 94–5
world, developing 675
  clinician, challenges 677–8
world, developed, *H. pylori* in the 21st
    century 675–7

X chromosome 242

z-line 301(table), 302
zinc 10
Zollinger–Ellison syndrome 341